Handbook of
SOCIALIZATION

Theory and Research

SECOND EDITION

edited by

Joan E. Grusec
Paul D. Hastings

THE GUILFORD PRESS
New York   London

© 2015 The Guilford Press
A Division of Guilford Publications, Inc.
370 Seventh Avenue, Suite 1200, New York, NY 10001
www.guilford.com

Paperback edition 2016

Printed in the United States of America

This book is printed on acid-free paper.

Last digit is print number: 9 8 7 6 5 4 3 2

Library of Congress Cataloging-in-Publication Data

Handbook of socialization : theory and research / edited by Joan E. Grusec, Paul D. Hastings.—Second edition.
    pages cm
  Includes bibliographical references and index.
  ISBN 978-1-4625-1834-0 (hardback)
  ISBN 978-1-4625-2582-9 (paperback)
  1. Socialization. I. Grusec, Joan E. II. Hastings, Paul D. (Paul David), 1966–
HM686.H36 2015
303.3′2—dc23

                                        2014014446

About the Editors

Joan E. Grusec, PhD, is Professor Emerita in the Department of Psychology at the University of Toronto. Her research interests center on socialization in the family, with a particular focus on differentiating among domains of socialization as well as exploring underlying motivations for different forms of prosocial action. Dr. Grusec has authored and edited numerous research papers, chapters, and books, and served as Associate Editor of *Developmental Psychology*.

Paul D. Hastings, PhD, is Chair and Professor of Psychology at the University of California, Davis, where he is also a member of the Center for Mind and Brain. His research focuses on examining the contributions of neurobiological regulation and parental socialization to adaptive and maladaptive socioemotional development in children and adolescents. Dr. Hastings has authored more than 90 research articles, chapters, and books.

Contributors

Craig A. Anderson, PhD, Department of Psychology, Iowa State University, Ames, Iowa

Jeffrey Jensen Arnett, PhD, Department of Psychology, Clark University, Worcester, Massachusetts

Reut Avinun, MSc, Department of Psychology, Hebrew University of Jerusalem, Jerusalem, Israel

Hideko H. Bassett, PhD, Department of Psychology, George Mason University, Fairfax, Virginia

John E. Bates, PhD, Department of Psychological and Brain Sciences, Indiana University, Bloomington, Indiana

Talya N. Bauer, PhD, School of Business Administration, Portland State University, Portland, Oregon

David A. Beaulieu, PhD, Department of Psychology, Tomball College, Tomball, Texas

John W. Berry, PhD, Department of Psychology, Queen's University, Kingston, Ontario, Canada; National Research University Higher School of Economics, Moscow, Russia

Mara Brendgen, PhD, Department of Psychology, University of Quebec at Montreal, Montreal, Quebec, Canada

Stephanie C. Brown, BA, Department of Psychology, Iowa State University, Ames, Iowa

Daphne Blunt Bugental, PhD, Department of Psychology, University of California, Santa Barbara, Santa Barbara, California

William M. Bukowski, PhD, Centre for Research in Human Development, Department of Psychology, Concordia University, Montreal, Quebec, Canada

Melisa Castellanos, MA, Department of Psychology, Concordia University, Montreal, Quebec, Canada

Xinyin Chen, PhD, Applied Psychology and Human Development Division, Graduate School of Education, University of Pennsylvania, Philadelphia, Pennsylvania

Pamela M. Cole, PhD, Department of Psychology, The Pennsylvania State University, University Park, Pennsylvania

Randy Corpuz, BA, Department of Psychology, University of California, Santa Barbara, Santa Barbara, California

Maricela Correa-Chávez, PhD, Department of Psychology, California State University, Long Beach, Long Beach, California

Maayan Davidov, PhD, Department of Social Work, Hebrew University of Jerusalem, Jerusalem, Israel

Susanne A. Denham, PhD, Department of Psychology, George Mason University, Fairfax, Virginia

Amy L. Dexter, PhD, Department of Psychology, Roosevelt University, Chicago, Illinois

Judy Dunn, PhD, Social, Genetic, and Developmental Psychiatry Research Centre, Institute of Psychiatry, King's College, London, United Kingdom

Jacquelynne S. Eccles, PhD, School of Education, University of California, Irvine, Irvine, California

Allison M. Ellis, MS, Department of Psychology, Portland State University, Portland, Oregon

Berrin Erdogan, PhD, School of Business Administration, Portland State University, Portland, Oregon

Timea Farkas, MA, Department of Psychology, University of California, Santa Cruz, Santa Cruz, California

Rachel H. Farr, PhD, Department of Psychology, University of Massachusetts at Amherst, Amherst, Massachusetts

Karen L. Fingerman, PhD, Department of Human Development and Family Sciences, University of Texas at Austin, Austin, Texas

Nathan A. Fox, PhD, Institute for Child Study, Department of Human Development and Quantitative Methodology, University of Maryland, College Park, Maryland

Jennifer A. Fredricks, PhD, Department of Human Development, Connecticut College, New London, Connecticut

Tahl I. Frenkel, PhD, Institute for Child Study, Department of Human Development and Quantitative Methodology, University of Maryland, College Park, Maryland

Jill Froimson, MS, Department of Psychology, Lehigh University, Bethlehem, Pennsylvania

Rui Fu, MA, Applied Psychology and Human Development Division, Graduate School of Education, University of Pennsylvania, Philadelphia, Pennsylvania

Mary Gauvain, PhD, Department of Psychology, University of California, Riverside, Riverside, California

Douglas A. Gentile, PhD, Department of Psychology, Iowa State University, Ames, Iowa

Christopher L. Groves, MS, Department of Psychology, Iowa State University, Ames, Iowa

Joan E. Grusec, PhD, Department of Psychology, University of Toronto, Toronto, Ontario, Canada

Sam A. Hardy, PhD, Department of Psychology, Brigham Young University, Provo, Utah

Paul D. Hastings, PhD, Center for Mind and Brain, University of California, Davis, Davis, California

Ariel Knafo-Noam, PhD, Department of Psychology, Hebrew University of Jerusalem, Jerusalem, Israel

Leon Kuczynski, PhD, Department of Family Relations and Applied Nutrition, University of Guelph, Guelph, Ontario, Canada

Deborah Laible, PhD, Department of Psychology, Lehigh University, Bethlehem, Pennsylvania

Campbell Leaper, PhD, Department of Psychology, University of California, Santa Cruz, Santa Cruz, California

Gloria Luong, PhD, Max Planck Research Group "Affect Across the Lifespan," Max Planck Institute for Human Development, Berlin, Germany

Eleanor E. Maccoby, PhD, Department of Psychology, Stanford University, Stanford, California

Jonas G. Miller, MA, Center for Mind and Brain, University of California, Davis, Davis, California

Leslie C. Moore, PhD, Department of Teaching and Learning, Ohio State University, Columbus, Ohio

C. Melanie Parkin, MSc, Department of Psychology, University of Guelph, Guelph, Ontario, Canada

Charlotte J. Patterson, PhD, Department of Psychology, University of Virginia, Charlottesville, Virginia

Susan M. Perez, PhD, Department of Psychology, University of North Florida, Jacksonville, Florida

Gregory S. Pettit, PhD, Department of Human Development and Family Studies, Auburn University, Auburn, Alabama

Robyn Pitman, PhD, Department of Family Relations and Applied Nutrition, University of Guelph, Guelph, Ontario, Canada

Michael W. Pratt, EdD, Department of Psychology, Wilfrid Laurier University, Waterloo, Ontario, Canada

Sara Prot, MA, Department of Psychology, Iowa State University, Ames, Iowa

Antje Rauers, PhD, Max Planck Research Group "Affect Across the Lifespan," Max Planck Institute for Human Development, Berlin, Germany

Rena L. Repetti, PhD, Department of Psychology, University of California, Los Angeles, Los Angeles, California

Bridget M. Reynolds, PhD, Department of Psychology, University of California, Los Angeles, Los Angeles, California

Jessica Robinson, BS, Department of Clinical and Social Sciences in Psychology, University of Rochester, Rochester, New York

Theodore F. Robles, PhD, Department of Psychology, University of California, Los Angeles, Los Angeles, California

Barbara Rogoff, PhD, Department of Psychology, University of California, Santa Cruz, Santa Cruz, California

Wendy M. Rote, PhD, Department of Clinical and Social Sciences in Psychology, University of Rochester, Rochester, New York

Muniba Saleem, PhD, Department of Communications and Research Center for Group Dynamics, Institute for Social Research, University of Michigan, Ann Arbor, Michigan

Sandra D. Simpkins, PhD, J. Denny Sanford School of Social and Family Dynamics, Arizona State University, Tempe, Arizona

Judith G. Smetana, PhD, Department of Clinical and Social Sciences in Psychology, University of Rochester, Rochester, New York

Patricia Z. Tan, PhD, Department of Psychiatry, Western Psychiatric Institute and Clinic, University of Pittsburgh, Pittsburgh, Pennsylvania

Ross A. Thompson, PhD, Department of Psychology, University of California, Davis, Davis, California

Natalie R. Troxel, MA, Department of Psychology, University of California, Davis, Davis, California

Frank Vitaro, PhD, Research Unit on Children's Psychosocial Maladjustment, School of Psychoeducation, University of Montreal, Montreal, Quebec, Canada

Wayne Warburton, PhD, Department of Psychology, Macquarie University, Sydney, Australia

Kathryn R. Wentzel, PhD, Department of Human Development, University of Maryland, College Park, Maryland

Todd Wyatt, PhD, Department of Psychology, George Mason University, Fairfax, Virginia

Siman Zhao, MA, Applied Psychology and Human Development Division, Graduate School of Education, University of Pennsylvania, Philadelphia, Pennsylvania

Preface

It has been a great pleasure to work on the second edition of the *Handbook of Socialization*. Since 2007, the first edition's publication date, much has happened in a field that is central to the understanding of human development. Nevertheless, most of the basic questions remain the same. Some answers that might have been tentative a few years ago have become more certain. Others have become even more tentative or have been shown to be wrong. But researchers are making definite progress in understanding socialization processes—that much is clearly evident.

We begin with a brief discussion of the nature of the socialization process, taken directly from the introduction to the first edition. We then move to an overview of the structure of the present edition.

What Is Socialization?

In the broadest terms, *socialization* refers to the way in which individuals are assisted in becoming members of one or more social groups. The word *assist* is important because it implies that socialization is not a one-way street but that newer members of the social group are active in the socialization process and selective in what they accept from older members of the social group. In addition, newer members may attempt to socialize older members.

Socialization involves a variety of outcomes, including the acquisition of rules, roles, standards, and values across the social, emotional, cognitive, and personal domains. Some outcomes are deliberately hoped for on the part of agents of socialization, while others may be unintended side effects of particular socialization practices (e.g., low self-esteem, anger and reactance, and aggression to peers as a function of harsh parenting). Socialization can also occur through many paths (e.g., discipline after deviation, modeling, proactive techniques, routines, rituals, and as a function of styles of interaction between the agent of socialization and the individual participating in the socialization process). Socialization is ongoing throughout the life course and can be accomplished by a variety of individuals, including parents, teachers, peers, and siblings, as well as by schools, the media, the Internet, the workplace, and general cultural institutions. Finally, and most important, we note that socialization cannot be adequately understood without a consideration of how biological and sociocultural factors interact in a complex and intertwined manner.

The field of socialization research, always an important area in psychology, has made considerable advances in recent years. These advances are partially attributable to more sophisticated methodological, conceptual, and statistical tools, as well as to the inclusion of a wide variety of theoretical perspectives and approaches. For example, although evolutionary theory has been part of the thinking of socialization theorists, particularly attachment theorists, since at least the 1970s, it is having an increased impact on how socialization is conceptualized. Advances in genetics are helping to shed light on the impact of environmental experiences on children, and new work on biological and hormonal regulatory systems, as well as brain function, is enriching analyses of socialization experiences and the nature of their impact on children. In a time when massive immigration is the norm and global interconnections grow ever stronger, researchers have enlarged their focus of interest from middle-class participants of Western European extraction to people all over the world. All of these exciting changes are represented in this handbook.

What are some of the themes that emerge from contemporary research on socialization? The first has to do with the interdependence of biology and experience. As just noted, evolutionary, cultural, genetic, neurological, and biological approaches are currently prominent, and one of the major tasks for future researchers will be to map the interrelationships among these various approaches to the socialization process. The second theme, which emerges in most of the chapters in this volume, has to do with the fact that socialization involves bidirectionality, with targets of socialization having an impact on the actions of agents of socialization. Indeed, the complexity of the interaction is underlined by the fact that it occurs in a developmental context—each member of the dyad or group is responding to the constantly changing behavior of the other members. The third theme has to do with the many contributing factors that interact to produce multiple socialization processes and pathways. The issue is raised in a number of different forms in many of the chapters. The impact of socialization experience is moderated by genetic predispositions and the child's temperament. Interactions between socialization strategies also occur as a function of a whole host of other variables, including the age, sex, and mood of the child; the nature of the parent–child relationship; the domain of behavior under consideration; and the cultural context. Context gives meaning to much of what goes on during the socialization process, and as a result, socialization cannot be understood independent of that context.

The Structure of the Book

Nearly all the chapters in the second edition address the same content areas as in the first edition. Some have had their original content updated and others have been thoroughly reworked with new perspectives and a different focus. Additional chapters have been added on socialization during adolescence, socialization in the workplace, neuroscience, and moral development.

Chapter 1, on the history of socialization research, remains virtually unchanged. We are indebted to Eleanor E. Maccoby, a pioneer in the area, for an insightful overview of the history of socialization research that was up to date as of 2007. We present that chapter again, because it still provides an excellent backdrop for the material that follows.

In 2007, after looking at socialization across the life span, we grouped chapters into those that concentrated on events in the family and those that concentrated on events outside the family. This distinction has been more difficult to make in the second edition: Although most contributors still maintain that the family, parents in particular, are the most important agents of socialization, they are also more likely to include in their chapters material on the influence of other agents of socialization. Thus, we can no longer maintain the intra- and extrafamily division. Accordingly, after a section that focuses on different problems and issues that seem more prevalent at certain points in the life span (early childhood, adolescence, emerging adulthood, old age), we move to a section with chapters that address socialization in the context of different relationships and settings (socialization involving equal agency, different domains or relationships, siblings, diverse family structures, peers, school, the media, and the workplace).

We struggled with the ordering of sections in the first edition, particularly with where to insert the material on biological approaches. In the first edition, we placed them at the beginning, just after history. In this second edition, we have inserted biological approaches immediately after those chapters that focus on core principles of the socialization of behavior, cognition, and affect over the life span and across relationships and settings. This ordering is meant to reflect that, to a considerable extent, findings with respect to action, thought, and feeling drive the kinds of questions that biological researchers address. We have placed the section on culture immediately after that on biology, noting that biology and culture are two framing contexts for understanding behavior, cognition, and affect. Within the section on biology, we have included evolutionary and genetic approaches, as well as work on temperament, hormones, and the brain. Within the section on culture, we have included discussion of processes accounting for cultural variation in socialization, the development of cultural repertoires, the role of culture in emotion socialization, and acculturation.

Finally, we present chapters that focus on the socialization of specific outcomes: gender, cognition, emotion, achievement, prosocial behavior, and moral development. In some sense, this last section serves as an overview of the book, because it calls on principles and mechanisms that have been discussed in earlier chapters as they are applied to specific behavioral challenges facing agents of socialization.

In conclusion, the study of socialization remains an active and exciting area of research. We are grateful to the writers of the chapters gathered together in this book for capturing that activity and excitement.

JOAN E. GRUSEC
PAUL D. HASTINGS

Contents

PART IV. BIOLOGICAL ASPECTS OF SOCIALIZATION

PART V. CULTURAL PERSPECTIVES ON SOCIALIZATION

PART VI. TARGETS OF SOCIALIZATION

PART I

HISTORICAL PERSPECTIVE ON SOCIALIZATION

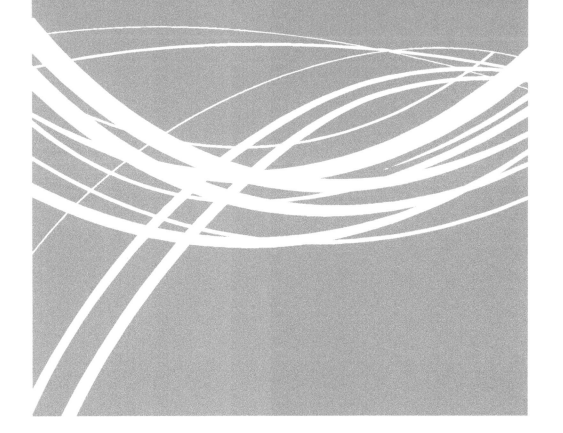

CHAPTER 1

Historical Overview
of Socialization Research and Theory

Eleanor E. Maccoby

The term *socialization* refers to processes whereby naive individuals are taught the skills, behavior patterns, values, and motivations needed for competent functioning in the culture in which the child is growing up. Paramount among these are the social skills, social understandings, and emotional maturity needed for interaction with other individuals to fit in with the functioning of social dyads and larger groups. Socialization processes include all those whereby culture is transmitted from each generation to the next, including training for specific roles in specific occupations. To speak of cross-generational cultural transmission might imply that "culture" is something static, encapsulated, and that the new generation is being rubber-stamped in the image of its predecessors. But, of course, cultures can and do undergo rapid change under the impact of new technology, warfare, climate change, pestilence, and, in recent generations, contraception.

When new generations adopt social structures and modes of social behavior that are different from those of the parent generation, does this mean that socialization processes have failed? Yes and no. Certainly the transmission of specific patterns of behavior has been disrupted, as in the case of Japanese youth who no longer bow to elders as their parents did. But in the larger sense, individuals can be socialized to adapt to changing circumstances. Training regimens can have much broader objectives than teaching specific behavior patterns, as in the case of K–12 schools whose objective is to produce individuals who are broadly educated in ways that will help to fit them for participation in a wide range of social enterprises, including innovative ones. And then there is the broadest socialization of all: to instill *character* or the internalization of certain enduring social norms, which are presumably still relevant however social structures change, and however different from the parent generation's circumstances the new circumstances are in which a new generation must function. Through such socialization, the trainee is presumably led to behave responsibly toward, and refrain from injuring, a large variety of interaction partners the individual will encounter in a variety of social settings. Presumably, in times of rapid cultural change, the importance of broad socialization for adaptation increases.

While a deep and lasting socialization is often assumed to occur primarily in childhood, socialization does, of course, go on throughout the life span, as individuals enter new social settings where new patterns of social behavior may be needed. Many agents are involved in the socialization of an individual, but parents (and religious teachers in some societies) have been thought to be the primary agents responsible for the broad "moral" socialization of the growing child.

We can conceive of socialization, then, as a succession of processes occurring at successive stages of development, with the child's family of origin being the first, and in many cases the most enduring, socializing institution, joined by peer groups, schools, religious institutions, and, in adulthood, employers and intimate partners as sources of norms for social behavior. The reader will note that socialization, as I have described it so far, is a normative concept. A given child can be said to be either well or poorly socialized. Certain families can be described as well functioning, providing effective parenting, if the child emerging from the family adjusts well to the social requirements of major settings encountered later (e.g., the Army, the workplace, marriage, and parenthood), while other families are "dysfunctional" in the sense that they fail to socialize the child to become able to take on these various adult roles, or to become a law-abiding citizen who is reasonably free of pathology.[1] For some time now, we have seen children as playing an active part in the construction of their own standards, so socialization should not be seen as the child's simply taking on the standards of others (Bugental & Goodnow, 1998; Bugental & Grusec, 2006). But I would urge that we can still apply some sort of normative yardstick to whatever standards children self-construct, as to how compatible they are with the likely future requirements of the social contexts in which children will live their lives. We cannot, and need not, take an entirely relativist position, or free the idea of socialization from its normative connotations.

In this chapter I focus primarily on in-family socialization and the processes of parenting. The nature of research on these processes underwent a number of deep changes during the 20th century—changes stemming from changes in the conceptual viewpoints guiding the research, as well as from some technological advances that expanded the menu of methods that could be used to study parenting and its effects. A number of historical reviews already exist in which the major viewpoints are described in detail (see Baldwin, 1955; Bugental & Goodnow, 1998; Goslin, 1969; Grusec, 1997; Maccoby, 1992; Maccoby & Martin, 1983; Parke & Buriel, 1998). This chapter does not go over in detail the ground already covered in these sources but traces a number of salient ideas concerning socialization, and the ways in which they have been modified or metamorphosed over time.

Socialization as the Teaching of Good Habits

A dominant point of view in the mid-20th century was that socialization is a process of instilling in a child a set of desired behavioral habits. Parents and other adults serve as teachers, the children as learners. Young children need to learn table manners, how to dress themselves, habits of personal hygiene, proper ways to speak to older people, and myriad other things—things that increase in complexity as children grow older. From the "socialization as habit-building" point of view, a well-socialized child is one who has accumulated a large store of the habits needed for acceptable social behavior and acceptable levels of skills, while not having acquired bad (antisocial or nonfunctional) habits. By making progress with the acquisition of good habits, the child is presumably enabled to become more and more self-reliant.

Skinnerian and Hullian learning theories placed *reinforcement* (i.e., learned connections between stimuli and responses) as the central process in the formation of habits. It was not always clear what could be considered a "response": Was it always a single action, or could it be something as global as a personality trait? In early work, the definition of responses was quite narrow. Initially, all stimulus–response (S–R) connections were thought to be equally easy to learn, but the possibility that certain connections might be "privileged" did begin to emerge as some of the work on "imprinting" by German ethologists became well known, and Chomsky's (1959) claims about innate processes in children's language acquisition entered the discourse about learning processes in the 1960s (Gewirtz, 1969).

S–R learning theories were progressively incorporated into thinking about parenting and its effects. Parents could "shape" their children's development by judiciously reinforcing desired behavior and punishing or withholding reward for undesired behaviors. Parents might, of course, unwittingly reinforce undesired behavior. In early writings it was noted that during the first year infants began to cling to their parents and protest separation from them. J. B. Watson, early in his career, said such "bad habits" could be avoided if parents would only refrain from kissing, cuddling, and holding their infants. Sears, Maccoby, and Levin (1957) regarded the development of "dependency" on mothers (i.e., clinging, following, and protesting separation) as inevitable because the reinforcing power of the mother herself becomes so great due to her role in feeding, comforting, and helping the child. However, the dependent behavior was thought to be "change-worthy," a habit appropriate only for early childhood, and one that must be weakened or eliminated through socialization pressures from the parents as the child grows older. Learned habits can be unlearned, and reinforcement theories did not assign any greater importance to habits learned early versus those learned at a later age. The theories were thus not developmental. They had little to say about any differences between younger and older children in what could be learned or in *how* learning occurred. However, early learned habits, such as using table utensils in a prescribed way, could persist for very long periods, indeed for a lifetime.

An important research program that emerged during the 1970s from the behavioral perspective on parenting is the one organized and led by Gerald Patterson at the Oregon Social Learning Center (Patterson, 1982). Patterson and colleagues focused on the families of aggressive children, comparing the interactive sequences between parent and child that occurred in these families to those in the families of nonaggressive children. They noted that parents could inadvertently build children's aggression by backing away from their control efforts when the child was aggressively defiant (they termed this process *negative reinforcement*). Patterson and colleagues stressed that parents needed to provide consequences (i.e., reward or punishment) for desired or undesired child behavior, and noted that in order to do so, parents needed to be vigilant in detecting infractions and keeping track of whether children have complied with parental directives. Thus, parental "monitoring" was a crucial element in parental management of children—a variable that has since been adopted by many other researchers studying parent–child interaction. The thinking by Patterson and his colleagues quickly moved beyond a simple Skinnerian paradigm in that it increasingly focused on dyads and two-way influence rather than on a simple "shaping" of children by parents.

In the 1950s and 1960s, Skinnerian ideas were brought to bear on the treatment of children with behavior problems (see summary in Alexander & Malouf, 1983), and behavioral therapy models based on reinforcement principles continue in active use to the present day. In general, however, developmental psychologists began to turn away from simple reinforcement accounts of parenting effects. Skinner's effort to explain language acquisition in reinforcement terms was notably unsuccessful (Chomsky, 1959). The concept of reward itself proved to be problematic: Children differed in what parental responses they found rewarding. Customary (expected) levels of reward or praise were adapted to, so that they lost their efficacy.

Perhaps the most powerful critique of reinforcement learning theory came from the work on observational learning, initiated in the 1960s by Bandura, Mischel, and their colleagues. Experimental evidence showed that children could learn without ever having performed, or been reinforced for, the responses in question, merely by observing models perform them. Bandura called this "no trial learning." He made a crucial distinction: Performance, he claimed, was governed by reinforcement contingencies; learning was not (Bandura, 1969).

Socialization as the Regulation of Impulses

Pychodynamic views of socialization emerged concurrently with the "learned habits" view described earlier. The two streams of thought were similar in that they were both "drive" theories, but they differed in fundamental respects. Beginning with Freud, psychodynamic theorists saw behavior in infancy and early childhood as the free expression of instinctual impulses, including aggressive and sexual impulses. Impulsive behavior was not just elicited by external stimuli. Rather, it was driven by strong intrinsic energy. The young child's impulses inevitably came into conflict with the requirements of social living, and adults—especially parents—had the responsibility for curbing and directing the child's impulsive behavior, channeling the energy according to what was allowed and what was not allowed in the culture in which a child was growing up. These adult constraints inevitably generated resistance and anger on the part of the young child, and controlling this anger itself then necessarily became a focus of adult control. Freud's writings were interpreted as meaning that harsh parental blocking of children's impulses would carry long-term risks, and the roots of many forms of adult psychopathology were thought to lie in the early childhood relationship of children with their parents and other socialization agents (Whiting & Child, 1953). A basic psychodynamic tenet was that socialization moves from a process of external control by parents to self-control by the child, and that self-control is achieved through a child's identifying with parents and internalizing their controls, thus developing a *superego* (i.e., conscience). The twin concepts of "internalization" and "identification" have continued to influence socialization research over many decades, though some of the psychodynamic theories about the psychosexual stages of early life have faded into what is, in my view, well-deserved oblivion. Unlike habit formation theories, psychodynamic theories were strongly developmental, with an early set of behavioral tendencies being transformed at a particular stage of development—around age 4 or 5, when the Oedipus complex was presumably being resolved—and great gains in children's self-control and social maturity would then become possible.

Beginning in the 1930s, an interdisciplinary group at Yale University asked whether it would be possible to bring Hullian learning theory to bear on psychoanalytic concepts. The Freudian concept of identification was operationally defined as imitation, and imitation was explained as a generalized habit of imitation, formed as a consequence of children's being reinforced so often for doing things as adults do them (Miller & Dollard, 1941). Anxieties acquired through punishment were conceptualized as learned motivational states whose reduction could then reinforce the learning of new habits.

In the 1950s, Robert Sears and colleagues (Sears et al., 1957; Sears, Rau, & Alpert, 1965; Sears, Whiting, Nowlis, & Sears, 1953) brought this line of thinking into the field of socialization research, studying childrearing practices and their relation to a set of children's personality traits. Their objective was to translate psychoanalytic hypotheses into the language of Hullian learning theory, and to develop a set of hypotheses that could be objectively assessed (see Grusec, 1997, for fuller exposition of some of these translations). Freudian theory held that children resolved their psychosexual conflicts with their parents by identifying with the same-sex parent. Successful identification would presumably bring about a coherent set of developments toward greater maturity. Although all children were thought to go through these developmental processes, individual children differed in how quickly and how successfully they would do so, and variations in parenting were thought to have a central role in determining how individual children would progress.

In this work, the choice of variables was governed largely by psychoanalytic theory, drawing on learning theory mainly in its relevance to punishment and anxiety. Thus, parenting attributes such as severity of weaning and toilet training, punishment for aggression, permissiveness for dependency, and the use of withdrawal of love as a technique of discipline were chosen for assessment. The "outcome" variables for the children included sex typing, adult role taking, aggression, dependency, and manifestations of "conscience" (e.g., resistance to temptation and feelings of guilt over transgressions).

The results of these studies were disappointing. A major problem was that the set of child characteristics that included presumably all the outcomes of successful identification with the same-sex parent cohered only slightly (i.e., weakly for girls and not at all for boys; Sears et al., 1965). On the whole, these studies did not confirm the idea that children achieved self-controlling levels of maturity through identification with the same-sex parent. The measured variations in parenting were not found to be consistent predictors of the child attributes that were chosen for study. The weak results of these studies called for rethinking the theories that underlay them. Nevertheless, the work by Sears and colleagues was important in giving impetus to the empirical study of parenting, specifically to the ways in which variations in the quality of parenting might be related to children's developing attributes.

Some psychodynamic concepts received strong support in objective studies. Bandura, Mischel, and colleagues conducted several studies of imitation in which the hypotheses were drawn from the psychoanalytic concepts of anaclitic and defensive identification. They found that children were indeed more likely to imitate adult models who were shown to be nurturant and also to imitate powerful models (those in a position to dispense desired rewards), by comparison with models who did not have these characteristics

(Bandura, Ross, & Ross, 1963; Mischel & Liebert, 1967). Because parents are typically both powerful and nurturant, their children would presumably be motivated to emulate them preferentially. Bandura and colleagues, however, did not see imitation as a process of "taking over" whole personality qualities from models. Indeed, they stressed that children learn from many models, and the "final common path" of their behavior may involve a blending of what they have learned observationally from many sources. This formulation puts the child's own agency at center stage, involving a considerable degree of self-socialization on the part of the child (see, e.g., Bandura, 1986).

As we see later, the Freudian idea that successful socialization must involve children's coming to be able to control their own impulses—to self-regulate—is very much alive, and in fact has received increasing emphasis in recent work. The processes that lead to self-regulation, however, have come to be seen very differently from the processes Freud proposed.

Good Parenting as Democracy

During the 1930s and early 1940s, a number of distinguished European intellectuals came as refugees to the United States and established research programs relevant to socialization. Else Frenkel-Brunswik came to Berkeley, bringing a strong psychoanalytic orientation; she joined with a group of colleagues (Adorno, Frenkel-Brunswik, Levinson, & Sanford, 1950) to study the roots of "authoritarian" personality structures. They concluded that harsh and threatening parenting was a key element in the formation of such personalities.

Kurt Lewin, also a refugee from Europe, brought a very different theoretical orientation. He was a "configurational" theorist, and his field theory, like Gestalt theories, emphasized holistic concepts such as the contextual and organizational properties of environments, rather than focusing on specific "stimuli." During the 1930s, Lewin joined with American colleagues in a set of studies on the effects of group atmospheres and leadership styles on the functioning of task-oriented groups. Most pertinent for developmental psychology was the study of groups of 10- and 11-year-old boys, who undertook a variety of tasks under the leadership of adults who had been trained to create one of three different kinds of "group atmospheres": authoritarian, democratic, or laissez-faire (Lewin, Lippitt, & White, 1939). They found, as expected, that when working under a democratic leadership regimen, the boys became more involved in the tasks, more able to carry on with the work when the leader was out of the room, and more competent in accomplishing their tasks successfully, than boys in either the authoritarian or laissez-faire groups.

It was a natural step to apply these concepts to families, which could be seen as small groups with adult leaders, and to ask whether some families could be identified as having an authoritarian group atmosphere, while others functioned more democratically. A further question was what effect such different atmospheres might have on the children growing up in these families. As it happened, Alfred Baldwin was a graduate student at Harvard during the 1930s, at a time when Lewin came there as a visiting faculty member. Baldwin was greatly impressed by the work on group atmospheres. When he left Harvard to set up his own research enterprise at the Fels Institute, he organized a longitudinal study of parenting styles. He and his colleagues made successive visits to the homes of young children over a period of several years, interviewing the mothers and at the same time making detailed notes of the interaction of the mother and child. Baldwin and colleagues were able to identify several different parenting styles, one of which corresponded closely to the democratic style Lewin had identified. They found it important, however, to distinguish "scientific democracy," which involved emotional detachment from the child, and "warm democracy," which entailed more affectionate behavior toward the child and more empathy for both the child's point of view and the child's emotional reactions to parental socializing efforts. Other parental patterns were labeled passive–neglectful, actively hostile, and possessive–indulgent. Baldwin and colleagues reported that warm-democratic parenting was associated with stronger intellectual development in children, more spontaneity, and less anxiety than the other parenting styles. The warm-democratic parents allowed the child a great deal of freedom, and this was associated with many positive developments but also with more antisocial behavior on the part of the child (see Baldwin, 1955).[2]

Both the Baldwin work and the work of the Berkeley group on authoritarian personalities pointed to undesired outcomes of authoritarian childrearing, implying that parents should be less strict, less focused on getting obedience and deference from their children, and more willing to express unconditional acceptance and love toward their children. To many, this seemed to amount to recommending unconditional permissiveness.

There was a backlash. Diana Baumrind was convinced that both authoritarian and laissez-faire leadership styles were ineffective in promoting optimal functioning of groups, and became concerned about the ways in which the authoritarian personality findings were being interpreted. In the 1960s, she and her colleagues began studying parenting styles, and their connections with a variety of characteristics of preschool-age children. As is now well known, she developed a three-part typology of parenting styles: an *authoritarian* style, a *permissive* style, and an *authoritative* style (Baumrind & Black, 1967). This latter style involved parents' making age-appropriate demands on children and setting up firmly enforced rules for their behavior. At the same time, authoritative parents were responsive to their children's needs, willing to listen to them and take their viewpoint into account, involving them in decisions whenever possible. They used reasoning and gave children explanations for parental demands. They both assigned responsibilities and made room for children's autonomy. They were affectionate and supportive of the child's enterprises. This could be seen as a form of democratic parenting, but it was combined with a level of strictness not found in Baldwin's "warm democracy" group. Comparing the nursery school behavior of children from these three kinds of homes, Baumrind and colleagues reported that it was the children from authoritative households who were most mature and competent, being assertive in pursuing their own ends but also considerate toward other children and cooperative with teachers.

The Baumrind work was stronger conceptually than it was empirically. A considerable number of families could not be classified as belonging to any one of the three groups. The connections between parenting styles and child behaviors were not robust. And later studies showed that most parents employed all three styles at one time or another, depending on a variety of contextual factors, such as the nature of the child's infraction, the parents' socialization goal, and the child's current mood (Grusec & Goodnow, 1994). The Baumrind work did call attention to the importance of parental authority as well as parental sensitivity, but more recent research has turned away from the goal of classifying parents according to some dominant parenting type, focusing instead on the nature of interactive relationships (see below).

Socialization by Parents as a Product of Evolution

In 1969, a groundbreaking book was published. It was the first of a three-volume series, *Attachment and Loss*, by John Bowlby. It described the development of the emotional attachment of young infants and toddlers to their mothers (or other primary caregivers) as *instinctive* behavior.[3] Bowlby's perspective was strongly evolutionary. Drawing on the work of Tinbergen and Lorenz, he described the way in which, in some species of birds, newly hatched chicks imprinted on the first moving creature they saw (usually the maternal bird) but considered this to be only roughly analogous to attachment in human children because birds have been on a separate evolutionary track from mammals for a very long time. However, Bowlby was unequivocal about human kinship with other mammals, and particularly with nonhuman primates. He said: "Whatever behaviour is found in sub-human primates we can be confident is truly homologous with what obtains in man" (Bowlby, 1969, p. 183). He described in detail the early appearance of a primate mother's greater orientation toward her own infant than toward other infants, and the appearance of a matching own-mother bias in the infant. Bowlby described how attachment behavior in monkeys, and in several species of great apes, waxes and wanes during the early phases of development. He said that attachment behavior in the human infant develops more slowly than it does in other primates, but that the nature of the behavior, the conditions that elicit it, and its time course relative to species-specific maturity were remarkably similar across primate species. Bowlby noted that the caregiving behavior of primate mothers changed in synchrony with the developmental status of the infant, but that even when the young animal had become fairly independent, mother and offspring would quickly move toward one another in the presence of threat.

Work by Harry Harlow and colleagues in Wisconsin showed quite clearly that infant monkeys' attachment to their mothers was not a by-product of feeding by her but should be seen as a separate behavioral system. The Harlows believed that the analogy to human infant attachment was clear (Harlow & Harlow, 1965). The bidirectional nature of the mother–infant attachment was underscored by stress-hormone work showing that in both monkeys and humans, stress levels in both mother and infant diminish when a separated pair is reunited. Bowlby (1969) saw attachment in primates as a reciprocal system in which evolution had equipped both child and mother with prepared readinesses to form a mutual bond.[4] He saw the bonding process as a *species* characteristic. That is, in both humans and other primates, some degree of attachment between the mother and her own infant must occur if the infant is to survive. Individual differences would have to be seen within this larger framework. Bowlby noted, however, that at least in humans, there were striking individual differences among mother–child pairs in the nature and closeness of the bond that developed over the first year. He thought that these differences stemmed partly from variations among the infants in their temperamental predispositions but also from variations in maternal involvement with, and responsiveness and sensitivity to, the infant. Bowlby's work was important, too, in emphasizing the emotional as well as the behavioral components of socialization.

Suomi (2002) has summarized extensive observational data on the interactions of maternal monkeys with their infants, showing how the nature of mothering changes as the infant matures. He points to individual variations in maternal styles, ranging from highly protective and restrictive to more "laissez-faire." These variations are related to the mother's social status, to the birth order of the infant, the size of the troupe in which the mother and infant live, and the occurrence of environmental perturbations. Naturally occurring variations in maternal style are associated with certain outcomes for the infants (e.g., their subsequent social status is affected).

The biological factors in the readiness of mothers and infants for bonding with one another begin much earlier than the appearance of attachment behaviors. Recent research has shown that the hormones of pregnancy and parturition contribute to mothers' close caregiving attention to their infants, and both mothers and infants appear to be predisposed for quick selective learning of their own partner's distinctive vocalizations and facial features (see review by Bugental & Grusec, 2006). Interestingly, fathers who are present during the pregnancy and involved in infant care also undergo some hormonal changes (though more limited than for mothers) that support bonding to infants.

Of course, attachment is not the only behavioral domain in which strong similarities have been noted between human children and the young of nonhuman primates. For example, these similarities exist with respect to many aspects of gender differentiation (Maccoby, 1998), social dominance and aggressive behavior, even sympathy and altruism (de Waal, 1996). These similarities serve to underscore the evolutionary roots of many aspects of human behavior and development, but they have also pointed to ways in which environmental inputs affect the ways in which evolved predispositions are overtly expressed.

Socialization as Support for Children's Capacities to Self-Regulate

Research interest in the development of self-regulation has a long history, and increasingly, the development of self-regulatory abilities is seen as a building block, a necessary precursor, for a set of subsequent developmental achievements. Traditional learning theory had little to say about self-regulation. When children acquired and performed a habit, no intervening regulatory process between the stimulus and response was invoked, nor thought to be needed. Psychoanalytic theory, by contrast, was centrally concerned with self-regulation. We have already seen that, in psychoanalytic views, infants and young children have strong instinctive drives that impel them to impulsive behavior that must be curbed and directed by adults, but eventually must come under the child's own control. I have selected three research programs on self-regulation to illustrate how self-regulation has been conceptualized and how socialization practices might affect self-regulatory development in children.

In psychoanalytic theory, two intrapsychic structures were thought to be involved in a child's controls: the *superego*, an internalized representation of the controlling parent, and the *ego*, a self-controlling entity that guides efforts to avoid fearful situations, deal with new circumstances, and regulate impulses. Beginning in the 1970s, Jack and Jeanne Block reformulated the psychoanalytic views of self-regulation. They distinguished between *ego control* (conceptualized as the degree of impulse control and modulation, ranging from undercontrol to overcontrol, with midscale scores representing an "appropriate" level of control) and *ego resiliency* (conceptualized as "the dynamic capacity of an individual to modify his/her modal level of ego-control, in either direction, as a function of the demand characteristics of the environmental context"; see Block & Block, 1980). Working with a longitudinal sample, they traced distinctive developmental trajectories for children varying on their two dimensions.

Walter Mischel and his colleagues, beginning in the 1960s, mounted an extensive program of research on a different aspect of self-regulation, namely, *postponement of gratification* (Mischel & Grusec, 1967; Mischel & Metzner, 1962). In typical studies, a child would be offered a choice between obtaining a small or relatively unattractive reward immediately, or waiting some time in order to receive a larger or more desirable reward. The studies showed that the ability to postpone gratification varies with a number of conditions (e.g., the trustworthiness of the promise of future reward, the length of time the child has to wait, and the cognitive strategies the child brings to bear during the waiting period). Self-regulation of attention deployment was shown to be a central component of successful delay.

Another approach to the development of self-regulation came out of studies of temperament. In this tradition, the focus has been on attempts to identify distinctive dimensions of temperament, such as sociability or fearfulness, thought to be constitutionally based. Rothbart and colleagues, in studying the temperamental characteristics of infants and young children, identified a set of characteristics that cluster together into a single dimension that they labeled "effortful control." In infancy, this control is manifest primarily in the form of being able to inhibit a dominant response in order to perform a subdominant response, as in the Piagetian A-not-B task (Rothbart & Bates, 1998). As the child grows into toddlerhood and preschool age, the ability to detect his or her own errors and engage in planning becomes part of the "effortful control" cluster. Engaging in effortful control means that a child must exercise control over the deployment of attention (i.e., maintain attentional focus and resist distraction) as well as inhibit impulsive behavior. Researchers have developed an impressive battery of measures for assessing children's ability to exercise effortful control (Kochanska, Murray, & Harlan, 2000; Posner & Rothbart, 1998), and have explored related aspects of brain function (Rothbart & Rueda, 2005).

Although these three streams of research have been conducted independently over many years, there have been some notable convergences. In all three, there is demonstrable stability of individual differences over a number of years. In all three, there are documented increases with age. Especially important is the fact that in all these research programs, self-regulatory abilities have been shown to presage the future development of a variety of "outcomes" that can be qualitatively quite distinct from, but conceptually linked with, self-regulation (Block & Block, 1980; Kochanska, Coy, & Murray, 2001; Mischel, Shoda, & Peake, 1988; Shoda, Mischel, & Peake, 1990).

For present purposes, the important question is: What is the impact of parenting on the kind and degree of self-regulation children develop? Block (1971) was among the first to address this question. He reported that undercontrolled people came from chaotic, conflict-ridden households in which parents often neglected their teaching responsibilities. The mothers and fathers of ego-resilient children, by contrast, had good relations with one another and agreed on values, were both loving and fair in their dealings with their children, and encouraged free interchange concerning feelings and problems. At the same time they were concerned with firmly transmitting values. Above all, they were seriously committed to their parenting responsibilities and devoted sustained effort and attention to childrearing. We can see links between the parenting clusters described by the Blocks and the trio of clusters described by Baumrind.

With rare exceptions, researchers in the Mischel tradition have not focused on what the possible socialization antecedents of the individual differences in abilities to postpone gratification might be. But inferences can be made from the experimental conditions that have been shown to affect children's ability to postpone gratification. For example, children are more willing to wait if they have experience with an experimenter who has kept a promise to provide a larger reward later, as compared with an experimenter whose promise proved unreliable (Mischel & Grusec, 1967). The implication for parenting would be that parents who follow through on their promises will support children's ability to postpone gratification.

Eisenberg, Smith, Sadovsky, and Spinrad (2004) have summarized a substantial research literature on the socialization of emotional self-regulation. They adopt Rothbart's term *effortful control* for the set of self-regulatory processes they review but define the term somewhat more broadly as the ability to "manage attention, motivation and behavior voluntarily," and they do not adopt the assumptions about primarily constitutional foundations that underlie the work on temperament. Eisenberg and colleagues report that children's development of strong self-regulatory capacities in early childhood is linked to parental responsiveness, parental warmth and emotional support, and a minimum of interference and intrusion into the child's autonomous activities, along with an absence of disciplinary practices that frighten the child unduly.

Students of moral development have noted that "moral" behavior involves the regulation of impulse (i.e., children must inhibit immediately gratifying, self-serving behavior to make way for more reasoned consideration of social obligations to others). Such self-regulation depends on a set of values with respect to which children evaluate and guide their own behavior. Grolnick, Deci, and Ryan (1997) say: "Whereas socializing agents can 'teach' their children the values and attitudes they hold dear, the important thing is having the children 'own' those attitudes and values" (p. 135)—in other words, to internalize them. In an influential chapter, Hoffman (1970) distinguished among several aspects of parental discipline, noting that while withdrawal of love did not appear to be an effective technique for building children's internalization of moral values, there was evidence for the importance of parental use of "induction" (explaining, and appealing to children's pride in being more grown up), and especially "other-oriented induction" (calling children's attention to the effects of their behavior on others). Hoffman also stressed the minimal use of parental power assertion as a factor in moral internalization.

Socialization as Specific to Contexts and Domains

In much of the socialization research done through the 1960s, 1970s, and 1980s, the primary interest was in the variation *between* parents, in terms of trait-like attributes that characterized their parenting. Many studies used factor analysis and other statistical techniques to try to identify major dimensions of parenting, and issues arose as to whether it was more productive to keep major dimensions separate in analyses, or combine them into Baumrind-like typologies (see review by Darling & Steinberg, 1993). But whether dimensions or typologies were used, the assumption was that individual parents, or individual children, could be characterized as having some degree of a fairly stable property or set of properties which they habitually manifested in their interactions with each other. Some researchers, although not dismissing these trait-like approaches as unimportant, began to find them to be too limited. Beginning in the early 1980s, Grusec began to produce evidence of considerable *within parent* variability. In their 1994 review paper, Grusec and Goodnow summarized the evidence, noting that the techniques parents typically use with their children depend on the nature and seriousness of the infraction and the context in which it has occurred, as well as the age and momentary emotional state of the child. And, Grusec and Goodnow claimed, the effect of a given kind of discipline would be different, depending on these same contextual conditions. They urged further that we have paid too little attention to the *content* of parental messages to children: their consistency and clarity, their "truth value" (i.e., there verifiability), and their direct relevance to the issue at hand. These things determine not only how well a parental message will be understood by the child but also the child's judgment about whether to believe and accept the message as being fair.

Building on the fact that individual parents do vary considerably from one context to another, Bugental and Goodnow (1998; Bugental, Corpuz, & Beaulieu, Chapter 14, this volume) propose a domain-specific account of socialization. The domains they identify are (1) protective care, which encompasses attachment and nurturance; (2) coalitional groups, the avenue whereby a child acquires a sense of ingroup belonging (more pertinent to the interactions in peer groups but still relevant to family membership); (3) hierarchical power, encompassing disciplinary encounters, and involving continuing renegotiation of power relationships as children mature; and (4) reciprocity/mutuality. Any given parent will function within each of these domains from time to time, depending on the issue or parental task involved. For each domain, they say, distinctive parenting patterns are called into play, and they argue that these have an evolutionary basis in both parent and child that prepare the dyad for interaction within a given domain. Sensitive parenting, then, means that a parent uses the parenting that is appropriate to the domain of interaction that is occurring at a given time. Thus, if a child is distressed, a sensitive parent soothes, an insensitive one might try to initiate a game or become power assertive; at a moment when a child is angrily defiant, hierarchical power comes into play and power assertion is appropriate and should be seen as reflecting parent sensitivity, while soothing would be inappropriate to the domain.

Children as Agents in Their Own Socialization

We have already seen that children are active agents in observational learning, as they choose preferred models for imitation and deploy attention toward some kinds of modeled activities rather than others. But their agency is much broader than this: They can *elicit* or even control some of the directive, controlling, and nurturing activity that parents direct toward them, and select which parental directives they will give more credence to.

The role of children in their own socialization has been underscored in studies that emphasize the role of children's genetic predispositions in determining how they will be socialized. For many decades, psychologists have been aware of genetic influences on children's development. There were early intensive studies of maturation, which were seen as evidence that there is an inborn developmental timetable driving changes in the child. The implication was that socialization must be organized around this timetable, changing as the child changes. And twin and adoption studies were widely cited, pointing to genetically based individual differences in children's temperaments and abilities. As we have seen in the review so far, however, most of the early socialization research focused on the kind of impact parenting processes might have on the developing child, with little regard to any genetic characteristics individual children might bring to parent–child encounters. Researchers were looking for general laws governing parenting effects, and when they found connections between parenting methods and children's "outcomes," these were usually interpreted as showing that parents were influencing children in predictable ways.

There were voices warning about possible reverse effects (Bell & Harper, 1977). Some excellent studies followed showing how children's behavior could determine the way adults treated them (e.g., Bugental, Corporael, & Shennum, 1980; Grusec & Kuczynski, 1980). Challenges to claims about strong parenting effects continue to the present day. For example, researchers studying adolescents have repeatedly found that weak, erratic monitoring by parents is associated with a number of problematic adolescent outcomes, including juvenile delinquency, drug use, and risky sexual activity (see Kerr & Stattin, 2003, for a review). These risky behaviors have been interpreted as "outcomes" of poor parental monitoring. Kerr and Stattin have strongly challenged this interpretation, arguing that parents can monitor effectively only if their adolescents are willing to talk to them openly about their activities, so that successful parental monitoring is driven by properties of the child (see review of this debate throughout this volume).

The strongest demand for reinterpretation of the direction of effects has come from behavior geneticists (see Moffitt, & Caspi, 2007; Avinun & Knafo-Noam, Chapter 15, this volume). What behavior geneticists reported in work appearing through the 1980s and early 1990s was sobering to people who had been stressing top-down effects from parent to child. Strong heritability coefficients, clustering around 50% or higher, were found with respect to many child characteristics. Especially startling was the claim that shared environmental effects were weak, indeed often close to zero (Plomin & Daniels, 1987), while *unshared* environmental effects were often substantial. The inference that was drawn from such findings was that variations in parenting could hardly be having much effect on children's development. These arguments were elaborated by Rowe (1994) and given a more popular treatment by Harris (1998). Sandra Scarr (1992), in her presidential address to the Society for Research in Child Development, argued that while extreme parental abuse or neglect could of course harm children, in the vast majority of families parenting was "good enough" to support children's development, and that other factors—children's genetics, nonfamilial environmental influences—were more important in determining individual differences in how children turned out. The extreme version of this point of view would be that parents hardly socialize their children at all—children socialize themselves, aided by a variety of nonparental influences. A more nuanced version would be that all parents do manage to socialize their children up to some base level regardless of their methods, but variations in parenting above this level account for very little variance in child outcomes.

There were strong reactions against these claims, and vigorous efforts to rebut them were mounted, along with presentations of studies with demonstrable parenting effects (see Borkowski, Ramey, & Bristol-Power, 2002; Collins, Maccoby, Steinberg, &

Hetherington, 2000; Maccoby, 2000; Turkheimer, 2000). Several of the behavior geneticists' strongest points have been widely accepted (if sometimes reluctantly!) and have greatly influenced more recent socialization research. One is the simple fact that children's genetic endowments do have an influence on the kind of parent–child relationship that is likely to develop, so that in attempting to evaluate parenting influences, it is important to take into account children's initial variations in temperament and abilities and the influence these things may have on what parents do and what effects they can have. Another is that parenting researchers have often overclaimed for the strength of their effects. And a third is that siblings growing up together can be very different, and in fact usually are. Until the 1980s, socialization researchers almost always studied only one child per family. Now it is understood that given the importance of so-called unshared rather than shared environmental factors, it must be the case that parental influence is often not the same for different children in the same family, and indeed that parental influence probably rarely functions to make siblings more alike with respect to the outcomes that are commonly measured.

These things being said, it must be noted that there have been widespread misinterpretations of some of the behavior geneticists' claims, and corrections have been called for. They define *shared environment* as any aspect of the environment that makes coresident children more alike. However, important parental influences that do not make children in the same family more alike can nevertheless serve to shape the development of individual children. It is important to note, too, that in interpreting behavior genetic studies, much depends on the magnitudes of the genetic (G), shared environmental (E), and nonshared E effects. All these, of course, depend on the original estimates of heritability, since E effects have been defined as the residual when heritability coefficients are subtracted from 100%. And these estimates of heritability turn out to be unstable (see Shonkoff & Phillips, 2001, for fuller exposition). In particular, they depend on the range of variation in G and E factors within the particular population studied, and they are highly responsive to data source. Comparisons of heritability estimates based on observational reports of mother–child interaction are almost always lower than such estimates based on parent report or child report, so that observational data allow more room for shared and unshared environmental effects to be shown. A recent example can be found in Neiderhiser and colleagues (2004), where the child's genetic contribution to mother's positivity is estimated at 48% from mother reports, 19% from child reports, and 0% from observer reports. Clearly, very large brackets must be put around any estimate of heritability, until the method variance in these estimates can be more fully understood.

To many researchers, the problem has remained one of trying to identify the causal contributions of each party in the parent–child dyad. And certainly if the larger agenda is to trace the ways in which parents pass culture on to the next generation of children, it would seem to make sense to focus on the kind and degree of influence parents can have, net of any contribution the child and nonparental environmental factors make to the process. Several methods have been pursued for covarying genetic and parenting variables so that their respective contributions can be independently assessed. These methods include (1) using longitudinal data, and assessing the connections of parenting at time 1 with child behavior at time 2 or 3, net of the child's initial time 1 behavior—in other words, to study *change* in children's behavior as predicted from earlier parenting; (2) using measures of temperament as proxies for genetic variations, allowing researchers to control for these variations and identify independent parent effects; (3) adopting "genetically sensitive" research designs in which variations in the degree of genetic relatedness among family members is known, and entered into multivariate analyses along with parenting variables; (4) ruling out genetic differences by studying pairs of identical twins, to assess the differences in parenting and estimating their effects; (5) cross-fostering experiments with animals in which littermates are placed for rearing with mothers differing in parenting behaviors; and (6) intervention studies, in which families are randomly assigned to parent-training or no-training groups—with randomization controlling for initial variation in a large range of both genetic and environmental factors—and testing for the effects of intervention-produced changes in parenting behavior (e.g., Brody et al., 2004; Martinez & Forgatch, 2001).

A detailed assessment of the strengths and weaknesses of these and other approaches to identifying the causal power of G and E risk factors can be found in Rutter, Pickles, Murray, and Eaves (2001). A number of these approaches permit the evaluation of G × E interactions—something that was seldom done in the early behavior genetics research—and it has been shown that a given parental action can have a different effect on children of different temperament but be an important source of influence nonetheless (e.g., Bates, Pettit, Dodge, & Ridge, 1988; Kochanska, 1995). Current work on molecular genetics stresses G × E interactions much more heavily than statistical behavior–genetic work has done (Moffitt, Caspi, & Rutter, 2006). There is now abundant evidence that from the moment of conception on, environmental inputs affect which genes will be activated at successive points in development. Some genes remain inactive unless triggered by specific environmental inputs. Environmental inputs help to guide brain development, and specifically the neuroendocrine system, in ways that will affect behavior. The usefulness of the "additive assumption" (that G and E effects, taken separately, add up to 100% of the forces controlling variance in any trait) is being widely challenged (Bugental & Grusec, 2006; Cairns, Elder, & Costello, 1996; Maccoby, 2000; Shonkoff & Phillips, 2001). It is now widely understood that feedback loops pervade parent–child interactions, so that whatever eliciting powers the genetic predispositions of parent or child might have had in initiating an interaction, these are quickly enmeshed in mutual influence. Within this bidirectional perspective, emphasis on the child's agency in the socialization process is now a central aspect of theory and research (e.g., Grolnick et al., 1997).

Parenting as a Bidirectional, Reciprocal Process

In 1951, Sears urged that parent and child be studied as a dyad in which each influenced the other. For a number of years this idea lay dormant, but from the publication of Bowlby's work and the early work of G. R. Patterson and colleagues, there has been increasing recognition of the reciprocal nature of parent–child interaction. But as this shift in focus occurred, researchers became increasingly aware of methodological issues that plagued the study of reciprocal interactions. While earlier research had relied heavily on parent interviews and questionnaires as the source of information about parenting, it became evident that parents were often not able to report accurately on some aspects of the dynamics of day-to-day interaction between parent and child. Researchers turned to a greater use of direct observation of parent–child interaction, and they were immediately struck by the way in which each responds to the other, and adapts his or her own behavior to that of the other. They encountered issues that were both methodological and conceptual: How could the behavior of each partner be coded in real time so that sequential dependencies could be detected? Should successive behaviors be separated into event units or time units? What is the optimum length of time units that will best capture the realities of a stream of interaction?

Methodological Advances

Technological developments helped to answer these questions. The Patterson research group in Oregon pioneered the recording of observed parent–child interaction in real time. They used an accordion-like keyboard that would allow the concurrent coding of parent and child behavior into predetermined categories. The growth of videotaping technology greatly enhanced the ability of researchers to code interaction reliably, and to reexamine interaction sessions for elements not originally selected for study. From videotapes it was possible to identify sequential dependencies of parents' and children's behavior on the other's prior actions, by coding the behavior of each in successive units of time. Or, more global ratings and behavioral scores could be derived from longer interaction segments.

A second major technological advance was in the computer processing of data. Beginning in the 1980s, computer programs were developed to carry out microanalytic analyses of sequential dependencies in real-time interaction data, and to compare several strategies for doing so (see Martin, Maccoby, Baran, & Jacklin, 1981). Enhanced computer power was especially important in handling the snowballing amounts of data accumulated in large longitudinal studies. Sophisticated structural modeling became feasible.

Microanalytic studies of interactive sequences have been intended to reveal the extent to which the behavior of each participant is contingent upon the prior behavior of the partner. Studies with infants and toddlers have shown that mother and infant do indeed influence one another's moment-to-moment behavior (with mothers, early in the child's life, adapting more to the behavior of their infants than vice versa). And, importantly, the reciprocation of affect—with parent and young child responding in kind to the other's positive or negative emotional signals—emerged as ubiquitous during parent–child interaction. While microanalytic studies have thus produced useful information, students of socialization have generally been more interested in understanding the longer-term influences of parents and children on one another than in the moment-to-moment give and take between them. In the 1980s, a number of short-term longitudinal studies extended the logic of sequential analysis over longer periods, by using cross-lagged analyses with longitudinal data to trace effects of parent on child and child on parent over several months or even years. In more recent years, such analyses have largely been replaced by structural modeling.

Mutual Responsiveness

In their 1983 chapter on parent–child interaction, Maccoby and Martin noted that while the importance of parental responsiveness to children's bids had been extensively studied, much less attention had been paid to children's responsiveness to parental signals or demands. They distinguished between *receptive* compliance and *situational* compliance, the former occurring without coercion, the latter occurring with parental bribery or power assertion. Receptive compliance has since been called *willing* compliance, or *committed* compliance (Kochanska & Askan, 1995; Kochanska & Thompson, 1997). Regardless of the label chosen, the distinction between the two different motivations underlying compliance has continued to be recognized as an important one. Kochanska and colleagues note that willing compliance is associated with young children's readiness to imitate the mother (i.e., with readiness to learn observationally from her), and they regard this "teachability" as another aspect of a child's receptive stance toward parental socialization (Forman & Kochanska, 2001).

Maccoby and Martin (1983) noted the mutuality of compliance, pointing to some suggestions in the literature that when a parent complied with a child, the likelihood of the child's complying to the parent increased. Following up on this theme, Parpal and Maccoby (1985) trained a group of mothers in responsive play. They showed that responsive maternal compliance with child directives did elevate the children's subsequent compliance with maternal directives. Lay, Waters, and Park (1989) showed that children's mood was elevated during mother-responsive play and showed further that experimentally elevating a child's mood would increase children's subsequent compliance, even in the absence of maternal responsive play. This work emphasizes once again the importance of affective reciprocity in mother–child interaction.

This theme also appears in the work of Martinez and Forgatch (2001), who report that children's willing compliance with parental directives improves when the mothers have been trained to engage in "positive parenting." Such parenting includes not only warmth, support, and concern for the child's interests but also *politeness*—in other words, a cluster of parenting features which imply some parental respect for the child's autonomy, as well as the creation of a pleasant family atmosphere. In this work, training in positive parenting proved to be even more important than training mothers not to yield to their children's coercion, although that too was important.

Maccoby and Martin (1983) proposed that if a state of positive mutual responsiveness prevails during much of infancy and early childhood, it will create a foundation for a well-functioning socialization relationship at a later time. Over a period of nearly two decades, Kochanska and colleagues have carried out a set of longitudinal studies of several cohorts of children, exploring the early dyadic relationship between mother–child pairs and looking to see what connections (if any) can be found between this relationship and the child's subsequent "internalized" compliance (i.e., ability to resist temptation and carry out a required task in the parent's absence) (see summary in Kochanska & Thompson, 1997). Among other findings, Kochanska and her colleagues have shown that measures of shared positive affect and mutual responsiveness taken at 33 months predict the child's ability, a year later, to persist in a task and resist temptation when the mother is out of the room. They have found, too, that willing face-to-face compliance by a young toddler or preschooler is a stepping-stone to a cluster of measures of "conscience" at a later age.

The reciprocity between parent and child was initially studied largely at the level of behavioral interaction, but as we have seen, reciprocity at the level of affect quickly emerged as a central feature of interaction. The study of reciprocity broadened further as it began to include the cognitive level. There is not space here to discuss the reciprocities that are made possible by the child's development of language. But several points emerging from socialization research in the 1980s and more recently deserve special notice: Parent and child develop expectancies about how the other will respond, based on the cumulating history of their interactions through time (see Lollis, 2003). Expectancies can become firmly established and embedded in automated, scripted interactive sequences. While such sequences can greatly smooth daily interaction, they can short-circuit needed communication when they run their course inflexibly, without regard to relevant contextual factors.

The success of parent and child in communicating with one another depends on the clarity of the messages each sends to the other, and on the openness of each to the other's messages. Grusec and Ungerer (2003) note that these things in turn frequently depend on emotional states. An angry child, or one who suffers from chronic anxiety or dysphoria (conditions which can stem from a history of dysfunctional interactions with parents), has difficulty taking in and digesting parental messages and indeed may fend them off defensively. Reciprocally, some parents tend to have distorted cognitions about their children's needs and to misinterpret their children's emotional cues, especially in ignoring or denying signs of children's negative affect. These cognitive distortions are bound up with parental depression and a low sense of parental efficacy. By contrast, when parent and child have a history of good cognitive synchrony in their interactions, each partner's sense of efficacy is enhanced.

Clearly, there must be serious consequences for the self-concepts of one or both members of the dyad if either resists the influence of the other. Bugental (1992) has focused on the minority of parents who feel that their children have more control over parent–child interactions than the parents themselves do. She documents how dysfunctional parenting can become in such families. Feelings of inefficacy are closely associated with maternal depression, and maternal depression, in turn, is associated with poor outcomes for children (Byrne, 2003). The causal connections between these things are of course complex, but recent work suggests that in some families a dynamic sequence starts with a difficult child, leading to a maternal sense of lacking control, which induces or exacerbates maternal depression and deteriorates parenting, followed by increased child misbehavior. This sequence is suggested by longitudinal intervention work in which teaching the mother to deal with child misbehavior firmly but not harshly leads to improvements in the child's behavior, which is then followed by a lessening of maternal depression (DeGarmo, Patterson, & Forgatch, 2004). Of course, initially dysfunctional parents do not all benefit equally from such training—some cannot muster sufficient self-regulation to become effective regulators of children.

Developmental Change in Parent–Child Interaction

A theme emerging strongly from the mid-1980s through the 1990s was a focus on developmental change—that is, on in-family socialization as a sequential process in which the parent–child relationship changes dramatically as children grow older, with each new phase growing out of the parent–child relationship established earlier. Although for many years studies of attachment mainly considered attachment to be a property of the child (i.e., the child is described as being either securely or insecurely attached), it has been evident from the beginning that the mother is reciprocally attached to the child. Developmental changes in the nature of this reciprocal relationship became a focus for study. Sroufe and Fleeson (1986) said: "The infant–caretaker attachment relationship is the womb from which the incipient person emerges. The first organization is dyadic, and it is from that organization, and not from inborn characteristics of the infant, that personality emerges" (p. 67). In his 1996 book on early emotional development, Sroufe integrated the developmental changes in children's attachment behavior with reciprocal changes in parenting. In this book, he drew on the decades-long work on attachment and its sequelae that he and his colleagues carried out. He saw the development of ego controls as central to emotional development. Sroufe said: "The evolving attachment relationship is conceptualized as progressive changes in the dyadic regulation of emotions, with an increasingly active role for the infant at each phase" (p. 10). He saw the acquisition of ego controls (self-regulation) as emerging out of this dyadic regulation, and as being central to emotional development. Sroufe has offered a beautifully detailed time-table, showing the successive changes that occur in the role of the mother (or other primary caregiver) in supporting the child's development of self-regulation through infancy and toddlerhood. Following this, at preschool age, Sroufe said that the child must be centrally concerned with managing impulses and maintaining acceptable behavior outside the immediate control of adults, while learning to interact with other children. During this time, the parent shifts from direct and immediate controls—prohibitions, interventions, demonstrations—to more indirect controls and the encouragement of the child's internalization of standards. This involves transmission of values, increasingly through reasoning and persuasion.

In their review of earlier work on developmental change in parenting, Collins and Madsen (2003) note that as children grow older, there is a progressive decrease in the amount of time parent and child spend together; physical displays of affection lessen, as do the frequency of disciplinary encounters and the direct expressions of anger between parent and child. Furthermore, the actions of parent and child increasingly depend on how they interpret one another's intentions. As children grow older, parents are more and more likely to view misbehavior as knowing and intentional, responding accordingly (Dix, Ruble, Grusec, & Nixon, 1986). With the decrease in direct, face-to-face interaction, cognitive aspects of the parent–child relationship become central. Parent–child reciprocity increasingly takes the form of coordinating cognized plans and agendas, and such coordination depends on the flow of information between parent and child, and how each codes the other's messages.

In 1994, Grusec and Goodnow said that the success of intergenerational transmission of values depended on two things: the accuracy of the child's perception of the parent's message, and the child's acceptance or rejection of the perceived message. With respect to the *accuracy* of children's understanding of parental messages, they note the importance of parents fitting their messages to the child's existing schemas. They note too that children's changing cognitive abilities affect what kind of parental reasoning they can digest, whether they can read the intent behind other' reactions, and whether they can interpret affective cues (especially when these are not consistent with what parents are saying). Children's *acceptance* depends on whether the child sees the parent's action as appropriate to the child's misdeed, whether the parent's message is believable (i.e., verifiable), and whether threats to the child's autonomy are minimized.

Research on the changes in parent–child interaction as children enter adolescence has brought into central focus the issue of how well the parent and child synchronize their ideas about the child's autonomy. Early adolescence is a time when parents' and children's perspectives concerning the rights of each diverge most strongly. Breakdowns in communication exacerbate this disjunction. Kerr and Stattin (2003) describe families in which an adolescent is defiant and secretive at home—a stance sometimes stemming from a history in which parents have reacted badly to disclosures. The youth may have confided about negative things that have happened away from home, only to have the parents respond with ridicule, blame, or punishment, or use the confided information against the adolescent on future occasions. The young person becomes wary, no longer confiding in the parents; they, in turn, worry about what might be going on behind their backs, lose trust, and show diminished affection and support, leading the adolescent to become more and more closed to communication with the parent. Parents, for their part, become reluctant to start up a conflict and diminish their efforts at control. We may suspect that such a dysfunctional spiral did not spring into being de novo in adolescence but may be traceable in part to missed opportunities in early childhood for forming a mutually responsive orientation.

Presenting a picture of more functional interaction between parents and adolescents, Youniss and Smollar in their groundbreaking 1985 book stressed the point that adolescence need not be—and usually is not—a time of *sturm and drang*—at least not within the economically comfortable two-parent families included in their research. Youniss and Smollar found that adolescents typically continue to recognize parental authority, while parents grant increasing freedom in synchrony with their children's increasing competence, so that conflict need not escalate. They did note, however, that children discriminate between domains of decision making, appropriating some domains (e.g., choice of clothes, hairstyles, friends—the "personal" domain) more than others as belonging to their own proper sphere of influence, not their parents'.

Socialization as a Family System Function

From the mid-1980s through the 1990s, as more and more researchers studied parent–child interaction longitudinally, there was a shift from a focus on the actions of individual parents and children—and on how each influenced the other—to a focus on their coaction and the nature of the relationship between them. At least from the time of Gestalt psychologists' early writings about development there have been claims about the holistic qualities of behaving organisms, with some thinking about how these change developmentally. From a family systems perspective, a family can be seen as composed of individuals, but also as a higher-level system with several dyadic subsystems, with systems and subsystems having properties of their own over and above the properties of the individuals making them up. In the 1980s, formulations from the work on adult close relationships began to percolate into developmental psychology, a landmark publication being Hartup and Rubin's (1986) *Relationships and Development*. This book began to bring thinking about the dynamic properties of within-family dyads into central focus, and research has burgeoned since that time (see Kuczynski, 2003).

An important aspect of dynamic systems theories as applied to family functioning is that systems are seen to be self-equilibrating. Parent and child both act in such a way as to keep the partner's behavior within acceptable boundaries. When one person in the system goes beyond the boundaries within which the family normally functions, the other members will react in such a way as to restore the balance. Though, of course, family dynamic systems can and do change over time, this self-corrective property of systems is a conservative force, serving to dampen change.

The Parent–Child Dyad

In the foregoing discussion of reciprocity I have already considered some dynamic properties of the parent–child subsystem within the family. Here I need only note that some researchers have studied properties of the dyad over and above the contributions to interaction that each participant makes. Kochanska and Aksan (1995) have used dyadic scores such as "shared positive affect," in which the score is not merely a sum of instances in which the child or the parent displays positive affect but a count of the number of instances in which the interactive pair displayed positive affect *simultaneously*. Other researchers have noted that while the nature of the relationship between an interacting pair is partly accounted for by the individual characteristics of the two persons involved, there is a large interactive component not attributable to either participant but to the pair jointly (Coie et al., 1999). William Cook (2003), studying the relationships between parents and their young-adult children, notes that the flow of mutual influence is to a large degree unique to specific pairs, so that the relationships between a mother and child 1 may involve quite a different pattern of mutual influence than that between this mother and child 2, and this same child 1 may have a different reciprocal relation with the mother than with the father. A unique interaction resides in the dyad.

The Parental Dyad

Much of the research on the parental dyad has examined the nature of the emotional relationships between the two parents, and the effect that harmony or discord in the parental relationship has on children (see review by Parke & Buriel, 1998) and on the parenting behavior of each (see summary in Katz, Kramer, & Gottman, 1995), but the importance of the parental dyad goes much beyond these issues. Minuchin (1974) was among the first to call attention to the importance of what he called the "executive subsystem" within the family (i.e., the importance of cooperation, communication, and coordination between two or more adults as they are involved in the joint rearing of a child). In recent years, a body of research has grown up on the functioning of the two as a coparental team (see review in McHale et al., 2002). These authors ask whether the quality of coparenting has effects on children's adjustment, over and above the effects of the conflict or harmony prevailing in the relation of the two parents to one another. Their review indicates that indeed there are real incremental effects of the way the two function as coparents.

   A basic coparental issue has to do with the way in which child care and childrearing responsibilities shall be apportioned between the two parents. In early studies of childrearing, role differentiation between the parents in childrearing was a built-in feature of the different economic roles of the two parents, with fathers being the almost exclusive breadwinners and mothers responsible for child care and home management. Later studies included many more families in which the mothers worked, and the feminist movement that burgeoned in the 1970s energized wide-ranging research on the effects of mothers' outside employment on the childrearing responsibilities of the two parents and on the interparental relationships (see summary in Maccoby, 1998). In modern societies in which mothers commonly have been working outside the home, the birth of the first child makes the question of how child care responsibilities will be divided between mother and father a major one. Through a program of research beginning in the mid-1980s, Phillip and Carolyn Cowan have shown how these issues are renegotiated after the birth of the first child, with mothers usually assuming a considerably larger proportion of the child care (and housework) than had been planned by the couple, with the fathers in many families increasing their hours of out-of-home work to compensate for losses of the mother's earnings (C. P. Cowan et al., 1985).

As McHale and colleagues (2002) note, a family's executive subsystem can vary in the quality of its functioning quite independently of how much division of labor there is between the parents; that is, a family can function effectively whether or not the two parents have equal and similar roles in daily childrearing. There are multiple ways in which parents can cooperate. A traditional mode is for one parent to specialize in providing economic support while the other cares for the children on a daily basis. But the less involved parent can nevertheless step in to defuse tensions between a child and the other parent, take over child care responsibilities when the other parent is tired or ill, or back up the other's authority. And most parents, regardless of their division of labor, discuss their childrearing objectives and practices in an effort to achieve consistency. Belsky, Crnic, and Gable (1995) have documented ways in which parents of a toddler son support or undermine one another's parenting activities. They note that a high level of daily hassles can amplify elements of dysfunctional coparenting that are otherwise minor in degree.

The quality of coparenting may depend on the gender of the parent or that of the child, or both. McHale (1995) notes, in observations of mother and father jointly interacting with their infant, that when the two parents have a conflicted relationships with one another, the father tends to engage in hostile undermining of the mother's interaction with an infant son, while he tends to withdraw if the infant is a girl. Other studies have found different pathways from coparenting to child outcomes for mothers than for fathers (see summary in P. A. Cowan & McHale, 1996). But in most observational studies of coparenting, samples have been too small to analyze fully for gender effects, so the findings to date remain only suggestive.

Issues of coparenting come to the fore in families in which the parents have divorced but continue to share responsibility for raising the children. Some work has focused on the interparental transactions that must occur when parents share custody of the children or when regular visitation occurs (Hetherington, Cox, & Cox, 1982; Maccoby & Mnookin, 1992). These studies have shown that if divorced parents are able to coodinate rules between the two households, avoid open conflict with one another, and communicate with one another about the children, the children benefit. However, these kinds of coparental cooperation diminish over time. Divorced parents become progressively more disengaged from each other even if the children continue to spend time in both households, especially if either parent has a new partner.

The Whole-Family System

A number of the coparenting studies discussed earlier have involved observations of two parents who were both present and interacting with their child—for example, studies of the parent–parent–child *triad* (see monograph edited by P. A. Cowan & McHale, 1996). Several aspects of all-family atmospheres or modes of interaction that might affect children's development have also been studied. These include family "climate," family paradigms, family coordinated practices, and family myths and rituals (see review by Parke & Buriel, 1998). *Residential stability* and *level of household organization* have emerged as important family-level characteristics (Adam, 2004; Buchanan, Maccoby, & Dornbusch,

1996; Hetherington et al., 1982; Weisner, Matheson, Coots, & Bernheimer, 2004). Both have been linked to children's achievement and positive adjustment. Asbury, Dunn, Pike, and Plomin (2003) have shown that the more chaotic a household is, the greater the connection between harsh parenting and children's maladjustment.

To date, research on family systems and subsystems is culturally limited. The work on coparenting and family triads of necessity deals almost exclusively with two-parent families, and these studies, along with those on family atmospheres and household organization, have included mainly middle-class families in industrialized Western societies. Thus, we do not know how closely the research described earlier applies in families in which a broader kinship network is involved in childrearing.

Where We Stand

Clearly, there have been great changes in the way we think about and carry out research on in-family socialization. Evolutionary thinking has been incorporated into accounts of parent–child roles and relationships. The early emphases on reinforcement, impulse control, and democratic and "authoritative" parenting have not been lost; they have simply been reconceptualized. For example, no one doubts that children's behavior is greatly influenced by the consequences of certain actions, through directly experiencing reward or discipline for these actions or observing these consequences experienced by others. But this is no longer thought of as a process of reinforcement whereby the habit strength of specific responses to specific stimuli is increased. Rather, a child's knowledge about the probability of receiving reward or punishment for certain actions in a specific context is now thought to enter into the child's moment-to-moment weighing of many possible short-term and long-term risks, benefits, and goals.

"Democratic" parenting has morphed into reciprocal responsiveness and has been incorporated into analyses of interactive processes between parents and children. "Internalization" continues to be a central process for study, but it is no longer seen as a product mainly of identification with parents. Rather, it is increasingly conceptualized as the development of self-regulation. There has been a shift away from the earlier almost exclusive focus on the *behavior* of parent and child to a greater concern with the ways in which each cognizes the other, and with the emotional valence that pervades parent–child interaction (i.e., with the balance between positive and negative affect in their encounters).

There has been a shift, too, away from the earlier studies of parental "traits," with greater recognition of situational variability in parent practices. Although certain parental traits such as "warmth," "responsiveness," or "power-assertiveness" have continued to hold up as useful concepts for describing individual differences among parents, our understanding of them has been greatly augmented by seeing them as reciprocal properties of parent–child dyads. This shift is part of the more general change from the top-down perspective of early behaviorist and psychoanalytic theories to interactive viewpoints which place increasing emphasis on the agency of the child as well as the parent in socialization processes.

There has been increasing interest in the sequential properties of socialization—in the way parenting must change with the development of the child, and the way in which early interactive processes undergird the later phases of parent–child relationships. Evidence has been accumulating for the importance of establishing a "good socializing relationship" with a child early in life. A major element in such a relationship appears to be the young child's growing willingness to be guided by parent directives and to accept parental values—something which is itself fostered by a parent's emotional reciprocity and positive affect. There is now increasing reason to believe that such an early relationship does facilitate the successful negotiation by parent and child of the issues concerning control and autonomy that pervade later childhood and adolescence. What is not known is how firm a foundation this is—how vulnerable it is to the vicissitudes of later episodes in family interaction, or to the pressures of the free-wheeling and highly commercialized adolescent culture the child encounters outside the family.

Theorizing about parental authority is perhaps the arena in which the most interesting and subtle shifts have taken place. Early studies pointed to deleterious effects of authoritarian childrearing, and a strong body of evidence grew up concerning the undesired side effects of parental power assertion. Yet, at the same time, there was increasing evidence for the benefits of parental "firm control." Several writers have noted that the parent–child relationship is intrinsically a hierarchical one, in that parents do have the responsibility for teaching and directing their children and reining in their impulsive or destructive behavior. Parents who do not succeed in these managerial functions begin to lose their sense of parenting efficacy, and in a negative feedback loop this further undermines their parental control functions (DeGarmo et al., 2004; Patterson & Forgatch, 1990).

How then do parental firm control and parental power assertion differ? How can their opposing effects be reconciled? Research has dealt with this issue in a number of ways. In rejecting authoritarian parenting, Baumrind offered instead a parenting pattern which combined responsive, supportive parenting with "firmness" (i.e., holding children to rules and standards). In the work of G. R. Patterson and colleagues, there has been an unwavering emphasis on rule setting, monitoring, and following up infractions with discipline, but in recent years there has been increasing emphasis on the importance of balancing these parental control functions with "positive parenting" (i.e., warmth, humor, responsiveness, and politeness to children). In the studies by Grusec (1997) and colleagues on disciplinary strategies, effective parents are seen to maintain their management goals while adapting their strategies to constantly changing contexts. Kochanska and colleagues have never doubted that parents must be able to induce their children to comply with parental directives; however, they have shown that it matters whether the children can be led to do so willingly or only under coercion, in that children's willingness allows parents to exercise control benignly rather than coercively. Barber and Olson (1997) distinguish between parental *regulation* of their children's behavior (setting fair and consistent limits) and parents' exercising *psychological control* (not permitting children to experience, value and express their own thoughts and emotions). They report that the highest levels of adjustment and competence are found in children coming from families that combine strong parental regulation with rare use of psychological control, along with a relationship of close emotional connectedness between parent and child.

The question underlying much modern parenting research, then, is not *whether* parents should exercise authority and children should comply but, rather, *how* parental control can best be exercised so as to support children's growing competence and self-management. Thus, it is increasingly understood that strong parent agency and strong child agency are not incompatible. Both can be maintained within a system of mutually understood realms of legitimate authority, though this understanding must be progressively renegotiated as children grow older. The agency of both parties can be encompassed within the bidirectional perspective that is now so widely accepted.

NOTES

1. A child who is "well socialized" is not necessarily one who is "well adjusted," but both are normative ideas that are central to distinguishing "good" parenting (or "good enough" parenting) from generally unsuccessful parenting.

2. It is worth noting that although the Baldwin work was going on at the same time as the studies of authoritarian personalities at Berkeley, the two groups did not cite each other and seemed to be entirely independent of one another.

3. Bowlby rejected any simple antithesis between "innate" and "acquired" behavior, noting that situational variations determined whether an instinctive system would be activated (see summary in Maccoby & Masters, 1970).

4. Recent work with animals (Hofer, 2006) has separated the concept of attachment or mother–infant bond into several elements, each infant component being regulated by a distinct feature of maternal contact.

REFERENCES

Adam, E. K. (2004). Beyond quality: Parental and residential stability and children's adjustment. *Current Directions in Psychological Science, 13,* 210–213.

Adorno, T., Frenkel-Brunswik, E., Levinson, D., & Sanford, R. (1950). *The authoritarian personality.* New York: Harper.

Alexander, J. F., & Malouf, R. E. (1983). Intervention with children experiencing problems in personality and social development. In P. H. Mussen & E. M. Hetherington (Eds.), *Handbook of child psychology* (4th ed., Vol. 4, pp. 913–981). New York: Wiley.

Asbury, K., Dunn, J. F., Pike, A., & Plomin, R. (2003). Nonshared environmental influences on individual differences in early behavioral development: A monozygotic twin differences study. *Child Development, 74,* 933–943.

Baldwin, A. L. (1955). *Behavior and development in childhood.* New York: Dryden Press.

Bandura, A. (1969). Social-learning theory of identificatory processes. In D. A. Goslin (Ed.), *Handbook of socialization theory and research* (pp. 213–262). Chicago: Rand McNally.

Bandura, A. (1986). *Social foundations of thought and action: A social-cognitive theory.* Englewood Cliffs, NJ: Prentice-Hall.

Bandura, A., Ross, D., & Ross, S. A. (1963). A comparative test of the status-envy, social power and secondary reinforcement theories of identificatory learning. *Journal of Abnormal and Social Psychology, 67,* 527–534.

Barber, B. K., & Olsen, J. A. (1997). Socialization in context: Connection, regulation and autonomy in the family, school, and neighborhood, and with peers. *Journal of Adolescent Research, 12,* 287–315.

Bates, J., Pettit, G., Dodge, K., & Ridge, B. (1998). Interaction of temperamental resistance to control and restrictive parenting in the development of externalizing behavior. *Developmental Psychology, 34,* 982–995.

Baumrind, D., & Black, A. E. (1967). Socialization practices associated with dimension of competence in preschool boys and girls. *Child Development, 38,* 291–327.

Bell, R. Q., & Harper, L. V. (1977). *Child effects on adults.* Hillsdale, NJ: Erlbaum.

Belsky, J., Crnic, K., & Gable, S. (1995). The determinants of coparenting in families with toddler boys: Spousal differences and daily hassles. *Child Development, 66,* 629–642.

Block, J. (1971). *Lives through time*. Berkeley, CA: Bancroft Books.

Block, J. H., & Block, J. (1980). The role of ego-control and ego-resiliency in the organization of behavior. In W. A. Collins (Ed.), *The Minnesota Symposia on Child Psychology: Vol. 13. Development of cognitions, affect, and social relations* (pp. 39–101). Hillsdale, NJ: Erlbaum.

Borkowski, J. G., Ramey, S. L., & Bristol-Power, M. (Eds.). (2002). *Parenting and the child's world: Influences on academic, intellectual and social-emotional development*. Mahwah, NJ: Erlbaum.

Bowlby, J. (1969) *Attachment and loss: Vol. 1. Attachment*. New York: Basic Books.

Brody, G. H., Murry, V. M., Gerard, M., Gibbons, F. X., Molgaard, V., & McNair, L. (2004). The strong African-American family program: Translating research into prevention programming. *Child Development, 75*, 900–917.

Buchanan, C. M., Maccoby, E. E., & Dornbusch, S. M. (1996). *Adolescents after divorce*. Cambridge, MA: Harvard University Press.

Bugental, D. B. (1992). Effective and cognitive processes within threat-oriented family systems. In I. E. Sigel, A. McGielicuddy-DiLise, & J. Goodnow (Eds.), *Parental relief systems: The psychological consequences for children* (pp. 219–248). Hillsdale, NJ: Erlbaum.

Bugental, D. B., Corporael, L., & Shennum, W. A. (1980). Experimentally induced child uncontrollability: Effects on the potency of adult communication patterns. *Child Development, 51*, 520–528.

Bugental, D. B., & Goodnow, J. J. (1998) Socialization processes. In W. Damon & N. Eisenberg (Eds.), *Handbook of child psychology* (5th ed., Vol. 3, pp. 389–462). New York: Wiley.

Bugental, D. B., & Grusec, J. E. (2006). Socialization processes. In N. Eisenberg (Vol. Ed.), *Handbook of child psychology* (6th ed., Vol. 3, pp. 366–428). Hoboken, NJ: Wiley.

Byrne, C. (2003). Parental agency and mental health: Construction and proaction in families with a depressed parent. In L. Kuczynski (Ed.), *Handbook of dynamics in parent–child relations* (pp. 229–244). Thousand Oaks, CA: Sage.

Cairns, R. B., Elder, G. H., & Costello, E. J. (Eds.). (1996). *Developmental science*. Cambridge, UK: Cambridge University Press.

Chomsky, N. (1959) Verbal behavior (Review of *Verbal behavior* by B. F. Skinner). *Language, 35*, 26–58.

Coie, J. D., Cillessen, A. H. N., Dodge, K. A., Hubbard, J. A., Schwartz, D., Lemarise, A., et al. (1999). It takes two to fight: A test of relational factors and a method for assessing aggressive dyads. *Developmental Psychology, 35*, 1179–1188.

Collins, W. A., Maccoby, E. E., Steinberg, L., & Hetherington, E. M. (2000). Contemporary research on parenting: The case for nature *and* nurture. *American Psychologist, 55*, 218–232.

Collins, W. A., & Madsen, S. D. (2003). Developmental change in parenting interactions. In L. Kuczynski (Ed.), *Handbook of dynamics in parent–child relations* (pp. 49–66). Thousand Oaks, CA: Sage.

Cook, W. L. (2003). Quantitative methods for deductive (theory-testing) research on parent–child dynamics. In L. Kuczynski (Ed.), *Handbook of dynamics in parent–child relations* (pp. 347–372). Thousand Oaks, CA: Sage.

Cowan, C. P., Cowan, P. A., Heming, G., Garrett, E., Coysh, W. S., Curtis-Boles, H., et al. (1985). Transitions to parenthood. *Journal of Family Issues, 6*, 451–481.

Cowan, P. A., & McHale, J. P. (1996). Coparenting in a family context: Emerging achievements, current dilemmas, and future directions. In J. P. McHale & P. A. Cowan (Eds.), *New directions for child development: Vol. 74. Understanding how family-level dynamics affect children's development* (pp. 93–106). San Francisco: Jossey-Bass.

Darling, N., & Steinberg, L. (1993). Parenting style as context: An integrative model. *Psychology Bulletin, 113*, 487–496.

DeGarmo, D. S., Patterson, G. R., & Forgatch, M. S. (2004). How do outcomes in a specified parent-training intervention maintain or wane over time? *Prevention Science, 5*, 73–89.

de Waal, F. (1996). *Good natured: The origins of right and wrong in humans and other animals*. Cambridge, MA: Harvard University Press.

Dix, T., Ruble, D. N., Grusec, J. E., & Nixon, S. (1986). Social cognitions in parents: Inferential and affective reactions to children of three age levels. *Child Development, 57,* 879–894.

Eisenberg, N., Smith, C. L., Sadovsky, A., & Spinrad, T. L. (2004). Effortful control: Relations with emotion regulation, adjustment, and socialization in childhood. In R. R. Baumeister & K. D. Vohs (Eds.), *Handbook of self-regulation: Research, theory, and applications* (pp. 259–282). New York: Guilford Press.

Forman, D. R., & Kochanska, G. (2001). Viewing imitation as child responsiveness: A link between the teaching and discipline dimensions of socialization. *Developmental Psychology, 37,* 198–206.

Gewirtz, J. L. (1969) Mechanisms of social learning: Some roles of stimulation and behavior in human development. In D. A. Goslin (Ed.), *Handbook of socialization theory and research* (pp. 57–213). Chicago: Rand McNally.

Goslin, D. A. (Ed.). (1969). *Handbook of socialization theory and research.* Chicago: Rand McNally.

Grolnick, W. S., Deci, E. L., & Ryan, R. M. (1997). Internalization within the family: The self-determination theory perspective. In J. E. Grusec & L. Kiczynski (Eds.), *Parenting and children's internalization of values* (pp. 135–161). New York: Wiley.

Grusec, J. E. (1997). A history of research on parenting strategies and children's internalization of values. In J. E. Grusec & L. Kuczynski (Eds.), *Parenting and children's internalization of values* (pp. 3–22). New York: Wiley.

Grusec, J. E., & Goodnow, J. J. (1994). Impact of parental discipline on the child's internalization of values: A reconceptualization of current points of view. *Developmental Psychology, 30,* 4–13.

Grusec, J. E., & Kuczynski, L. (1980). Direction of effects in socialization: A comparison of the parent's versus the child's behavior as determinants of disciplinary techniques. *Developmental Psychology, 16,* 1–9.

Grusec, J. E., & Ungerer, J. (2003). Effective socialization as problem solving and the role of parenting cognitions. In L. Kuczynski (Ed.), *Handbook of dynamics in parent–child relations* (p. 211–228). Thousand Oaks, CA: Sage.

Harlow, H. F., & Harlow, M. K. (1965). The affectional systems. In A. M. Schrier, H. F. Harlow, & F. Stollnitz (Eds.), *Behavior of non-human primates* (Vol. 2, pp. 287–334). New York: Academic Press.

Harris, J. R. (1998). *The nurture assumption: Why children turn out the way they do.* New York: Free Press.

Hartup, W. W., & Rubin, Z. (1986). *Relationships and development.* Hillsdale, NJ: Erlbaum.

Hetherington, E. M., Cox, M., & Cox, R. (1982). Effects of divorce on parents and children. In M. Lamb (Ed.), *Nontraditional families: Parenting and child development* (pp. 233–288). Hillsdale, NJ: Erlbaum.

Hofer, M. A. (2006). Psychobiological roots of early attachment. *Current Directions in Psychological Science, 15,* 84–88.

Hoffman, M. L. (1970). Moral development. In P. H. Mussen (Ed.), *Carmichael's manual of child psychology* (Vol. 2, pp. 261–359). New York: Wiley.

Katz, L. F., Kramer, L., & Gottman, J. M. (1995). Conflict and emotions in marital, sibling and peer relationships. In C. U. Shantz & W. W. Hartup (Eds.), *Conflict in child and adolescent development* (pp. 142–149). Cambridge, UK: Cambridge University Press.

Kerr, M., & Stattin, H. (2003). Parenting of adolescents: Action or reaction? In A. C. Crouter & A. Booth (Eds.), *Children's influence on family dynamics* (pp. 121–152). Mahwah, NJ: Erlbaum.

Kochanska, G. (1995). Children's temperament, mothers' discipline, and security of attachment: Multiple pathways to emerging internalization. *Child Development, 66,* 597–615.

Kochanska, G., & Aksan, N. (1995). Mother–child mutually positive affect, the quality of child compliance to requests and prohibitions, and maternal control as correlates of early internalization. *Child Development, 66,* 236–254.

Kochanska, G., Coy, K. C., & Murray, K. T. (2001). The development of self-regulation in the first four years of life. *Child Development, 72,* 1091–1111.

Kochanska, G., Murray, K. T., & Harlan, E. T. (2000). Effortful control in early childhood: Continuity and change, antecedents, and implications for social development. *Developmental Psychology, 36,* 220–232.

Kochanska, G., & Thompson, R. A. (1997). The emergence and development of conscience in toddlerhood and early childhood. In J. Grusec & L. Kuczynski (Eds.), *Parenting and children's internalization of values* (pp. 53–77). New York: Wiley.

Kuczynski, L. (2003). *Handbook of dynamics in parent–child relations.* Thousand Oaks, CA: Sage.

Lay, K., Waters, E., & Park, K. A. (1989). Maternal responsiveness and child compliance: The role of mood as a mediator. *Child Development, 60,* 1405–1411.

Lewin, K., Lippitt, R., & White, R. K. (1939). Patterns of aggressive behavior in experimentally created "social climates." *Journal of Social Psychology, 10,* 271–299.

Lollis, S. (2003). Conceptualizing the influence of the past and the future in parent–child relationships. In L. Kuczynski (Ed.), *Handbook of dynamics in parent–child relations* (pp. 67–88). Thousand Oaks, CA: Sage.

Maccoby, E. E. (1992). The role of parents in the socialization of children: An historical overview. *Developmental Psychology, 28,* 1006–1017.

Maccoby, E. E. (1998). *The two sexes: Growing up apart, coming together.* Cambridge, MA: Harvard University Press.

Maccoby, E. E. (2000). Parenting and its effects on children. *Annual Review of Psychology, 51,* 1–27.

Maccoby, E. E., & Martin, J. A. (1983). Socialization in the context of the family: Parent–child interaction. In P. H. Mussen & E. M. Hetherington (Eds.), *Handbook of child psychology* (4th ed., Vol. 4, pp. 1–102). New York: Wiley.

Maccoby, E. E., & Masters, J. C. (1970). Attachment and dependency. In P. H. Mussen (Ed.), *Carmichael's manual of child psychology* (4th ed., Vol. 2, pp. 73–158). New York: Wiley.

Maccoby, E. E., & Mnookin, R. H. (1992). *Dividing the child: Social and legal dilemmas of custody.* Cambridge, MA: Harvard University Press.

Martin, J. A., Maccoby, E. E., Baran, K., & Jacklin, C. N. (1981). Sequential analysis of mother–child interaction at 18 months: A comparison of microanalytic methods. *Developmental Psychology, 17,* 146–157.

Martinez, C. R., & Forgatch, M. S. (2001). Preventing problems with boys' noncompliance: Effects of a parent training intervention for divorcing mothers. *Journal of Consulting and Clinical Psychology, 69,* 416–428.

McHale, J. (1995). Co-parenting and triadic interactions during infancy: The roles of marital distress and child gender. *Developmental Psychology, 31,* 985–996.

McHale, J., Khazan, I., Erera, P., Rotman, T., DeCourcey, W., & McConnell, M. (2002). Coparenting in diverse family systems. In M. H. Bornstein (Ed.), *Handbook of parenting* (2nd ed., Vol. 3, pp. 75–108). Mahwah NJ: Erlbaum.

Miller, N. E., & Dollard, J. (1941). *Social learning and imitation.* New Haven, CT: Yale University Press.

Minuchin, S. (1974). *Families and family therapy.* Cambridge, MA: Harvard University Press.

Mischel, W., & Grusec, J. (1967). Waiting for rewards and punishments: Effects of time and probability on choice. *Journal of Personality and Social Psychology, 5,* 24–31.

Mischel, W., & Liebert, R. M. (1967). The role of power in the adoption of self-reward patterns. *Child Development, 38,* 673–684.

Mischel, W., & Metzner, R. (1962). Preference for delayed reward as a function of age, intelligence, and length of delay interval. *Journal of Abnormal and Social Psychology, 64,* 425–431.

Mischel, W., Shoda, Y., & Peake, P. (1988). The nature of adolescent competencies predicted by preschool delay of gratification. *Journal of Personality and Social Psychology, 54,* 687–696.

Moffitt, T. E., & Caspi, A. (2007). Evidence from behavioral genetics for environmental contributions to antisocial conduct. In J. E. Grusec & P. D. Hastings (Eds.), *Handbook of socialization: Theory and research* (pp. 96–123). New York: Guilford Press.

Moffitt, T. E., Caspi, A., & Rutter, M. (2006). Measured gene–environment interactions in psychopathology: Concepts, research strategies, and implications for research, intervention and public understanding of genetics. *Perspectives in Psychology Science, 1,* 5–27.

Neiderhiser, J. M., Reiss, D., Pedersen, N. L., Lichenstein, P., Spotts, E. L., Hansson, K., et al. (2004). Genetic and environmental influences on mothering of adolescents: A comparison of two samples. *Developmental Psychology, 40,* 335–351.

Parke, R. D., & Buriel, R. (1998). Socialization in the family: Ethnic and ecological perspectives. In W. Damon & N. Eisenberg (Eds.), *Handbook of child psychology* (5th ed., Vol. 3, pp. 463–552). New York: Wiley.

Parpal, M., & Maccoby, E. E. (1985). Maternal responsiveness and subsequent child compliance. *Child Development, 56,* 1326–1334.

Patterson, G. R. (1982). *Coercive family process,* Eugene, OR: Castalia.

Patterson, G. R., & Forgatch, M. S. (1990). Initiation and maintenance of processes disrupting single-mother families. In G. R. Patterson (Ed.), *Depression and aggression in family interaction* (pp. 209–245). Hillsdale, NJ: Erlbaum.

Plomin, R., & Daniels, D. (1987). Why are children in the same family so different from each other? *Behavioral and Brain Sciences, 10,* 1–16.

Posner, M. L., & Rothbart, M. K. (1998). Attention, self-regulation and consciousness. *Philosophical Transactions of the Royal Society of London B, 353,* 1915–1927.

Rothbart, M. K., & Bates, J. E. (1998). Temperament. In W. Damon & N. Eisenberg (Eds.), *Handbook of child psychology* (5th ed., Vol. 3, pp. 105–176). New York: Wiley.

Rothbart, M. K., & Rueda, M. R. (2005). The development of effortful control. In U. Mayr, E. Awh, & S. W. Keele (Eds.), *Developing individuality in the human brain: A festschrift honoring Michael I. Posner—May, 2003* (pp. 167–188). Washington, DC: American Psychological Association Press.

Rowe, D. C. (1994). *The limits of family influence: Genes, experience, and behavior.* New York: Guilford Press.

Rutter, M., Pickles, A., Murray, R., & Eaves, L. (2001). Testing hypotheses on specific environmental causal effects on behavior. *Psychological Bulletin, 127,* 291–324.

Scarr, S. (1992). Developmental theories for the 1990s: Development and individual differences. *Child Development, 63,* 1–19.

Sears, R. R. (1951). A theoretical framework for personality and social behavior. *American Psychologist, 6,* 476–483.

Sears, R. R., Maccoby, E. E., & Levin, H. (1957). *Patterns of child rearing.* Evanston, IL: Row, Peterson.

Sears, R. R., Rau, L., & Alpert, R. (1965). *Identification and child rearing.* Stanford, CA: Stanford University Press.

Sears, R. R., Whiting, J. W. M., Nowlis, V., & Sears, P. S. (1953). Some child-rearing antecedents of aggression and dependency in young children. *Genetic Psychology Monographs, 47,* 135–234.

Shoda, Y., Mischel, W., & Peake, P. (1990). Predicting adolescent cognitive and self-regulatory competencies from preschool delay of gratification: Identifying diagnostic conditions. *Developmental Psychology, 26,* 978–986.

Shonkoff, J. P., & Phillips, D. A. (Eds.). (2001). *From neurons to neighborhoods: The science of early childhood development.* Washington, DC: National Academy Press.

Sroufe, L. A. (1996). *Emotional development.* Cambridge, UK: Cambridge University Press.

Sroufe, L. A., & Fleeson, J. (1986). Attachment and the construction of relationships. In W. Hartup & Z. Rubin (Eds.), *Relationships and development* (pp. 51–71). Hillsdale, NJ: Erlbaum.

Suomi, S. J. (2002). Parents, peers, and processes of socialization in primates. In J. G. Borkowski, S. L. Ramey, & M. Bristol-Power (Eds.), *Parenting and the child's world* (pp. 265–282). Mahwah, NJ: Erlbaum.

Turkheimer, E. (2000). Three laws of behavior genetics and what they mean. *Current Directions in Psychological Science, 9*, 160–164.

Weisner, T. S., Matheson, C., Coots, J., & Bernheimer, L. P. (2004). Sustainability of daily routines as a family outcome. In A. Maynard & M. Martini (Eds.), *Learning in cultural context: Family, peers and school* (pp. 41–73). New York: Kluwer Academic/Plenum Press.

Whiting, J. W. M., & Child, I. L. (1953). *Child training and personality.* New Haven, CT: Yale University Press.

Youniss, J., & Smollar, J. (1985). *Adolescent relations with mothers, fathers and friends.* Chicago: University of Chicago Press.

PART II

SOCIALIZATION ACROSS THE LIFE SPAN

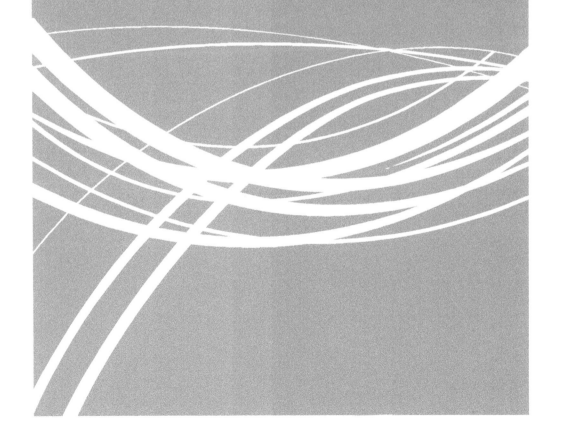

CHAPTER 2

Early Socialization
The Influence of Close Relationships

Deborah Laible
Ross A. Thompson
Jill Froimson

The importance of close relationships for a young child's acquisition of culturally rel-evant knowledge, skills, and behaviors has long been acknowledged. Early theories of socialization highlighted the importance of a warm, nurturing relationship for foster-ing socialization (e.g., Sears, Maccoby, & Levin, 1957), but these early views of both the relationship and its influences were too simplistic. For example, many early theo-ries of socialization (e.g., Baldwin, 1949) took a relatively unidirectional approach to socialization (e.g., knowledge was transmitted from parent to child) and took a rather one-dimensional approach to assessing the quality of parent–child relationships. More modern relational approaches to socialization (e.g., Thompson, 2006), however, appreci-ate the bidirectional influences of close relationships, recognizing that the qualities of children (e.g., their temperament) influence the type of care that they receive, and appre-ciate that relationships are multifaceted; for example, a relationship imbued with warmth may not be one that involves trust or security (Goldberg, Grusec, & Jenkins, 1999; Gru-sec & Davidov, 2010). Thus, a modern relational approach to socialization focuses on how children develop a unique set of social skills in the context of close relationships, acknowledging that skills are the result of the behavioral, emotional, and representa-tional contingencies that emerge between two people who know each other well (e.g., Collins & Laursen, 1999; Dunn, 1993).

Taking a *relational* perspective to socialization can be useful because of some of the defining features of relationships. First, each relationship is unique because it is created from the mutual contributions of both partners over time, and each partner's behavior toward the other is influenced by not only the partner's current behavior but also the meaning of that behavior based on the shared history of the dyad. Thus, each partner's behavior is also influenced by the mental representations (and the expectations, relational schemes, and affective biases) that are in part based on their relational history.

Second, relationships are dynamic and affective. They change over time owing to developmental changes in each partner, the growth of the relationship, and the influences of other events in both partners' lives (e.g., the birth of a sibling). Relationships are also colored by the emotion inherent in them, which makes each partner's behaviors salient to the other and in turn influences each partner's interpretation of the other. It is not surprising, as a result, that the emotional quality of the relationship (e.g., warmth) has both direct (e.g., influencing the child's willingness to cooperate) and moderating (e.g., influencing the effectiveness of discipline) effects on children's behavior and outcomes.

Finally, relationships encompass both broad (e.g., warmth) and immediate (e.g., rewards) influences that interact to determine children's outcomes. Thus, for example, the security inherent in the relationship supports the child's engagement in conversational discourse (especially surrounding negatively charged events), which influences the impact of this discourse on the child's growing socioemotional understanding (Laible, Murphy, & Augustine, 2013b; Laible & Panfile, 2009). This suggests that early socialization entails dyadic interactions that are meaningful only within their broader relational context, and that the impact of specific socialization practices depends on the quality of the relationships in which they are embedded.

Our goal is to examine both the broad relational qualities and the more immediate processes involved in early socialization. We begin by considering the broad indices of relational quality, including warmth, security, and mutual reciprocity, that are important because of how they affect each partner's receptiveness to the influence of the other. We then examine a number of more immediate relational processes that are influential in socialization, including reinforcement, modeling, sensitive responsiveness, proactive regulation, emotional communication, routines and rituals, and parent–child discourse. Next, we highlight characteristics of children that impact the socialization process, including their construction of experience, their self-understanding, and their temperamental and genetic susceptibility to relational influences. Finally, we examine recent work from both animal and human studies that suggest close relationships not only influence children's behavioral outcomes but may also modify their biology, including stress reactivity and gene expression. We conclude by discussing the importance of examining socialization from a relational perspective.

The Quality of Close Relationships

The quality of relationships has both direct consequences for a child's socialization and consequences that are more complex and indirect. Many aspects of the quality of close relationships concern their affective impact on each partner. Warm, reciprocal relationships, for example, enhance motivation for children to cooperate with relational partners (see Grusec & Davidov, 2010; Thompson & Meyer, 2007). Ultimately, children who are part of warm, secure, and mutually responsive relationships enthusiastically embrace parental values and are eager participants in their own socialization (Kochanska, Aksan, & Carlson, 2005). Several studies also demonstrate, however, that the affective quality of the relationship between parents and children moderates the influence of immediate relational processes, such as discipline (Deater-Deckard, Ivy, & Petrill, 2006) and shared conversation (Laible & Song, 2006). Thus, specific relational processes, such as corporal punishment, may have entirely different consequences if applied in the context of a warm relationship versus in a more coercive relationship. Finally, the affective quality of the relationship might also influence the types of practices that parents use in socialization. For example, Kochanska, Askan, Prisco, and Adams (2008) found that mothers who were part of mutually responsive relationships with their toddlers used less power assertion with their children. These researchers conclude that mothers who are part of a mutually responsive relationship need to rely less on forceful discipline techniques to accomplish their socialization goals, in part because of children's willingness to embrace maternal values. Thus, over time, the affective quality of the relationship may influence the specific relational processes that parents enlist for socialization.

Warmth

Warmth involves noncontingent displays of affection and positive emotion. Cultural values vary in their emphasis on expressions of warmth, but infant survival requires some expressions of parental solicitude and care through which warmth is manifested. In the socialization literature, warmth has most frequently been studied as a characteristic of caregivers that promotes relational harmony, and the child's developing socioemotional competence. Warmth has also been conceived as a relational construct, especially in the context of research on early conscience development (see Kochanska, 2002). A relational approach to warmth underscores the bidirectional quality of positive affect and its influence on overall relational quality. Thus, although warmth has often been portrayed as a characteristic of specific relational partners, it is easily conceived as a *relational* construct that indicates the shared positive affect of each partner toward the other.

Warmth has a number of important influences on early socialization. First, warm relationships with caregivers provide children with a sense that they are loved and respected. As a result, children are more likely to identify with caregivers and are motivated to please them, thereby enhancing their receptiveness to be socialized (Grusec, Goodnow, & Kuczynski, 2000). Second, the intrinsic pleasure that children experience in the context of positive affect encourages them to share experiences with relational partners, which expands children's opportunities to be socialized. Finally, warm relationships often also provide children with appropriate models of regulation of emotions (e.g., Spinrad et al., 2012), which in turn enhance children's abilities to self-regulate. High levels of self-regulation influence children's abilities to comply with parental requests and to attend to, reflect upon, and process parental messages.

Security

Attachment theory argues that young children's needs for security in the context of threat derive from biologically based motives that are deeply rooted in species evolution (Ainsworth, Blehar, Waters, & Wall, 1978; Bowlby, 1969/1982). In times of threat, the sensitive responsiveness of a caregiver served a highly adaptive function by enabling human young to survive in the savannah grasslands of human evolution. Children's confidence in the sensitivity of caregivers to protect and comfort them has numerous consequences for socialization, which include facilitating children's active exploration of the environment (and therefore their learning), as well as coloring their interactions with caregivers and with others.

Attachment security derives from and further influences the harmony of the parent–child relationship (see Thompson, 2008, for a review). As a result, secure children are more receptive, cooperative, and responsive to the socialization attempts of caregivers, and are more likely to comply with parental requests, participate in shared activities, and internalize parental values (Thompson, Meyer, & McGinley, 2006). Thus, similar to warmth, a secure attachment relationship lays the groundwork for a reciprocal, harmonious relationship that enhances the child's future willingness to be socialized (Kochanska et al., 2010).

Security also influences socialization in other ways that are different than warmth. Attachment theory also proposes that through these early interactions with caregivers, children create internal working models of attachment figures themselves, and relationships that color how children experience subsequent relationships (Thompson, 2008). These internal working models constitute interpretive filters through which children construct their experiences of new relationships in ways that are consistent with the expectations they have formed from their relational history. Internal working models also bias children's mental representations in ways that are relevant to socialization efforts, including their understanding of the caregiver, other people (e.g., emotional understanding), relationships (e.g., social informational processing), and the self (e.g., self-concept). Research has suggested that secure children have more positive representations of the caregiver (Toth, Rogosch, Sturge-Apple, & Cicchetti, 2009) and more advanced conscience development (Kochanska, 1995; Laible & Thompson, 2000), are less prone to a hostile attribution bias (Raikes & Thompson, 2008), exhibit higher levels of emotional understanding (Laible & Thompson, 1998), and have more positive representations of self and relationships (Goodvin, Meyer, Thompson, & Hayes, 2008). Thus, secure children are more receptive to the socialization initiatives of parents than are insecure children in part because of their positive representations of the parent and their tendency to attribute good intent to relational partners. Moreover, secure children have the ability (owing to their more sophisticated sociomoral understanding) to reflect upon and internalize parental values.

The effects of attachment on socialization may not always involve simple direct effects. Attachment security may have both mediational and moderation effects that influence the nature of future developmental cascades (Kochanska & Kim, 2012). Early security or insecurity might set children on trajectories that are both complex and conditional. Therefore, the effects of attachment security on socialization might be easily missed by researchers (Thompson, 2008). Kochanska and her colleagues have recently demonstrated the cascading effects of attachment security on children's developmental pathways, especially for children who were anger-prone toddlers (Kochanska & Kim, 2012). The parents of insecure dyads were more likely to be involved in coercive interactions with their anger-prone toddlers and to use increased levels of power-assertive discipline. Power assertion, in turn, led to less internalization of values, less self-regulation, and more oppositional and aggressive behavior from insecure anger-prone children. The same cascade of effects was not found in secure dyads. For secure dyads, there was no link between children's anger proneness and the parent's use of power assertion or between the parent's power assertion and children's antisocial outcomes. Ultimately, attachment insecurity acted as a catalyst that created an adversarial relationship between parent and child that sets the child on the path to antisocial outcomes (Kochanska & Kim, 2012).

Mutual Reciprocity

An important dimension of relational quality that emerged from some of the early work on socialization is that of mutual reciprocity. Maccoby and Martin (1983) emphasized that, at its best, the parent–child relationship introduces young children into a relational system that involves the mutual obligations of each partner to the other. More recently, Kochanska and colleagues (Aksan, Kochanska, & Ortmann, 2006; Kochanska et al., 2008) have emphasized that a mutually responsive orientation (MRO) is a truly dyadic construct that characterizes dyads that are highly cooperative, show high levels of shared positive affect, and engage in harmonious communication. Parents and young children in high-MRO relationships show an enhanced level of cooperation that reflects both their generally receptive stance toward one another and their invested interest in maintaining a positive relationship (Aksan et al., 2006). In an MRO relationship, children feel an obligation to respond positively to parental socialization initiatives and accept parental values, which makes them eager and willing to be socialized. Moreover, parents in MRO relationships do not need to use coercive or punitive methods to ensure children's cooperation because simple requests by the parent are usually sufficient to elicit compliance.

Kochanska and colleagues have demonstrated that an MRO is a relatively stable characteristic of both mother–child and father–child relationships (see, e.g., Aksan et al., 2006; Kochanksa, Forman, Aksan, & Dunbar, 2005) that has consequences for children's conscience development. Children of dyads with high MRO demonstrate more advanced levels of early conscience development both concurrently and longitudinally (see Kochanska, Forman, et al., 2005; Laible & Thompson, 2000). Several mechanisms have been shown to mediate the links between MRO and conscience development, including children's committed compliance and parent's diminished use of power-assertive discipline (Kochanska et al., 2008). Thus, children from dyads with high MRO in infancy show more committed compliance as toddlers and have mothers who, across time, use decreasing amounts of power-assertive discipline. Committed compliance and lower levels of power assertion, in turn, are associated with higher levels of conscience development.

Relational Processes

In addition to these broad relational qualities are the immediate (and specific) relational processes that influence children's socialization. We begin by exploring a number of processes that are traditionally conceived as being primarily under the control of the caregiver, including reinforcement–punishment, sensitive responsiveness, proactive regulation, emotional communication, and the establishment of routines and rituals. There is growing recognition, however, that even though parents may have considerable control over these specific socialization processes, the characteristics and behaviors of children influence parents' adoption of specific socialization strategies; thus, the links that they share with child outcomes are truly bidirectional (Choe, Olson, & Sameroff, 2013;

Newton, Laible, Carlo, Steele, & McGinley, in press; Verhoeven, Junger, van Aken, Deković, & van Aken, 2010). In addition to exploring the specific socialization processes that have traditionally been conceived as being under the influence of parents, we also consider one specific process that is clearly dyadic in nature: parent–child discourse.

Reinforcement, Rewards, and Punishment

The significance of rewards and reinforcement provided by the parent has long been recognized in the developmental literature. Attitudes toward the use of tangible rewards by parents to socialize children's competencies, however, have a mixed history. A number of theorists have argued that tangible reinforcement undermines intrinsic motivation. For example, in an influential early study, Lepper (1981) found that preschool children who initially experienced pleasure in drawing pictures were less motivated to continue to draw at posttest if they had been rewarded previously. Similarly, in a more recent study, Warneken and Tomasello (2008) found that young children's willingness to provide instrumental help to an experimenter decreased if they previously received a tangible reward for helping. In stark contrast, however, recent studies indicate that tangible rewards can be helpful in socializing healthy eating habits (Cooke et al., 2011). Ultimately, the effectiveness of tangible rewards in influencing a child's behavior depends on many factors, including how substantial the reward is, how and by whom the reward is offered, and the child's initial intrinsic motivation to engage in the behavior.

It seems important that children respond to internal incentives (e.g., a desire to be kind to others) rather than just to external reinforcement of competent conduct; thus, parental use of incentives (both praise and material rewards) must be subtle enough to ensure that children attribute their compliance to internal rather than external motives. For example, mothers help to provide a foundation for prosocial motivation when they provide their young children with emotionally powerful messages concerning the distress of another person and also clarify, when relevant, the child's culpability for that distress (Zahn-Waxler & Robinson, 1995). By focusing on the other person's distress, mothers encourage the child to respond prosocially based on the emotional needs of the other.

There continues to be a lively debate about the effects of physical punishment, primarily spanking, on outcomes relevant to socialization. In a meta-analytic review, Gershoff (2002) concluded that corporal punishment has few positive effects besides inducing immediate compliance and has mostly harmful effects, including later increased aggression and parent–child relationship erosion. In contrast, other researchers argue that prior research has failed to distinguish between the effects of harsh discipline and the mild use of spanking as a backup discipline method, and that the research has overstated the case against spanking (see Baumrind, Larzelere, & Cowan, 2002). Moreover, family factors that tend to co-occur with physical discipline, such as poverty and the negative affectivity of the caregiver, may contribute to the negative effects that spanking is thought to have on children, and the links between corporal punishment and child outcomes depend in part on race, ethnicity, and the degree to which the discipline is perceived as culturally normative (see Benjet & Kazdin, 2003; Critchley & Sanson, 2006).

Recent work on spanking has not ended the debate, but it has suggested that the effects of corporal punishment on child outcomes are complex. First, contrary to prior conclusions, race and ethnicity do not seem to moderate the influence of spanking on children's externalizing behavior, although the extent to which corporal punishment is perceived as normative does (Gershoff et al., 2010; Gershoff, Lansford, Sexton, Davis-Kean, & Sameroff, 2012). However, it is important to point out that even though the negative effects of corporal punishment were diminished when it was perceived as more culturally normative, it still was associated with externalizing behavior in children. At the same time, recent work also suggests that many of the negative effects of spanking on children substantially diminish when other contextual risk factors (e.g., family stress and socioeconomic status) are accounted for (MacKenzie, Nicklas, Waldfogel, & Brooks-Gunn, 2012).

Moreover, there is growing evidence that the meaning of physical discipline to children varies depending on the quality of the relationship in which it is applied. Several studies have found that the strength of the relation between physical discipline and children's externalizing problems substantially diminishes in the context of a warm parent–child relationship (Deater-Deckard et al., 2006; Towe-Goodman & Teti, 2008). This work suggests that the effects of spanking depend on the broader emotional context of the relationship in which it is applied. It is also important to acknowledge that in these studies, parental responsiveness (including warmth and sensitivity) and spanking are often negatively correlated, supporting the idea that parents' use of physical discipline is associated with decreased relational quality.

Finally, it is important to point out that cross-lagged longitudinal studies have demonstrated consistent links between children's early behavioral problems and parents' greater use of physical discipline across time (see Choe et al., 2013; Sheehan & Watson, 2008). Thus, children with behavioral problems tend to evoke harsh, physical discipline from parents, which serves to increase their behavioral problems. Clearly, the links between corporal punishment and child outcomes are bidirectional in nature.

Modeling

Because recent theoretical views have highlighted the importance of early imitation for a child's emergent understanding of others and the self (Meltzoff, 2002; Olineck & Poulin-Dubois, 2007), interest in empirically examining modeling and imitative processes in socialization has emerged afresh. One reason is the realization that even early imitative activity is cognitively complex, involving sophisticated inferences of the intentional activity of the model, including the model's desires and goals (e.g., Carpenter, Akhtar, & Tomasello, 1998; Huang, Heyes, & Charman, 2002); thus, young children perceive the behavior of a model with considerable psychological depth (Wellman, 2002).

Individual differences in young children's imitative activity may reflect broader relational influences, such as the child's identification with the other person and his or her generally receptive stance to socialization (Forman & Kochanska, 2001). Forman and his colleagues (Forman, Aksan, & Kochanska, 2004; Forman & Kochanska, 2001) have argued that young children who are eager to imitate are also motivated to cooperate with and learn from their parents. In their research, Forman and Kochanska (2001) found that individual differences in 14-month-olds' willingness to imitate their mothers in a teaching task were longitudinally stable (from 14 to 22 months) and predicted children's compliance with the mother in disciplinary assessments and conscience nearly 2 years later (Forman et al., 2004). Thus, imitative activity may also reflect a child's broader responsiveness to the parent's socialization initiatives.

Sensitive Responsiveness

Sensitivity is characterized by responsiveness that is contingent and appropriate to a child's signals. A social partner who is sensitive is attuned to the other's needs, responds in a timely manner, and is effective in meeting their needs (Lohaus, Keller, Ball, Voelker, & Elben, 2004). Sensitive caregiving is assumed to be not only a central predictor of the child's attachment security but also a central contributor to other important developmental outcomes, including attentional and cognitive skills, language acquisition, affect regulation, and social competence (Leerkes, Blankson, & O'Brien, 2009; Tamis-LeMonda & Bornstein, 2002). Sensitive caregiving is presumed to have its effects by creating in young children a sense of control over their social environment and providing them with a sense of the self as a competent interaction partner (Bornstein, Hendricks, Haynes, & Painter, 2007).

The context of sensitive responding is important, however. Parental sensitivity in the context of distress is important for attachment security, affect regulation, and related socioemotional outcomes, such as empathy and behavioral problems (Davidov & Grusec, 2006; Leerkes et al., 2009; McElwain & Booth-LaForce, 2006). Sensitive responding to children's negative emotions likely helps them learn to self-regulate (Thompson, 2011) and gives them a sense of confidence in their ability to control emotion and to access parental assistance when needed, which creates in children greater trust and security in the caregiver's responsiveness in contexts of stress. In contrast, maternal sensitivity in nondistress situations likely fosters competence in play, positive expressivity, and cognitive development (see, e.g., Leerkes et al., 2009; Tamis-LeMonda & Bornstein, 2002). In this context, sensitive responding affirms the intentionality and goal-directedness of the child's efforts at mastery and communication, and contributes to the growth of cognitive and linguistic competence.

Proactive Regulation

Relationships afford opportunities for partners to have proactive influence, that is, to structure circumstances to create desired outcomes for the other person. Parents often employ proactive techniques with young children. Childproofing a home to prevent accidents is one type of proactive regulation, and immunizations, pediatric health care, and nutrition have similarly proactive functions. Another form of proactive regulation consists of the anticipatory prevention of discipline confrontations. Holden (1983) reported that mothers use a variety of strategies in the supermarket to avoid child misbehavior, such as circumventing aisles with tempting items and distracting the child. Mothers who used such techniques had children who misbehaved less frequently than did the children of mothers who used only reactive control (i.e., responding after misbehavior) (see also Holden & West, 1989). Holden has argued that proactive control techniques have several benefits for parent–child relationships. First, proactive regulation minimizes conflict between parents and children and enhances relational quality. Second, by structuring the environment in a manner that encourages children to behave appropriately, parents scaffold children's understanding of appropriate conduct.

Since Holden's original work in 1983, there has been limited research on this topic. Some studies have examined how minority parents prepare children for discrimination (Barr & Neville, 2008). There has also been some work with older children on how parents monitor children in an effort to prevent misbehavior (see, e.g., Lansford et al., 2006), and research highlights the anticipatory processes that parents use to prevent misbehavior, including redirecting, teaching, and involvement in their activity (Gardner, Ward, Burton, & Wilson, 2003; Putnam, Spritz, & Stifter, 2002). In addition, parents also proactively manage children's activities by regulating access to peers (e.g., through transportation). Parents' use of these types of proactive regulation has been associated with fewer behavioral problems and better self-control in children (Pettit, Keiley, Laird, Bates, & Dodge, 2007).

Emotional Communication

Nonverbal displays of emotion are a central feature of close relationships. Emotional communication from caregivers exerts its influence on children in a number of venues, including (but not limited to) parent–infant face-to-face play, social referencing, and communication among family members (e.g., spouses). These processes of emotional communication influence important socialization outcomes, including the development of young children's emotional expression and regulation, social expectations, and psychological well-being. Thus, although early relational quality can be broadly characterized in terms of warmth and other features, immediate processes of emotional communication are also important to socialization.

The influence of emotional communication between parent and child begins in infancy, with the emergence of episodes of face-to-face play at 2–3 months of age. Studies have indicated that infants respond animatedly to the contingency in an adult's behavior and readily share in the positive affect of their parent, and from these encounters acquire general social expectations that others will be responsive and interactive (Bigelow & Rochat, 2006; Markova & Legerstee, 2006). The importance of the emotional reciprocity of these exchanges is also reflected in studies of babies whose mothers are not well attuned their babies' signals in these face-to-face interactions, such as mothers who are depressed. Depressed mothers are less responsive and emotionally more negative in face-to-face play with their infants than typical mothers, and their offspring become less responsive and express less negative affect when faced with noncontingent interactions (e.g., Field et al., 2007; Friedman Beebe, Jaffe, Ross, & Triggs, 2010). These studies, combined with those on highly critical and anxious mothers, suggest that early misattunement in emotional communication leads to infants adopting similar dysfunctional styles of communication (Field, Diego, & Hernandez-Reif, 2009).

By the end of the first year, infants are good consumers of the emotional signals they detect in others, and they use the affirmative or cautionary messages they receive to alter their subsequent behavior. This phenomenon, called *social referencing*, is especially apparent when infants are uncertain about how to interpret novel situations (see G. Kim & Kwak, 2011), and through this mode of communication, caregivers influence the young child's emotional interpretation of events and children's response to them. Although social referencing is particularly important in communicating danger to infants in hazardous situations, it is also a broader means of conveying expectations through emotional cues. Thus, parents often exhibit cues of disapproval as toddlers are about to engage in forbidden activity. Parents' emotional signals also convey evaluations of other people (e.g., when a sibling misbehaves) and of the child's behavior (e.g., a parent who displays disappointment when a child fails to comply) (Thompson & Newton, 2010). In this way, social referencing imbues certain behaviors, objects, and people with emotional significance and becomes one way in which young children learn about prohibited and permitted activities.

Young children and parents are also influenced by the broader emotional climate of the family (Halberstadt, Crisp, & Eaton, 1999). For example, high levels of maternal distress color the mother's interpretation of the child's behavior and lead to less maternal sensitivity (Yoo, Popp, & Robinson, 2014). Similarly, children are affected by the emotional communication between parents, especially when the communication involves conflict (see Cummings & Davies, 2010). Children's broader emotional security is affected by the parents' approaches to handling conflict. Parents who constructively address marital conflict using problem solving and perspective taking increase children's emotional security (McCoy, Cummings, & Davies, 2009). Parents' frequent, destructive marital conflict undermines children's feelings of security and leads to less optimal outcomes in children (e.g., behavioral problems; Cummings & Davies, 2010). Moreover, the impact of marital conflict on children's perceptions of threat is also moderated by the broader emotional climate of the family. Children perceive marital conflict as less threatening in the context of otherwise cohesive families (Lindahl & Malik, 2011). Ultimately, parents' negative expressiveness toward each other in conflict provides young children with especially salient lessons in how disturbing feelings such as anger are resolved.

Routines and Rituals

Family routines and rituals provide children with a predictable structure to their everyday lives, guide children's behavior, and shape the broader emotional climate of the family (Fiese et al., 2002; Spagnola & Fiese, 2007). Routines involve recurrent patterns of family activity in which some or all family members participate, such as practices associated with mealtimes and bedtimes. Routines often have instrumental goals (e.g., getting the child into bed) (Fiese et al., 2002) and most families with young children report using routines to organize daily lives. *Rituals* are routines that assume metacognitive meaning for family members because of their symbolic and affective significance, such as birthdays, and such rituals contribute to family identity (Fiese et al., 2002; Spagnola & Fiese, 2007). Although family routines and rituals are unique to each family, and in some cases may reflect family dysfunction, they often share common positive cultural elements and are one important way children acquire culturally appropriate conduct (Spagnola & Fiese, 2007). Routines and rituals give both parents and children feelings of control because of their predictable nature and defined roles, and they promote a sense of family cohesiveness (Spagnola & Fiese, 2007). Family routines and rituals are an important way that children are socialized regarding the responsibilities of family members and about family identity and values.

Routines and rituals might be especially important for socialization in early childhood because of how they are represented by young children. Research on early memory shows that young children bootstrap their recall of unique events on their representations of familiar recurrent routines (Hudson, 1993; Nelson, 1978). Thus, everyday routines are a foundation for how young children represent and think about their experiences. In the context of everyday routine events, parents often convey to children moral and conventional standards, including prohibitions, sharing, simple manners, self-care standards (e.g., teeth brushing), and appropriate conduct (Smetana, Kochanska, & Chuang, 2000).

Because of young children's sensitivity to normative obligations (Wellman & Miller, 2008), these behavioral expectations are likely to become incorporated into their scripts for routine events.

Parent–Child Discourse

Another important avenue through which children are socialized is within the context of everyday conversations about shared experiences. These conversations begin as soon as children are verbal, and both parents and children contribute to the quality of these early conversations. Although parents might provide much of the structure of these conversations, there is growing evidence that children's willingness to participate in these conversations has consequences for the meaning that is co-constructed in them (see Laible et al., 2013b). Research indicates that these early conversations with caregivers are significant catalysts to children's developing psychological understanding and that differences in the quality of these conversations have important consequences for children's social cognitive development (Fivush, 2006; Laible & Panfile, 2009).

Traditional views of socialization emphasized the role of parental reasoning in the context of the discipline encounter for fostering children's internalization of parental values (Hoffman, 2000). It seems likely that such inductive techniques, especially those that help to clarify the feelings and motivations of those involved in the transgression, are influential in promoting children's conscience (Thompson & Newton, 2010) Research on inductive discipline provides support for these ideas (Hastings, Utendale, & Sullivan, 2007). However, there are reasons to believe that conversations in the context of discipline may not be the most productive avenues for fostering children's sociomoral understanding. In the context of discipline, children's cognitive resources might be otherwise occupied with managing the negative emotion inherent in these encounters, and as a result, children might not process or attend to the messages that are conveyed by caregivers. Conversations about the transgression later in the day (and once children's negative affect has dissipated) might be more potent contexts for socialization (Laible & Thompson, 2000). Reminiscent conversations, especially those that center on issues of the child's cooperation, harmful behavior, and emotional experiences are therefore important contexts in which children are socialized (for reviews, see Laible & Panfile, 2009; Thompson, 2006).

In the context of these reminiscent conversations, parents do several things that help promote children's psychological understanding. First, parents discuss with children the emotions, intentions, and beliefs of people involved in the shared experience (see, e.g., Fivush & Nelson, 2006; Laible & Panfile, 2009). Such discussions give children psychological insight into their own and others' behavior. Second, when conversing about shared experiences, both the adult and the child have their own representation of the event, and often these representations do not agree (Fivush & Nelson, 2006). When they differ, shared conversation becomes a tutorial in divergent mental representations of the same event and fosters children's perspective taking.

One of the most consistent predictors of children's socioemotional outcomes has been the degree to which parents elaborate during reminiscence. Mothers who elaborate during reminiscence provide the child with rich background detail and ask frequent open-ended questions. The elaboration that mothers use during reminiscence has been associated with children's emotional understanding, early conscience development, and more positive representations of relationships (Laible, 2004a, 2004b; Laible & Panfile, 2009). By providing children with rich detail about their personal experiences, mothers help them to understand better the causes and consequences of their actions and feelings, and give insight into their reasons for certain expectations. In addition to elaboration, other, important aspects of conversational discourse may not be so well explored in the literature. For example, it seems likely that how caregivers morally evaluate the behavior of their children and others, the attributions they make about culpability, and the characteristics they attribute to the child likely have important consequences for a child's early moral and self-understanding (Laible & Murphy, 2014).

Other discourse contexts besides reminiscence are also important contexts for children's socialization, including (but not limited to) conversations about future events, conversations that happen during storybook reading, and conversations that occur in the frequent conflicts that divide parents and children. For example, by talking about the future, parents prepare children for upcoming events (e.g., trips to the doctor) and provide them with anticipatory event representations that create feelings of predictability about the future (Hudson, 2002). In the context of storybook reading, mothers and children frequently discuss story characters' intentions and feelings, which in turn fosters children's social cognitive understanding (e.g., LaBounty, Wellman, Olson, Lagattuta, & Liu, 2008). Finally, in the context of conflict with children, parents justify their side of an argument and clarify their reasons for taking a particular stance (Laible & Thompson, 2002).

It is important to realize that these early conversations are also shaped by children. Young children contribute to the content and style of parent–child conversation in many ways: by their willingness or resistance to participate (especially when discussing difficult or sensitive topics), by their topic switching, by disputing the mother's interpretation of events, by their emotional demeanor during conversations, and by their capacities to put into words their emotional or psychological experience. Moreover, children's engagement in these dialogues influences the overall quality of the meaning that is constructed in the conversation (in part because it allows parents to explore themes in more depth) and influences the impact of these conversations on children's developing understanding (see Laible, Murphy, & Augustine, 2013a). Research has shown that children's engagement is affected, in part, by the mother's validation of the child's perspective and the security of their relationship (Waters et al., 2010). In addition to engagement, there is growing evidence that other characteristics of children, such as temperament, are also related to the quality of these conversations. For example, children's effortful control has been related to the amount of maternal elaboration, collaboration, and intersubjectivity, and children's discussion of emotion in reminiscence (Laible, 2004a; Laible et al., 2013b).

Children's Influence

Children are active participants in their own socialization; for example, children negotiate their roles in routines and rituals, and influence parental discourse by their willingness to discuss sensitive or threatening topics. Research also highlights how characteristics of the child (e.g., temperament) influence specific relational processes (e.g., discourse; Laible et al., 2013b) and suggests that children's genetic and temperamental profiles may even influence how susceptible children are to relational influences (Belsky & Pluess,

2009). In this section we highlight the ways that characteristics of the child influence the socialization process.

Constructing Social Experience

Children are active constructors of social knowledge. As a result, how children respond to a caregiver's socialization initiatives depends on how they perceive the meaning of the adult's behavior, which is based on the clarity and relevance of the parent's message, whether the parent's intervention is perceived as appropriate, whether the parent's behavior is experienced as a threat to the child's autonomy, and other factors, such as the quality of the relationship (Grusec & Goodnow, 1994). In addition, children's judgments about the appropriateness and relevance of the parent's message are also related to the child's conceptual skills, which develop quickly in early childhood.

During early childhood there are remarkable advances in social cognition, which influence how young children interpret parental initiatives. There is growing evidence that children can infer the goals and intentions of others well before their first birthday (e.g., Brandone & Wellman, 2009; Woodward, 1998), and this likely contributes to the development of social referencing and social expectations for the behavior of parents and familiar partners (Thompson, 2006). Perceiving others as intentional agents also influences toddlers' social behavior, especially in their efforts to alter the parent's subjective, intentional orientation through communicative gestures and sounds (e.g., pointing to a desired object that is out of reach).

There are also remarkable developments in children's theory of mind in early childhood that are related to understanding of parental socialization initiatives. Recent work suggests that by midway through their second year of life, toddlers have an implicit understanding of the beliefs and desires of others (Onishi & Baillargeon, 2005; Song, Onishi, Baillargeon, & Fisher, 2008), although these studies remain controversial (Ruffman & Perner, 2005). By the age of 3, children seem to have a more explicit theory of mind, and they begin to interpret the actions of others in terms of emotions and desire. By age 4–5 years, children also have a more explicit understanding of the representational nature of mental phenomena. This contributes to young children's dawning awareness of the privacy of mental experience (i.e., that one can hide one's feelings and thoughts from others), developing capacities for deception, and growing ability to enlist display rules for emotional expressions in social situations (Thompson, 2006). As children develop a more sophisticated theory of mind, they are able to interpret the reasons for others' behavior in more psychologically complex ways, influencing their expectations for social partners and their behavior toward them. It also permits children to reflect on the intentions behind parents' socialization messages.

Closely related to children's developing theory of mind is their developing conceptions of obligations, which also allow them to have more insight into parent's socialization initiatives. Preschoolers strive to comprehend normative standards for everything from their appearance to expectations for conduct (Thompson, 2006; Wellman & Miller, 2008). Moreover, parents strive to get children to adhere to deontic rules (e.g., "If you are outside playing, an adult must be with you"); thus, children need to be able to determine which actions are allowed or prohibited (Cummins, 1996). Preschool children can easily understand and apply prescriptive rules (e.g., "Painting is permitted if a smock is worn") (Cummins, 1996). Young children's deontic reasoning, however, is more heavily influenced by context than is adult reasoning (Dack & Astington, 2011). Preschoolers can also understand that an actor's intentions are important when evaluating rule violations, but despite this, they have trouble coordinating moral evaluations with an understanding of the transgressor's intentions and actions (Wainryb & Brehl, 2006). Young children also become proficient at distinguishing between types of obligations (e.g., moral vs. social conventional; Smetana et al., 2012) and these important distinctions become the building blocks of a more mature moral understanding.

Taken together, these studies indicate that by age 5 (if not earlier), young children are likely attuned to the psychological motivations underlying parents' actions, know that parents can be mistaken or deceived, and understand that behavioral standards involve obligations, and why certain standards of conduct are more obligatory than others. Much more research is needed to understand how these developing facets of theory of mind and domain understanding are applied in the everyday contexts in which socialization occurs (e.g., in how mothers discuss transgressions with children), but together they suggest that young children enlist formidable conceptual resources in their interpretation of the parent's message and behavior.

Self-Understanding

Infancy and early childhood also witness remarkable advances in the development of self-related processes, including self-awareness, self-regulation, and self-understanding. These skills have important consequences for a child's socialization. First, children's developing self-awareness and self-understanding contribute to their awareness of the self as a causal agent and that their behavior is evaluated by others. Beginning late in the second year, toddlers begin to develop conceptual self-representations that are manifested in verbal self-referential behavior, assertions of competence and responsibility, self-assertiveness, assertions of ownership, and greater sensitivity to the evaluative standards of others (see Thompson, 2006). Moreover, young children's incentives to cooperate with parents are enhanced by their striving to be perceived as competent because of how their sense of self has become strongly linked with behaviors that evoke caregiver approval or disapproval (Stipek, Recchia, & McClintic, 1992).

Second, children's self-regulatory and self-control capacities, which develop rapidly across the preschool years, are important for socialization (Kochanska, Philibert, & Barry, 2009). Self-regulation is closely tied with children's ability to control affect, which is important in their ability to attend to parental messages in the context of negatively charged situations (e.g., during a discipline encounter). Moreover, self-regulatory capacities also allow children to exercise constraint over their immediate desires and to comply with the wishes of caregivers. Ultimately, children's self-regulatory capacities are fundamental for socialization.

Young children also begin to experience social emotions (e.g., guilt and pride) that enhance the affective incentives to comply with parents' socialization initiatives. During the second year, young children begin to exhibit signs of pride when their behavior elicits praise from adults, and guilt or shame when their behavior violates explicit or internal standards of conduct (Jennings, 2004; Kochanska & Aksan, 2006; Lewis, 2000). Caregivers enlist these feelings in their discipline practices and in their conversations with children by explicitly discussing the transgression, by invoking salient attributions of responsibility, and often by directly evaluating the child's behavior (e.g., "That was naughty"). Young children often have trouble reflecting on and understanding their past transgressions (especially those related to the psychological consequences of doing harm; see Pasupathi & Wainryb, 2010), and such discussions about the child's transgressions give them a structure to evaluate the misbehavior.

These remarkable advances in self-related processes in early childhood underscore how much the efficacy of socialization depends on children's developing self-image and capacities for self-control, and suggest that variations in young children's self-concept, self-regulation, and proneness toward experiencing self-conscious emotions may significantly moderate the influence of parental socialization initiatives. Research examining the moderating influence of self-awareness, self-concept, and self-control on socialization practices is lacking.

Temperamental and Genetic Influences

There is growing evidence that the influence of early relationships on children's socialization is in part determined by the child's temperament and genetic individuality. Current thinking extends traditional views of the organismic specificity of environmental influences and goodness-of-fit models of the interaction of temperament and care. In particular, research suggests that the temperamental and genetic profiles of the child interact with relational processes and in some cases may make children more susceptible to the influence of relational processes and qualities (see Belsky & Pluess, 2009). Research supports the idea that children with certain temperamental profiles, particularly children who are high in negative emotionality, are more likely to succeed in sensitive responsive relationships but at the same time are more at risk in the event of insensitive or poor parenting (e.g., S. Kim & Kochanksa, 2012; Van Aken, Junger, Verhoeven, Van Aken, & Deković, 2007). For example, S. Kim and Kochanska (2012) found that for children who were high in negative emotionality, the quality of the mother–child relationship was associated with children's levels of self-regulation. For those who were low in negative emotionality, the quality of the relationship did not matter. Children high in negative emotionality were well regulated when they were in a mutually responsive relationship but less regulated when they were in an unresponsive relationship.

Second, there is also work that suggests that relational influences interact with particular genes. Although a number of genes have been studied in humans, several are noteworthy with regards to their interaction with relational influences. The monoamine oxidase A (*MAOA*) gene, located on the X chromosome, produces the MAOA enzyme that metabolizes neurotransmitters such as serotonin, dopamine, and norepinephrine, and renders them inactive. In an influential study, Caspi and colleagues (2002) followed individuals from childhood into adulthood and found that the presence of the gene with low MAOA activity led young adults who had experienced risk for child maltreatment to become violence prone. Interestingly, those with a high MAOA activity allele were significantly less influenced by a history of maltreatment risk.

Also studied has been a polymorphism of the dopamine receptor D4 (*DRD4*) gene, which has variants that differ by 48-base pairs in the exon III area of the ribonucleic acid (RNA) molecule. The 7-repeat allele is associated with low dopaminergic efficiency and has been linked with novelty-seeking behavior (Kluger, Siegfried, & Ebstein, 2002). Several studies suggest that this gene interacts with maternal sensitivity to produce both positive and negative outcomes for children. In a longitudinal study, maternal insensitivity in infancy predicted toddler externalizing behavior, but only for children carrying the 7-repeat *DRD4* allele (Bakermans-Kranenburg & van IJzendoorn, 2006). Children with the allele who had insensitive mothers had the most externalizing problems, but those with the allele and who had sensitive mothers had the lowest levels of externalizing behaviors. Similar findings have emerged with regards to children's prosocial behavior. For example, children with the *DRD4* 7-repeat allele were more prosocial as a result of maternal positive parenting than were children without this gene who also experienced positive parenting (Knafo, Israel, & Ebstein, 2011).

Biological Consequences of Early Relationships

Over the last 10 years, researchers have begun to illuminate the complex interplay of biological factors and environmental experience, especially parenting, in shaping children's development. What has emerged from this research is the idea that early relational processes not only interact with the child's genotype but may also influence children's developmental biology in complex ways (see Thompson, in press). In particular, we discuss several recent lines of work that highlight these new ways of thinking about the biological consequences of early relationships, including work that focuses on how early relational experiences shape stress neurobiology and research that highlights developmental epigenetic models. These lines of work have important consequences for thinking about the influence of parent–child relationships because they suggest that the quality of parent–child relationships is one of the most important elements of environmental influence on gene expression and stress neurobiology (Thompson, in press). Ultimately, these lines of research suggest that the quality of early relationships not only has important behavioral and cognitive consequences but also important consequences for a child's biological functioning.

Stress Neurobiology

The hypothalmic–pituitary–adrenocortical (HPA) axis is a stress-related neurobiological system that prepares the body for stressors by producing cortisol. Recent studies suggest that the quality of early relationships can alter the reactivity of the HPA axis to stressors (Gunnar & Donzella, 2002). For example, in a study of families living in rural poverty, toddlers' persistent exposure to domestic violence was associated with elevated levels of cortisol in challenging tasks at 24-months. However, sensitive mothering (observed in earlier assessments) buffered the effects of domestic violence on toddlers' cortisol reactivity (Hibel, Granger, Blair, Cox, & the Family Life Project Key Investigators, 2011). Similarly, children who experienced social deprivation in orphanages often show hypo-reactive HPA axis functioning (Carlson & Earls, 1997; Gunnar, Morison, Chisholm, & Schuder, 2001), which has the potential of improving after adoption into caring families if institutional deprivation was not extreme or enduring (Dozier, Peloso, Lewis, Laurenceau, & Levine, 2008; Fisher, Stoolmiller, Gunnar, & Burraston, 2007). Finally, securely attached children have been shown to have lower levels of salivary cortisol when accompanied by their mothers to the first few days of child care than do insecurely attached children accompanied by their mothers (Ahnert, Gunnar, Lamb, & Barthel, 2004). These, and similar studies, suggest that variations in parent–child relationship quality can influence the functioning of neurohormonal regulation and HPA axis functioning.

Epigenetics

Epigenetics involves the study of heritable changes in gene expression that result without changes to the DNA sequence. For genes to be expressed, gene transcription must be activated by the *epigenome* (a biochemical regulatory system that changes, activates, or silences genes without changing the DNA sequence). This happens as a result of chemical processes that alter DNA's protective chromatin layer (i.e., the protein structure surrounding the DNA molecule), and alter transcription through DNA methylation or other processes. Some modifications of the genome are influenced by environmental experiences, and there is growing evidence from animal studies that these processes are influenced by differences in the caregiving environment (Thompson, in press).

The influence of early relational experiences on epigenetic processes has been best examined in animal studies. In one of the most relevant studies, Meaney and his colleagues have demonstrated that differences in maternal care are associated with epigenetic processes in rodents (see Meaney, 2010, for a review). Differences in maternal licking and grooming (LG) are associated with enduring differences in the stress reactivity and neurocognitive functioning of pups. Offspring of low-LG mothers demonstrate heightened HPA reactivity, for example, compared to those high-LG mothers because maternal LG alters the chromatin that regulates, among other things, glucocorticoid receptor gene expression in hippocampal neurons, which are in turn associated with differences in synaptic density and plasticity in the hippocampus. The offspring of high-LG mothers show increases in synaptic density and synaptic plasticity in the hippocampus as a result of less methylation of glucocorticoid receptors. Thus, these epigenetic processes influence the neurocognitive and, through other biochemical processes, the stress reactivity of offspring and likely have other consequences on behavior as well (e.g., D. L. Champagne et al., 2008). These epigenetic marks are preserved (under normal environmental conditions), which leads to enduring differences in the HPA axis stress reactivity and other behaviors of the high-LG and low-LG pups.

Moreover, there appear to be intergenerational effects of early maternal care. Epigenetic changes are inherited as a result of epigenetic markers in the germ line being passed on to offspring. In addition, low maternal LG results, for female offspring, in greater methylation of estrogen receptor gene expression in the hypothalamus, less dopamine release during nursing bouts, and decreased oxytocin levels, which contributes to less LG when these offspring have their own pups (F. A. Champagne, 2011). As a result of epigenetic changes in the brain caused by earlier levels of LG by mothers, low-LG pups grow up to be low-LG mothers.

There has been little work on how epigenetic processes influence human development as the result of differences in maternal care. However, it seems likely that the quality of parental care has an important influence on gene expression that not only influences children's behavior, but also is potentially heritable (Thompson, in press). Thus, early relationships contribute to heritable differences in the phenotype that are epigenetic in origin. Preliminary research supports these ideas. For example, Naumova and colleagues (2012) found that children who experienced institutional care had greater DNA methylation in areas associated with brain development, stress reactivity, and immune functioning (consistent with the behavioral deficits that these children have shown in past studies) compared to children raised by biological parents. In addition, McGowan and colleagues (2009) found that a history of child abuse was associated with a decreased hippocampal glucocorticoid gene expression in suicide victims compared to both controls and suicide victims without a history of abuse.

Conclusion

A relational approach to socialization highlights the diversity of relational processes and qualities that contribute to important socialization outcomes. Most importantly, a relational approach highlights the complex nature of the influences involved in socializing a young child. Children are embedded in significant emotional relationships that are more than the sum of their parts. Both the parent and the child are influential in shaping these unfolding relational processes and the broader relational qualities that influence socialization. This is complicated by the fact that the specific relational processes are mutually influential and compounding across time.

Research suggests that children influence their relational partners in diverse and sophisticated ways. Earlier theories of socialization that assumed parents (and other socialization agents) shape children missed the tremendous influence that children's behavior, temperament, and genetics have on shaping the socialization process. Children's early social behavior (including both their aggressive and prosocial behavior) influences parental sensitivity and the discipline approaches that parents use (Choe et al., 2013; Newton et al., in press; Verhoeven et al., 2010). Children's growing conceptual sophistication influences the way they interpret the behavior and messages of parents, and this in turn influences children's acceptance and internalization of parental values. Children's developing self-regulation influences their abilities to comply with parental requests and rules, which in turn may change the tactics that parents use to socialize children (e.g., parents may need less power assertion as children become more self-regulated). Moreover, children's willingness to engage in conversations with caregivers, especially surrounding challenging issues (e.g., misbehavior) influences the quality of these conversations and influences their construction of understanding. Equally important are child temperament and genetic individuality, which not only influence the parent's use of specific relational processes (e.g., discipline) but may also determine the extent to which children are even influenced by relational qualities and processes.

Moreover, according to a relational approach to socialization, children are motivated by far more than avoidance of punishment and/or self-interest. Young children have a desire to maintain warm and close relationships with people who are significant to them, and this provides them with an eagerness and willingness to be socialized. In addition, young children's growing understanding of the feelings and needs of others, coupled with a desire to be perceived as competent, mature, and cooperative, provides children with stronger incentives to be guided by relational partners. Thus, close relationships with others provide children's motivation to be socialized.

In addition, parents and other socialization agents do far more than just enforce behavioral standards through direct instructions and discipline; parents contribute to socialization by fostering warm mutual relationships, by responding sensitively to children's initiatives, by proactively regulating events to promote children's cooperation, and by structuring routines and rituals within which behavioral standards are integrated.

They contribute to a child's socialization by directing verbal and nonverbal communication toward both the child and others in the household. The warmth, mutuality, and security of the relationships parents share with children moderates the effects of specific socialization processes by giving meaning to parents' initiatives.

These processes have broad consequences for children. They influence children's internalization of values, self-conception, conscience development, capacities for self-regulation and self-control, emotion understanding, empathy development, and psychological understanding of others. More profoundly, however, there is growing evidence that these relational processes and qualities also have biological consequences for children through the impact that they have on the developing brain, stress regulation system, and children's gene expression. Therefore, these early relational experiences may have lasting and profound influences on children's development through these biological consequences. We may have vastly underestimated the impact that these early relationships have on children's outcomes. In many respects, the research on how early relationships influence biological and brain development is one of the most exciting new directions of relational science.

REFERENCES

Ahnert, L., Gunnar, M. R., Lamb, M. E., & Barthel, M. (2004). Transition to child care: Associations with infant–mother attachment, infant negative emotion, and cortisol elevations. *Child Development, 75,* 639–650.

Ainsworth, M. D. S., Blehar, M., Waters, E., & Wall, S. (1978). *Patterns of attachment.* Hillsdale, NJ: Erlbaum.

Aksan, N., Kochanska, G., & Ortmann, M. R. (2006). Mutually responsive orientation between parents and their young children: Toward methodological advances in the science of relationships. *Developmental Psychology, 42,* 833–848.

Bakermans-Kranenburg, M. J., & van IJzendoorn, M. H. (2006). Gene–environment interaction of the dopamine D4 receptor (*DRD4*) and observed maternal insensitivity predicting externalizing behavior in preschoolers. *Developmental Psychobiology, 48,* 406–409.

Baldwin, A. L. (1949). Socialization and the parent–child relationship. *Child Development, 19,* 127–136.

Barr, S. C., & Neville, H. A. (2008). Examination of the link between parental racial socialization messages and racial ideology among Black college students. *Journal of Black Psychology, 34,* 131–155.

Baumrind, D., Larzelere, R., & Cowan, P. (2002). Ordinary physical punishment: Is it harmful?: Comment on Gershoff. *Psychological Bulletin, 128,* 580–589.

Belsky, J., & Pluess, M. (2009). Beyond diathesis–stress: Differential susceptibility to environmental influences. *Psychological Bulletin, 135,* 885–908.

Benjet, C., & Kazdin, A. E. (2003). Spanking children: The controversies, findings, and new directions. *Clinical Psychology Review, 23,* 197–224.

Bigelow, A. E., & Rochat, P. (2006). Two-month-old infants' sensitivity to social contingency in mother–infant and stranger–infant interaction. *Infancy, 9,* 313–325.

Bornstein, M. H., Hendricks, C., Haynes, O. M., & Painter, K. M. (2007). Maternal sensitivity and child responsiveness: Associations with social context, maternal characteristics, and child characteristics in a multivariate analysis. *Infancy, 12,* 189–223.

Bowlby, J. (1982). *Attachment and loss: Vol. 1. Attachment* (2nd ed.). New York: Basic Books. (Original work published 1969)

Brandone, A. C., & Wellman, H. M. (2009). You can't always get what you want: Infants understand failed goal-directed actions. *Psychological Science, 20,* 85–91.

Carlson, M., & Earls, F. (1997). Psychological and neuroendocrinological sequelae of early social deprivation in institutionalized children in Romania. *Annals of the New York Academy of Sciences, 807*, 419–428.

Carpenter, M., Akhtar, N., & Tomasello, M. (1998). Fourteen- to 18-month-old infants differentially imitate intentional and accidental actions. *Infant Behavior and Development, 21*, 315–330.

Caspi, A., McClay, J., Moffitt, T., Mill, J., Martin, J., Craig, I., et al. (2002). Role of genotype in the cycle of violence in maltreated children. *Science, 297*, 851–854.

Champagne, D. L., Bagot, R. C., van Hasselt, F., Ramakers, G., Meaney, M. J., de Kloet, R., et al. (2008). Maternal care and hippocampal plasticity: Evidence for experience-dependent structural plasticity, altered synaptic functioning, and differential responsiveness to glucocorticoids and stress. *Journal of Neuroscience, 28*, 6037–6045.

Champagne, F. A. (2011). Maternal imprints and the origins of variation. *Hormones and Behavior, 60*, 4–11.

Choe, D. E., Olson, S. L., & Sameroff, A. J. (2013). Effects of early maternal distress and parenting on the development of children's self-regulation and externalizing behavior. *Development and Psychopathology, 25*, 437–453.

Collins, W. A., & Laursen, B. (Eds.). (1999). *The Minnesota Symposia on Child Psychology: Vol. 30. Relationships as developmental contexts*. Mahwah, NJ: Erlbaum.

Cooke, L. J., Chambers, L. C., Añez, E. V., Croker, H. A., Boniface, D., Yeomans, M. R., et al. (2011). Eating for pleasure or profit: The effect of incentives on children's enjoyment of vegetables. *Psychological Science, 22*, 190–196.

Critchley, C. R., & Sanson, A. V. (2006). Is parent disciplinary behavior enduring or situational?: A multilevel modeling investigation of individual and contextual influences on power assertive and inductive reasoning behaviors. *Journal of Applied Developmental Psychology, 27*, 370–388.

Cummings, E. M., & Davies, P. T. (2010). *Marital conflict and children: An emotional security perspective*. New York: Guilford Press.

Cummins, D. (1996). Evidence of deontic reasoning in 3- and 4-year-old children. *Memory and Cognition, 24*, 823–829.

Dack, L. A., & Astington, J. W. (2011). Deontic and epistemic reasoning in children. *Journal of Experimental Child Psychology, 110*, 94–114

Davidov, M., & Grusec, J. E. (2006). Untangling the links of parental responsiveness to distress and warmth to child outcomes. *Child Development, 77*, 44–58.

Deater-Deckard, K., Ivy, L., & Petrill, S. A. (2006). Maternal warmth moderates the link between physical punishment and child externalizing problems: A parent–offspring behavior genetic analysis. *Parenting: Science and Practice, 6*, 59–78.

Dozier, M., Peloso, E., Lewis, E., Laurenceau, J. P., & Levine, S. (2008). Effects of an attachment-based intervention on the cortisol production of infants and toddlers in foster care. *Development and Psychopathology, 20*, 845–859.

Dunn, J. (1993). *Young children's close relationships: Beyond attachment*. Newbury Park, CA: Sage.

Field, T., Diego, M., & Hernandez-Reif, M. (2009). Depressed mothers' infants are less responsive to faces and voices. *Infant Behavior and Development, 32*, 239–244.

Field, T., Hernandez-Reif, M., Diego, M., Feijo, L., Vera, Y., Gil, K., et al. (2007). Still-face and separation effects on depressed mother–infant interactions. *Infant Mental Health Journal, 28*, 314–323.

Fiese, B. H., Tomcho, T. J., Douglas, M., Josephs, K., Poltrock, S., & Baker, T. (2002). A review of 50 years of research on naturally occurring family routines and rituals: Cause for celebration? *Journal of Family Psychology, 16*, 381–390.

Fisher, P. A., Stoolmiller, M., Gunnar, M. R., & Burraston, B. O. (2007). Effects of a therapeutic intervention for foster preschoolers on diurnal cortisol activity. *Psychoneuroendocrinology, 32*, 892–905.

Fivush, R. (2006). Scripting attachment: Generalized event representations and internal working models. *Attachment and Human Development, 8*, 283–289.

Fivush, R., & Nelson, K. (2006). Parent–child reminiscing locates the self in the past. *British Journal of Developmental Psychology, 24*, 235–251.

Forman, D., Aksan, N., & Kochanska, G. (2004). Toddlers' responsive imitation predicts preschool-age conscience. *Psychological Science, 15*, 699–704.

Forman, D., & Kochanska, G. (2001). Viewing imitation as child responsiveness: A link between teaching and discipline domains of socialization. *Developmental Psychology, 37*, 198–206.

Friedman, D. D., Beebe, B., Jaffe, J., Ross, D., & Triggs, S. (2010). Microanalysis of 4-month infant vocal affect qualities and maternal postpartum depression. *Clinical Social Work Journal, 38*, 8–16.

Gardner, F., Ward, S., Burton, J., & Wilson, C. (2003). The role of mother–child joint play in the early development of children's conduct problems: A longitudinal observational study. *Social Development, 12*, 361–378.

Gershoff, E. T. (2002). Corporal punishment by parents and associated child behaviors and experiences: A meta-analytic and theoretical review. *Psychological Bulletin, 128*, 539–579.

Gershoff, E. T., Grogan-Kaylor, A., Lansford, J. E., Chang, L., Zelli, A., Deater-Deckard, K., et al. (2010). Parent discipline practices in an international sample: Associations with child behaviors and moderation by perceived normativeness. *Child Development, 81*, 487–502.

Gershoff, E. T., Lansford, J. E., Sexton, H. R., Davis-Kean, P., & Sameroff, A. J. (2012). Longitudinal links between spanking and children's externalizing behaviors in a national sample of white, black, Hispanic, and Asian American families. *Child Development, 83*, 838–843.

Goldberg, S., Grusec, J. E., & Jenkins, J. M. (1999). Confidence in protection: Arguments for a narrow definition of attachment. *Journal of Family Psychology, 13*, 475–483.

Goodvin, R., Meyer, S., Thompson, R. A., & Hayes, R. (2008). Self-understanding in early childhood: Associations with child attachment security and maternal negative affect. *Attachment and Human Development, 10*, 433–450.

Grusec, J. E., & Davidov, M. (2010). Integrating different perspectives on socialization theory and research: A domain-specific approach. *Child Development, 81*, 687–709.

Grusec, J., & Goodnow, J. (1994). Impact of parental discipline methods on the child's internalization of values: A reconceptualization of current points of view. *Developmental Psychology, 30*, 4–19.

Grusec, J., Goodnow, J., & Kuczynski, L. (2000). New directions in analyses of parenting contributions to children's internalization of values. *Child Development, 71*, 205–211.

Gunnar, M. R., & Donzella, B. (2002). Social regulation of the cortisol levels in early human development. *Psychoneuroendocrinology, 27*, 199–220.

Gunnar, M. R., Morison, S., Chisholm, K., & Schuder, M. (2001). Salivary cortisol levels in children adopted from Romanian orphanages. *Development and Psychopathology, 13*, 611–628.

Halberstadt, A., Crisp, V., & Eaton, K. (1999). Family expressiveness: A retrospective and new directions for research. In P. Philippot, R. Feldman, & E. Coats (Eds.), *The social context of nonverbal behavior* (pp. 109–155). Cambridge, UK: Cambridge University Press.

Hastings, P. D., Utendale, W. T., & Sullivan, C. (2007). The socialization of prosocial development. In J. E. Grusec & P. D. Hastings (Eds.), *Handbook of socialization: Theory and research* (pp. 638–664). New York: Guilford Press.

Hibel, L., Granger, D. A., Blair, C., Cox, M. J., & the Family Life Project Key Investigators. (2011). Maternal sensitivity buffers the adrenocortical implications of intimate partner violence exposure during early childhood. *Development and Psychopathology, 23*, 689–701.

Hoffman, M. (2000). *Empathy and moral development*. Cambridge, UK: Cambridge University Press.

Holden, G. W. (1983). Avoiding conflict: Mothers as tacticians in the supermarket. *Child Development, 54*, 233–240.

Holden, G. W., & West, M. J. (1989). Proximate regulation by mothers: A demonstration of how differing styles affect young children's behavior. *Child Development, 60*, 64–69.

Huang, C. T., Heyes, C., & Charman, T. (2002). Infants' behavioral reenactment of "failed attempts": Exploring the roles of emulation learning, stimulus enhancement, and understanding of intentions. *Developmental Psychology, 38*, 840–855.

Hudson, J. (1993). Understanding events: The development of script knowledge. In M. Bennett (Ed.), *The child as psychologist: An introduction to the development of social cognition* (pp. 142–167). New York: Harvester Wheatsheaf.

Hudson, J. A. (2002). "Do you know what we're going to do this summer?": Mothers' talk to young children about future events. *Journal of Cognition and Development, 3*, 49–71.

Jennings, K. D. (2004). Development of goal-directed behaviour and related self-processes in toddlers. *International Journal of Behavioral Development, 28*, 319–327.

Kim, G., & Kwak, K. (2011). Uncertainty matters: Impact of stimulus ambiguity on infant social referencing. *Infant and Child Development, 20*, 449–463.

Kim, S., & Kochanska, G. (2012). Child temperament moderates effects of parent–child mutuality on self-regulation: A relationship-based path for emotionally negative infants. *Child Development, 83*, 1275–1289.

Kluger, A. N., Siegfried, Z., & Ebstein, R. P. (2002). A meta-analysis of the association between *DRD4* polymorphism and novelty seeking. *Molecular Psychiatry, 7*, 712–717.

Knafo, A., Israel, S., & Ebstein, R. P. (2011). Heritability of children's prosocial behavior and differential susceptibility to parenting by variation in the dopamine receptor D4 gene. *Development and Psychopathology, 23*, 53–67.

Kochanska, G. (1995). Children's temperament, mothers' discipline, and security of attachment: Multiple pathways to emerging internalization. *Child Development, 66*, 597–615.

Kochanska, G. (2002). Committed compliance, moral self, and internalization: A mediated model. *Developmental Psychology, 38*, 339–351.

Kochanska, G., & Aksan, N. (2006). Children's conscience and self-regulation. *Journal of Personality, 74*, 1587–1618.

Kochanska, G., Aksan, N., & Carlson, J. J. (2005). Temperament, relationships, and young children's receptive cooperation with their parents. *Developmental Psychology, 41*, 648–660.

Kochanska, G., Aksan, N., Prisco, T. R., & Adams, E. E. (2008). Mother–child and father–child mutually responsive orientation in the first 2 years and children's outcomes at preschool age: Mechanisms of influence. *Child Development, 79*, 30–44.

Kochanska, G., Forman, D. R., Aksan, N., & Dunbar, S. B. (2005). Pathways to conscience: Early mother–child mutually responsive orientation and children's moral emotion, conduct, and cognition. *Journal of Child Psychology and Psychiatry, 46*, 19–34.

Kochanska, G., & Kim, S. (2012). Toward a new understanding of legacy of early attachments for future antisocial trajectories: Evidence from two longitudinal studies. *Development and Psychopathology, 24*, 783–806.

Kochanska, G., Philibert, R. A., & Barry, R. A. (2009). Interplay of genes and early mother–child relationship in the development of self-regulation from toddler to preschool age. *Journal of Child Psychology and Psychiatry, 50*, 1331–1338.

Kochanska, G., Woodard, J., Kim, S., Koenig, J. L., Yoon, J. E., & Barry, R. A. (2010). Positive socialization mechanisms in secure and insecure parent–child dyads: Two longitudinal studies. *Journal of Child Psychology and Psychiatry, 51*, 998–1009.

LaBounty, J., Wellman, H. M., Olson, S., Lagattuta, K., & Liu, D. (2008). Mothers' and fathers' use of internal state talk with their young children. *Social Development, 17*, 757–775.

Laible, D. (2004a). Mother–child discourse surrounding a child's past behavior at 30 months: Links to emotional understanding and early conscience development at 36 months. *Merrill–Palmer Quarterly, 50*, 159–180.

Laible, D. (2004b). Mother–child discourse in two contexts: Links with child temperament, attachment security, and socioemotional competence. *Developmental Psychology, 40*, 979–992.

Laible, D., & Murphy, T. (2014). Constructing moral, emotional, and relational understanding in the context of mother–child reminiscing. In C. Weinraub & H. Recchia (Eds.), *Talking about right and wrong: Parent–child conversations as contexts for moral development* (pp. 98–122). New York: Cambridge University Press.

Laible, D., Murphy, T., & Augustine, M. (2013a). Constructing emotional and relational understanding: The role of mother–child reminiscing about negatively-valenced events. *Social Development, 22,* 300–318.

Laible, D., Murphy, T., & Augustine, M. (2013b). Predicting the quality of mother–child reminiscing surrounding negative emotional events at 42- and 48-months. *Journal of Cognition and Development, 14,* 270–291.

Laible, D., & Panfile, T. (2009). Mother–child reminiscing in the context of secure attachment relationships: Lessons in understanding and coping with negative emotion. In J. Quas & R. Fivush (Eds.), *Emotion and memory in development: Biological, cognitive, and social considerations* (pp. 166–195). Oxford, UK: Oxford University Press.

Laible, D., & Song, J. (2006). Constructing emotional and relational understanding: The role of affect and mother–child discourse. *Merrill–Palmer Quarterly, 52,* 44–69.

Laible, D. J., & Thompson, R. A. (1998). Attachment and emotional understanding in preschool children. *Developmental Psychology, 34,* 1038–1045.

Laible, D. J., & Thompson, R. A. (2000). Mother–child discourse, attachment security, shared positive affect, and early conscience development. *Child Development, 71,* 1424–1440.

Laible, D. J., & Thompson, R. A. (2002). Mother–child conflict in the toddler years: Lessons in emotion, morality, and relationships. *Child Development, 73,* 1187–1203.

Lansford, J. E., Malone, P. S., Stevens, K. I., Dodge, K. A., Bates, J. E., & Pettit, G. S. (2006) Developmental trajectories of externalizing and internalizing behaviors: Factors underlying resilience in physically abused children. *Developmental Psychopathology, 18,* 35–55.

Leerkes, E. M., Blankson, A. N., & O'Brien, M. (2009). Differential effects of maternal Sensitivity to infant distress and nondistress on social–emotional functioning. *Child Development, 80,* 762–775.

Lepper, M. R. (1981). Intrinsic and extrinsic motivation in children: Detrimental effects of superfluous social controls. In W. A. Collins (Ed.), *Minnesota Symposia on Child Psychology: Vol. 14. Aspects of the development of competence* (pp. 155–181). Hillsdale, NJ: Erlbaum.

Lewis, M. (2000). Self-conscious emotions: Embarrassment, pride, shame, and guilt. In M. Lewis & J. M. Haviland-Jones (Eds.), *Handbook of emotions* (pp. 563–573). New York: Guilford Press.

Lindahl, K. M., & Malik, N. M. (2011). Marital conflict typology and children's appraisals: The moderating role of family cohesion. *Journal of Family Psychology, 25,* 194–201.

Lohaus, A., Keller, H., Ball, J., Voelker, S., & Elben, C. (2004). Maternal sensitivity in interactions with three- and 12-month-old infants: Stability, structural composition, and developmental consequences. *Infant and Child Development, 13,* 235–252.

Maccoby, E., & Martin, J. (1983). Socialization in the context of the family: Parent–child interaction. In P. Mussen (Ed.) & E. Hetherington (Vol. Ed.), *Handbook of child psychology: Vol. IV. Socialization, personality, and social development* (pp. 1–101). New York: Wiley.

MacKenzie, M. J., Nicklas, E., Waldfogel, J., & Brooks-Gunn, J. (2012). Corporal punishment and child behavioural and cognitive outcomes through 5 years of age: Evidence from a contemporary urban birth cohort study. *Infant and Child Development, 21,* 3–33.

Markova, G., & Legerstee, M. (2006). Contingency, imitation, and affect sharing: Foundations of infants' social awareness. *Developmental Psychology, 42,* 132–140.

McCoy, K., Cummings, E. M., & Davies, P. T. (2009). Constructive and destructive marital conflict, emotional security and children's prosocial behavior. *Journal of Child Psychology and Psychiatry, 50,* 270–279.

McElwain, N. L., & Booth-LaForce, C. (2006). Maternal sensitivity to infant distress and nondistress as predictors of infant–mother attachment security. *Journal of Family Psychology, 20,* 247–255.

McGowan, P. O., Sasaki, A., D'Alessio, A. C., Dymov, S., Labonté, B., Szyf, M., et al. (2009). Epigenetic regulation of the glucocorticoid receptor in human brain associates with childhood abuse. *Nature Neuroscience, 12,* 342–348.

Meaney, M. J. (2010). Epigenetics and the biological definition of gene × environment interactions. *Child Development, 81,* 41–79.

Meltzoff, A. (2002). Elements of a developmental theory of imitation. In A. Meltzoff & W. Prinz (Eds.), *The imitative mind* (pp. 19–41). Cambridge, UK: Cambridge University Press.

Naumova, O., Lee, M., Koposov, R., Szyf, M., Dozier, M., & Grigorenko, E. L. (2012). Differential patterns of whole-genome DNA methylation in institutionalized children and children raised by their biological parents. *Development and Psychopathology, 24,* 143–155.

Nelson, K. (Ed.). (1978). *Event knowledge: Structure and function in development.* Hillsdale, NJ: Erlbaum.

Newton, E., Laible, D., Carlo, G., Steele, J., & McGinley, M. (in press). Do sensitive parents foster kind children, or vice versa?: Bidirectional influences between children's prosocial behavior and parental sensitivity. *Developmental Psychology.*

Olineck, K. M., & Poulin-Dubois, D. (2007). Imitation of intentional actions and internal state language in infancy predict preschool theory of mind skills. *European Journal of Developmental Psychology, 4,* 14–30.

Onishi, K. H., & Baillargeon, R. (2005). Do 15-month-old infants understand false beliefs? *Science, 308,* 255–258.

Pasupathi, M., & Wainryb, C. (2010). Developing moral agency through narrative. *Human Development, 53,* 55–80.

Pettit, G. S., Keiley, M. K., Laird, R. D., Bates, J. E., & Dodge, K. A. (2007). Predicting the developmental course of mother-reported monitoring across childhood and adolescence from early proactive parenting, child temperament, and parents' worries. *Journal of Family Psychology, 21,* 206–217.

Putnam, S. P., Spritz, B. L., & Stifter, C. A. (2002). Mother–child coregulation during delay of gratification at 30 months. *Infancy, 3,* 209–225.

Raikes, H. A., & Thompson, R. A. (2008). Attachment security and parenting quality predict children's problem-solving, attributions, and loneliness with peers. *Attachment and Human Development, 10,* 319–344.

Ruffman, T., & Perner, J. (2005). Do infants really understand false belief?: Response to Leslie. *Trends in Cognitive Sciences, 9,* 462–463.

Sears, R. R., Maccoby, E. E., & Levin, H. (1957). *Patterns of child rearing.* Evanston, IL: Row, Peterson.

Sheehan, M. J., & Watson, M. W. (2008). Reciprocal influences between maternal discipline techniques and aggression in children and adolescents. *Aggressive Behavior, 34,* 245–255.

Smetana, J. G., Kochanska, G., & Chuang, S. (2000). Mothers' conceptions of everyday rules for young toddlers: A longitudinal investigation. *Merrill–Palmer Quarterly, 46,* 391–416.

Smetana, J. G., Rote, W. M., Jambon, M., Tasopoulos-Chan, M., Villalobos, M., & Comer, J. (2012). Developmental changes and individual differences in young children's moral judgments. *Child Development, 83,* 683–696.

Song, H. J., Onishi, K. H., Baillargeon, R., & Fisher, C. (2008). Can an agent's false belief be corrected by an appropriate communication?: Psychological reasoning in 18-month-old infants. *Cognition, 109,* 295–315.

Spagnola, M., & Fiese, B. H. (2007). Family routines and rituals: A context for development in the lives of young children. *Infants and Young Children, 20,* 284–299.

Spinrad, T. L., Eisenberg, N., Silva, K. M., Eggum, N. D., Reiser, M., Edwards, A., et al. (2012). Longitudinal relations among maternal behaviors, effortful control and young children's committed compliance. *Developmental Psychology, 48,* 552–566.

Stipek, D., Recchia, S., & McClintic, S. (1992). Self-evaluation in young children. *Monographs of the Society for Research in Child Development, 57,* 1–98.

Tamis-LeMonda, C., & Bornstein, M. H. (2002). Maternal responsiveness and early language acquisition. In R. V. Kail & H. W. Reese (Eds.), *Advances in child development and behavior* (Vol. 29, pp. 89–127). San Diego, CA: Academic Press.

Thompson, R. A. (2006). The development of the person: Social understanding, relationships, self, conscience. In W. Damon & R. M. Lerner (Eds.) & N. Eisenberg (Vol. Ed.), *Handbook of child psychology: Vol. 3. Social, emotional, and personality development* (6th ed., pp. 24–98). New York: Wiley.

Thompson, R. A. (2008). Early attachment and later development: Familiar questions, new answers. In J. Cassidy & P. R. Shaver (Eds.), *Handbook of attachment: Theory, research, and clinical applications* (2nd ed., pp. 348–365). New York: Guilford Press.

Thompson, R. A. (2011). Emotion and emotion regulation: Two sides of the developing coin. *Emotion Review, 3,* 53–61.

Thompson, R. A. (in press). Relationships, regulation, and early development. In R. M. Lerner (Ed.) & M. E. Lamb & C. Garcia Coll (Vol. Eds.), *Handbook of child psychology: Vol. 3. Social, emotional, and personality development* (7th ed.). New York: Wiley.

Thompson, R. A., & Meyer, S. (2007). The socialization of emotion regulation in the family. In J. J. Gross (Ed.), *Handbook of emotion regulation* (pp. 249–268). New York: Guilford Press.

Thompson, R. A., Meyer, S., & McGinley, M. (2006). Understanding values in relationship: The development of conscience. In M. Killen & J. Smetana (Eds.), *Handbook of moral development* (pp. 267–297). Mahwah, NJ: Erlbaum.

Thompson, R. A., & Newton, E. K. (2010). Emotion in early conscience. In W. Arsenio & E. Lemerise (Eds.), *Emotions, aggression, and morality: Bridging development and psychopathology* (pp. 6–32). Washington, DC: American Psychological Association.

Toth, S. L., Rogosch, F. A., Sturge-Apple, M., & Cicchetti, D. (2009). Maternal depression, children's attachment security, and representational development: An organizational perspective. *Child Development, 80,* 192–208.

Towe-Goodman, N. R., & Teti, D. M. (2008). Power assertive discipline, maternal emotional involvement, and child adjustment. *Journal of Family Psychology, 22,* 648–651.

Van Aken, C., Junger, M., Verhoeven, M., Van Aken, M. A. G., & Deković, M. (2007). The interactive effects of temperament and maternal parenting on toddlers' externalizing behaviours. *Infant and Child Development, 16,* 553–572.

Verhoeven, M., Junger, M., van Aken, C., Deković M., & van Aken, M. A. (2010). Parenting and children's externalizing behavior: Bidirectionality during toddlerhood. *Journal of Applied Developmental Psychology, 31,* 93–105.

Wainryb, C., & Brehl, B. A. (2006). "I thought she knew that would hurt my feelings": Developing psychological knowledge and moral thinking. *Advances in Child Development and Behavior, 34,* 131–171.

Warneken, F., & Tomasello, M. (2008). Extrinsic rewards undermine altruistic tendencies in 20-month-olds. *Developmental Psychology, 44,* 1785–1788.

Waters, S., Virmani, E., Thompson, R. A., Meyer, S., Raikes, A., & Jochem, R. (2010). Emotion regulation and attachment: Unpacking two constructs and their association. *Journal of Psychopathology and Behavioral Assessment, 32,* 37–47.

Wellman, H. (2002). Understanding the psychological world: Developing a theory of mind. In U. Goswami (Ed.), *Handbook of childhood cognitive development* (pp. 167–187). Oxford, UK: Blackwell.

Wellman, H. M., & Miller, J. G. (2008). Including deontic reasoning as fundamental to theory of mind. *Human Development, 51,* 105–135.

Woodward, A. L. (1998). Infants selectively encode the goal object of an actor's reach. *Cognition, 69,* 1–34.

Yoo, Y. S., Popp, J., & Robinson, J. (2014). Maternal distress influences young children's family representations through maternal view of child behavior and parent–child interactions. *Child Psychiatry and Human Development, 45*(1), 52–64.

Zahn-Waxler, C., & Robinson, J. (1995). Empathy and guilt: Early origins of feelings of responsibility. In J. P. Tangney & K. W. Fischer (Eds.), *The self-conscious emotions: Theory and research* (pp. 143–173). New York: Guilford Press.

CHAPTER 3

Socialization in Adolescence

Judith G. Smetana
Jessica Robinson
Wendy M. Rote

Broadly, *socialization* refers to the process by which youth are helped to acquire the skills necessary to function competently and successfully as members of their social group or culture. Much of the theorizing and psychological research on socialization has focused on early and middle childhood because, depending on one's theoretical predilections, this is when children are seen as most malleable in response to environmental influences, when innate predispositions are manifested, or when, through biopsychosocial processes, trajectories toward different developmental endpoints are firmly established. But socialization continues in the second decade of life and in ways continuous with childhood on many dimensions. At the same time, and as we elaborate below, there are unique aspects to socialization during adolescence. Particularly, parenting increasingly occurs at a distance as children become more independent, as new forms of peer relationships emerge, and as different developmental issues assume prominence.

Before turning to these issues, we address several conceptual and methodological issues. Early theoretical models viewed socialization as a largely unidirectional process whereby parents transmitted cultural norms and standards to their children, with the goal of reproducing them in successive generations. Thus, assessments focused largely on children's compliance with parental expectations or their acquisition of culturally valued goals and behaviors (see Smetana, 2002, 2011). However, most researchers, including those from different theoretical vantage points, now agree that socialization is considerably more complex than this model suggests.

There has been an increasing emphasis on bidirectional processes and children's active role in their own development. For instance, Kuczynski, Parkin, and Pitman (Chapter 6, this volume) have focused on socialization as a reciprocal dynamic process and on children's agency in parent–child relationships. Grusec (2002) and her colleagues (Grusec, Goodnow, & Kuczynski, 2000) have raised questions about the conditions under which children accept or reject parental messages and the goals beyond compliance that parents have for children. In addition, there is substantial evidence that children and adolescents interpret, negotiate, and respond to adults' (as well as peers') efforts to control, guide, or influence their behavior (Smetana, 2011). Indeed, adolescents do not unthinkingly adopt adult values; they challenge and sometimes resist those that they consider to be inappropriate, immoral, or illegitimate (Smetana, 2011). Thus, effective socialization depends, in part, on adolescents' evaluations of the messages communicated—for instance, whether or not the behavior being prescribed is culturally normative, or whether adolescents believe that adults are acting out of concern or support, as opposed to being intrusive and controlling. As we illustrate in this chapter, there is ample evidence that socialization processes are dynamic and reciprocal and that teens actively participate and exert agency in their development.

In addition, there has been a profound shift over the past few decades in the samples employed in research on adolescent socialization and development. In a relatively short span of time, the field has moved beyond Graham's (1992) observation that "most of the subjects of research were white and middle class" (p. 629) to studying normative processes in much more diverse populations of youth. Initially, this was reflected in studies from the United States focusing primarily on African American adolescents (Steinberg & Morris, 2001) and in studies from other Western societies with selected immigrant groups. Recently, however, research has become more broadly inclusive, giving increased attention to the development of youth from different racial and ethnic backgrounds, as well as different countries and cultures (Chao & Otsuki-Clutter, 2011). There also has been increased recognition of the heterogeneity among adolescents from different ethnic groups and therefore more attention to specifying their national origins or backgrounds (e.g., Mexican Americans or Puerto Ricans rather than the broader category of Latino/ Latinas or Chinese Canadians as compared to Mainland Chinese). In addition, reflecting demographic trends around the globe, research has increasingly considered how immigration, acculturation, ethnicity, and social class interact to influence adolescents' developing values, beliefs, and behavior. This has resulted in a dramatic increase over the past decade in studies of immigrant youth and processes of acculturation, ethnic identity development, and experiences of discrimination (Chao & Otsuki-Clutter, 2011; Fuligni, Hughes, & Way, 2009), as well as a much richer and more complex understanding of adolescent socialization in different contexts.

We begin by briefly describing several features that are unique to the second decade of life or that distinguish socialization during adolescence from processes occurring in childhood. Then we turn to different contexts of socialization, which provide the organizational framework for the rest of the chapter. Although researchers have recognized that various agents, including siblings, adult relatives, peers, social institutions, and the media, all are important influences, socialization research has focused heavily on parents. This is because society views parents as primarily responsible for raising children, and parents typically have the most time and opportunity to influence them (Grusec, 2002). Here, we discuss the role of parents, siblings, peers, and very briefly, out-of-school settings, but in keeping with previous scholarship, we focus most heavily on the family.

Adolescence as a Distinct Developmental Period

The second decade of life is a period of enormous growth and change. The transformations of puberty result in a growth spurt that is second only to that in infancy (Archibald, Graber, & Brooks-Gunn, 2003), and this presents significant challenges, not only for adolescents' adaptation, but also for those around them. In addition, teenagers' understanding of their physical and social worlds changes significantly. Adolescents become better able to plan, make decisions, and think about the future; they also face new psychosocial challenges around issues of identity, autonomy, intimacy, and sexuality. As we describe below, these result in major transformations in how much time adolescents spend with parents and peers, and in the quality and type of relationships they have.

Changing Contexts of Adolescent Socialization

How Adolescents Spend Their Time

Research on how and with whom adolescents spend their time provides important insights into the socialization opportunities and developmental contexts that youth experience. Larson and his colleagues (Larson, Richards, Moneta, Holmbeck, & Duckett, 1996; Larson, Richards, Sims, & Dworkin, 2001) have conducted several longitudinal studies using the experience sampling method (ESM), in which adolescents report their activities, interactions, and moods at random moments during the day when contacted by pager or cell phone. These studies demonstrate that there are dramatic changes—at least for some youth—in the amount of time spent with parents versus peers. For instance, there is a sharp decrease from early to late adolescence in how much time European American teens spend with family members (from 35% of waking hours in fifth grade to 14% by 12th grade; Larson et al., 1996). Similar decreases with age have been observed among Mexican American adolescents (as assessed in nightly phone calls to families spread over several weeks; Updegraff, McHale, Whiteman, Thayer, & Crouter, 2006). However, poor and working-class urban African American fifth to eighth graders appear to interact much more with relatives than do European American adolescents (Larson et al., 2001), in part because many African American youth live with extended family. This pattern is much like what has been observed in non-Western cultures such as India (Larson et al., 2001). Thus, for some ethnic minority youth, like youth in non-Western cultures, extended kin are potential sources of socialization and support.

As they grow older, teens spend less leisure time with parents but increase slightly (particularly girls) in the amount of time they spend talking with parents (although more so for mothers than fathers; Larson et al., 1996). They also spend more time alone in their bedrooms and with friends (Larson et al., 1996, 2001). Because the latter frequently occurs in unstructured contexts, it is associated with more problem behavior (Larson, 2001). However, as Larson notes, U.S. teens spend less time on schoolwork and in school than do youth in most other industrialized countries, and they therefore have more time for leisure. Ethnic socialization also has an impact; for instance, youth whose parents have a stronger orientation to Mexican culture spend more time with peers who share their Mexican heritage than with more heterogeneous peers (Updegraff et al., 2006).

Changes in Relationships with Parents during Adolescence

Relationships with parents change during adolescence in ways that may influence adolescents' receptiveness to parental socialization. Numerous studies, both cross-sectional and longitudinal, and employing different methods, have demonstrated that among youth from diverse ethnic backgrounds and cultures, positive aspects of parent–teen relationships, including support, closeness, warmth, cohesion, and intimacy, decline during adolescence (Fuligni, 1998; Furman & Buhrmester, 1985; Shanahan, McHale, Crouter, & Osgood, 2007), although the timing varies (Fuligni, 1998).

These declines appear to level off in late adolescence and become more stable. For instance, in a recent 8-year longitudinal study following a large and diverse sample of U.S. youth, Tsai, Telzer, and Fuligni (2013) found that feelings of cohesion with both mothers and fathers normatively declined during adolescence but then, for mothers, stabilized in young adulthood. There were surprisingly few differences among Latino, Asian, and European American youth in the trajectories of continuity and change over time. Furthermore, Shanahan, McHale, Crouter, and Osgood (2007) found that warmth toward mothers but not fathers increased after age 18, whereas other research indicates that closeness increases in late adolescence, but only after teens leave home for college (Acquilino, 1997). Most researchers agree that normative changes in family relationships during adolescence reflect adolescents' attempts to individuate from the family and develop greater autonomy. This contrasts with young adulthood, in which the orientation is toward maintaining and strengthening family ties (Tsai et al., 2013).

Studies also consistently show that across adolescence and into young adulthood, adolescents are closer and spend more time interacting with mothers than with fathers (Larson et al., 1996, 2001; Tsai et al., 2013); adolescent females also generally report closer relationships with parents, and especially their mothers, than do adolescent males. Although such studies are rare, there is also some evidence pointing to within-family differences in closeness. For instance, Shanahan, McHale, Crouter, and Osgood (2007) found that firstborn offspring reported warmer relationships with mothers across adolescence and with fathers in early adolescence than did second-born offspring. This difference was attributed to older siblings' greater maturity, although other factors, such as the time or attention given to first-born versus later-born offspring, or the latter's greater need to individuate from the family, also could have accounted for these effects.

Reciprocally, negative affect and conflict with parents increase during adolescence (see Smetana, 2011, for a review). There is some consensus among researchers that moderate levels of conflict with parents in early adolescence are a normative and temporary perturbation that lead to transformations toward greater mutuality in family relationships (Holmbeck, 1996). The frequency of conflict peaks in early adolescence and then declines, whereas conflict intensity increases from early to middle adolescence (Laursen, Coy, & Collins, 1998). As with closeness, these patterns are strikingly similar among youth of different ethnicities and in other cultures (Fuligni et al., 2009). Furthermore, Shanahan, McHale, Osgood, and Crouter (2007) found "spillover" between siblings in the developmental timing of conflict with parents. That is, conflicts between second-born offspring and their parents were found to increase in frequency when firstborns transitioned to adolescence, rather than when second-borns transitioned.

Changes in Adolescents' Relationships with Peers

The changes in relationships with parents during adolescence are paralleled by changes in adolescents' relationships with peers, signaling the increasing importance of peers as a context for adolescent socialization. During childhood, children's play and organized activities are typically adult-supervised and are often at or in close proximity to home. But during adolescence, teenagers become more independent, and their peer interactions increasingly occur away from home and adult supervision (Dijkstra & Veenstra, 2011). Thus, rather than being able to observe their children's activities directly or have other watchful adults keep them informed, parents must supervise and monitor from a distance. In turn, this results in new parental strategies and ways of obtaining information about teenagers' activities and associates (more about this later).

In addition, friendships and the structure of adolescent peer groups change during adolescence. Adolescents' friendships become closer and more intimate, disclosing, and supportive with age (Collins & Steinberg, 2006). Adolescents also congregate in larger groupings of peers, including *cliques*. These are small groups of same-age, same-sex (at least in early adolescence), and similar socioeconomic-status peers that are based on friendship and shared activities (Collins & Steinberg, 2006). Although present in childhood, cliques become particularly prominent in early adolescence, helping to define the social hierarchy (both within and between cliques) and establish certain peers as leaders of the social system. Cliques remain present throughout adolescence and beyond but become more fluid with age, with increasing membership turnover and more individuals not belonging at all or belonging to multiple cliques (Brown & Klute, 2003). In early to midadolescence, youth also begin to affiliate with *crowds*, or loose, reputation-based groupings derived from perceived attitudes, interests, and behaviors (Collins & Steinberg, 2006). Similar to cliques, the shared reputations of crowd members help to locate adolescents in the social hierarchy, channeling them toward different pathways and friendships, and allowing them to "try on" different identities (Brown & Larson, 2009). Although teens may not spend much time with other crowd members, crowd membership is important for friendship and identity formation. Thus, friendships, cliques, and crowds become increasingly central contexts for adolescent socialization.

Changes in Measures of Socialization in Adolescence

There is a great deal of continuity from childhood to adolescence in the behaviors, values, and attitudes that adults view as important for mature, competent functioning and that are used to measure successful socialization. But there are some changes in emphasis as well. For instance, adolescence is widely seen as a developmental period reflecting preparation for adult roles and responsibilities. Consequently, it becomes important to prepare youth to become independent and care for themselves, and autonomy development becomes increasingly important.

Likewise, issues of ethnic identity development and cultural socialization become particularly salient in adolescence (Hughes et al., 2006). A positive ethnic identity and adherence to the values of one's cultural, ethnic, or racial group have been found to enhance well-being and serve a protective function (Fuligni et al., 2009; Hughes et al., 2006). Also, ethnic minority parents typically wait until adolescence to broach more challenging and sensitive issues, such as coping with discrimination and unequal treatment

(Fuligni et al., 2009; Hughes et al., 2006). Thus, there has been increasing emphasis on how parents transmit cultural practices and values, convey information regarding race and ethnicity, and prepare minority youth to cope with the unique ecological challenges that they may face.

Research on socialization also focuses on risky behaviors that are on the rise during adolescence. For instance, experimentation and regular use of alcohol, illegal drugs, abuse of prescription medications, and cigarettes increase during adolescence for U.S. (Johnston, O'Malley, Bachman, & Schulenberg, 2012) and Canadian teens (Leatherdale & Burkhalter, 2012). The incidence of these risky behaviors is extremely low at the onset of adolescence, but by the end of adolescence the vast majority of contemporary U.S. adolescents have tried alcohol, and about 40% have smoked marijuana and cigarettes, although rates of regular use are substantially lower. Among Canadian teens, 51% report having drunk alcohol, 29% have used marijuana, and 16% have used tobacco by 12th grade (Leatherdale & Burkhalter, 2012).

In addition, about 65% of all U.S. teens have had sexual intercourse by the end of high school, much of it unprotected (although estimates vary). By age 15, 25% of European youth have had sexual intercourse, with rates substantially higher in some countries (e.g., 38% in Denmark) and much lower in others (e.g., Slovakia, where 10% of females and 15% of males report having had intercourse; Currie et al., 2012). Furthermore, research suggests that early sexual debut (before age 14) carries substantial risks for maladjustment (Diamond & Savin-Williams, 2009). Thus, researchers have examined these various behaviors as indicators of risk or poor socialization. Likewise, although much antisocial behavior has its roots in childhood, a certain amount of less serious antisocial behavior may be normative during adolescence (Moffitt, 2006). Not surprisingly then, many researchers have focused on both life-course-persistent and "adolescence-limited" antisocial behavior and the socialization of each.

Finally, there has been increased interest over the last decade in studying adolescent civic engagement as a positive indicator of successful socialization during adolescence (Sherrod, Torney-Purta, & Flanagan, 2010). Research on civic engagement focuses on the varying factors that result in adolescents' engagement in their communities and political institutions, as a step toward becoming good adult citizens of their society. During adolescence, this includes becoming politically active (e.g., by voting and staying informed about current events), participating in community organizations, and engaging in volunteering and service. Although these behaviors surely have their origins in childhood, research on civic engagement has focused almost entirely on the emergence and maintenance of these behaviors during adolescence.

Summary

Research reviewed in this section indicates that how much time teens report spending with parents overall or in certain activities, and the quality of parent–child relationships decline during adolescence, resulting in more limited opportunities for parental socialization and less receptivity to parental influence than at earlier ages. Correspondingly, friendships become closer and more intimate, and cliques and crowds become important sources of influence. Finally, research often focuses on risky behaviors that increase during adolescence but in recent years, there also has been more attention paid to positive indicators of socialization, such as ethnic identity and civic engagement.

Parenting as a Context for Adolescent Socialization

Although adolescence is a time of transformation in both social relationships and socialization goals, the contexts of socialization are similar in childhood and adolescence, with parents, siblings, peers, and out-of-school activities serving as important influences. Parenting styles, more specific parenting practices, and the interplay of parenting and adolescent beliefs during adolescence have all received particular attention.

The Influence of Parenting Styles

Baumrind's research on parenting styles has been the most influential approach to parental socialization of social competence and psychological adjustment during adolescence. Baumrind and her colleagues (Baumrind, 1971; Baumrind, Larzelere, & Owens, 2010) have championed the use of pattern-based analyses, arguing that parenting is a gestalt, or "a totality made up of integrated practices that interact in such a way as to confer properties that are not possessed by a sum of its component practices" (p. 185). In her original work, Baumrind classified parenting into various categories, which were grouped into three broad parenting styles: authoritative, authoritarian, and permissive. Subsequently, Maccoby and Martin (1983) characterized parenting styles according to two orthogonal dimensions of demandingness and responsiveness and added a fourth category, rejecting–neglecting parenting, which reflected low levels of both dimensions. Baumrind believes that parenting styles are functionally continuous from childhood to adolescence, although the specific behaviors parents deploy may change as children grow older.

Numerous studies have shown that adolescents raised in authoritative homes (where parents are both highly demanding and responsive) are more competent, as assessed on a wide range of outcomes, than adolescents raised in authoritarian, permissive, or rejecting–neglecting homes (Sorkhabi & Mandara, 2013). Most of the evidence comes from cross-sectional research, or studies focused on the short-term longitudinal effects of parenting across adolescence. This research shows that parenting influences adolescent adjustment, although bidirectional models typically have not been tested (but see Kerr, Stattin, & Ozdemir, 2012, who found that adolescent behavior has a much stronger effect on parenting style than the reverse).

Recently, Baumrind and colleagues (2010) reanalyzed their original data to examine the influence of parenting styles assessed in early and middle childhood on competence (examined in terms of cognitive competence, individuation, self-efficacy, and absence of problem behavior) in middle adolescence. These researchers found that parenting in early childhood had unique effects on early adolescent adjustment, over and above the effects of parenting assessed both in middle childhood and concurrently. Authoritative parenting resulted in the greatest competence, followed by permissive and then authoritarian parenting. These analyses also distinguished between detrimental (e.g., coercive) and positive (e.g., what Baumrind referred to as "confrontive") forms of power assertion as well as between demandingness and responsiveness.

Baumrind's longitudinal sample comprised primarily European American and middle-class participants. But research consistently has demonstrated that European American parents and those from higher socioeconomic statuses are more likely to employ authoritative parenting than are parents from ethnic minority, lower socioeconomic status, and non-Western cultures, where authoritarian parenting prevails. Nevertheless, some have claimed that in contemporary industrialized societies and because of the nurturance and parental involvement, authoritative parenting benefits most youth (Sorkhabi & Mandara, 2013). Asian American youth experience higher levels of authoritarian parenting but have higher levels of academic achievement than youth from other ethnic backgrounds; this been attributed to the value placed on academic achievement in Chinese culture (Mason, Walker-Barnes, Tu, Simons, & Martinez-Arrue, 2004).

Some have asserted, however, that Baumrind's parenting styles reflect distinctively European American values and that parenting in other groups should be assessed in terms of relevant, more indigenous cultural values. For instance, Chao (2001) has claimed that Chinese parenting is often described as authoritarian, punitive, and adult-centered, whereas she believes it actually reflects a Confucian, child-centered emphasis on the importance of strictness in the service of training (*guan*). Moreover, there is some evidence that the positive effects of authoritative parenting, at least for immigrant Chinese youth, reflect the influence of greater exposure to American society (Chao, 2001). At issue here is how adolescents of different ethnicities interpret parental control, as discussed in the following section.

Dimensional Approaches to Parenting

Researchers have increasingly unpacked parenting styles by employing dimensional approaches, which are seen as providing greater specificity. For instance, rather than viewing parental control as a single dimension, researchers have distinguished between psychological and behavioral control. *Psychological control* refers to parenting behaviors that manipulate adolescents' thoughts and feelings, thereby violating adolescents' sense of self through intrusiveness, guilt induction, and love withdrawal and resulting in poorer adjustment (Barber, Stolz, & Olsen, 2005). In contrast, *behavioral control* refers to parents' attempts to regulate adolescents' behavior by setting high standards, and regulating and enforcing them through supervision and monitoring. It is considered to be a more positive form of control because it provides adolescents with a clear set of parental expectations and the structure and guidance needed for the development of competent, autonomous, and responsible behavior. This distinction in forms of control is particularly relevant for parental socialization in adolescence because psychological control impinges on individuals' sense of self and their ability to develop personal identity, both of which are crucial developmental processes in adolescence.

Parental Psychological Control

Although researchers agree that parental psychological control involves undue socialization pressure, there are disagreements about how best to conceptualize and measure it (Chao & Otsuki-Clutter, 2011). Recently, Barber and his colleagues (2012) identified parental disrespect as the underlying dimension that leads to adverse effects on adolescent adjustment. In contrast, from a self-determination theory perspective, Soenens and Vansteenkiste (2010) have proposed that psychological control needs to be conceptualized narrowly in terms of parenting that pressures internally (e.g., conditional approval by manipulating feelings of guilt, shame, and separation anxiety) rather than externally through the use of threats of physical punishment and contingencies such as controlling rewards or removal of privileges.

Numerous factors have been associated with parental psychological control, including single parenthood, less maternal education, and ethnicity (with greater psychological control found among African American than among European American parents; Laird, 2011). Some personality attributes, including parental neuroticism and maladaptive perfectionism, also have been identified (Laird, 2011), as has parents' use of harsh discipline with young children (Pettit, Laird, Bates, Dodge, & Criss, 2001). High levels of adolescent depression and antisocial behavior are reciprocally associated with feeling psychologically controlled (Laird, 2011; Pettit et al., 2001). Parents are also seen as more psychologically controlling when they control issues that teens believe should be under their personal jurisdiction (Smetana & Daddis, 2002), and feeling overcontrolled, in turn, is associated with greater internalizing distress (Hasebe, Nucci, & Nucci, 2004).

Barber and his colleagues (2005, 2012) claim that parental psychological control has adverse effects on adjustment for all youth and have provided extensive cross-cultural evidence to that effect. However, this has been subject to debate because variations in findings have been observed in different ethnic and racial groups (Chao & Otsuki-Clutter, 2011). There is evidence to suggest that the cultural meaning of psychological control moderates its negative effects. For instance, American adolescents from African, European, and Hispanic backgrounds have been found to vary as to whether they interpret controlling behavior as reflecting parents' love and concern (Mason et al., 2004) or whether, instead, it arouses feelings of anger (Chao & Acque, 2009). More specifically, the latter investigators found that feeling angry moderated the negative effects of psychological control on problem behavior for European American youth but not American youth from various Asian backgrounds. In contrast, interpreting parental psychological control as reflecting love and concern, which was more likely among African American than among European American youth, led to less adverse (but still negative) outcomes (Mason et al., 2004).

Parental Behavioral Control

Behavioral control and the guidance it provides are considered important for socialization. Much research has shown that greater parental behavioral control is associated with higher academic achievement and better adjustment for adolescents of different ethnicities (Lamborn, Dornbusch, & Steinberg, 1996, Pettit et al., 2001).

Behavioral control is a broad construct that has been defined in many different ways. Grolnick and Pomerantz (2009) have proposed that the term *control* should be used only in reference to parental psychological control and that *structure* should replace *behavioral control*. These researchers define structure as "parents' organization of children's environment to facilitate children's competence" (p. 167); this involves providing clear and consistent guidelines, rules, and expectations, as well as predictable consequences and clear feedback for behavior. This distinction between structure and control is important because, according to self-determination theory, children have basic needs for psychological autonomy (which may be violated by parental control) and competence (which may be satisfied by parental structuring), but they do not have a basic psychological need to be regulated. However, Baumrind and colleagues (2010) countered that parenting can be both behaviorally controlling and autonomy-supportive if it is confrontive, or "firm, direct, forceful, and consistent" (e.g., authoritative, p. 158) but not coercive (i.e., peremptory, domineering, arbitrary, and hierarchical—e.g., authoritarian).

In addition to this definitional confusion, many different measures have been employed to assess behavioral control. Monitoring is considered one of the most important practices in parents' toolkit because, as noted earlier, parenting during the adolescent years increasingly occurs at a distance. Monitoring allows parents to keep track of their teens while permitting greater autonomy. Numerous studies have shown that too little parental monitoring is associated with externalizing problems such as drug use, truancy, and antisocial behavior (Collins & Steinberg, 2006). Furthermore, parental monitoring has been found to have beneficial effects among ethnically diverse youth in the United States and elsewhere (Chao & Otsuki-Clutter, 2011).

These positive effects have been attributed to both contextual and cultural factors. For instance, there are clear benefits to strict parental supervision for adolescents living in dangerous neighborhoods (which is more often the case for minority than for majority youth), as this may help to protect adolescents and keep them safe (Lamborn et al., 1996). In addition, supervision, strictness, and protectiveness are part of Latino (e.g., familism) and Chinese (e.g., *guan*) cultural values, as Chao and Otsuki-Clutter (2011) have noted. Indeed, in the study by Chao and Acque (2009) discussed earlier, Chinese adolescents who were immigrants to the United States (but not other Asian immigrant youth) felt less anger in response to parental strictness than did European American adolescents. However, consistent with Grolnick and Pomerantz's (2009) conceptual analysis, Chao and Acque's factor analysis revealed empirical distinctions between "Provides Structure" and "Strictness" (both dimensions of behavioral control). Unlike the findings for strictness, providing structure was more negatively associated with problem behavior in European than in Asian American (particularly Filipino) youth. Indeed, for Filipinos, providing structure was associated with increased internalizing and externalizing symptoms, suggesting that Filipino parents may employ this form of control only when youth exhibit problem behavior. More generally, the findings suggest that parental structure and strictness are conceptually distinct.

Monitoring versus Parental Knowledge

Problems also have been identified in how parental monitoring has been operationalized in research. As Stattin and Kerr (2000) observed, monitoring typically has been assessed in terms of parents' knowledge of adolescents' away-from-home activities rather than parents' active tracking and surveillance. Research has shown that parents have different strategies for learning about teens' activities. Compared to fathers, mothers use more active methods, such as asking their offspring directly or asking informed others (e.g., teachers or spouses), and actively participating in activities, such as driving the child to events (Waizenhofer, Buchanan, & Jackson-Newsom, 2004). In contrast, fathers rely more exclusively on their spouses for information, particularly about their daughters (Crouter, Bumpus, Davis, & McHale, 2005; Waizenhofer et al., 2004). However, Crouter and colleagues (2005) found that a relational style involving high levels of adolescent voluntary disclosure, as well as parental observation and listening, led to greater parental knowledge, which in turn was associated with lower levels of risky behavior, including less involvement with deviant peers, problem behavior, truancy, and drug use. Along with several other risk factors, lower levels of parental knowledge are also associated with an increasing risk of substance use, anxiety, and depression for a range of youth, including those growing up in highly affluent communities.

Much research has now confirmed that adolescents' willing disclosure is more strongly associated with parental knowledge than is parental monitoring (e.g., parents' solicitation of information or behavioral control) (Crouter et al., 2005; Kerr, Stattin, & Burk, 2010; Stattin & Kerr, 2000). These findings highlight the importance of considering adolescents' agency in their development because adolescents actively manage the information they permit parents to have. Even when relationships are warm, close, and trusting, adolescents' disclosure to parents and parents' knowledge of adolescents' activities normatively decline from childhood levels (Smetana & Daddis, 2002), and secrecy and concealment increase. Information management has been described as a way of gaining greater autonomy from parents while maintaining positive relationships (Marshall, Tilton-Weaver, & Bosdet, 2005). But some forms of information management have positive functions, while others do not. Laird and Marrero (2010) have shown that telling parents only if asked is associated with better family relationships and adjustment, whereas concealment strategies generally have adverse effects, although less so for acts of omission, such as omitting details and avoidance, than for outright lying (Marshall et al., 2005).

While adolescents clearly control the flow of information to parents, good parenting can contribute to adolescent disclosure. Parenting that is authoritative, responsive, accepting, and trusting and low in levels of psychological control all have been found to increase adolescents' willingness to keep parents informed about their activities (Darling, Cumsille, Caldwell, & Dowdy, 2006; Smetana, Villalobos, Tasopoulos-Chan, Gettman, & Campione-Barr, 2009). Furthermore, when parents respond to disclosure negatively or punitively, adolescents report feeling more controlled and less connected to parents, which in turn results in increased secrecy and decreased disclosure over time (Tilton-Weaver et al., 2010). In addition, there is some evidence that parental solicitation of information in early adolescence (as reported by teens) reduces antisocial behavior, but only for adolescents who are likely to be noncompliant and uncooperative because they spend more time unsupervised and tend to challenge the legitimacy of their parents' authority (Laird, Marrero, & Sentse, 2010). Because unsupervised time and low legitimacy beliefs are predictors of antisocial behavior, it appears that parental solicitation may work for teens who need it most.

Perceptions of Parenting and Judgments of the Legitimacy of Parental Authority

Legitimacy of Parental Authority

Despite claims that behavioral and psychological control are distinct parenting dimensions, research also has demonstrated that they may become blurred for some youth and under certain conditions, such as when behavioral control is applied at high levels or used to control issues that adolescents view as personal. For instance, teens do not differentiate between psychological control and high levels of behavioral control (parents' prohibiting behaviors) as assessed in hypothetical vignettes; both were seen as reflecting greater parental intrusiveness and beliefs that teens matter less to parents than was moderate behavioral control (setting limits and conditions; Kakihara & Tilton-Weaver, 2010). And high levels of parental control—of different types—are interpreted negatively when applied to personal issues (Kakihara & Tilton-Weaver, 2010; Smetana & Daddis, 2002).

Personal issues have been defined within social domain theory (Smetana, 2011; Turiel, 1983) as issues that are outside of the realm of legitimate external regulation and up to the individual to decide because they pertain to privacy, control over one's body, and personal preferences and choices regarding friends, appearance, and leisure time pursuits. Control over personal issues satisfies psychological needs for autonomy, agency, and self-efficacy; therefore, its existence is seen as universal (Nucci, 1996). However, the breadth and content of the personal domain may vary both within and between cultures. For instance, for many North American youth, career choices and eligible dating and marriage partners are treated as personal issues, but for some North American ethnic minority youth or youth in other cultures, these behaviors are not.

The findings of research on conceptions of parental authority are important for adolescent socialization because they indicate that adolescents' willingness to endorse parental values and expectations varies by domain. A great deal of research has shown that teens and parents agree that parents have the legitimate authority to regulate *moral* concerns regarding others' welfare and rights (although parents are not seen as having the right to make rules that inflict harm or cause injustice to others), and *social-conventional* norms, and throughout much of adolescence, *prudential* issues of health, comfort, and safety, including risky behaviors (Smetana, 2011). Additionally, the personal domain expands during adolescence, with issues that are seen as legitimately regulated by parents in early adolescence increasingly coming under teens' control with age (see Smetana, 2002, 2011). However, for a variety of reasons—for instance, because parents are concerned about their child's welfare or believe that he or she is not yet responsible or competent enough to make independent decisions—parents may not grant their teen as much personal jurisdiction as he or she desires (Smetana, 2011).

Discrepancies between adolescents' and parents' views of legitimate parental authority lead to conflicts in their relationships and potentially to adolescents' nondisclosure and secrecy with parents (Smetana, 2011). Conflicts and nondisclosure often occur over multifaceted issues (e.g., issues that teens view as personal but that parents treat as conventional or prudential; Smetana, 2011). Indeed, research suggests that there may be an inverse association between the extent to which open disagreement is tolerated or permitted in different cultures and ethnic groups (Fuligni, 1998), and the extent to which teens resort to secrecy and information management to get their way (Yau, Tasopoulos-Chan, & Smetana, 2009).

There are also individual differences in adolescents' beliefs about parents' legitimate authority. Studying transitions to adolescence, Kuhn and Laird (2011) found that relative to same-age peers, preadolescents who were European American rather than African American, less advanced in their pubertal development, less resistant to parental control, less autonomous in their family's decision making, and who experienced less psychologically controlling parents had stronger beliefs in parents' legitimate authority over personal and friendship issues.

Other studies have shown that there are normative changes in levels of and beliefs about parental authority, and that they have implications for healthy adjustment. Too much autonomy over personal issues in early adolescence is maladaptive (Wray-Lake, McHale, & Crouter, 2010) and leads to greater involvement in antisocial behavior (Darling et al., 2006; Laird & Marrero, 2010), more depression, and lower self-worth in late adolescence (Smetana, Campione-Barr, & Daddis, 2004). Indeed, premature autonomy combined with the belief that parents do not have legitimate authority has been associated with trajectories of antisocial behavior (Dishion, Nelson, & Bullock, 2004). The most adaptive pattern for adolescent well-being appears to involve increased autonomy over personal and multifaceted issues between middle and late adolescence (Smetana et al., 2004).

Normative Context of Parenting

The varying effects of psychological control for some groups of youth (Chao & Acque, 2009; Mason et al., 2004) discussed previously suggest that when harsh, coercive, or psychologically controlling parenting is more normative, its negative effects may be reduced. Indeed, the cultural normativeness of different disciplinary practices (e.g., spanking or slapping, grabbing, shaking, and beating), examined in diverse countries, has been found to moderate the link between parenting practices and adjustment (e.g., Gershoff et al., 2010; Lansford et al., 2005). This research clearly shows that physical discipline, particularly in its more extreme forms, has adverse effects. But when physical discipline is perceived as more normative in a particular setting, children and teens are more likely to attribute it to good and caring parenting, and its adverse effects on outcomes are less extreme. Although the normativeness of psychological control has not been examined as a moderator, psychological control is more common among Asian and African American parents and is more likely to be viewed as indicating love and concern (Mason et al., 2004; Ng, Pomerantz, & Deng, 2014). This suggests that cultural or ethnic differences in the effects of psychological control on adjustment are at least in part due to the context of parenting. Thus, this research, like the research on conceptions of the legitimacy of parental authority, highlights the importance of considering how the meaning adolescents give to different socialization practices alters their effects.

Cultural, Ethnic, and Racial Socialization

As noted earlier, there has been a dramatic increase over the past decade in studies of the practices parents use to transmit cultural values and teach youth about their ethnic and racial background. In response to the conceptual confusion in how cultural, racial, and ethnic socialization have been defined, Hughes and colleagues (2006), in their comprehensive review, have proposed that researchers employ the term *cultural socialization* to refer to parental practices that are intended to teach youth about their history and cultural heritage, their cultural customs and traditions, and to instill cultural, ethnic, or racial pride. The majority of U.S. parents from ethnic minority groups report using these types of practices (Fuligni et al., 2009; Hughes et al., 2006); U.S. parents who are recent immigrants are more likely to engage in cultural socialization, focusing on their native language, customs, and traditions, than are more acculturated parents or those who have been in the United States longer. We know of very little comparable research on immigrants to other countries.

Some evidence also suggests that parents who are better educated and have higher socioeconomic status engage in more cultural socialization than their less educated, lower socioeconomic status counterparts (Hughes et al., 2006). This may be partly due to neighborhood context because minority families with higher socioeconomic status are more likely to reside in more heterogeneous communities and may therefore feel a greater need to engage in cultural socialization with their offspring. Cultural socialization has been consistently associated with a range of positive developmental outcomes among youth of different ethnicities, including more exploration and achievement of ethnic identity, greater self-esteem, more positive ingroup attitudes, and less externalizing behavior (Berry, Chapter 22, this volume; Fuligni et al., 2009), although the effects of cultural socialization on academic achievement are inconsistent (Hughes et al., 2006).

Ethnic minority parents, and particularly African American parents, also consciously socialize their adolescents to cope with discrimination and unequal treatment (Hughes et al., 2006). These efforts focus on teaching children about racial bias in the broader society and "pre-arming" them with strategies to cope with prejudice (see Chapter 8 in Smetana, 2011, for qualitative examples from middle-class African American parents). As with cultural socialization, parents with more schooling, higher incomes, or more professional or managerial jobs are more likely to prepare their adolescents for bias. Socialization regarding bias also increases in frequency as teens grow older, but girls are more likely to receive messages regarding racial pride, whereas boys more often are prepared for discrimination and given messages about barriers (Chao & Otsuki-Clutter, 2011). This is no doubt because, at least among African Americans, males are more often victims of discrimination than are females.

Preparation for bias has been distinguished from more negative parental practices that are designed to promote wariness and distrust in interactions with other groups or cautions about barriers to success (Chao & Otsuki-Clutter, 2011; Fuligni et al., 2009; Hughes et al., 2006). Adolescents whose parents prepare them for bias have been found to use more proactive strategies in their coping and have better mental health outcomes than those of parents who do not address these issues with their teens. There is some evidence, however, that there can be negative effects (e.g., greater depression and conflict with parents) when parents stress the potential for discrimination (Hughes et al., 2006). Studies examining links between these two aspects of racial socialization (preparation for bias and promotion of distrust) and adolescent development have yielded mixed results depending on the socialization measures employed and the particular adjustment measures studied (Chao & Otsuki-Clutter, 2011; Hughes et al., 2006). Fuligni and colleagues (2009) suggest that this is partly because research has not adequately distinguished between the positive aspects of preparing for bias and the negative aspects of instilling distrust. Furthermore, relatively few studies have examined how ethnic minority and cultural groups other than African Americans socialize their adolescents to handle experiences with discrimination. Thus, there is a need for more research on diverse samples of youth.

A further positive racial socialization strategy that parents of different ethnic groups have been found to employ is referred to as *egalitarianism* (Hughes et al., 2006). These messages orient youth away from their minority status or native culture to emphasize the development of skills and abilities needed to thrive in the dominant or mainstream culture. Research also suggests that a small percentage of ethnic minority parents are silent about race or ethnicity and do nothing to teach their children about these issues (Hughes et al., 2006). This can be considered a socialization strategy in that it communicates values and perspectives about race.

Summary

While authoritative parenting generally has beneficial effects on adolescent adjustment, debate continues about the meaning and role of different parenting styles for diverse youth, leading to a focus on dimensional approaches to parenting. Psychological control is seen as having adverse effects on adjustment, whereas behavioral control has beneficial effects. But these findings are complicated because these two parenting dimensions may overlap under certain conditions, and the negative effects of harsh parenting and psychological control may be lessened when they are culturally normative. Furthermore, recent research demonstrates the importance of adolescent disclosure (rather than parenting) in influencing adjustment through its effect on parental knowledge. These findings, as well as research on teens' evaluations of legitimate parental authority, point to the importance of adolescents' interpretations of parenting and their agency in socialization. Ethnic minority parents also seek to prepare their offspring to cope with discrimination and unequal treatment.

Sibling Relationships as a Context for Adolescent Socialization

Interest in the role of older siblings as socialization influences has increased substantially over the past decade. This increased attention is due to both the greater prominence of family systems theories (e.g., Minuchin, 2002), with their focus on how different subsystems of the family interact to influence behavior, and to increased research on how the role of shared versus nonshared environmental influences in the family affect adolescents' attitudes and behavior. Moreover, sibling relationships are highly salient in adolescence, as early adolescents have more conflicts with siblings than with anyone else (e.g., fathers, grandparents, friends, or teachers; Furman & Buhrmester, 1985) except maybe mothers (Laursen & Collins, 2009). Sibling conflicts occur primarily over invasions of siblings' personal domains and moral issues of fairness and equality (Campione-Barr, Greer, & Kruse, 2013). Conflicts over the former are associated with poorer quality sibling relationships, but both types of conflicts are longitudinally associated with poorer emotional adjustment (Campione-Barr et al., 2013). Beyond conflict, however, relationships with brothers and sisters are also important sources of companionship, affection, and intimacy (see Dunn, Chapter 8, this volume).

Siblings are often similar in their involvement in various risky behaviors such as alcohol and substance use, delinquency, and sexual attitudes and behavior, and these similarities cannot be attributed only to shared parenting or genetics (see McHale, Updegraff, & Whiteman, 2012). Accordingly, different socialization processes have been examined. For instance, older siblings may serve as role models for younger siblings, but only if younger siblings perceive their older siblings as likable and nurturing, so that younger siblings want to be around and learn from them (Whiteman & Buchanan, 2002). Siblings can also influence each other through shared friends and introduction to deviant peer networks (McHale et al., 2012); this, as well as modeling and siblings' shared genetic background, can account for convergence between siblings.

In contrast, sibling deidentification accounts for potential divergence. The notion is that siblings respond to parents' differential treatment by defining themselves as different from each other. They pursue different domains of competence and interest to avoid comparison and rivalry. Sibling deidentification is more frequent and intense among siblings who are more similar in gender, age, and birth order (Schachter & Stone, 1987), and it has been found to influence risky behaviors, adjustment, and psychosocial development.

Sibling differentiation is seen as especially relevant during adolescence because of the developmental salience of identity development (McHale et al., 2012).

A recent study that compared modeling, introduction to peer networks, and sibling deidentification in a sample of sibling pairs who were, on average, 15 and 17 years of age, found that different profiles involving combinations of all three processes emerged (Whiteman, Jensen, & Maggs, 2014). Similarities in alcohol use and delinquency were found in two groups of siblings: one group that reported high levels of shared friends and mutual modeling, and another group characterized by younger siblings' high levels of admiration for and modeling of the older siblings' behavior and low levels of differentiation (the latter pattern was more likely among siblings characterized by larger age differences). Differences in alcohol use and delinquency were found in members of a third group of siblings with high differentiation processes. Another study also employing person-centered analyses of siblings of roughly similar ages (14- and 16-year-olds) also obtained deidentification and modeling groups (peer influences were not examined), but their third cluster reflected an apparent lack of investment in the sibling relationship (Whiteman, McHale, & Crouter, 2007).

Siblings also have been found to influence parent–adolescent relationships. That is, parents' childrearing experiences with their firstborns influence their expectations for their younger child's adolescence, even when researchers controlled for temperament (Whiteman & Buchanan, 2002). Furthermore, parents have less conflict with and greater knowledge of daily activities for later-born than for firstborn adolescents (Whiteman, McHale, & Crouter, 2003), and, as we noted earlier, changes in conflict with second-born children correspond to the firstborn child's entry into adolescence (Shanahan, McHale, Osgood, & Crouter, 2007). These studies highlight the importance of considering the broader family social system. Not only do siblings have unique effects on adolescent behavior and values over and above the effects of parents, but parents also learn from their experiences, modifying and fine-tuning their parenting practices with subsequent children. This fine-tuning also varies according to sibling gender constellation (Shanahan, McHale, Crouter, & Osgood, 2007; Shanahan, McHale, Osgood, & Crouter, 2007; Wray-Lake et al., 2010), demonstrating the complexity of sibling relationships as socialization contexts.

Summary

Older siblings serve as socialization influences. Modeling and introduction to older siblings' friends and deviant peer networks may lead to similarities between siblings, whereas sibling deidentification accounts for divergence. Siblings also influence parent–teen relationships because parents' experiences with their firstborn influence how they parent subsequent offspring.

Peer Relationships as a Context for Adolescent Socialization

Research on peer socialization has largely emphasized the negative effects of peers in encouraging teen deviance and involvement in risky activities. But, as we discuss in the following section, peers also may have positive effects. Additionally, although teens increasingly identify with peers, there is also considerable evidence that parents remain influential overall in socialization, as well as in adolescents' peer relationships.

Peer Selection and Socialization

Both peer selection (adolescents' tendency to befriend individuals who are similar to themselves; Dishion, Patterson, Stoolmiller, & Skinner, 1991), and peer socialization (increases in similarity between friends over time; Dishion & Owen, 2002) have been posited to account for peer influence on adolescent behavior. Research comparing these processes has focused heavily on delinquency. For instance, peer selection approaches highlight the fact that risk-taking youth seek each other out, whereas peer socialization emphasizes the role of deviancy training. Evidence suggests that the two processes are complementary. For example, Dishion and colleagues (1991) found that substance use in early adulthood is a joint product of socialization and peer selection processes throughout adolescence, although parenting also may moderate some of these effects: Parental monitoring reduced selection of delinquent friends in early adolescence, but only for teens who did not feel overcontrolled by parents (Tilton-Weaver, Burk, Kerr, & Stattin, 2013).

As these studies suggest, risk taking (e.g., drinking, driving, and delinquency) during adolescence occurs primarily in the presence of peers rather than when the adolescent is alone or in the company of parents. Researchers (Albert, Chein, & Steinberg, 2013; Casey, Jones, & Somerville, 2011; Steinberg, 2008) have marshaled neurodevelopmental evidence to account for these contextual effects. They have focused on the maturational gap between structural changes in the dopaminergic system that occur at puberty and lead to increases in sensation seeking, and the prolonged amount of time it takes for the brain's cognitive control system to strengthen and mature. This research has shown that over time, increased coordination between these affective and cognitive processes results in better self-regulation in affectively arousing situations and, accordingly, increased capacity to resist peer influence.

Apart from the extensive focus on delinquency and risk taking, research also suggests that peers may have positive effects on adolescent development, especially for majority youth (e.g., European Americans in the United States), who spend more time with peers than do ethnic minority youth. Positive peer pressure, or peers' perceived efforts to encourage positive behavior, has been linked with positive outcomes such as empathic responding. This is especially true when peers' positive values indirectly influence teens' behavior (Padilla-Walker & Bean, 2009).

Peers also have been shown to influence adolescents' autonomy development, serving as a metric by which adolescents measure acceptable or normative levels of autonomy (Daddis, 2008). Friends are seen as influencing adolescents' views as to how much autonomy they should have. When they perceive their friends as having more autonomy than they do, adolescents desire increased autonomy, specifically, over issues that are not clearly within the personal domain (Daddis, 2011). Peer selection effects have also been demonstrated. Adolescents have been shown to be more similar to friends than to nonfriends in their beliefs about the acceptable boundaries of personal authority and in their justifications regarding the legitimacy of parental authority. Indeed, supporting selection more than socialization effects, similarities between friends were greater among younger than among older adolescents, and direct discussion of autonomy issues between friends was related to less agreement (Daddis, 2008).

Parental Influence and Management of Peer Relationships

Current research suggests that parents continue to play an important role in influencing peer relationships. Such influence comes through two avenues: directly, through parenting behaviors designed to affect peer relationships, and indirectly, through structuring teens' environments. Direct influences include monitoring, mediating teens' peer relationships, and consulting (giving advice). Mounts (2008) has shown that parents' greater use of monitoring and consulting promotes adolescents' selection of less delinquent peers, as well as more positive peer relationships. On the other hand, certain consulting behaviors (e.g., forbidding adolescents to associate with delinquent peers), make adolescents more likely to select delinquent peers as friends (Keijsers et al., 2012). Indirect parental influences on peer relationships include the selection of neighborhoods and afterschool activities. Safer neighborhoods with higher quality extracurricular activities facilitate interaction with nondelinquent peers (Mounts, 2008). In addition, parenting styles influence adolescent–peer relationships directly, through their links with specific parenting practices, and indirectly, by creating an emotional climate that affects how teens interpret such behaviors (Darling & Steinberg, 1993; Mounts, 2002). Both authoritative and authoritarian parents display high levels of monitoring, but only authoritative parents offer more support for teens' peer relationships (Mounts, 2002). In turn, for youth with authoritative parents, high levels of monitoring were found to be linked with lower levels of drug use 1 year later. However, among teens with authoritarian parents, high levels of monitoring did not have this salutary effect, perhaps because monitoring is seen as more intrusive in the absence of the warmth that accompanies authoritative parenting (Mounts, 2002).

The effects of culture and ethnicity on parents' management of peer relationships have also been examined. Updegraff, Killoren, and Thayer (2007) found that generational differences in Mexican American parents' identification with traditional Mexican values were associated with their parental peer management practices. Parents who more strongly identified with traditional Mexican values placed more restrictions on adolescents' peer relationships and encouraged relationships with the family more than those with peers (perhaps accounting for the differences in time spent with peers noted earlier). Ethnicity is also associated with the types of goals parents endorse and the practices they use to achieve them. In a study of European American, African American, and Latino parents, Mounts and Kim (2007) found that African American parents were more concerned with peer management goals related to preventing problem behavior—and used more mediating and consulting strategies, and granted teens less autonomy over their peer relationships—than did other parents. Latino parents also engaged in more mediating but in less consulting behaviors than did European American and African American parents. Additionally, as might be expected, ethnic minority parents were more likely to have ethnically oriented peer management goals, and, for example, to worry about their child being exposed to racist peers or encourage the child to choose same-ethnicity friends.

Parents often worry that their teen will hang out with "the wrong crowd" or with friends of whom they disapprove. However, research shows that parenting behaviors indirectly influence crowd affiliation through adolescent behavior. In a study examining a large, diverse sample of U.S. youth, Brown, Mounts, Lamborn, and Steinberg (1993) demonstrated that specific parenting practices such as monitoring and encouragement of achievement were positively associated with adolescents' self-reliance and academic achievement, and negatively associated with their drug use, all of which in turn were associated with adolescents' membership in different peer crowds. As noted earlier, peer crowds channel teens in different directions (e.g., joining a "druggie" crowd may lead to increasing drug use). Although the links need to be tested longitudinally, this research shows the importance of parents' values and parenting practices relative to these pathways.

Summary

Peers influence adolescent attitudes and behavior both through peer selection and peer socialization. The focus has been mostly on negative influences, including increased deviance and risk-taking. The maturational gap between the brain's reward system and the cognitive control system, which predisposes adolescents to sensation seeking through risky behavior and which occurs primarily in the company of peers, has been identified as a potential explanation for these negative effects. Although less studied, friends also have positive effects on adolescent competence and serve as metrics for teens' autonomy seeking. Parents influence peer relationships both directly and indirectly, and this varies as a function of culture and ethnicity.

Adolescents' Out-of-School Activities

How adolescents spend their time outside of school has a considerable impact on their development (Mahoney, Vandell, Simpkins, & Zarrett, 2009). Out-of-school activities include those that lack adult supervision, as well as teens' involvement in organized activities, which have been found to offer significant opportunities for positive youth development (Mahoney et al., 2009). The success of youth programs has been attributed partially to the positive influence of adult mentors, who may provide some of the structure and responsiveness that may be missing from adolescents' home environments (Mahoney et al., 2009).

However, mentoring in youth programs has uneven and quite modest effects, due to substantial variability in the quality of programs (Rhodes & Lowe, 2009). More structured programs with clear expectations, support for mentors, and instrumental goals fared best in yielding positive outcomes for vulnerable youth (Rhodes & Lowe, 2009). Thus, there is reason to be optimistic about the potential of such programs to enhance important developmental outcomes. Indeed, the characteristics of programs that produce positive developmental outcomes—opportunities for belonging, skills building, appropriate structure, positive social norms, and supportive relationships with adults and peers— mirror the types of parenting that facilitate positive trajectories in adolescent development.

Conclusions

Against a backdrop of significant continuity between childhood and adolescence, we have described some of the distinctive features of socialization during adolescence, including changes in time spent with parents versus peers, more parenting at a distance, changes in the structure of peer relationships and their influence, and risky behaviors that increase during adolescence. Adolescent socialization must be considered in the context of adolescents' interpretation of their social world and social relationships. Teens begin to move into a world where they are less under the control of their parents, and where their conceptions of acceptable parental behavior and control change rapidly. Adolescents push for more autonomy, resulting in increased conflict, nondisclosure, and secrecy in adolescent–parent relationships and normative declines in closeness. On the bright side, however, closeness rebounds during young adulthood, as youth seek to reestablish family ties. And although the world of peers looms large for adolescents and poses risks for deviant behaviors, parents continue to exert both direct and indirect effects on peer relationships. Furthermore, adolescents may obtain the support and mentoring they need in other contexts, such as in their out-of-school activities. Indeed, among researchers there is an emerging consensus as to the parenting, peer management practices, and out-of-school programs that facilitate better outcomes for youth of diverse ethnicities. Positive socialization experiences with family and peers can help facilitate adolescents' involvement and engagement in the broader society as they become competent, mature young adults and citizens of diverse societies.

REFERENCES

Acquilino, W. S. (1997). A prospective study of parent–child relations during the transition to adulthood. *Journal of Marriage and the Family, 59*, 670–686.

Albert, D., Chein, J., & Steinberg, L. (2013). The teenage brain: Peer influences on adolescent decision-making. *Current Directions in Psychological Science, 22*, 114–120.

Archibald, A., Graber, J., & Brooks-Gunn, J. (2003). Pubertal processes and physiological growth in adolescence. In G. R. Adams & M. D. Berzonsky (Eds.), *Blackwell handbook of adolescence* (pp. 24–47) Oxford, UK: Blackwell.

Barber, B. K., Stolz, H. E., & Olsen, J. A. (2005). Parental support, psychological control, and behavioral control: Assessing relevance across time, method, and culture. *Monographs of the Society for Research in Child Development, 70*(4), 1–137.

Barber, B. K., Xia, M., Olsen, J. A., Stolz, H. E., McNeely, C. A., & Bose, K. (2012). Feeling disrespected by parents: Refining the measurement and understanding of psychological control. *Journal of Adolescence, 35*, 273–287.

Baumrind, D. (1971). Current patterns of parental authority. *Developmental Psychology Monographs, 4*(I, Pt. 2), 1–103.

Baumrind, D., Larzelere, R. E., & Owens, E. B. (2010) Effects of preschool parents' power assertive patterns and practices on adolescent development, *Parenting: Science and Practice, 10*, 157–201.

Brown, B. B., & Klute, C. (2003). Friendships, cliques, and crowds. In G. R. Adams & M. D. Berzonsky (Eds.), *Blackwell handbook of adolescence* (pp. 330–348). Oxford, UK: Blackwell.

Brown, B. B., & Larson, J. (2009). Peer relationships in adolescence. In R. L. Lerner & L. Steinberg (Eds.), *Handbook of adolescent psychology* (3rd ed., Vol. 2, pp. 74–103). New York: Wiley.

Brown, B. B., Mounts, N., Lamborn, S., & Steinberg, L. (1993). Parenting practices and peer group affiliation in adolescence. *Child Development, 64*, 467–482.

Campione-Barr, N., Greer, K. B., & Kruse, A. (2013). Differential associations between domains of sibling conflict and adolescent emotional adjustment. *Child Development, 84*, 938–954.

Casey, B. J., Jones, R., & Somerville, L. (2011). Braking and accelerating of the adolescent brain. *Journal of Research on Adolescence, 21*, 21–33.

Chao, R. (2001). Extending research on the consequences of parenting style for Chinese Americans and European Americans. *Child Development, 72*(6), 1832–1843.

Chao, R., & Acque, C. (2009). Interpretations of parental control by Asian immigrant and European American youth. *Journal of Family Psychology, 23*, 342–354.

Chao, R., & Otsuki-Clutter, M. (2011). Racial and ethnic differences: Sociocultural and contextual explanations. *Journal of Research on Adolescence, 21*, 47–60.

Collins, W. A., & Steinberg, L. (2006). Adolescent development in interpersonal context. In N. Eisenberg (Ed.) & W. Damon (Series Ed.), *Handbook of child psychology: Vol. 3. Social, emotional, and personality development* (6th ed., pp. 1003–1067). New York: Wiley.

Crouter, A. C., Bumpus, M. F., Davis, K. D., & McHale, S. M. (2005). How do parents learn about adolescents' experiences?: Implications for parental knowledge and adolescent risky behavior. *Child Development, 76*, 869–882.

Currie, C., Zanotti, C., Morgan, A., Currie, D., de Looze, M., Roberts, C., et al. (2012). *Social determinants of health and well-being among young people: Health Behaviour in School-Aged Children (HBSC) Study: International Report from the 2009/2010 survey* (Health Policy for Children and Adolescents, No. 6). Copenhagen: WHO Regional Office for Europe.

Daddis, C. (2008). Influence of close friends on the boundaries of adolescent personal authority. *Journal of Research on Adolescence, 18*, 75–98.

Daddis, C. (2011). Desire for increased autonomy and adolescents' perceptions of peer autonomy: "Everyone else can; why can't I?" *Child Development, 82*, 1310–1326.

Darling, N., Cumsille, P., Caldwell, L. L., & Dowdy, B. (2006). Predictors of adolescents' disclosure to parents and perceived parental knowledge: Between- and within-person differences. *Journal of Youth and Adolescence, 35*, 667–678.

Darling, N., & Steinberg, L. (1993). Parenting style as context: An integrative model. *Psychological Bulletin, 113*, 487–496.

Diamond, L., & Savin-Williams, R. (2009). Sexuality. In B. Brown & M. Prinstein (Eds.), *Encyclopedia of adolescence* (Vol. 2, pp. 314–321). New York: Academic Press.

Dijkstra, J. K., & Veenstra, R. (2011). Peer relations. In B. Brown & M. Prinstein (Eds.), *Encyclopedia of adolescence* (Vol. 2, pp. 255–259). New York: Academic Press.

Dishion, T., Patterson, G., Stoolmiller, M., & Skinner, M. (1991). Family, school, and behavioral antecedents to adolescent involvement with antisocial peers. *Developmental Psychology, 27*, 172–180.

Dishion, T. J., Nelson, S. E., & Bullock, B. M. (2004). Premature adolescent autonomy: Parent disengagement and deviant peer process in the amplification of problem behavior. *Journal of Adolescence, 27*, 515–530.

Dishion, T. J., & Owen, L. D. (2002). A longitudinal analysis of friendships and substance use: Bidirectional influence from adolescence to adulthood. *Developmental Psychology, 38*, 480–491.

Fuligni, A. J. (1998). Authority, autonomy, and parent–adolescent conflict and cohesion: A study of adolescents from Mexican, Chinese, Filipino, and European backgrounds. *Developmental Psychology, 34*, 782–792.

Fuligni, A. J., Hughes, D. L., & Way, N. (2009). Ethnicity and immigration. In R. M. Lerner & L. Steinberg (Eds.), *Handbook of adolescent psychology* (Vol. 2, 3rd ed., pp. 527–569). Hoboken, NJ: Wiley.

Furman, W., & Buhrmester, D. (1985). Children's perceptions of the personal relationships in their social networks. *Developmental Psychology, 21*, 1016–1024.

Gershoff, E. T., Grogan-Kaylor, A., Lansford, J. E., Chang, L., Zelli, A., Deater-Deckard, K., et al. (2010). Parent discipline practices in an international sample: Associations with child behaviors and moderation by perceived normativeness. *Child Development, 81*, 487–502.

Graham, S. (1992). Most of the subjects were white and middle class: Trends in published research on African-Americans in selected APA journals, 1970–1989. *American Psychologist, 47*, 629–639.

Grolnick, W., & Pomerantz, E. M. (2009). Issues and challenges in studying parental control: Toward a new conceptualization. *Child Development Perspectives, 3,* 165–170.

Grusec, J. E. (2002). Parental socialization and children's acquisition of values. In M. H. Bornstein (Ed.), *Handbook of parenting: Vol. 5. Practical issues* (2nd ed., pp. 143–167). Mahwah, NJ: Erlbaum.

Grusec, J. E., Goodnow, J. J., & Kuczynski, L. (2000). New directions in analyses of parenting contributions to children's acquisition of values. *Child Development, 71,* 205–211.

Hasebe, Y., Nucci, L., & Nucci, M. S. (2004). Parental control of the personal domain and adolescent symptoms of psychopathology. *Child Development, 75,* 815–828.

Holmbeck, G. N. (1996). A model of family relational transformations during the transition to adolescence: Parent–adolescent conflict and adaptation. In J. A. Graber, J. Brooks-Gunn, & A. C. Petersen (Eds.), *Transitions through adolescence: Interpersonal domains and context* (pp. 167–199). Mahwah, NJ: Erlbaum.

Hughes, D., Rodriguez, J., Smith, E. P., Johnson, D. J., Stevenson, H. C., & Spicer, P. (2006). Parents' ethnic–racial socialization practices: A review of research and directions for future study. *Developmental Psychology, 42,* 747–770.

Johnston, L. D., O'Malley, P. M., Bachman, J. G., & Schulenberg, J. E. (2012). Monitoring the future: 2012 overview: Key findings on adolescent drug use. Retrieved from *www.monitoringthefuture.org/pubs/monographs/mtf-overview2012.pdf.*

Kakihara, F., & Tilton-Weaver, L. (2010). Adolescents' interpretations of parental control: Differentiated by domain and types of control. *Child Development, 80,* 1722–1738.

Keijsers, L., Branje, S., Hawk, S. T., Schwartz, S. J., Frijns, T., Koot, H. M., & Meeus, W. (2012). Forbidden friends as forbidden fruit: Parental supervision of friendships, contact with deviant peers, and adolescent delinquency. *Child Development, 83*(2), 651–666.

Kerr, M., Stattin, H., & Burk, W. J. (2010). A reinterpretation of parental monitoring in longitudinal perspective. *Journal of Research on Adolescence, 20,* 39–64.

Kerr, M., Stattin, H., & Ozdemir, M. (2012). Perceived parenting style and adolescent adjustment: Revisiting direction of effects and the role of parental knowledge. *Developmental Psychology, 48,* 1540–1553.

Kuhn, E. S., & Laird, R. D. (2011). Individual differences in early adolescent' beliefs in the legitimacy of parental authority. *Developmental Psychology, 47,* 1353–1365.

Laird, R. D. (2011). Correlates and antecedents of parental psychological control in early adolescence. *Parenting: Science and Practice, 11,* 72–86.

Laird, R. D., & Marrero, M. D. (2010). Information management and behavior problems: Is concealing misbehavior necessarily a sign of trouble? *Journal of Adolescence, 33,* 297–308.

Laird, R. D., Marrero, M. D., & Sentse, M. (2010). Revisiting parental monitoring: Evidence that parental solicitation can be effective when needed most. *Journal of Youth and Adolescence, 39,* 1431–1441.

Lamborn, S. D., Dornbusch, S. M., & Steinberg, L. (1996). Ethnicity and community context as moderators of the relations between family decision making and adolescent adjustment. *Child Development, 67,* 283–301.

Lansford, J. E., Chang, L., Dodge, K. A., Malone, P. S., Oburu, P., Palmerus, K., et al. (2005). Physical discipline and children's adjustment: Cultural normativeness as a moderator. *Child Development, 76,* 1234–1246.

Larson, R. W. (2001). How U.S. children and adolescents spend time: What it does (and doesn't) tell us about their development. *Current Directions in Psychological Science, 10,* 160–164.

Larson, R. W., Richards, M. H., Moneta, G., Holmbeck, G., & Duckett, E. (1996). Changes in adolescents' daily interactions with their families from ages 10 to 18: Disengagement and transformation. *Developmental Psychology, 32,* 744–754.

Larson, R. W., Richards, M. H., Sims, B., & Dworkin, J. (2001). How urban African American young adolescents spend their time: Time budgets for locations, activities, and companionship. *American Journal of Community Psychology, 29,* 565–597.

Laursen, B., & Collins, W. A. (2009). Parent–child relationships during adolescence. In R. L. Lerner & L. Steinberg (Eds.), *Handbook of adolescent psychology* (3rd ed., Vol. 2, pp. 3–42). New York: Wiley.

Laursen, B., Coy, K., & Collins, W. A. (1998). Reconsidering changes in parent–child conflict across adolescence: A meta-analysis. *Child Development, 69*, 817–832.

Leatherdale, S. T., & Burkhalter, R. (2012). The substance use profile of Canadian youth: Exploring the prevalence of alcohol, drug, and tobacco use by gender and grade. *Addictive Behaviors, 37*, 318–322.

Maccoby, E. E., & Martin, J. A. (1983). Socialization in the context of the family: Parent–child interaction. In E. M. Hetherington (Ed.), *Handbook of child psychology: Vol. 4. Socialization, personality, and social development* (pp. 1–102). New York: Wiley.

Mahoney, J. L., Vandell, D. L., Simpkins, S., & Zarrett, Z. (2009). Adolescents' out-of-school activities. In. L. Lerner & L. Steinberg (Eds.), *Handbook of adolescent psychology* (3rd ed., Vol. 2, pp. 228–269). New York: Wiley.

Marshall, S. K., Tilton-Weaver, L. C., & Bosdet, L. (2005). Information management: Considering adolescents' regulation of parental knowledge. *Journal of Adolescence, 28*, 633–647.

Mason, C., Walker-Barnes, C. J., Tu, S., Simons, J., & Martinez-Arrue, R. (2004). Ethnic differences in the affective meaning of parental control behaviors. *Journal of Primary Prevention, 25*, 59–79.

McHale, S. M., Updegraff, K. A., & Whiteman, S. D. (2012). Sibling relationships and influences in childhood and adolescence. *Journal of Marriage and Family, 74*, 913–930.

Minuchin, P. (2002). Looking toward the horizon: Present and future in the study of family systems. In S. McHale & W. Grolnick (Eds.), *Retrospect and prospect in the psychological study of families* (pp. 259–278). Mahwah, NJ: Erlbaum.

Moffitt, T. (2006). Life-course persistent versus adolescence-limited antisocial behavior. In D. Cichetti & D. Cohen (Eds.), *Developmental psychopathology* (2nd ed., pp. 570–598). New York: Wiley.

Mounts, N. S. (2002). Parental management of adolescent peer relationships in context: The role of parenting style. *Journal of Family Psychology, 16*, 58–69.

Mounts, N. S. (2008). Linkages between parenting and peer relationships: A model for parental management of adolescents' peer relationships. In M. Kerr, H. Stattin, & R. Engels (Eds.), *What can parents do?: New insight into the role of parents in adolescent problem behavior* (pp. 163–189). West Sussex, UK: Wiley.

Mounts, N. S., & Kim, H. S. (2007). Parental goals regarding peer relationships and management of peers in multiethnic samples. In B. B. Brown & N. S. Mounts (Eds.), *Linking parents and family to adolescent peer relations: Ethnic and cultural considerations* (pp. 17–34). San Francisco: Jossey-Bass.

Ng, F. F.-Y., Pomerantz, E., & Deng, C. (2014). Why are Chinese mothers more controlling than American mothers?: "My child is my report card." *Child Development, 85*(1), 355–367.

Nucci, L. P. (1996). Morality and personal freedom. In E. S. Reed, E. Turiel, & T. Brown (Eds.), *Values and knowledge* (pp. 41–60). Mahwah, NJ: Erlbaum.

Padilla-Walker, L. M., & Bean, R. A. (2009). Negative and positive peer influence: Relations to positive and negative behaviors for African American, European American, and Hispanic adolescents. *Journal of Adolescence, 32*, 323–337.

Pettit, G. S., Laird, R. D., Bates, J. E., Dodge, K. A., & Criss, M. M. (2001). Antecedents and behavior-problem outcomes of parental monitoring and psychological control in early adolescence. *Child Development, 72*, 583–598.

Rhodes, J. E., & Lowe, S. R. (2009). Mentoring in adolescence. In R. M. Lerner & L. Steinberg (Eds.), *Handbook of adolescent psychology* (Vol. 2, 3rd ed., pp. 152–190). Hoboken, NJ: Wiley.

Schachter, F. F., & Stone, R. K. (1987). Comparing and contrasting siblings: Defining the self. *Journal of Children in Contemporary Society, 19*, 55–75.

Shanahan, L., McHale, S. M., Crouter, A. C., & Osgood, D. W. (2007). Warmth with mothers and fathers from middle childhood to late adolescence: Within- and between-families comparisons. *Developmental Psychology, 43,* 551–563.

Shanahan, L., McHale, S. M., Osgood, D. W., & Crouter, A. C. (2007). Conflict frequency mothers and fathers from middle childhood to late adolescence: Within- and between-families comparisons. *Developmental Psychology, 43,* 539–550.

Sherrod, L. R., Torney-Purta, J., & Flanagan, C. A. (2010). *Handbook of research on civic engagement in youth.* New York: Wiley.

Smetana, J. G. (2002). Culture, autonomy, and personal jurisdiction in adolescent–parent relationships. *Advances in Child Development and Behavior, 29,* 51–87.

Smetana, J. G. (2011). *Adolescents, families, and social development: How teens construct their worlds.* West Sussex, UK: Wiley-Blackwell.

Smetana, J. G., Campione-Barr, N., & Daddis, C. (2004). Developmental and longitudinal antecedents of family decision-making: Defining health behavioral autonomy for African American adolescents. *Child Development, 75,* 1418–1434.

Smetana, J. G., & Daddis, C. (2002). Domain-specific antecedents of psychological control and parental monitoring: The role of parenting beliefs and practices. *Child Development, 73,* 563–580.

Smetana, J. G., Villalobos, M., Tasopoulos-Chan, M., Gettman, D. C., & Campione-Barr, N. (2009). Early and middle adolescents' disclosure to parents about activities in different domains. *Journal of Adolescence, 32,* 693–713.

Soenens, B., & Vansteenkiste, M. (2010). A theoretical upgrade of the concept of parental psychological control: Proposing new insights on the basis of self-determination theory. *Developmental Review, 30,* 74–99.

Sorkhabi, N., & Mandara, J. (2013). Are the effects of Baumrind's parenting styles culturally specific or culturally equivalent? In R. E. Larzelere, A. S. Morris, & A. W. Harrist (Eds.), *Authoritative parenting: Synthesizing nurturance and discipline for optimal child development* (pp. 113–135). Washington, DC: American Psychological Association.

Stattin, H., & Kerr, M. (2000). Parental monitoring: A reinterpretation. *Child Development, 71,* 1072–1085.

Steinberg, L. (2008). A social neuroscience perspective on adolescent risk-taking. *Developmental Review, 28,* 78–106.

Steinberg, L., & Morris, A. S. (2001). Adolescent development. *Annual Review of Psychology, 52,* 83–110.

Tilton-Weaver, L., Kerr, M., Pakalniskeine, V., Tokic, A., Salihovic, S., & Stattin, H. (2010). Open up or close down: How do parental reactions affect youth information management? *Journal of Adolescence, 33,* 333–346.

Tilton-Weaver, L. C., Burk, W. J., Kerr, M., & Stattin, H. (2013). Can parental monitoring and peer management reduce the selection or influence of delinquent peers?: Testing the question using a dynamic social network approach. *Development Psychology, 49*(11), 2057–2070.

Tsai, K. M., Telzer, E. H., & Fuligni, A. J. (2013). Continuity and discontinuity in perceptions of family relationships from adolescence to young adulthood. *Child Development, 84,* 471–484.

Turiel, E. (1983). *The development of social knowledge: Morality and convention.* Cambridge, UK: Cambridge University Press.

Updegraff, K., Killoren, S., & Thayer, S. (2007). Mexican-origin parents' involvement in adolescent peer relationships: A pattern analytic approach. In B. Brown & N. S. Mounts (Eds.), *Linking parents and family to adolescent peer relations: Ethnic and cultural considerations* (pp. 51–65). San Francisco: Jossey-Bass.

Updegraff, K. A., McHale, S. M., Whiteman, S. D., Thayer, S. M., & Crouter, A. C. (2006). The nature and correlates of Mexican-American adolescents' time with parents and peers. *Child Development, 77,* 1479–1486.

Waizenhofer, R. N., Buchanan, C. M., & Jackson-Newsom, J. (2004). Mothers' and fathers' knowledge of adolescents' daily activities: Its sources and its links with adolescent adjustment. *Journal of Family Psychology, 18,* 348–360.

Whiteman, S. D., & Buchanan, C. M. (2002). Mothers' and children's expectations for adolescence: The impact of perceptions of an older sibling's experience. *Journal of Family Psychology, 16,* 157–171.

Whiteman, S. D., Jensen, A. C., & Maggs, J. L. (2014). Similarities and differences in adolescent siblings' alcohol-related attitudes, use, and delinquency: Evidence for convergent and divergent influence processes. *Journal of Youth and Adolescence, 43*(4), 687–697.

Whiteman, S. D., McHale, S. M., & Crouter, A. C. (2003). What parents learn from experience: The first child as a first draft? *Journal of Marriage and Family, 65,* 608–621.

Whiteman, S. D., McHale, S. M., & Crouter, A. C. (2007). Competing processes of sibling influence: Observational learning and sibling deidentification. *Social Development, 16,* 642–661.

Wray-Lake, L., McHale, S., & Crouter, N. (2010). Developmental patterns in decision-making autonomy across middle childhood and adolescence: European American parents' perspectives. *Child Development, 81,* 636–651.

Yau, J. Y., Tasopoulos-Chan, M., & Smetana, J. G. (2009). Disclosure to parents about everyday activities among American adolescents from Mexican, Chinese, and European backgrounds. *Child Development, 80,* 1481–1498.

CHAPTER 4

Socialization in Emerging Adulthood

*From the Family to the Wider World,
from Socialization to Self-Socialization*

Jeffrey Jensen Arnett

Emerging adulthood is a period of life that has developed in recent decades in industrialized societies, lasting from the late teens through most of the 20s. A number of influences led to the rise of this new period (Arnett, 2014). Economic changes from a manufacturing to an information-based world economy increased the need for and desirability of obtaining additional education and training beyond secondary school. A scientific advance, the invention of the birth control pill, made it relatively easy for young people to become sexually active in their late teens without a high risk of pregnancy. Corresponding social changes, specifically, increased acceptance of premarital sexuality and cohabitation, further weakened the traditional belief that marriage must be entered before sexual activity begins. Median ages of entering marriage and parenthood rose into the late 20s.

Thus, the period of life from the late teens through the 20s changed in less than half a century from a period of entering and settling into adult roles of marriage, parenthood, and long-term work to a period when young people typically focus on their self-development as they gradually lay the foundation for their adult lives. During this time, they gradually attain a subjective sense that they have reached adulthood and are ready to take on the full range of adult responsibilities (Arnett, 1998). It has been proposed that, developmentally, emerging adulthood can be characterized as *the age of identity explorations, the age of instability, the self-focused age, the age of feeling in between,* and *the age of possibilities* (Arnett, 2006a, 2014). These features have received empirical support (Reifman, Arnett, & Colwell, 2006). Further empirical investigation may change our understanding of the specific features that characterize this age period developmentally and reveal important variations according to socioeconomic status, ethnic/cultural group, and other characteristics, but this much seems clear: Full adulthood is reached later than in the past, and a new life stage has opened up in recent decades, as reflected in broader participation in higher education and later ages of marriage and parenthood (Arnett, 2014). I proposed applying a new term, *emerging adulthood*, to this new period of life, and to distinguish it from the adolescence that precedes it and the young adulthood that follows it.

The question of the nature of socialization in emerging adulthood presents a variety of intriguing problems and challenges. The focus of most theory and research on socialization has been on the family—that is, on how parents socialize their children. But most emerging adults leave their parents' household and consequently are much less exposed to parental socialization than they were at younger ages. Even those who remain home or return home tend to be much more autonomous than they were in adolescence, as both parents and emerging adults adjust in response to emerging adults' increasing capabilities (Aquilino, 2006). So the first challenge for a conception of socialization in emerging adulthood is to assess how socialization changes during this period.

What Is the Nature of Socialization in Emerging Adulthood?

Because the focus of socialization theory and research has been on childhood and adolescence, there is little to draw on directly to conceptualize socialization in emerging adulthood. Some previous theoretical ideas have indirect implications. Erikson (1950, 1968), in his psychosocial theory of development across the life course, described early adulthood as a time when the focus of development is on the capacity for forming an intimate partnership. In discussing the challenge of intimacy versus isolation, Erikson implied that family socialization is largely over by this time; the challenge is to risk one's identity, newly formed in the course of the socialization experiences of childhood and adolescence, by forming a committed intimate relationship with another person. Erikson also discussed the concept of a "psychosocial moratorium" during this period, which is the idea that some young people delay forming an intimate relationship for some years after adolescence and spend this time exploring various possibilities for their future. Here again, however, there was no suggestion that socialization is a major part of development during these years. The young person experiencing the psychosocial moratorium was depicted as an independent agent, guided by individual choice.

Other theorists have also contributed ideas that have limited application to socialization in emerging adulthood. Keniston (1971) described a period of "youth" between adolescence and young adulthood. However, Keniston viewed youth as a time of "refusal of socialization" (p. 9) and rejection of what the adult world has to offer the young. His views were based on the student protesters of the 1960s and have an anachronistic quality by now. Levinson (1978) called ages 17–33 the "novice phase" of development, and argued that the central task of this phase is to move into the adult world and build a stable life structure. He emphasized the primacy of mentors as socialization influences during these years.

Thus, the question of how socialization takes place in emerging adulthood remain wide open and in need of a fresh conceptualization that would apply to contemporary emerging adults. This question can be addressed by focusing on what socialization entails. According to Grusec (2002), socialization is how "individuals are assisted in the acquisition of skills necessary to function as members of their social group" (p. 143). In this process, "elders" (i.e., teachers, professors, trainers, employers, and experienced workers) and novices collaborate. The elders help the novices to develop the values, behaviors, and motives necessary to becoming a part of the social community. By this standard, socialization clearly continues through emerging adulthood. In fact, as noted, one of the social changes that has led to the development of emerging adulthood is the increased pervasiveness of postsecondary education and training, in which emerging adults acquire from elders the skills that will enable them to participate in the modern economy. This process involves acquiring not only knowledge and behaviors but also values, such as reliability, and motives, such as the attainment of self-sufficiency (Arnett, 2014).

Grusec (2002) further proposes that socialization involves three specific outcomes: (1) the development of self-regulation of emotion, thinking, and behavior; (2) the acquisition of a culture's standards, attitudes, and values, including appropriate and willing conformity with the direction of authority figures; and (3) the development of role-taking skills, strategies for resolving conflicts, and ways of viewing relationships. I have proposed a similar framework of three goals of socialization (Arnett, 1995b), but here I use Grusec's conceptualization, as it applies especially well to socialization in emerging adulthood. However, I prefer *goals* to *outcomes* because the term implies intentionality and volition. All cultures have a conception of what it means to become an adult (Arnett, 1998), and the adults in a culture typically socialize the young toward gradually developing the beliefs and behavior they believe an adult should have. As part of the socialization process, adults convey to young people whether or not they are making adequate progress toward those goals.

In industrialized cultures, all three of the goals of socialization arguably continue to be developed in emerging adulthood. Self-regulation, for most people, is by no means attained by the end of adolescence. With respect to emotional self-regulation, mood fluctuations are greater in adolescence than in childhood or adulthood, and depressed moods are common (Arnett, 1999; Larson & Richards, 1994). Emotional self-regulation improves substantially in the course of emerging adulthood; consequently, overall emotional well-being rises steadily from age 18 to 25 (Schulenberg & Zarrett, 2006). With respect to behavioral self-regulation, emerging adulthood is a period when a variety of types of risky behavior are highest, including substance use, driving while intoxicated, and unprotected sex (Arnett, 2000, 2005). However, toward the end of emerging adulthood, in the mid-to-late 20s, frequencies of risky behavior decline substantially, suggesting the attainment of behavioral self-regulation.

With respect to the second goal of socialization—the acquisition of a culture's standards, attitudes, and values—here, too, socialization is incomplete at the end of adolescence and continues into emerging adulthood. Most notably, in Western societies, a central cultural standard is that in order to attain adult status, young people should learn to become self-sufficient, to accept responsibility for themselves (Arnett, 1998). In numerous studies, across a variety of socioeconomic classes, ethnic groups, and nationalities, accepting responsibility for oneself has been found consistently to be the top criterion for reaching adulthood (see Nelson, in press, for a review). Furthermore, this criterion is rarely met by the end of adolescence; in these studies, few adolescents believe they have reached adulthood. It is during emerging adulthood that the cultural standard of accepting responsibility for oneself is gradually attained and people move from feeling that they are in between adolescence and adulthood to feeling that they have reached adulthood.

Emerging adulthood may also be a key time for the development of the third goal of socialization, that of learning role-taking skills, strategies for resolving conflicts, and ways of viewing relationships. Emerging adults become notably more adept at role taking, and their relationships with parents improve in part because they are better at taking their parents' perspectives (Arnett, 2014). Whether parents actually teach (explicitly or implicitly) role-taking skills that promote this change or whether the skills simply develop as a consequence of other social and cognitive changes in emerging adults is uncertain. It also seems likely that emerging adults change in their methods for resolving conflicts and in their ways of viewing relationships. Certainly, in their romantic relationships, emerging adults become capable of a greater degree of interpersonal intimacy with a romantic partner than they had as adolescents (Collins & van Dulmen, 2006). However, whether this is due to advances in the way one resolves conflicts and views relationships or to some other factor is an intriguing but heretofore unexamined research question.

Overall, it seems clear that socialization is not complete by the end of adolescence, and important developments in socialization take place in emerging adulthood. This leads to a second key problem in conceptualizing socialization in emerging adulthood: If parents play less of a role in the socialization of emerging adults than they do for children or adolescents, what are the sources of socialization in emerging adulthood? Most of this chapter is devoted to this question. First, however, I summarize my socialization theory and offer a few comments on the contexts of socialization.

Cultural, Historical, and Developmental Contexts

As a framework for the remainder of the chapter, I use my theory of broad and narrow socialization (Arnett, 1995b), in which I specify seven levels on which socialization takes place: the cultural belief system, the family, peers (including friends and romantic partners), neighborhood/community, school/work, media, and the legal system. The cultural belief system is the level that underlies all the others. Cultures tending toward broad socialization have cultural beliefs that value individualism, independence, and self-expression. Cultures tending toward narrow socialization have cultural beliefs that prize obedience, duty, and conformity. These beliefs then influence how parents parent, how teachers teach, and so on.

This basic contrast in socialization, between an emphasis on individualism and self-expression on the one hand and conformity and obedience on the other, has been a staple of theory and research on parenting in the United States for decades, accompanied by a variety of terminologies. Two other characteristics distinguish the theory of broad and narrow socialization. First, it is a cultural theory, meaning that the focus is on the cultural beliefs that underlie socialization rather than on the parenting practices that reflect cultural beliefs. Second, the theory emphasizes the range of individual differences that cultures allow or encourage—relatively broad in the case of broad socialization, relatively narrow in the case of narrow socialization. In my view, the heart of socialization lies in the boundaries cultures set on the development of individuals. As Scarr (1993) observed, "Cultures set a range of opportunities for development; they define the limits of what is desirable, 'normal' individual variation. . . . Cultures define the *range* and *focus* of personal variation that is acceptable and rewarded" (pp. 1335, 1337; original emphasis). Similarly, Child described socialization as "the whole process by which an individual born with behavioral potentialities of enormously wide range, is led to develop actual behavior which is confined within a much narrower range—the range of what is customary and acceptable for him according to the standards of his group" (quoted in Clausen, 1966, p. 3).

It is important to emphasize that broad and narrow socialization are not two homogeneous categories but two points at either end of a continuum. Most cultures are not either broad or narrow, as pure types, but are somewhere along the continuum, relatively broad or relatively narrow. Furthermore, in some cultures, socialization is relatively broad on some levels, relatively narrow on others. Still, the various levels are interrelated and tend to reinforce one another because the cultural belief system underlies and influences all the others. For example, if socialization in the family is narrow, it is likely to be partly because the cultural belief system is narrow. However, because each culture may be evaluated for the extent to which it is broad or narrow on each of the seven levels, the theory makes it possible to accommodate the great diversity in socialization practices of different cultures, while also making a useful distinction between different general types of socialization.

The range of acceptable individual differences can vary between cultures, across history, and through the life course. Cultures differ in the degree of restrictiveness they impose, based on their cultural beliefs. Across history, as cultural beliefs change, socialization changes as well. Through the life course, socialization changes as people become more subject to or more exempt from the prohibitions and restrictions of others.

All three of these considerations—culture, history, and life course period—are important for understanding the socialization of emerging adults today. Culturally, emerging adulthood exists mainly in cultures that allow their young people a substantial amount of freedom from their late teens through at least their mid-20s—that is, cultures with relatively broad socialization. Emerging adulthood is a period in which people focus on their self-development as they consider the possible life paths available to them and gradually move toward making the choices that will structure their adult lives (Arnett, 2014). This requires a cultural belief system that values individual development over obligations and duties to others, especially the family (Arnett, 2011). Such individualistic beliefs tend to develop mainly in cultures that are industrialized enough that economic interdependence among kin is not necessary for daily survival (Schlegel & Barry, 1991). Table 4.1 shows median marriage ages in various countries and suggests that emerging adulthood is experienced by the majority in economically developed countries but is not normative in developing countries.

Historically, emerging adulthood developed only in the past half century, as young people began to focus on self-development in their late teens and early 20s; consequently, the median ages of marriage and parenthood rose. There is substantial evidence that socialization in the U.S. majority culture, for example, broadened in the second half of the 20th century, when the individualism that has long been part of Western cultural beliefs became substantially more pronounced (Alwin, 1988; Bellah, Madsen, Sullivan, Swidler, & Tipton, 1985).

Within cultures, socialization may vary among subgroups, including periods of the life course. Socialization tends to be notably broader in emerging adulthood than at any other age. Children have the boundaries for their behavior set by adults, even in a culture characterized by broad socialization. Adults generally decide what children will do and when they will do it, and adults communicate to children what is acceptable and unacceptable behavior in the culture, sometimes explicitly, sometimes by example. Adolescents, too, are under the authority of their parents. They may have greater autonomy

TABLE 4.1. Median Marriage Age (Females) in Selected Countries

Developed countries	Age	Developing countries	Age
United States	27	Egypt	19
Canada	29	Ethiopia	17
Germany	30	Ghana	20
France	30	Nigeria	18
Italy	30	India	18
Japan	29	Indonesia	21
Australia	29	Guatemala	19

Note. Data from United Nations (2009).

than children (although not necessarily; in cultures that value female virginity before marriage, socialization may become narrower for girls when they reach adolescence), but their parents still set the rules and boundaries for their daily lives. Beyond emerging adulthood, once the adult roles of spouse, parent, and long-term worker are entered, the roles set standards for behavior that adults are compelled to follow.

Socialization is broadest in emerging adulthood in the sense that this is when people have the most freedom to decide for themselves how to live, and what to do and when to do it. Parents no longer have as much power over one as they did in childhood and adolescence, and obligations to a spouse or long-term partner, children, and long-term employer have not yet been entered. Peers and friends are agents of socialization at all ages, but because emerging adults change residences so often (and consequently social groups), peers/friends may have less power during emerging adulthood than at other life stages (Barry, Madsen, & DeGrace, in press). Emerging adulthood is a self-focused age, when social control is at an ebb and people have the greatest freedom to focus on their self-development (Arnett, 2014). Consequently, emerging adulthood is the most diverse, heterogeneous period of the life course (Arnett, 2006a, 2006b). Nearly all children and adolescents live at home with one or both parents, and the great majority of adults live with a spouse or romantic partner, but emerging adults may live alone, with friends, in a college group setting, with a romantic partner, or with parents, and they change their living arrangements more often than persons at any other age period (Arnett, 2014). Nearly all children and adolescents in developed countries attend school, and the great majority of adults are employed, but emerging adults have a dizzying range of combinations of school and work, and are also more likely than persons in any other age group to be "disengaged" (i.e., neither working nor in school; Hamilton & Hamilton, 2006). Thus, the consequence of the self-focused freedom conferred by broad socialization in emerging adulthood is that the variance in living arrangements, school–work combinations, and other areas (to be discussed later) is greater than at any other age period.

The Rise of Individualization in the Socialization Process

An important sociological concept that can be applied here is *individualization*. According to sociologists and historians of the life course (Côté, 2000; Heinz, 2002; Mayer, 2004; Mills, 2007), the life course has become deinstitutionalized in recent decades.

Institutions (e.g., family and community) have lost their binding power, and individuals have gained more control of and responsibility for the direction of their lives. According to Heinz (2002), there has been "a shift from standardized, institutionalized life course patterns that constitute an age- and gender-bound temporal order of life towards the individualized biography" (p. 43). The result is individualization, which means that people are no longer as constrained or supported by institutions as they were in the past, and they must work out their life course choices for themselves.

Sociologists rarely frame individualization in developmental terms, instead applying it to the life course in general. Nevertheless, they discuss it especially in relation to life course transitions that pertain mainly to emerging adulthood, such as transitions related to education, employment, partnership/marriage, and parenthood (Heinz, 2002; Mayer, 2004; Mills, 2007). Applying individualization developmentally to emerging adulthood is useful for emphasizing that socialization is broader now than in the past and broader in emerging adulthood than in other age periods. As Heinz (2002) notes, due to individualization there has been "a de-standardization of the programmed trajectories, and *increasing variations* in the timing and duration of transitions in relation to the family, education, and employment" (p. 49, emphasis added).

Heinz (2002) makes an explicit connection between individualization and socialization with his concept of *self-socialization*. The self-socialization framework has two main principles:

> 1) Individuals construct their own life course by attempting to come to terms with opportunities and constraints concerning transition pathways and life stages. 2) Individuals select pathways, and act and appraise the consequences of their actions, in terms of their self-identity. (p. 58)

Thus, individualization requires people to construct their own life course, so that socialization is something that is done by the individual rather than imposed by outside social or institutional forces.

As with individualization, the self-socialization framework is not presented developmentally, but it is easy to see the developmental basis that underlies it and how it pertains especially to emerging adulthood. Children and adolescents have limited freedom to construct their life course and choose their socialization contexts because many of their choices are either structured by their parents or made by their parents directly. As for adults, once they select their pathways through the choices they make in work and family, the structure of adult life that is set up by those choices tends to perpetuate itself and resist change. It is during emerging adulthood that self-socialization is most pronounced because people have more freedom to choose their socialization contexts and construct their life course than they did before or will again once they enter the roles and responsibilities of young adulthood.

Let us now return to the question of where and how socialization takes place in emerging adulthood, with a focus on the levels of family, peers/friends, school–work, and media. Family is addressed (even though, as noted, family socialization usually wanes in emerging adulthood) because socialization theory and research have traditionally focused mainly on parenting, and important changes in parental socialization take place in emerging adulthood. Peers/friends, school–work, and media are addressed because these levels of socialization are especially important in emerging adulthood.

Family

If we accept that socialization takes place during emerging adulthood, to what extent do parents continue to be part of the socialization process? And to what extent does parental socialization in childhood and adolescence have effects that endure into emerging adulthood? There is no doubt that the parents' role in socialization diminishes from adolescence to emerging adulthood, as it diminishes from childhood to adolescence. Parents control nearly every aspect of their children's environment from birth through early to middle childhood. Adolescents begin to gain more autonomy from their parents; consequently, they spend a considerable proportion of their time with friends, unmonitored by their parents or other adults (B. B. Brown & Bakken, 2011). Emerging adults are even more different from adolescents than adolescents are from children with respect to autonomy from parents because they typically move out of their parents' household. Once they move out, their exposure to socialization from parents becomes voluntary to a large extent. Indeed, avoiding their parents' efforts to influence their lives on a daily basis is a primary motivation for moving out in emerging adulthood (Arnett, 2014). Once they move out, emerging adults are able to control the information their parents have about their lives and let them in on only what they want them to know.

Nevertheless, the continuing influence of parents continues to be evident in emerging adulthood on all three of Grusec's (2002) socialization outcomes. With respect to self-regulation, parents assist in the development of this quality to the extent that they support their emerging adults' increased capacity for it. This does not mean withdrawal of parental support, emotional and financial, once secondary school ends and emerging adulthood begins. On the contrary, it means flexibility in adjusting to emerging adults' needs for autonomy and dependency as the balance of these needs gradually moves more toward autonomy, perhaps in fits and starts, over the course of emerging adulthood (Aquilino, 2006). Most parents of emerging adults do quite well at supporting their emerging adults' development toward greater self-regulation. For example, in a national U.S. survey, only 30% of 18- to 29-year-olds agreed: "My parents are more involved in my life than I really want them to be" (Arnett & Schwab, 2012). However, some parents express anxiety or reluctance about their emerging adults' growing capacity for autonomy (Bartle-Haring, Brucker, & Hock, 2002).

Moving out promotes the development of self-regulation in emerging adults and also makes it easier for parents to support it. While emerging adults remain home, for most parents, the daily presence of their emerging adults in the household proves to be too much of a temptation, and they attempt to regulate their children's behavior more than most emerging adults believe they need or want. Emotional boundaries, physical privacy, and parental intrusiveness often become critical issues (Arnett, 2014). Parents' attempts to regulate their emerging adults' daily schedules, eating habits, financial practices, and sexuality become sources of conflict. Emerging adults' progress toward full self-regulation proceeds more smoothly for both parents and emerging adults if they do not live together.

The influence of parents is also evident with respect to the second socialization goal, the acquisition of the culture's standards, attitudes, and values. An important standard with respect to emerging adulthood is the expectation that emerging adults will move toward self-sufficiency, an expectation that reflects cultural values of independence and individualism (Arnett, 1998, 2011). Parents influence their emerging adults' progress toward this goal by communicating the values of independence and individualism long before their children reach emerging adulthood. By emerging adulthood, both parents and children usually concur that it is best for emerging adults to move toward independence from parents and learn to stand alone.

One area of research that has implications for this issue concerns perceptions of what it means to become an adult (Nelson, in press). Across numerous studies, in a variety of industrialized countries, the consistent finding has been that the top three criteria for adulthood are accepting responsibility for oneself, making independent decisions, and becoming financially independent. All three of these criteria reflect common underlying values of independence and individualism (Arnett, 2011).

Both parents and emerging adults—in fact, persons of all ages—favor these three criteria as being most important for adulthood (Arnett, 2001; Arnett & Schwab, 2013). Furthermore, all three criteria pertain to emerging adults' independence from parents. Accepting responsibility for oneself means not depending on one's parents to come to the rescue when unpleasant consequences result from one's actions. Making independent decisions means relying on one's own judgment rather than relying on parents for advice. Becoming financially independent means no longer requesting or accepting parents' financial help. By favoring the attainment of these three criteria for adulthood, parents may also communicate the importance of values of independence and individualism. However, studies indicating how much parents encourage the attainment of these markers in their emerging adult children, implicitly or explicitly, have yet to be conducted.

Of course, independence and (more generally) individualism are not universal values but are cultural values prevalent in industrialized societies, especially Western societies (Arnett, 2011). But even within these societies, some cultural groups have values that depart from the values of the majority culture. With respect to conceptions of what it means to be an adult, an interesting contrast exists between the values of the majority culture in American society and the values of Asian Americans (Arnett, 2003, 2014). Like European Americans, Asian Americans place a high value on the individualistic criteria of accepting responsibility for oneself, making independent decisions, and becoming financially independent. However, a criterion that is highly valued among Asian American emerging adults but almost never mentioned by European Americans is becoming capable of taking care of one's parents. This criterion is clearly derived from the traditional Asian value of *filial piety* (i.e., respecting, obeying, and revering one's parents). (Indeed, emerging adults in China have also been found to place high importance on becoming capable of taking care of their parents as a criterion of adulthood; Nelson, Badger, & Wu, 2004.) Thus, it can be reasonably presumed that Asian American parents (and perhaps others in the cultural community) convey the value of filial piety to their children in the course of childhood socialization, and it is expressed in emerging adulthood in the importance placed on becoming capable of taking care of one's parents.

The third goal of socialization, the development of role-taking skills, strategies for resolving conflicts, and ways of viewing relationships, is strikingly evident in relationships with parents during emerging adulthood. Relationships with parents typically improve greatly in emerging adulthood, compared to adolescence (Aquilino, 2006; Arnett, 2014). Conflict is lower, and warmth and closeness are higher. This is partly because emerging adults typically move out of their parents' household, and it is easier for them to get along well when the friction that results from day-to-day living together is avoided. As noted previously, emerging adults get along considerably better with their parents if they move out than if they remain at home (Dubas & Petersen, 1996).

However, there is more to the improved relations than simply seeing each other less. Another key contributor to improved relations is in precisely this area of emerging adults' enhanced role-taking skills and new ways of viewing relationships. Emerging adults are considerably less egocentric than adolescents, and considerably better at role taking with respect to their parents, which leads them to understand their parents as persons and not merely as parents (Arnett, 2014; Fingerman, 2000). They learn to view their relationships with their parents as more of a relationship among adults rather than strictly in terms of the roles of parents and children.

Whether this change in emerging adults is a consequence of parental socialization is unknown, and it seems unlikely that the direction of effects runs only from parents to children. Emerging adults may even drive the change in the relationship, through their development of new social cognitive skills (Labouvie-Vief, 2006). Parents welcome this change in their children, and parents change, too, becoming less didactic with their children and relating to them more as adults, or at least near-adults. Their role as monitor of their children's behavior and enforcer of household rules diminishes, and this results in a more relaxed and amiable relationship with their children. Thus, socialization with respect to relationships between parents and emerging adults appears to be bidirectional, with both changing and both responding to the changes in the other (Arnett, 2014; Fingerman, 2000).

Parental Socialization and Emerging Adults' Psychosocial Development

In addition to research on parental socialization that pertains directly to the three socialization outcomes discussed earlier, there is a considerable amount of research describing the association between relations with parents and psychosocial development in emerging adulthood. This research is mainly in three areas: parents' and emerging adults' psychological well-being, parents' and emerging adults' capacity for intimate relations with others, and emerging adults' responses to parental conflict and divorce.

With respect to psychological well-being, research pertaining to emerging adulthood confirms the long-standing finding of socialization research on childhood and adolescence, that the parenting combination of *demandingness* and *responsiveness* that characterizes the authoritative parenting style is consistently related to positive outcomes in children. For example, in a study of college students, Wintre and Yaffe (2000) found that authoritative parenting was related to higher academic achievement and successful adjustment to college life. Similarly, research on attachments to parents in emerging adulthood confirms findings from child and adolescent research that a secure attachment to parents is related to positive outcomes. For example, a 6-year national longitudinal study in the Netherlands extending through participants' 20s revealed that attachments to parents did not diminish over that period, and the association between attachment to parents and psychological well-being remained strong and positive (van Wel, Linssen, & Ruud, 2000).

Although authoritative parenting and secure attachment are positively related to favorable psychological outcomes in emerging adulthood, as they are in childhood and adolescence, the nature of authoritative parenting and secure attachment changes with the age of the children. Authoritative parenting for emerging adults involves a different kind of demandingness than that at earlier ages, with broader boundaries and less monitoring; parental responsiveness is likely to be on a less than daily basis, especially once emerging adults move out of their parents' household. Secure attachment, too, is likely to involve less frequent contact with parents in emerging adulthood than at earlier ages, and the "secure base" provided by parents is likely to be more psychological than literal (Allen & Land, 1999). With both authoritative parenting and secure attachment, competent parental socialization includes adapting to the new capacities that children develop in emerging adulthood and fostering their autonomy even as a strong emotional bond to parents is maintained (Allen, Hauser, O'Connor, & Bell, 2002; Aquilino, 2006).

With respect to parental socialization and relations with others in emerging adulthood, research indicates that parental socialization earlier in development is related to emerging adults' later intimate relationships. For example, in one longitudinal study that followed a rural sample from ages 12 to 21, authoritative parenting (high in warmth, support, and monitoring) in early adolescence was predictive of behavior toward romantic partners in emerging adulthood that was also warm and supportive (Conger, Cui, Bryant, & Elder, 2000). In another longitudinal study, beginning with participants ages 13–18 and following up 6 years later at ages 19–25, family cohesion in adolescence predicted self-reported happiness in romantic relationships in emerging adulthood, especially for women (Feldman, Gowen, & Fisher, 1998). These studies appear to indicate that socialization in the family affects the development of interpersonal skills, which are then later carried into emerging adults' romantic relationships (Conger & Conger, 2002).

With respect to the effects of parental divorce, substantial evidence indicates that emerging adults who experienced their parents' divorce during childhood are at risk for depression and other mental health problems in emerging adulthood (Amato, 2010). One study of a large national sample in Great Britain even showed evidence of a "sleeper effect" of divorce, with its negative influence on mental health becoming more evident in emerging adulthood than it was in childhood (Cherlin, Chase-Lansdale, & McRae, 1998). Furthermore, several studies have indicated that parental divorce in childhood is negatively related to emerging adults' capacity for intimacy and trust in romantic relationships (Jacquet & Surra, 2001; Summers, Forehand, Armistead, & Tannenbaum, 1998; Toomey & Nelson, 2001).

There is evidence that it is the parental conflict surrounding divorce, and not just divorce per se, that accounts for the relation between parental divorce and negative outcomes in childhood and adolescence, as well as emerging adulthood (Cui, Fincham, & Pasley, 2008). However, studies that control for parental conflict have found that the effects of divorce remain (Amato, 2010). Laumann-Billings and Emery (2000) noted that research on divorce typically focuses on disorders of behavior, such as how divorce affects functioning in school or work, whereas clinical case studies typically focus on the distress that results from divorce, such as how divorce feels to those affected by it. In two studies of emerging adults, one with college students and one with a low-income community sample, researchers found that emerging adults often reported painful feelings, beliefs, and memories concerning the divorce, even if in their behavior they seemed to have recovered from it.

The Question of Parental Influence

Like studies on parental socialization at other ages, studies of parental socialization in emerging adulthood must be examined with respect to questions of interpretation, specifically, the question of the extent to which an association between parental socialization and children's behavior represents the influence of parents on their children or is due instead to other factors. One of the most important considerations is the possibility of passive, evocative, and active genotype–environment processes (Plomin, 2009; Scarr & McCartney, 1983). Passive genotype–environment processes occur in biological families when parents provide both genes and environment for their children. This seems like a truism at first glance, but it has profound implications for interpreting socialization research. It means that in biological families, when an association is found between parents' behavior and children's outcomes, it is difficult to tell if this association is due to the environment the parents provided or the genes they provided because they provided both. In socialization research involving emerging adults, including virtually all the studies cited in the previous section, associations between parents' characteristics and emerging adults' characteristics are routinely described in terms of parental "effects" and "influences." However, this interpretation may be questionable because it ignores the role of passive genotype–environment processes.

Behavioral genetic studies have begun to address this problem in socialization research, mainly using twin and adoption studies to unravel the usual confound between genetics and environment that occurs in biological families (see Avinun & Knafo-Noam, Chapter 15, this volume). Few behavioral genetic studies on this topic have included emerging adults, but one might expect that parental socialization effects would be smaller in emerging adulthood than in childhood or adolescence, due to the fact that emerging adults are less likely to have daily contact with their parents (Aquilino, 2006; Arnett, 2014). However, it is also possible that parental socialization in childhood and adolescence has effects that endure into emerging adulthood.

Evocative genotype–environment processes exist when children's genetically based characteristics evoke responses from parents (and others), so that the children's socialization is due not simply to the effects of parents on children but to the children's effects on the parents. This is part of the broader idea of bidirectional effects (i.e., the idea that socialization is an interactive process in which the direction of effects goes not only from parents to children but from children to parents). There is substantial evidence for this in the literature on socialization in childhood and adolescence (e.g., Pardini, 2010; Reiss, Neiderhiser, Hetherington, & Plomin, 2000). In emerging adulthood, the child-to-parent effect might be expected to be even stronger because the relationship between emerging adults and their parents become closer to a relationship between equals (or at least near-equals) than that in childhood or adolescence (Arnett, 2004). But research on bidirectional effects in emerging adulthood is scarce.

Finally, the concept of active genotype–environment processes means that people pursue environmental niches on the basis of their genetically based characteristics (Plomin, 2009). One might expect that active genotype–environment processes would be more evident in emerging adulthood than at earlier ages because emerging adults have the freedom to leave the environment provided by their parents and seek out their own niches, to an extent that children and adolescents do not. Here, as with the other varieties of genotype–environment processes, few studies that have been conducted involve emerging adults.

There is substantial evidence that parental socialization influences development in childhood and adolescence, especially when parental socialization is at the negative extreme, and especially in the area of antisocial behavior (Pardini, 2010). It is also well established that parental socialization in childhood and adolescence is influenced by genotype–environment processes. However, the extent to which parental socialization is influential in emerging adulthood has yet to be investigated in a way that takes genotype–environment processes into account.

Peers and Friends

What kind of role do peers and friends play in the socialization of emerging adults? Because research on peers and friends in emerging adulthood is very limited, it may be useful to begin by examining the research on peer/friend socialization in adolescence, then consider how these findings might change from adolescence to emerging adulthood. The abundant research on peer/friend socialization in adolescence has led to several conclusions. First, peers and friends are highly important in the lives of adolescents. Adolescents are happiest in the company of friends (Larson & Richards, 1994, 1998), and are closer to friends than to parents in many respects (De Goede, Branje, Delsing, & Meeus, 2009; Youniss & Smollar, 1985). Over the course of adolescence, the amount of time adolescents spend with friends increases, whereas the time they spend with family decreases (Larson, Richards, Moneta, Holmbeck, & Duckett, 1996). Issues of popularity and unpopularity are prominent in secondary schools, and adolescents are acutely aware of how they and others rank with respect to popularity (Becker & Luthar, 2007). Thus, because of their importance in the lives of adolescents, peers and friends have a great deal of potential power in the socialization process.

Second, like people in other age groups, adolescents tend to choose friends who are similar to themselves in many ways, a process known as *selective association* (B. B. Brown & Larson, 2009). Consequently, when similarities are found among friends, it is likely that the similarities were there before they became friends, and in fact led to their friendship, rather than being produced by "peer pressure" or peer influence. Adolescent friends do influence one another, but those influences are complex. Although the influence of friends in adolescence is often assumed to be negative, tending toward violations of the socialization outcomes of self-regulation and conforming to authority figures (e.g., toward illicit substance use), in fact, adolescent friends tend to reinforce their preexisting similarities (Hamm, 2000). That is, adolescent friends who have a tendency toward deviant behavior encourage each other toward such deviance, whereas adolescent friends who tend to follow the rules reinforce that tendency in each other (Maxwell, 2002).

Third, intimacy in friendships is higher in adolescence than in childhood and rises over the course of adolescence (B. B. Brown & Larson, 2009). Prior to adolescence, friendships are based mainly on shared activities, but adolescents rate intimate features such as trust and loyalty as more important to friendship than do younger children, and adolescents are more likely to value their friends as persons who understand them and with whom they can share personal information (B. B. Brown & Bakken, 2011). Thus, with respect to the third socialization goal of teaching role-taking skills, strategies for resolving conflicts, and ways of viewing relationship, friends also play an important part.

Unfortunately, research on friendships is as sparse in the emerging adulthood literature as it is abundant in literature on adolescence (Barry et al., in press). Nevertheless, a number of contrasts can be drawn between the socialization role of peers and friends in adolescence and in emerging adulthood, based on what is known. First, peers and friends play a less prominent role in emerging adulthood than they did in adolescence. Emerging adults leave the peer-centered context of secondary school, so they are no longer part of a peer culture on a daily basis, and no longer are guaranteed to see their friends at least 5 days a week. Emerging adults who enter a residential college context may also have a wide circle of peers, but this is a minority of emerging adults even at ages 18–22 (National Center for Education Statistics, 2012), and after college the number of people in emerging adults' social support networks drops sharply (Barry et al., in press).

Emerging adults also spend more of their time alone than do adolescents; in fact, emerging adults spend more time alone than any group except older adults (Luong, Charles, & Fingerman, 2008). Furthermore, emerging adults are more likely than adolescents to be involved with a romantic partner, which typically leads to a selective withdrawal from friendships with peripheral friends, while retaining close friends (Barry et al., in press). Overall, it seems clear that the opportunities for socialization influence by peers and friends decreases from adolescence to emerging adulthood. With peers and friends, as with parents, emerging adults' relationships become more volitional; that is, emerging adults have more control over the extent to which they are exposed to the socialization influences of others.

Second, selective association in friendships may be even more pronounced in emerging adulthood than in adolescence. Although adolescents tend to seek out friends who are similar to themselves, parents are able to influence the friendship networks their adolescents are likely to experience and the pool of peers from which adolescents are likely to select their friends. Parents do this through their choices about where to live, where to send their adolescents to school (e.g., public vs. private school), and where (or whether) to attend religious services. Parental control in all these respects diminishes in emerging adulthood. Furthermore, emerging adults may be less responsive to the influence of their friends than they were as adolescents. Even in the course of adolescence the influence of friends diminishes, after peaking in early adolescence (B. B. Brown & Larson, 2009). In emerging adulthood, this decrease is likely to continue, as emerging adults see their friends less often and have more control over when and where they see them. In addition, emerging adults become very intent on learning to make their own decisions as part of becoming an adult (Arnett, 1998, 2003, 2014), which may make them even less responsive to the socialization attempts of their friends.

Third, with respect to intimacy in friendships, evidence indicates that intimacy increases from adolescence to emerging adulthood (Collins & van Dulmen, 2006). Friendships in emerging adulthood tend to be characterized by greater emotional depth and complexity, and greater communication about topics of personal importance. Thus, in contrast to the decline in friends' socialization influence that takes place in most respects, with respect to the socialization goal of learning role-taking skills, strategies for resolving conflicts, and ways of viewing relationships, friendships may rise in importance from adolescence to emerging adulthood (although little research has addressed this question directly).

What about romantic relationships as a source of socialization? There is a large literature on romantic relationships in emerging adulthood, mostly from studies of college students (Hatfield & Rapson, 2006). These studies generally focus on relationship quality and sexual issues. Although the results of the studies are rarely framed in terms of socialization effects, they pertain to the third goal of socialization, that of learning role taking, conflict resolution skills, and ways of viewing relationships. These are all things that emerging adults learn in the course of having romantic relationships (Collins & van Dulmen, 2006). As with friends, the relationship skills learned in romantic relationships occur bidirectionally, between equals, in contrast to the power differential that usually applies when parents are socializing children.

In addition to the research on romantic relationships in emerging adulthood, suggestions regarding romantic relationships as a source of socialization can be found in the literature on the socializing effects of cohabitation and marriage. It has long been established that marriage is positively related to a variety of aspects of physical and mental health (Waite & Gallagher, 2000). Emerging adulthood, the period just prior to marriage for most people, is a low-risk period for physical illness and disease, but it is the highest-risk period of the life span for a variety of disorders and injuries caused by behaviors such as substance use and risky sexual behavior (Schulenberg & Zarrett, 2006). Marriage has the effect of reducing the behaviors that lead to problems, thereby improving physical and mental health. It is single men who especially engage in high-risk behavior in emerging adulthood, so the change in their behavior once they enter marriage is especially striking (Waite & Gallagher, 2000). Although findings in studies on the effects of marriage rarely are framed in terms of socialization, it seems evident that the decline in emerging adults' risky behaviors following marriage reflects increased conformity to their culture's standards, attitudes, and values. It also seems evident that their behavior becomes better regulated after marriage, although this may be not so much self-regulation as mutual regulation in the marriage relationship.

The socializing effects of marriage presumably result at least in part from having a person around on a daily basis who monitors one's behavior and discourages behavior that reflects a lack of self-regulation or that violates cultural norms. It is surprising, then, that cohabitation appears to have little of the socializing influence of marriage. For example, with respect to substance use, the Monitoring the Future surveys have followed a sample from members' senior year of high school through the next 10 years (Bachman, Wadsworth, O'Malley, Johnston, & Schulenberg, 1997). Even in high school, the future cohabitors reported higher levels of drinking and marijuana use than those who had married or remained single a decade later. However, in the course of the decade following high school, the cohabitors reported very high and increasing levels of smoking, drinking, and other drug use, whereas those who married during that decade showed declines in all those substance use behaviors following marriage.

What explains these findings? Although emerging adults who cohabit are different in some ways from those who do not, such as being less religious and having higher rates of risky behavior in high school, these differences do not account for the differential effects of cohabitation and marriage. Even when these differences are taken into account statistically, the differential effects remain (Waite & Gallagher, 2000). Instead, there seems to be something about the institution of marriage itself that modifies the behavior of people who enter into it. Despite marked increases in cohabitation and divorce, young people continue to believe in what Waite and Gallagher (2000) call "the power of the vow" (i.e., in marriage as a permanent union that obligates those entering it to modify their behavior so that it is less risky and less in violation of cultural norms). Thus, the socializing influence of marriage may be derived mainly from the beliefs that people have about what marriage requires of them.

School and Work

Once adolescents finish secondary school, the main context of their daily experience becomes college, work, or some combination of the two (Hamilton & Hamilton, 2006). What kind of socialization takes place in these two contexts? Here, again, few studies have looked at this question explicitly in terms of socialization issues, but other evidence does have implications for socialization.

Let us examine school first. Although the majority of emerging adults in most industrialized countries are involved in some kind of schooling or occupational training in the first years of emerging adulthood, the nature of the school experience changes considerably from adolescence to emerging adulthood. The secondary school experience of adolescents is highly structured and closely monitored by adults. Adolescents are typically required by law to attend school (at least until sometime in their late teens, with the upper age varying among countries). They spend 4–7 hours a day in the classroom, where teachers record their attendance and monitor their behavior. Although they usually have some discretion in which courses to take, many of their courses are required as part of their general education. Thus, in addition to educating them, teachers and other school personnel are socializing adolescents to acquire cultural standards of doing what is required, and conforming to or at least cooperating with the direction of authority figures.

The role of school in socialization broadens considerably in emerging adulthood. Involvement in school at all is discretionary because there is no longer a legal requirement for attendance. There is a wider variety of schooling options from which to choose, including an array of colleges and universities, as well as vocational programs. For most of these options, the amount of time spent receiving direct instruction is relatively small compared to that in secondary school, and more learning is to be done through assigned work that students do on their own. Instructors are less likely to monitor whether the students come to class. Thus, schooling in emerging adulthood requires greater capacities for self-regulation in order to succeed.

Like school, work takes place in both adolescence and emerging adulthood, but the nature of it as a socialization context changes, especially in the United States. Unlike adolescents in most other developed countries, over 80% of U.S. adolescents have held a part-time job by the time they leave high school, and by their senior year of high school adolescents who are employed work over 15 hours a week on average (Staff, Schulenberg, & Bachman, 2010). However, the purpose of these jobs is mainly to obtain money to finance an active leisure life, not to obtain useful occupational training for the future: Most of the jobs U.S. adolescents hold are in restaurant work or retail sales and are unrelated to the work they expect to be doing as adults (Schneider & Stevenson, 1999).

This has important implications for socialization. Because they have no personal investment in the long-term future of their work, adolescents have little reason to cultivate self-regulation on the job or to learn cultural standards of behavior that may be desired by their employers. Thus, longitudinal studies have shown that although such adolescents say they learn culturally valued qualities on the job, such as responsibility, money management, and time management, in fact, the more they work, the more they tend to engage in deviant behavior such as substance use, fighting, and vandalism (Mortimer, 2003). Also, a majority of working adolescents report some form of "occupational deviance" in the workplace, such as stealing from employers or coworkers or giving away items for free or for less than their value (Apel & Paternoster, 2009; Ruggiero,

Greenberger, & Steinberg, 1982). Thus, working in adolescence often undermines rather than promotes the socialization process.

Work in emerging adulthood has a much different nature. The stakes are higher because most emerging adults are looking for employment not just to provide money for the moment, but as a way to build a foundation for the kind of work they will be doing in adulthood. This does not mean that they suddenly become more responsible and less deviant in the workplace than they were as adolescents. On the contrary, employers are often reluctant to hire applicants younger than age 25 who have not obtained a college education, regardless of their secondary school achievements, because of their experiences with emerging adults who have been irresponsible and did not prove to be worth the effort and expense involved in training them (Hamilton & Hamilton, 2006; Wilson, 1996). Nevertheless, most people gain in responsibility, future orientation, and planful competence over the course of emerging adulthood (Masten, Obradovic, & Burt, 2006; Roisman, Masten, Coatsworth, & Tellegen, 2004). The workplace rewards these qualities, so emerging adults have a strong incentive to respond to the socialization requirements of the workplace in order to succeed. If they fail to cultivate these qualities, they soon experience the painful consequences of being fired or failing to get the jobs and promotions they would like.

In European countries, there is not such a sharp contrast between work in adolescence and in emerging adulthood as there is in the United States. Work and school are more integrated because most adolescents receive education and training in secondary school that is directly related to the occupation they plan to have once they leave school. Many adolescents are involved in apprenticeship programs that combine work with schooling that pertains directly to their work (Flammer & Alsaker, 2001). Thus, in European countries, there is more continuity in workplace socialization from adolescence though emerging adulthood because self-regulation and cultural standards of responsibility and diligence are required and promoted consistently. However, this system is changing in response to economic changes resulting from globalization and the workplace becoming more flexible. The consequences of these changes for socialization in the workplace remain to be seen.

Media

Media have held a substantial and growing place in the socialization environment of industrialized societies in recent decades (Arnett, 1995a; Prot et al., Chapter 12, this volume). For today's emerging adults, the media environment is more diverse and complex than it has ever been before. They are the "new media generation" (J. D. Brown, 2006), that is, the first to grow up with the Internet, social media, virtual games, virtual friends (e.g., chat rooms), and make-your-own CDs, in addition to the traditional media of radio, television, recorded music, movies, newspapers, and magazines.

The importance of media in the socialization process can be seen with respect to the three goals of socialization. First, the goal of self-regulation pertains in part to sexuality and aggression, especially in emerging adulthood, when risky behavior in these areas tends to be high (Lefkowitz & Gillen, 2006), and a large proportion of media content, especially the content most popular among young people, contains sexual and aggressive themes. Second, the goal of learning cultural standards, attitudes, and values is communicated in the media through cognitive and social learning processes. Moral situations are depicted, certain behaviors are shown as rewarded and others as punished, and some characters are depicted as admirable and others as despicable. Also, values of materialism and consumerism are communicated through the abundant advertising that accompanies most media. Third, the goal of learning, knowledge, and skills concerning relationships is promoted through media depictions of relationships, including between parents and children, romantic partners, and friends (Ward, Gorvine, & Cytron-Walker, 2002).

However, media also differ in an important way from other socialization sources, especially parents, school, and work (Arnett, 1995a). The goal of these other social-izers is for children and young people to become socialized members of their culture, in the sense that they have attained adequate self-regulation; accepted mainstream cultural standards, attitudes, and values; and learned culturally appropriate ways of behaving in relationships. In contrast, the goal of most media is profit, the bigger the better. Thus, the goal of the media is not necessarily consistent with and in fact may undermine the goal of the other socializers. Media companies are generally willing to sell content with sexual and aggressive themes even if it undermines self-regulation, which most media research-ers believe it does (e.g., Cantor, 2000). Similarly, media content violating mainstream cultural standards, attitudes, and values will be sold if people will buy it, irrespective of whether it undermines that socialization goal.

What role, then, do media play in the socialization of emerging adults, in particular? A good framework for answering this question is the media practice model (J. D. Brown, 2006; J. D. Brown, Steele, & Walsh-Childers, 2002; Steele & Brown, 1995). As shown in Figure 4.1, this model portrays media use as a dynamic process between the person and the media environment. The person's Identity (and, more broadly, personality) leads to the Selection of some media products rather than others. Even among those who select the same media products, their Interaction with those products results in differences in how they experience and make sense of them. They also vary in the Application of the media messages (i.e., the extent to which they incorporate or resist the messages).

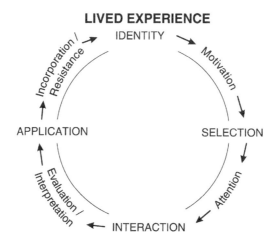

FIGURE 4.1. The media practice model. Copyright 1999 by Jeanne R. Steele, University of St. Thomas. Reprinted by permission.

Their acceptance of the messages contributes to the further development of their identity. "Lived Experience" refers to the interconnections between media use and other contexts (e.g., when friends gather to see a movie or listen to music, or when parents and children disagree about the media content the children should consume).

Each of the elements of the model takes a distinctive form in emerging adulthood. Although Identity has traditionally been associated with adolescence, today identity issues are perhaps even more central to development in emerging adulthood (Arnett, 2014; Côté, 2000, 2006). With respect to media and identity development, in one study, 70% of Canadian college students reported that they had a "celebrity idol," usually a movie star or musician (Boon & Lemore, 2001). More than half said their idols had influenced their attitudes and values, indicating the role of media with respect to that socialization goal. More than one-fourth said they had sought to change aspects of their personality to make it more like that of their favorite idol.

With respect to Selection, it is notable that media selection is less constrained in emerging adulthood than in any other age period. Children and adolescents have parents in the household who may disapprove, restrict, or prohibit their selection of certain media products. Beyond emerging adulthood, most adults have a spouse or live-in partner who may express disapproval or criticism of certain media choices. But in emerging adulthood, media choices are virtually unconstrained by any social influences. This may explain why the most avid audience for violent video games and Internet pornography is emerging adult men (J. D. Brown, 2006). Here, as in some other respects, socialization is never broader than it is in emerging adulthood.

However, the effects of media on emerging adults may be different than they are for children and adolescents, due to developmental differences in interaction and application. Although very few studies have compared adolescents' and emerging adults' responses to media, research on cognitive development has demonstrated that emerging adults think in ways that are more complex, reflective, and insightful (Labouvie-Vief, 2006), and this may mean that they are more capable than adolescents of stepping back from media content, evaluating it, and consciously resisting it. Even in adolescence, the effects of media are not as strong as they are in childhood (Huesmann, Moise-Titus, Podolski, & Eron, 2003), and it seems likely that the dilution of direct media effects continues into emerging adulthood. Even more than in earlier development, media effects in emerging adulthood are likely to be subtle and conditional. Nevertheless, media effects on college students have been reported in diverse areas, including aggression, body image, occupational choice, and political ideology (J. D. Brown, 2006). But more research is needed on non-college-educated emerging adults and comparison of adolescents and emerging adults. More research is also needed on potential positive effects of media use in emerging adulthood (see Prot et al., Chapter 12, this volume), such as providing information in areas of education and occupation.

Conclusion

In industrialized societies, and in the growing middle class of developing countries, adulthood is reached later today than in the past. Economic changes have made it more desirable for young people to obtain education and training past secondary school in order to qualify for jobs in the new information-based world economy. Even more important, growing individualism has allowed young people greater freedom to decide when to enter adult roles of marriage, parenthood, and long-term work, and given this freedom, many of them wait until at least their mid-20s before doing so. As a result, in between adolescence and young adulthood, a new period of the life course, emerging adulthood, has developed.

For emerging adults, the socialization goals of self-regulation, developing a set of beliefs and values, and learning roles and relationship skills are still very much in progress but not yet reached. However, the nature of the socialization process changes from adolescence to emerging adulthood. Parents and peers/friends are still involved in socialization for emerging adults, but to a lesser extent than they were in adolescence. School remains a socialization context for emerging adults, but in a broader, less restrictive form, and only for *some* emerging adults. Thus, institutional frameworks weaken in the socialization process, and emerging adults experience individualization, because they are left on their own to make their way to adulthood through self-socialization. This freedom can be exhilarating, but some find it disconcerting and disorienting. Socialization can become so broad that it provides inadequate support and guidance, so that the goals of socialization may remain elusive. The extent to which emerging adults thrive or struggle under their exceptionally broad socialization is still largely unknown.

The field of emerging adulthood is new, and the study of socialization in emerging adulthood is in a nascent stage. Although quite a bit is known about parental socialization in emerging adulthood, research on socialization with respect to peers/friends, school and work, and the media is sparse. This limits the extent to which a full picture of socialization in emerging adulthood can be drawn, but it presents great opportunities for creative theory and research for scholars seeking to contribute to this growing field.

REFERENCES

Allen, J., Hauser, S., O'Connor, T., & Bell, K. (2002). Prediction of peer-rated adult hostility from autonomy struggles in adolescent–family interactions. *Development and Psychopathology, 14*, 123–137.

Allen, J., & Land, P. (1999). Attachment in adolescence. In J. Cassidy & P. R. Shaver (Eds.), *Handbook of attachment: Theory, research, and clinical applications*. New York: Guilford Press.

Alwin, D. F. (1988). From obedience to autonomy: Changes in desired traits in children, 1928–1978. *Public Opinion Quarterly, 52*, 33–52.

Amato, P. R. (2010). Research on divorce: Continuing trends and new developments. *Journal of Marriage and the Family, 72*, 650–666.

Apel, R., & Paternoster, R. (2009). Understanding "criminogenic" corporate culture: What white-collar crime researchers can learn from studies of the adolescent employment–crime relationship. In S. S. Simpson & D. Weisburd (Eds.), *The criminology of white-collar crime* (pp. 15–33). New York: Springer.

Aquilino, W. S. (2006). Family relationships and support systems in emerging adulthood. In J. J. Arnett & J. L. Tanner (Eds.), *Coming of age in the 21st century: The lives and contexts of emerging adults* (pp. 193–217). Washington, DC: American Psychological Association.

Arnett, J. J. (1995a). Adolescents' uses of media for self–socialization. *Journal of Youth and Adolescence, 24*, 519–533.

Arnett, J. J. (1995b). Broad and narrow socialization: The family in the context of a cultural theory. *Journal of Marriage and the Family, 57*, 617–628.

Arnett, J. J. (1998). Learning to stand alone: The contemporary American transition to adulthood in cultural and historical context. *Human Development, 41*, 295–315.

Arnett, J. J. (1999). Adolescent storm and stress, reconsidered. *American Psychologist, 54*, 317–326.

Arnett, J. J. (2000). Emerging adulthood: A theory of development from the late teens through the twenties. *American Psychologist, 55*, 469–480.

Arnett, J. J. (2001). Conceptions of the transition to adulthood: Perspectives from adolescence to midlife. *Journal of Adult Development, 8*, 133–143.

Arnett, J. J. (2003). Conceptions of the transition to adulthood among emerging adults in American ethnic groups. *New Directions in Child and Adolescent Development, 100*, 63–75.

Arnett, J. J. (2004). *Adolescence and emerging adulthood: A cultural approach* (2nd ed.). Upper Saddle River, NJ: Prentice Hall.

Arnett, J. J. (2005). The developmental context of substance use in emerging adulthood. *Journal of Drug Issues, 35*, 235–253.

Arnett, J. J. (2006a). Emerging adulthood: Understanding the new way of coming of age. In J. J. Arnett & J. L. Tanner (Eds.), *Coming of age in the 21st century: The lives and contexts of emerging adults* (pp. 3–19). Washington, DC: American Psychological Association.

Arnett, J. J. (2006b). The psychology of emerging adulthood: What is known, and what remains to be known? In J. J. Arnett & J. L. Tanner (Eds.), *Coming of age in the 21st century: The lives and contexts of emerging adults* (pp. 303–330). Washington, DC: American Psychological Association.

Arnett, J. J. (2011). Emerging adulthood(s): The cultural psychology of a new life stage. In L. A. Jensen (Ed.), *Bridging cultural and developmental psychology: New syntheses in theory, research, and policy* (pp. 255–275). New York: Oxford University Press.

Arnett, J. J. (2014). *Emerging adulthood: The winding road from the late teens through the twenties.* New York: Oxford University Press.

Arnett, J. J., & Schwab, J. (2012). *The Clark University Poll of Emerging Adults: Thriving, struggling, and hopeful.* Worcester, MA: Clark University.

Arnett, J. J., & Schwab, J. (2013). *The Clark University Poll of Parents of Emerging Adults: Moving toward a new equilibrium.* Worcester, MA: Clark University.

Bachman, J. G., Wadsworth, K. N., O'Malley, P. M., Johnston, L. D., & Schulenberg, J. E. (1997). *Smoking, drinking, and drug use in young adulthood: The impacts of new freedoms and new responsibilities.* Mahwah, NJ: Erlbaum.

Barry, C. M., Madsen, S. D., & DeGrace, A. (in press). Friends and peers. In J. J. Arnett (Ed.), *Oxford handbook of emerging adulthood.* New York: Oxford University Press.

Bartle-Haring, S., Brucker, P., & Hock, E. (2002). The impact of parental separation anxiety on identity development in late adolescence and early adulthood. *Journal of Adolescent Research, 17*, 439–450.

Becker, B. E., & Luthar, S. S. (2007). Peer-perceived admiration and social preference: Contextual correlates of positive peer regard among suburban and urban adolescents. *Journal of Research on Adolescence, 17*(1), 117–144.

Bellah, R. N., Madsen, R., Sullivan, W. M., Swidler, A., & Tipton, S. M. (1985). *Habits of the heart: Individualism and commitment in American life.* New York: Harper & Row.

Boon, S. D., & Lemore, C. D. (2001). Admirer–celebrity relationships among young adults: Explaining perceptions of celebrity influence on identity. *Human Communication Research, 27*, 432–465.

Brown, B. B., & Bakken, J. P. (2011). Parenting and peer relationships: Reinvigorating research on family–peer linkages in adolescence. *Journal of Research on Adolescence, 21*(1), 153–165.

Brown, B. B., & Larson, J. (2009). Peer relationships in adolescence. In R. M. Lerner & L. Steinberg (Eds.), *Handbook of adolescent psychology* (Vol. 2, 3rd ed., pp. 74–103). Hoboken, NJ: Wiley.

Brown, J. D. (2006). Emerging adults in a mediated world. In J. J. Arnett & J. L. Tanner (Eds.), *Coming of age in the 21st century: The lives and contexts of emerging adults* (pp. 279–299). Washington, DC: American Psychological Association.

Brown, J. D., Steele, J., & Walsh-Childers, K. (Eds.). (2002). *Sexual teens, sexual media*. Mahwah, NJ: Erlbaum.

Cantor, J. (2000). Violence in films and television. In R. Lee (Ed.), *Encyclopedia of international media and communications*. New York: Academic Press.

Cherlin, A. J., Chase-Lansdale, P. L., & McRae, C. (1998). Effects of parental divorce on mental health throughout the life course. *American Sociological Review, 63*, 239–249.

Clausen, J. A. (1966). *Socialization and society*. Boston: Little, Brown.

Collins, W. A., & van Dulmen, M. (2006). Friendships and romance in emerging adulthood: Assessing distinctiveness in close relationships. In J. J. Arnett & J. L. Tanner (Eds.), *Coming of age in the 21st century: The lives and contexts of emerging adults* (pp. 219–234). Washington, DC: American Psychological Association.

Conger, R., & Conger, K. (2002). Resilience in midwestern families: Selected findings from the first decade of a prospective, longitudinal study. *Journal of Marriage and Family, 64*, 361–373.

Conger, R., Cui, M., Bryant, C., & Elder, G. (2000). Competence in early adult romantic relationships: A developmental perspective on family influences. *Journal of Personality and Social Psychology, 79*, 224–237.

Cooper, C. R., & Ayers-Lopez, S. (1985). Family and peer systems in early adolescence: New models of the role of relationships in development. *Journal of Early Adolescence, 5*, 9–22.

Côté, J. (2000). *Arrested adulthood: The changing nature of maturity and identity in the late modern world*. New York: New York University Press.

Côté, J. (2006). Emerging adulthood as an institutionalized moratorium: Risks and benefits to identity formation. In J. J. Arnett & J. L. Tanner (Eds.), *Coming of age in the 21st century: The lives and contexts of emerging adults* (pp. 85–116). Washington, DC: American Psychological Association.

Cui, M., Fincham, F. D., & Pasley, K. B. (2008). Young adults' romantic relationships: The role of parents' marital problems and relationship efficacy. *Personal and Social Psychology Bulletin, 34*, 1226–1235.

De Goede, I. H. A., Branje, S. J. T., Delsing, M. J. M. H., & Meeus, W. H. J. (2009). Linkages over time between adolescents' relationships with parents and friends. *Journal of Youth and Adolescence, 38*(10), 1304–1315.

Dubas, J. S., & Petersen, A. C. (1996). Geographical distance from parents and adjustment during adolescence and young adulthood. *New Directions for Child Development, 71*, 3–19.

Erikson, E. H. (1950). *Childhood and society*. New York: Norton.

Erikson, E. H. (1968). *Identity: Youth and crisis*. New York: Norton.

Feldman, S., Gowen, L., & Fisher, L. (1998). Family relationships and gender as predictors of romantic intimacy in young adults: A longitudinal study. *Journal of Research on Adolescence, 8*, 263–286.

Fingerman, K. L. (2000). "We had a nice little chat": Age and generational differences in mothers' and daughters' descriptions of enjoyable visits. *Journal of Gerontology, 55B*, 95–106.

Flammer, A., & Alsaker, F. D. (2001). Adolescents in school. In L. Goossens & S. Jackson (Eds.), *Handbook of adolescent development: European perspectives*. Hove, UK: Psychology Press.

Grusec, J. (2002). Parental socialization and children's acquisition of values. In M. Bornstein (Ed.), *Handbook of parenting* (pp. 143–168). Mahwah, NJ: Erlbaum.

Hamilton, S. F., & Hamilton, M. A. (2006). School, work, and emerging adulthood. In J. J. Arnett & J. L. Tanner (Eds.), *Coming of age in the 21st century: The lives and contexts of emerging adults* (pp. 257–277). Washington, DC: American Psychological Association.

Hamm, J. V. (2000). Do birds of a feather flock together?: The variable bases for African American, Asian American, and European American adolescents' selection of similar friends. *Developmental Psychology, 36*, 209–219.

Hatfield, E., & Rapson, R. L. (2006). *Love and sex: Cross-cultural perspectives*. Boston: Allyn & Bacon.

Heinz, W. R. (2002). Self-socialization and post-traditional society. *Advances in Life Course Research, 7*, 41–64.

Huesmann, L. R., Moise-Titus, J., Podolski, C., & Eron, L. D. (2003). Longitudinal relations between children's exposure to TV violence and their aggressiveness in young adulthood. *Developmental Psychology, 39*, 201–221.

Jacquet, S., & Surra, C. (2001). Parental divorce and premarital couples: Commitment and other relationship characteristics. *Journal of Marriage and the Family, 63*, 627–638.

Keniston, K. (1971). *Youth and dissent: The rise of a new opposition.* New York: Harcourt Brace Jovanovich.

Labouvie-Vief, G. (2006). Emerging structures of adult thought. In J. J. Arnett & J. L. Tanner (Eds.), *Coming of age in the 21st century: The lives and contexts of emerging adults* (pp. 59–84). Washington, DC: American Psychological Association.

Larson, R., & Richards, M. H. (1994). *Divergent realities: The emotional lives of mothers, fathers, and adolescents.* New York: Basic Books.

Larson, R., & Richards, M. H. (1998). Waiting for the weekend: Friday and Saturday nights as the emotional climax of the week. *New Directions for Child and Adolescent Development, 82*, 37–52.

Larson, R. W., Richards, M. H., Moneta, G., Holmbeck, G., & Duckett, E. (1996). Changes in adolescents' daily interactions with their families from ages 10 to 18: Disengagement and transformation. *Developmental Psychology, 32*, 744–754.

Laumann-Billings, L., & Emery, R. E. (2000). Distress among young adults from divorced families. *Journal of Family Psychology, 14*, 671–687.

Lefkowitz, E. S., & Gillen, M. M. (2006). "Sex is just a normal part of life": Sexuality in emerging adulthood. In J. J. Arnett & J. L. Tanner (Eds.), *Coming of age in the 21st century: The lives and contexts of emerging adults* (pp. 235–255). Washington, DC: American Psychological Association.

Levinson, D. J. (1978). *The seasons of a man's life.* New York: Ballantine.

Luong, G., Charles, S. T., & Fingerman, K. L. (2008). Better with age: Social relationships across adulthood. *Journal of Social and Personal Relationships, 23*, 9–28.

Masten, A. S., Obradovic, J., & Burt, K. B. (2006). Resilience in emerging adulthood. In J. J. Arnett & J. L. Tanner (Eds.), *Coming of age in the 21st century: The lives and contexts of emerging adults* (pp. 173–190). Washington, DC: American Psychological Association.

Maxwell, K. A. (2002). Friends: The role of peer influence across adolescent risk behaviors. *Journal of Youth and Adolescence, 31*, 267–277.

Mayer, K. U. (2004). Whose lives?: How history, societies, and institutions define and shape life courses. *Research in Human Development, 1*, 161–187.

Mills, M. (2007). *Individualization and the life course: Towards a theoretical model and empirical evidence.* Toronto: Palgrave Macmillan.

Mortimer, J. T. (2003). *Working and growing up in America.* Cambridge, MA: Harvard University Press.

National Center for Education Statistics. (2012). *The condition of education, 2012.* Washington, DC: U.S. Department of Education.

Nelson, L. J. (in press). Conceptions of adulthood. In J. J. Arnett (Ed.), *Oxford handbook of emerging adulthood.* New York: Oxford University Press.

Nelson, L. J., Badger, S., & Wu, B. (2004). The influence of culture in emerging adulthood: Perspectives of Chinese college students. *International Journal of Behavioral Development, 28*, 26–36.

Pardini, D. A. (2010). Novel insights into longstanding theories of bidirectional parent–child influences: Introduction to the special issue. *Journal of Abnormal Child Psychology, 36*, 627–631.

Plomin, R. (2009). The nature of nurture. In K. McCartney & R. A. Weinberg (Eds.), *Experience and development: A festschrift in honor of Sandra Wood Scarr* (pp. 61–80). New York: Psychology Press.

Reifman, A., Arnett, J. J., & Colwell, M. J. (2006). *The IDEA: Inventory of Dimensions of Emerging Adulthood*. Manuscript submitted for publication.

Reiss, D., Neiderhiser, J., Hetherington, E. M., & Plomin, R. (2000). *The relationship code: Deciphering genetic and social influences on adolescent development*. Cambridge, MA: Harvard University Press.

Roisman, G. I., Masten, A. S., Coatsworth, J. D., & Tellegen, A. (2004). Salient and emerging developmental tasks in the transition to adulthood. *Child Development, 75*, 1–11.

Ruggiero, M., Greenberg, E., & Steinberg, L. (1982). Occupational deviance among first-time workers. *Youth and Society, 13*, 423–448.

Scarr, S. (1993). Biological and cultural diversity: The legacy of Darwin for development. *Child Development, 64*, 1333–1353.

Scarr, S., & McCartney, K. (1983). How people make their own environments. *Child Development, 54*, 424–435.

Schlegel, A., & Barry, H. (1991). *Adolescence: An anthropological inquiry*. New York: Free Press.

Schneider, B., & Stevenson, D. (1999). *The ambitious generation: America's teenagers, motivated but directionless*. New Haven, CT: Yale University Press.

Schulenberg, J. E., & Zarrett, N. R. (2006). Mental health in emerging adulthood: Continuity and discontinuity in courses, causes, and functions. In J. J. Arnett & J. L. Tanner (Eds.), *Coming of age in the 21st century: The lives and contexts of emerging adults* (pp. 135–172). Washington, DC: American Psychological Association.

Staff, J., Schulenberg, J. E., & Bachman, J. G. (2010). Adolescent work intensity, school performance, and academic engagement. *Sociology of Education, 83*(3), 183–200.

Steele, J. R., & Brown, J. D. (1995). Adolescent room culture: Studying media in the context of everyday life. *Journal of Youth and Adolescence, 24*, 551–576.

Summers, P., Forehand, R., Armistead, L., & Tannenbaum, L. (1998). Parental divorce during early adolescence in Caucasian families: The role of family process variables in predicting the long-term consequences for early adult psychosocial adjustment. *Journal of Consulting and Clinical Psychology, 66*, 327–336.

Toomey, E., & Nelson, E. (2001). Family conflict and young adults' attitudes toward intimacy. *Journal of Divorce and Remarriage, 34*, 49–69.

United Nations. (2009). *World fertility report, 2009: Country profiles*. Department of Economic and Social Affairs, Population Division. Retrieved from *www.un.org/esa/population/publications/wfr2009_web/data/countryprofiles_wfr2009.pdf*.

van Wel, F., Linssen, H., & Ruud, A. (2000). The parental bond and the well-being of adolescents and young adults. *Journal of Youth and Adolescence, 29*, 307–318.

Waite, L. J., & Gallagher, M. (2000). *The case for marriage: Why married people are happier, healthier, and better off financially*. New York: Doubleday.

Ward, L. M., Gorvine, B., & Cytron-Walker, A. (2002). Would that really happen?: Adolescents' perceptions of sexual relationships according to prime-time television. In J. D. Brown, J. R. Steele, & K. Walsh-Childers (Eds.), *Sexual teens, sexual media: Investigating media's influence on adolescent sexuality* (pp. 95–123). Mahwah, NJ: Erlbaum.

Wilson, W. J. (1996). *When work disappears: The world of the new urban poor*. New York: Knopf.

Wintre, M., & Yaffe, M. (2000). First-year students' adjustment to university life as a function of relationships with parents. *Journal of Adolescent Research, 15*, 9–37.

Youniss, J., & Smollar, J. (1985). *Adolescent relations with mothers, fathers, and friends*. Chicago: University of Chicago Press.

The Multifaceted Nature
of Late-Life Socialization
Older Adults as Agents and Targets of Socialization

Gloria Luong
Antje Rauers
Karen L. Fingerman

Old age is a unique period in life. Individuals enter old age with the knowledge that most of their years of life, although not necessarily their best years, have passed. "Old age" is not a unified stage of life, but scholars generally demarcate the start of this period at around 60 to 65 years of age and lasting until the end of life. Adults often experience relatively good health and active engagement during the early period of old age (young old age, 60–75 years) followed by accumulated health problems and social losses toward the end of life (oldest old age, older than 85 years (P. B. Baltes, 1997; Smith, Borchelt, Maier, & Jopp, 2002). Thus, in later life, although there may be continuity and growth in areas of prior strength, older adults may also have to navigate biological and social changes and detriments. The need to adapt to these positive and negative changes, as well as the accumulation of life experiences, make socialization in older age distinct from socialization in other phases of life.

During childhood and adolescence, individuals are often the targets of socialization by their parents and peers (e.g., Smetana, Campione-Barr, & Metzger, 2006). Socialization in early life is often future-oriented and focused on preparing youth to manage the tasks of social life in adulthood (Bugental & Grusec, 2006). For example, children are encouraged to acquire social skills and competence (Connell & Prinz, 2002), to develop an understanding of appropriate moral and social behavior (e.g., Smetana, 2006), and to form social bonds (e.g., Rubin, Bukowski, & Parker, 2006). From young adulthood through later life, individuals continue to build and maintain important social relationships, often by forming marital bonds or enduring romantic partnerships and raising children, and they may, in turn, become agents of socialization themselves. Socialization differs from that in other periods of life because the time perspective of socialization in old age is multifaceted. Older adults are concerned not only with the future but also with their past, and with present adaptation to challenges and gains. In addition, older adults serve as both targets and agents of socialization; that is, from childhood through later life, individuals continue to be socialized and shaped by their social environments. Moreover, after decades of serving as parents, grandparents, or mentors, older adults have likely acquired a view of themselves as socialization agents as well.

Gerontological studies suggest that social partners and cultural institutions influence the aging process, but studies are not framed in terms of socialization per se. Thus, in this chapter, we draw on scholarship in related topics to develop an understanding of socialization in old age. Our definition of *socialization* involves processes through which individuals internalize experiences from their social world in ways that alter their behavior, beliefs, health, and emotions. In this chapter, we first review how the challenges and gains in later life influence motivational goals and strivings that in turn shape *individual agency* (i.e., the extent to which individuals influence their own development). We discuss how older adults exercise their own individual agency to influence how and by whom they are socialized. Next, we review the major agents involved in socializing older adults: their social partners and the broader culture and society. We discuss how each of these agents influences older adults' behaviors, beliefs, emotions, and physical and cognitive health. Following that, we turn to the role of older adults as the agents of socialization in their social networks and review how older adults influence their social partners and subsequent generations (e.g., grandchildren). We conclude by summarizing the state of the literature and provide recommendations for future directions.

Individual Agency and Socialization in Later Life

First, we consider how individual agency shapes socialization in later life. For example, in earlier life, individuals may be more constrained in selecting their social environments. Children are subjected to the schools, communities, and neighborhoods that their parents choose for them and are generally limited to the social partners they encounter in these contexts. During adolescence, although decision-making opportunities generally increase and adolescents have greater control over the selection of their peer groups and friends, they may still have relatively little control over their specific school environments (e.g., they may be restricted to schools within their district; Barber & Olsen, 2004).

Across adulthood, however, individuals become increasingly responsible for their own socialization. Beginning in emerging adulthood in Western cultures, individuals are expected to make decisions and guide the course of their own development. Accordingly, Arnett (2001) found that Americans between ages 13 and 55 years viewed the onset of adulthood as involving responsibility for one's actions, deciding on one's beliefs and values, establishing an equal relationship with parents, and becoming financially independent. These shifts persist throughout adulthood, such that individuals attempt to shape their own behavior and adaptations to the aging process (e.g., Lerner, 2002).

One of the leading theories of adult development relevant to socialization pertains to how adults seek control over their lives (Heckhausen, Wrosch, & Schulz, 2010). Researchers distinguish between *primary control* (behavioral attempts to influence external circumstances) and *secondary control* (behavioral and cognitive responses to regulate internal experiences). Primary control increases dramatically throughout childhood and adolescence until midlife. In later life, primary control generally decreases due to limitations associated with physical health problems, disability, and cognitive decline, while reliance on secondary control increases. Despite these changes, however, older adults can still influence their social environments. Thus, individuals select and create environments that fit with their motivational goals and developmental needs and as a result may directly and indirectly shape how and by whom they become socialized across adulthood. Both theories of control and theories of social relationships suggest that older adults effectively regulate the social world to meet their needs.

Indeed, according to socioemotional selectivity theory (Carstensen, Isaacowitz, & Charles, 1999), older adults shape their interpersonal environments by maintaining ties with close social partners and limiting exposure to less meaningful ties. The theory posits that individuals prioritize different motivational goals as a function of their time perspective. When they perceive that their future is open-ended and expansive, as is generally true for healthy younger adults, they may focus on future-oriented goals, such as seeking information or making novel social connections. As their future time perspective becomes diminished, as in later life, however, individuals may shift their priorities to more present-oriented goals, such as finding emotional meaning and deriving satisfaction from their social partners. Thus, older adults may be especially motivated to restructure their social networks to retain emotionally meaningful ties to make the most of their remaining time. In fact, a recent meta-analysis confirmed that although older adults' social networks tend to be smaller than those of their younger counterparts, much of this decrease is associated with a reduction in the number of less close friends and acquaintances (Wrzus, Hänel, Wagner, & Neyer, 2013). In other words, older adults' networks comprise a larger proportion of emotionally close ties to those whom they have known for a longer duration (Antonucci, Birditt, & Ajrouch, 2010).

The available evidence suggests that the changes in network composition are largely due to individual agency, such that older adults play an active role in constructing their social environments. For example, when presented with hypothetical situations regarding a foreshortened future time perspective, such as situations in which one will be moving across the country alone and be out of contact with loved ones, younger individuals make similar social choices as older adults: They prefer to spend their remaining free time with close social partners rather than meeting new people (Fredrickson & Carstensen, 1990). In other words, manipulating one's time perspective to be shorter, in line with that of older adults, leads to social preferences that are consistent with those observed in later life. These findings suggest that age differences in social network composition are deliberate choices shaped by individual agency and future time perspective. That is, it is not merely a coincidence that older adults' social networks consist primarily of emotionally close ties; diminishing time perspective in later life shapes older adults' proactive choices to retain ties with close social partners and to reduce the effort they invest in less meaningful relationships (e.g., acquaintances). In further support of this interpretation, another study examined social network changes of older adults between 70 and 103 years of age (Lang, 2000). Older adults were asked to name all the individuals in their social networks at the beginning of the study and again 4 years later. Most of the changes in networks reflected the loss of peripheral ties rather than the loss of emotionally close, rewarding ties. Furthermore, in the cases in which a social partner was named at the baseline assessment but was omitted from the network at the second assessment, participants indicated why those social partners were no longer part of the network. Older adults reported that they deliberately chose to end the relationship with most omitted network partners (as opposed to other, nondeliberate reasons such as death). Specifically, older adults were more likely to end deliberately (or consciously allow to languish) relationships with non-kin and less close social partners. Thus, it appears that older adults actively mold their social network composition to fit their motivational goals and needs, in line with predictions from socioemotional selectivity theory (Lang, 2004).

Older adults' selective culling of their social partners suggests they are adept at optimizing emotional well-being within their social networks—a skill they have presumably learned across a lifetime of experiences (e.g., Charles, 2010). For example, compared to younger adults, older adults focus more on diagnostic information about moral behaviors (e.g., dishonesty) when evaluating prospective social partners (Hess & Kotter-Grühn, 2011). Older adults are therefore better at identifying social characteristics that might have important emotional consequences (e.g., that dishonest individuals would be vexing social partners).

Older adults have also learned how to manage social conflict effectively when it arises in the relationship. In general, for example, older adults prefer to avoid conflict with social partners or let the situation pass when another person does something annoying (e.g., Birditt & Fingerman, 2003). These conflict-avoidant strategies are deemed to be among the most effective ways of dealing with difficult interpersonal situations (Blanchard-Fields, Mienaltowski, & Seay, 2007). Furthermore, older adults also report less negative emotional reactivity as a result of avoiding conflict than do their younger counterparts (Charles, Piazza, Luong, & Almeida, 2009). Thus, when older adults avoid conflict, they also avoid getting upset.

In summary, older adults' ties are not part of their social networks by accident. Older adults selectively reduce contact with less-close social partners and continue to foster positive relations with people they consider to be emotionally close (Lang, 2000). As a result of this social selection, older adults reap benefits by influencing their socialization processes, particularly with respect to emotional well-being: By maintaining ties with close social partners, older adults surround themselves with individuals from whom they derive satisfaction and support. Indeed, older adults generally report being more satisfied with their social interactions and closer to their social partners than do younger individuals (see review by Luong, Charles, & Fingerman, 2011). Additionally, when conflicts do arise in their social relationships, older adults appraise these situations as less stressful than do younger individuals (Birditt, Fingerman, & Almeida, 2005). Thus, older adults effectively exercise individual agency to shape how and by whom they are socialized. In the following section, we discuss how agents of socialization—specifically, social partners, culture, and society—influence older adults' behaviors, beliefs, health, and emotions.

Agents of Socialization

Social Partners

As outlined earlier, close relationships become increasingly important in old age. The configuration of close social partners, however, is variable in late life. Some individuals enter old age married, with offspring and grandchildren; other individuals are embedded in a circle of friends; and still others are widowed and connected to siblings. Other patterns of relationships are also possible. As may be typical throughout adulthood, older individuals who are married typically list their spouse as their closest social partner, widowed older adults list a child, and never-married older adults may list a close friend (DePaulo & Morris, 2005; Fingerman, 2001). Systems of compensation and substitution allow older people who lack a given social partner (e.g., a grown child) to derive benefits from a different type of social partner (e.g., a church member; Chatters, Taylor, Lincoln, & Schroepfer, 2002). Of course, older adults also interact with people who are not emotionally close. They talk with health care personnel, live near neighbors, and interact with acquaintances through religious or community gatherings (Fingerman, 2004a, 2009).

The influence social partners have in later life unfolds in the context of the lifetime of experiences that precede this period. An account of socialization in old age needs to acknowledge that older adults' present and past socialization experiences are closely related: (1) Past relationship experiences may continue to influence individuals during their late years, and (2) interactions with current relationship partners can influence the way older adults construe their past, thus reshaping their life story and identity.

Past Influences on the Present

Past relationship experiences may continue to affect late-life adaptation. Such processes might be considered delayed effects of socialization partners. Older adults' close relationships may be distinct from close relationships involving younger people due to two features: (1) The relationships may have lasted for decades, and (2) the social partners may have infrequent contact. Family members and friends may have known the older adult for half a century or more. Older adults may have little contact with these social partners, however, particularly if they reside far away. Nonetheless, individuals who have been in relationships for decades may not require repeated interactions to retain strong ties. The prolonged nature of these relationships may permit socialization influences in late life, even in the absence of direct contact. For example, Fingerman and Griffiths (1999) examined adults' subjective interpretations of the holiday cards they received in December and January. Participants completed a survey for each card they received. Many older adults exchanged holiday greetings with people they had not seen in decades. From the perspective of a younger adult, these liaisons might not truly qualify as *relationships*. They do not provide interaction, emotional connection, or resources. Yet older adults reported that these relationships meant a great deal to them as connections to their personal past because, for example, they involved a last remaining relative from their youth, a college roommate, or a neighbor from a long-time residence.

Social partners with whom older adults no longer visit or communicate may continue to influence their decisions and beliefs, thus socializing them without direct engagement. Studies have not examined this issue empirically, but in situations in which older adults must apply values or make decisions, it would be worth investigating the extent to which they think about the viewpoints of social partners whom they no longer encounter on a daily basis. It is easy to imagine an older adult who considers social partners who are deceased: "How would my mother handle this situation?" or "What would my late husband have done?" Therefore, the scope of socialization agents in late life may be different than that in early life.

Theoretical work has also proposed going back even further by considering delayed effects of primary social experiences for late-life development. Theorists argue that early attachment (i.e., between parents and infants) may carry over into an individual's subsequent romantic relationship patterns (e.g., Hazan & Shaver, 1994; Shaver, Belsky, & Brennan, 2000). Similarly, it has been theorized that such early experiences may continue to shape late-life adaptation (e.g., Magai, Consedine, Gillespie, O'Neal, & Vilker, 2004). This literature suggests that social and emotional styles in old age have their roots in much earlier socialization. Empirical evidence for direct socialization effects from infancy to old age, however, is scant. Researchers have not examined infant attachment patterns and subsequent adaptation in old age longitudinally and must therefore rely on retrospective memories of relationships. Thus, it is not entirely clear whether presumed early effects reflect memories tainted by present circumstances or accurate portraits of the past. For example, in one study (Carpenter, 2001), adults' memories of relationships with parents in childhood shaped their relationships with those parents in old age; the ways in which adults cared for their parents in old age were associated with their earlier memories of how their parents treated them. In another study, memories of the relationship quality with one's parents during childhood were associated with daily psychological distress and emotional reactivity to stressors among adults between 25 and 74 years of age (Mallers, Charles, Neupert, & Almeida, 2010).

Other early life social experiences may also influence later life outcomes. For example, in an eight-decade longitudinal study, participants' lives were tracked from childhood onward (Friedman & Martin, 2012). Individuals whose parents divorced during childhood had greater mortality risk than individuals from intact families. Interestingly, the effect of parental divorce was partly explained by the fact that children from divorced families were more likely to become divorced themselves and engage in unhealthy behaviors as adults. In addition to relationships, sociologists who study life course theory have examined other early life precursors to patterns of adaptation in later life (for a review, see Elder, 1998). For example, the experience of economic hardships during the Great Depression as a young adult may differ depending on one's socioeconomic status at the time, and these experiences in turn, may uniquely influence later life emotional health and intellectual abilities (Elder & Liker, 1982).

Present Influences on the Past

Social relationships in old age may also change the way older adults see their past, which in turn shapes their identities. People reminisce about past experiences in their conversations with others, which may help them make sense of their own life stories and improve identity coherence (McLean, Pasupathi, & Pals, 2007). Importantly, both autobiographical stories and the memories to which they pertain are highly malleable. During collaborative reminiscing, the listener may contribute additions, opinions, and evaluations. The listener may further respond with particular interest to the story or individual aspects of it, which influences how the speaker (re)tells the story. This dynamic may also shape the speaker's own memory of the event. Social partners can therefore contribute to older adults' past and present identity by co-narrating their lives. These collaboratively generated construals may subsequently influence older adults' current and future behaviors, emotions, and beliefs (Pasupathi, 2001).

In summary, socialization in late life occurs after a lifetime of experiences, and older adults' perceptions of past and present experiences may mutually influence each other. In terms of delayed effects of socialization, past relationships with others may continue to influence socialization in old age. Current social partners may also influence older adults' construals of their personal past, thereby shaping their identities.

Interpersonal Dynamics: How Social Partners Socialize Older Adults

Socialization partners' interactions with older adults differ from interactions with younger recipients of socialization, and these patterns may shape socialization processes in old age. One important dynamic in this regard is outlined by the social input model (Fingerman & Charles, 2010). According to this model, social partners are motivated to treat older adults more kindly, avoid conflicts with them, and more easily forgive them for social transgressions. This implies that the input provided by socialization partners may differ depending on the age of the recipient. Building on propositions of socioemotional selectivity theory (Carstensen et al., 1999), the social input model posits that people become more aware of limited time horizons when age is made salient. Perceiving that the remaining time with the older adult is limited may also motivate social partners to avoid conflicts (e.g., negotiations about mutually acceptable behavior) and instead focus on more proximal emotional rewards (e.g., spending a harmonious afternoon together). People may also be more inclined to forgive if perceived lifetime is limited (Allemand, 2008). Furthermore, in some situations, social partners may behave in ways that are infantilizing rather than treat the older adult as an equal social partner with whom they can disagree. Similarly, at times social partners may avoid conflict with an older adult because they view him or her as stubborn or unchangeable. Thus, not all conflict avoidance is steeped in positive sentiments about the older adult. Nonetheless, not only are older adults motivated to avoid conflicts with their social partners, but their social partners may also be less likely to initiate conflict with older adults.

In one study, middle-aged daughters privately reported a situation in which they were irritated with their mother (Fingerman, 2003). Afterwards, daughters and their aging mothers were brought together and asked to discuss an irritating situation in their relationship. In their mothers' presence, over one-third of all daughters stated that they did not remember any irritating situation with their mothers, even though they had previously recalled such an event when interviewed alone. Thus, adult daughters may be creating more benign social environments for their aging mothers by avoiding topics of conflict in their relationship. This effect is not constrained to family ties. In another study, younger and older adult participants were asked how they would respond if their closest younger and older social partners said something hurtful to them (Fingerman, Miller, & Charles, 2008). Respondents more likely reported that they would use confrontational and direct behavior if the target was young. The study also included an experimental manipulation to attempt to understand reasons for these age differences, and sense of time remaining with the social partner partially explained why people provide preferential treatment toward older adults. Likewise, in another study, people were more likely to assume that an offended person would be forgiving of a social transgression if the transgressor was described as an older adult (vs. a younger adult; Miller, Charles, & Fingerman, 2009). In summary, people are less likely to engage in confrontational behavior with older adults and more likely to forgive an older person in the face of social *faux pas*.

However, the social input model outlines a second factor that may contribute to more lenient behaviors toward older adults, namely, stereotypes of aging. Negative aging stereotypes can directly influence social partners' behaviors and attitudes. For instance, social partners may attribute older adults' behaviors to aging-related deficiencies instead of intentional transgressions. These appraisals, in turn, evoke more sympathetic and forgiving responses toward older adults' transgressions and may reduce the likelihood of negative feedback. These effects were demonstrated in a study in which participants were presented with an ambiguous story about either a younger or older woman leaving a store without paying for a hat (Erber, Szuchman, & Prager, 2001). Participants were more likely to believe that the younger protagonist in the story intentionally stole the hat, whereas the older protagonist simply forgot to pay for the hat, and thereby endorsed harsher punishment for the younger than older woman. In these studies of hypothetical transgressions by younger and older close social partners, the participants rated the degree to which they believed these individuals could change their behaviors. Compared to their younger counterparts, older transgressors were viewed as being less culpable for their negative behaviors. Furthermore, ascribed blame was associated with the degree to which participants endorsed confronting the transgressor (Fingerman et al., 2008; Miller et al., 2009). Therefore, conflict avoidance vis-à-vis older adults may also be based on the perception that older transgressors cannot be blamed for their behaviors because they are difficult to change.

These studies suggest that participants' attributions about the targets' intentions were informed by aging stereotypes (e.g., not criminal, but forgetful) that led them to judge older targets' behaviors more leniently. Moreover, these more benign judgments resulted in preferential treatment for older adults. Concerning socialization processes in old age, the tenets outlined by the social input model suggest that both familiar and unfamiliar interaction partners are less likely to provide older as opposed to younger adults with negative feedback regarding their potentially inadequate behaviors. These dynamics may involve emotional benefits for social interactions, but potential drawbacks are also conceivable. For instance, one's reluctance to comment on a social transgression committed by an older adult may also imply a missed opportunity to encourage positive or adaptive changes.

Another factor contributing to this dynamic may be that socialization agents in late life tend to have known the older adult for many years. Many individuals who influence older adults' behaviors, emotions, and beliefs may themselves have been socialized *by* these older adults (e.g., a son or daughter). This factor may further reduce the need for controversial or negative feedback that social partners provide to older adults. Alternatively, after years of interactions, members of younger generations may have accepted older adults' flaws and difficult behaviors, and cease to engage in efforts to change them. Due to the mutual long-term influence between socialization agents and socialization targets over the years, older adults may often be provided with input that is already quite in line with their current behaviors or beliefs. In contrast, younger adults frequently interact with diverse peripheral social partners, who may challenge their current behaviors and beliefs.

In summary, the social input model proposes that older adults receive more positive input and more lenient feedback after social transgressions than do younger adults. In fact, older adults' social partners may even avoid pointing out or drawing attention to older adults' negative behaviors to avoid conflict situations. This effect may be additionally supported by the fact that older adults' interactions focus on long-term friendships and family members, with whom they have already negotiated values, beliefs, or social behaviors in earlier years, or who have come to accept the older adults' flaws. More empirical support is needed to test whether older adults' social partners may perceive efforts to socialize them to change long-standing behaviors as futile, and this may be an additional reason why social partners avoid conflict with older adults (e.g., Fingerman et al., 2008; Miller et al., 2009). Nevertheless, social ties continue to shape development well into old age. Although social partners may have good intentions when avoiding conflict with older adults, these behaviors could be interpreted in negative ways by older adults (e.g., as infantilizing behaviors). In the next section, we describe in greater detail how social partners may both positively and negatively influence older adults in the important domains of health and cognition, with crucial implications for late-life developmental challenges.

Important Domains of Influence: Health and Cognition

In late life, social contacts continue to shape ontogeny in multiple domains. In the following sections, we focus on two domains that are of particular importance in old age: physical health and cognitive functioning. In both domains, aging-related losses potentially threaten older adults' independence and quality of living. However, late-life trajectories in both health and cognition substantially differ between persons (Hertzog, 2008; Kern & Friedman, 2011). Research suggests that some of these individual differences are related to variation in social environments. Health and cognition trajectories may therefore be susceptible to the socializing influence of social partners.

Health

Both the quality and the quantity of social relationships appear to have important implications for health and mortality. Having a variety of social partners is related to better health-related behaviors, functional health, and mortality (Holt-Lunstad, Smith, & Layton, 2010; House, 2001; Thomas, 2012). The literature suggests, however, that loneliness and social isolation are particularly pernicious for poor cognitive, psychological, and physical health outcomes, more so than the social network composition (Antonucci et al., 2002; Cacioppo, Hawkley, & Thisted, 2010). Theorists have argued that these effects may be even more pronounced in late life, when physiological resilience decreases (Hawkley & Cacioppo, 2007). In one study, for example, younger and older lonely and not lonely adults were subjected to a social evaluative threat in the laboratory (Ong, Rothstein, & Uchino, 2012). The lonely older adults showed the steepest systolic blood pressure reactivity to the stressor, and more delayed systolic blood pressure recovery, compared to the other groups. These findings suggest that social isolation and loneliness may place older adults at greater physiological risk in the presence of stressors, which in turn negatively influences physical health processes.

Some researchers have suggested that social isolation represents a chronic stressor that places older adults at greater risk of experiencing heightened physiological reactivity to acute stressors (e.g., Charles, 2010). Another important factor explaining these links may be that socially isolated individuals lack social support, which in turn is related to various biological outcomes, such as poorer cardiovascular, neuroendocrine, or immune function (Uchino, 2006). A meta-analysis by Holt-Lunstad and colleagues (2010) has shown, for example, that social support is associated with a 50% lower mortality risk across numerous major diseases. Relatedly, older adults may derive social support benefits to their health via social partners' provision of health-related information. For example, studies suggest that older adults turn to close sons and daughters for information about health care (Fingerman, Hay, Kamp Dush, Cichy, & Hosterman, 2007). Social partners may also support older adults' efforts to engage in positive health-related behaviors, such as eating well, exercising, or complying with medical treatments (DiMatteo, 2004; Lewis & Rook, 1999).

Theoretical models also suggest that psychological processes may explain the association between social support and health and mortality. It is possible, for example, that social partners contribute to psychological and emotional well-being, which in turn improves older adults' health. Indeed, researchers have found links between engaging with diverse social partners in late life (i.e., with close and peripheral social partners) and better psychological well-being (Litwin & Stoeckel, in press). A recent empirical review, however, shows that the association between social support and physiological health is tenuously explained, if at all, by psychological mechanisms, such as emotional well-being (Uchino, Bowen, Carlisle, & Birmingham, 2012). More studies are needed to determine whether these inconclusive results are due to the current limitations in the literature of study design and statistical analyses, or whether theoretical models regarding how socialization influences physical health processes need revision.

As in any life phase, however, social relationships can also have negative effects on emotional adjustment, health-related behaviors, and physical health. For example, social partners can serve as a bad example via unhealthy diets and sedentary lifestyles. Furthermore, social partners may contribute to psychological stressors by eliciting ambivalent or negative emotions. Ambivalent or conflict-ridden relationships can have negative effects for late-life adjustment and health (Rook, Luong, Sorkin, Newsom, & Krause, 2012). For example, ambivalent social relationships, which comprise both positive and negative facets, are associated with shorter telomere length (Uchino, Cawthon, et al., 2012). Telomeres are similar to "caps" on the ends of chromosomes that become truncated with cell division. If telomere lengths become too short, the cell enters replicative senescence (i.e., stops dividing), which is why telomere length is sometimes considered a marker of cellular aging (Codd et al., 2013). Hence, apart from the sheer quantity of social contacts or social support, the quality of older adults' social contacts additionally shapes late-life development (Uchino, 2006).

Cognition

The social environment may also facilitate behaviors that promote favorable cognitive functioning in late life. Engaging in intellectually stimulating activities may protect against aging-related cognitive declines (Hertzog, Kramer, Wilson, & Lindenberger, 2008), and one's social environment can encourage the pursuit of such activities. For example, older adults may be more motivated to attend a local debating club if a close social partner joins them. Indeed, research has established that engaging in a socially active lifestyle is associated with better cognitive functioning in late adulthood, although the causal links may be bidirectional, with lifestyle influencing cognition, and vice versa (Small, Dixon, McArdle, & Grimm, 2012). Research also indicates that everyday collaborations with others may allow older adults to mitigate the detrimental effects of aging-related cognitive losses on everyday functioning (Martin & Wight, 2008). For example, older adults collaborate with close others to recall past events, or to make sure that they remember future appointments (Dixon, Rust, Feltmate, & See, 2007).

As outlined earlier, older adults spend much of their time with close individuals whom they have known for years. Some research suggests that close social partners may offer particular benefits for everyday collaborations. Apart from the emotional gains when spending time with a loved one, collaborating with a familiar individual may conserve cognitive resources, which becomes increasingly important as people age. Navigating a social interaction is cognitively demanding, but these demands can be reduced if the partners know each other. This familiarity effect promotes successful collaborations and has been shown especially to support individuals with low cognitive resources (Rauers, Riediger, Schmiedek, & Lindenberger, 2011). This potential benefit (for individuals with limited resources at their disposal) may, however, also imply disadvantages. Relying on established interaction patterns with a limited number of close individuals is less challenging than adjusting to various social partners, but may involve missed opportunities for cognitive stimulation, which could be detrimental in the long run.

In summary, social networks provide opportunities to remain active in late life, which benefits cognitive development. Collaborating with others, particularly with close social partners, may also offer a means to overcome individual cognitive limitations and to maintain one's level of functioning in spite of aging-related constraints. However, relying on others also has its caveats. It may increase interpersonal dependency and counteract the important developmental task of preserving one's autonomy in spite of losses in later life (M. M. Baltes & Horgas, 1997; Gardner & Helmes, 2006).

Socialization partners may even reinforce older adults' dependency by behaving in ways that convey age-related beliefs or stereotypes. Most aging stereotypes tend to emphasize negative characteristics (e.g., slow, absentminded, or incompetent; Kite, Stockdale, Whitley, & Johnson, 2005). Younger adults who perceive older people to be frail tend to engage in overhelping, patronizing behaviors (e.g., patting or winking) or "elderspeak" (i.e., talking more slowly, exaggerating individual words, and using shorter and less complex sentences or a patronizing tone; Hess, 2006). Importantly, this alleged adjustment to the older adults' assumed frailness is typically not supportive. Instead, it communicates to older adults that they are perceived as incompetent.

Indeed, social partners' behaviors toward older adults can lower their self-esteem and confidence in their own abilities, may be detrimental to their health and functioning, and may reinforce aging stereotypes (Hess, 2006; Pasupathi & Löckenhoff, 2002). Activating such aging stereotypes increases dependent behaviors such as help seeking (Coudin & Alexopoulos, 2010) and may affect older adults' cognitive performance. For example, highlighting negative aging stereotypes reduces memory performance in older adults, thereby exaggerating age differences in performance (Chasteen, Bhattacharyya, Horhota, Tam, & Hasher, 2005). In some cases, however, as noted in our discussion of the social input model, aging stereotypes may lead social partners to treat older adults more kindly and may in turn promote more positive social interactions. Similar to the physical health domain, social partners' influences on late-life cognition may be a mixed blessing. Although older adults' social partners may facilitate maintenance and even growth in cognitive function, social partners can interact with older adults in ways that negatively affect older adults' self-images and cognitive performance.

In essence, older adults spend most of their time with close social partners, but less close individuals also exert socialization pressures. These socialization processes occur over a lifetime of accumulated experiences. Present social relationships may therefore be influenced by earlier experiences. Conversely, social partners may also shape older adults' identities by influencing older adults' construal of their personal past. Socialization processes in late life may involve less conflict and negative feedback, and more lenient and forgiving behaviors. Among the life domains influenced by social partners, health and cognition take on a particularly important role in old age. Social partners influence older adults' behaviors and beliefs pertaining to health and cognition, with important implications for late-life adjustment.

Culture

Another major source of socialization in late life comes from the broader culture in which older adults are embedded. Individuals adopt views of aging, both positive and negative, throughout their life course. Unlike other personal characteristics that are stable across the life span (e.g., gender, race), people become "old" and need to reconcile their views of aging with their current life stage and newer identity as an older adult. Thus, socialization in older age may be strongly influenced by cultural norms, including prevalent stereotypes, views of aging, and social structures and hierarchies.

Stereotypes of Aging

Cultures vary in terms of attitudes toward older adults and aging in general, which in turn may influence how individuals in different cultures experience the aging process (Levy, 1999). Individuals within cultures appear to share stereotypes of older people (Hummert, Garstka, Shaner, & Strahm, 1994; Levy, 2003). Past research indicates that Asian cultures tend to endorse more positive views of aging than do Western cultures (Levy & Langer, 1994; Yoon, Hasher, Feinberg, Rahhal, & Winocur, 2000), but these findings may also depend on whether the perceiver is relatively young or old (e.g., Boduroglu, Yoon, Luo, & Park, 2006; Yun & Lachman, 2006). In any case, much of the research on stereotypes of aging, at least in Western contexts, suggests that older age is viewed negatively (e.g., Ellis & Morrison, 2005), as a life period plagued with poor physical health and disability, cognitive impairments, and loneliness (e.g., Ory, Hoffman, Hawkins, Sanner, & Mockenhaupt, 2003). Some aging stereotypes, however, can be positive. In a study of 26 countries, older age was associated with more positive personality traits, such as emotional stability (i.e., less impulsivity) and less antagonism (Chan et al., 2012).

Research by Levy and colleagues suggests that aging stereotypes are internalized by older adults and have profound influences on health and cognitive function, including cardiovascular reactivity to stress (Levy, Hausdorff, Hencke, & Wei, 2000), memory performance (Levy & Langer, 1994), will to live (Levy, Ashman, & Dror, 1999), and even longevity (Levy, Slade, Kunkel, & Kasl, 2002), with negative stereotypes exerting detrimental consequences, and positive stereotypes promoting more adaptive outcomes. Interestingly, social partners do not need to interact with older adults in ways that are consistent with aging stereotypes for these effects to persist. In fact, subtle cues and reminders (e.g., reading words related to aging stereotypes, such as "frail" and "slow") are sufficient to activate aging stereotypes among older adults. Thus, broader cultural views of older age can have a drastic influence on older adults' health and cognitive functioning.

Culture and Socialization Partners

Culture also influences the types of socialization partners individuals encounter in late life. Although size of the social network tends to diminish with age across cultures, as discussed (e.g., Antonucci et al., 2002), the configuration of the social network in late life varies across cultures. For example, in the United States, older adults are generally closer to and receive support from their daughters' families, whereas in East Asian nations such as China and Japan, the tendency is to align with a son's family and to receive support from a daughter-in-law (Antonucci, Akiyama, & Birditt, 2005).

Later life living arrangements and their consequences also vary by culture. Living alone is a risk factor for depression for Hispanic older adults but not for African American and non-Hispanic white older adults (Russell & Taylor, 2009), possibly because living alone represents a mismatch in Hispanic older adults' preferences to coreside with kin ties. Sereny (2011) found that older adults in China generally preferred to reside with their adult children, but individuals with more financial and family care resources preferred to live alone. Chinese older adults who preferred to live alone, and currently lived alone and independently, reported better health, whereas Chinese older adults who lived with their adult offspring were more likely to be disabled, even when accounting for their preference to live with their children. Thus, culture shapes not only normative living arrangements for older adults but also the support structure for older adults who require care.

Indeed, political systems differ considerably in the structure of their health care systems and long-term care models for older adults. In China, for example, older adults may primarily rely on support via filial piety, in which adult children are morally obligated and expected to care for their aging parents via emotional, instrumental, and financial support (e.g., Cheng & Chan, 2006). Given the rapid societal, economic, and familial shifts in China, however, some recent studies indicate that filial piety may be eroding in more modernized regions (Cheung & Kwan, 2009). In response to these societal changes, Family Support Agreements (FSAs) have been formed recently and monitored by the Chinese government (Chou, 2011). FSAs are contracts between aging parents and their adult children that outline how care will be provided to the parents. Although FSAs are voluntary and based on filial piety, failure to fulfill contractual obligations may result in legal repercussions (Chou, 2011). Therefore, in certain parts of China, especially rural areas that are less influenced by modernization, older adults may be socialized to be more dependent on kin ties for support. With the rise of rapidly aging populations, many nations, not just China, are struggling with how to provide and care for older adults.

In addition, in the United States, few states support home-based formal care for the older adult population. In the United States, there is a general emphasis on familial and institutional care (Feinberg & Newman, 2004). Although well-off older adults may be able to pay for assisted living facilities that offer some support for independent living, families often are the primary line of support and care until the older adult requires care in a nursing home setting and possibly qualifies for Medicaid. It is therefore possible that the American approach may increase dependency behaviors among older adults (M. M. Baltes & Horgas, 1997).

Possible Limitations in the Influence of Culture on Aging

Culture is an important socialization force throughout life, but it may have less impact on older individuals' development than it does on shaping behaviors and development in early life. Although the experience of old age differs across cultures, it does not necessarily mean that culture shapes the aging process per se. The cultural differences may arise from socialization during early life that simply persists through later adulthood. There are several reasons why this might be the case: (1) Cultural influences may be most pronounced during early stages of life, when individuals are seeking information about themselves and the positions they may hold in society; (2) older adults may attempt to sustain themselves relative to traditions rather than incorporating new elements of the culture; and (3) cultural media target younger individuals.

Culture may be most efficacious in shaping behaviors of young rather than older people. Previously, we described socioemotional selectivity theory and the processes through which individuals become increasingly invested in emotionally rewarding social partners as their future time perspective diminishes. This shift in motivation reflects a move away from seeking social partners who can provide information about the culture, toward emotional rewards (Carstensen et al., 1999). By reducing their social networks to close friends and family, older adults may decrease the chances of encountering new information from the culture. Consistent with this idea, mean-level personality trait changes across adulthood suggest that later life is associated with being less open to new experiences (e.g., Chan et al., 2012). Of course, younger relatives engage in behaviors that are culturally acceptable for their generation and cohort, and may socialize older relatives in doing so. For example, an older adult may grow to accept the idea of cohabitation after a beloved grandchild moves in with a partner. Older adults are not completely immune to the impact of cultural changes, but they may not actively seek out new information concerning cultural expectations.

In comparison to younger adults, older adults may also encounter less exposure to media that convey cultural messages (Roberts & Foehr, 2008). Young adults rely on cultural media such as popular music, movies, social media, and Internet blogs to help establish a sense of identity (Lefkowitz, Vukman, & Loken, 2012). The content and advertising in these media tend to target adolescents and young adults rather than older adults. Thus, when older adults go to the movies, surf websites, or watch television, they are unlikely to see older adults portrayed as models of cultural imperatives. Many of the images of older adults in the mass media are negative or comical (Carrigan & Szmigin, 1999). Some recent studies, however, indicate that although older adults are underrepresented in television commercials in general, when they were present, they may be characterized in a positive manner, such as socially engaged and open to new experiences (Kessler, Schwender, & Bowen, 2010), although not as positively as other age groups (Lee, Carpenter, & Meyers, 2007).

This is not to say that older adults avoid cultural media. In fact, older adults spend about one-third of their sampled time watching television—approximately three times the amount that younger adults watch television (Depp, Schkade, Thompson, & Jeste, 2010). Among adults over 65 years old, 50% use the Internet (Zickuhr & Madden, 2012). Many of these older adults are strong adherents of e-mail, with 86% of them reporting that they use it to stay in touch with social partners, and about one-third of older adults reporting that they use social networking sites such as Facebook or MySpace (Duggan & Brenner, 2013). In fact, in a study of age differences in the use of the online social networking website, MySpace, older adults' friend networks included a larger age distribution than that of adolescents, who generally have friends of the same age group (Pfeil, Arjan, & Zaphiris, 2009). Although more research is needed on the composition of online social networks, these studies suggest that older adults may use social media websites to connect with their grandchildren and other kin (Pfeil et al., 2009). This interpretation is consistent with socioemotional selectivity theory, which suggests that older adults may be more interested in communicating with relatives than with searching for information when they use the computer.

In summary, with regard to culture and socialization, cultural institutions that provide health care or other forms of support influence the aging process, such as dependency behaviors and expectations for care. Older adults may be more likely to view themselves as vehicles of traditions within their families and less likely to seek new information actively from media or social partners. Studies have not yet examined the extent to which older adults adopt attitudes and beliefs embraced by younger family members, but it is likely that such socialization occurs.

Older Adults as Agents of Socialization

So far, we have considered ways in which older adults are socialized by their social and cultural context. In the following section, we turn to a different perspective on aging and socialization: the ways in which older adults may act as agents of socialization of their social partners and subsequent generations (e.g., grandchildren).

Adults enter late life after spending decades as young and middle-aged adults. During these earlier years, healthy adults foster relationships with family members and friends (Antonucci et al., 2002), serve to maintain family traditions (see review by Fiese et al., 2002), and take on leadership and mentoring roles (Markus, Ryff, Conner, Pudberry, & Barnett, 2001). In summary, by the time they reach old age, most people have spent more time serving as "socialization agents" than as objects of socialization. Socialization in old age, therefore, involves forces that influence how older adults are socialized (as reviewed in the previous sections), as well as how older adults may continue to serve as agents of socialization for others. In the next section, we focus primarily on the role of generativity in motivating older adults to continue socializing others.

Erikson's (1950) concept of *generativity* helps explain the basis for older adults' continued involvement as socialization agents. Among Erikson's eight stages of life span development, generativity is expected to occur in midlife. Generativity involves investment in future generations and motivation to improve the world for the future. Although Erikson initially proposed this as a stage specific to midlife, he reframed this issue in late life, arguing that it is important for older adults to continue to give back to society to remain vital and engaged (Erikson, Erikson, & Kivnick, 1986). Considerable evidence has since confirmed that generativity remains a high priority for older adults (Ehlman & Ligon, 2012).

Older adults benefit in a variety of ways from remaining generative and serving as socialization agents. This includes viewing their life in more positive terms. McAdams and colleagues have found that middle-aged and older adults who score high on measures of generativity also frame their life stories in more positive ways (McAdams, 2011;

McAdams, Diamond, de St. Aubin, & Mansfield, 1997). That is, when individuals have a general desire to be involved in socializing others, they also tend to view their own lives more positively and to believe their past mistakes led them to be better people (what McAdams refers to as a "redemption" narrative) and to thrive psychologically.

Rather than taking the form of productivity and creativity characteristic of midlife, generativity and socialization in late life may reflect more altruistic tendencies, in which older adults are motivated to engage in behaviors that benefit others (e.g., Morrow-Howell, Hinterlong, Rozario, & Tang, 2003). In late life, individuals are often involved in helping friends, neighbors, and relatives. Following retirement, many individuals engage in formal community volunteer work (Mutchler, Burr, & Caro, 2003), although the choice to volunteer in later life may be related to past socialization (in terms of prior volunteering experience; Dye, Goodman, Roth, Bley, & Jensen, 1973). Older adults who engage in such volunteer work show a variety of psychological benefits, such as decreases in depressive symptoms (Hong & Morrow-Howell, 2010) and physical benefits, as demonstrated in prospective longitudinal studies, including diminished functional decline and lower mortality risk (Hong & Morrow-Howell, 2010; Okun, August, Rook, & Newsom, 2010).

Interestingly, researchers rarely frame involvement with grown children and grandchildren as generativity. Nonetheless, family may be the forum in which older adults invest their greatest efforts as agents of socialization. Many older adults are parents and have spent two or three decades (and sometimes four or five decades) engaged in socializing their children. A classic study has shown that although grandparents' political and religious attitudes were predictive of their middle-aged adult child's attitudes, the magnitude of this association was weaker in comparison to the influence of middle-aged parents' attitudes on their young adult child's attitudes, suggesting that parental socialization forces may decrease with age (Glass, Bengtson, & Dunham, 1986). Still, in late life, parents may persist in attempts to influence and help their grown children by, for instance, offering advice and providing emotional support (Fingerman, Miller, Birditt, & Zarit, 2009). Indeed, older mothers' unsolicited advice and continued attempts to socialize their middle-aged daughters can become a source of strain in their relationships (Fingerman, 2001). Thus, older adults' socialization efforts in the family may not always be effective or well received.

Similarly, the role of grandparent may involve highly generative activity. Research, however, suggests that not all grandparents actively find opportunities to socialize their grandchildren (Thiele & Whelan, 2006). In general, grandmothers are more likely to be actively involved with grandchildren than are grandfathers (Monserud, 2011; Roberto & Stroes, 1992). Older grandparents typically are less involved with grandchildren than are middle-aged grandparents, in part due to the ages of the grandchildren; older grandchildren are less involved with grandparents than are younger grandchildren. Many grandchildren view their grandparents as important family members (Roberto & Stroes, 1992) and grandparents typically find their family role very satisfying (Thiele & Whelan, 2006). Nonetheless, the extent to which older adults experience themselves as socialization agents varies as a function of time spent with grandchildren, as well as involvement with the middle generation (i.e., the parents; Fingerman, 2004b).

In summary, a discussion of socialization in late life would be remiss if we did not address the role of older adults as socialization agents in their own right and the implications for their well-being. In general, older adults thrive in contexts where they are able to engage with and influence younger generations, such as situations involving mentorship through volunteer work, family gatherings, and conveying the accumulated expertise of a life. Of course, under some conditions, older adults' socialization efforts may be viewed as ineffective or problematic, such as when providing unsolicited advice to their adult children or when disciplining grandchildren.

Conclusion

Although, traditionally, socialization and gerontology research have had limited conceptual overlap, the research reviewed in this chapter suggests that socialization indeed shapes late-life development, and that old age may offer unique perspectives for conceptualizing socialization. In old age, people exercise individual agency to shape their social world actively to fit their goals and needs by including an increasing proportion of close and meaningful social ties in their social network. They thereby select the social convoy that accompanies them throughout old age and will socialize them during their late years. Peoples' personal past plays an important role in late-life socialization. For example, past relationships may continue to influence how older adults adapt to late-life changes. Also, present relationships may influence how older adults construe their biography and identity. The type of feedback provided by socialization partners may change across adulthood, with social partners offering more lenient and less negative feedback for older adults than for younger social partners. In late life, socialization partners continue to influence beliefs and behaviors related to health and cognitive functioning. These two domains are of crucial importance in old age, due to the likelihood of declines in both physical well-being and cognitive performance. In these areas, the effects of socialization partners on the individual's late-life adaptation may be both beneficial and detrimental (e.g., social partners may provide social support and companionship but may also model poor health behaviors).

Above and beyond the proximal social environment, the aging individual is also socialized by the greater cultural context. Support patterns and living arrangements vary across cultures, as do health care systems, long-term care models, and views about aging. These factors may shape older adults' values and choices (e.g., about living arrangements), as well as their beliefs (e.g., regarding their own competence), with important implications for late-life health, independence, and emotional well-being. Apart from their role as targets of socialization, older adults also act as agents of socialization. For example, they influence their kin ties. Indeed, giving back to others and socializing partners continue to be important goals well into late life and may provide older adults with a source of meaning and purpose in life.

In essence, socialization across the life span is characterized by both continuity and change. There is continuity in that socialization is not completed at any given age; instead, it is a lifelong process. As people enter old age, social partners and the greater societal context continue to influence their identities, beliefs, behaviors, emotions, cognitive performance, and health. These influences can promote, but also impede, late-life adaptation. Given the rapidly aging population, the question of how socialization continues to shape late-life development becomes an increasingly important area of research. Notably, research on socialization across the life span also needs to acknowledge age-related discontinuities. Late life brings about new developmental tasks, and the effects of socialization may pertain to different life domains than socialization in younger phases in life. Socialization in old age may also imply different interpersonal dynamics, margins of malleability, and outcomes than in earlier phases of life. Emphasizing socialization as a lifelong process that includes late-life development may therefore provide new facets to conceptualizing the process.

REFERENCES

Allemand, M. (2008). Age differences in forgivingness: The role of future time perspective. *Journal of Research in Personality, 42*, 1137–1147.

Antonucci, T. C., Akiyama, H., & Birditt, K. S. (2005). Intergenerational exchange in the United States and Japan. In M. Silverstein (Ed.), *Intergenerational relations across time and place: Annual review of gerontology and geriatrics* (pp. 224–248). New York: Springer.

Antonucci, T. C., Birditt, K. S., & Ajrouch, K. (2010). Convoys of social relations: Past, present, and future. In K. L. Fingerman, C. Berg, J. Smith, & T. C. Antonucci (Eds.), *Handbook of life-span development* (pp. 161–182). New York: Springer.

Antonucci, T. C., Lansford, J. E., Akiyama, H., Smith, J., Baltes, M. M., Takahashi, K., et al. (2002). Differences between men and women in social relations, resource deficits, and depressive symptomatology during later life in four nations. *Journal of Social Issues, 58*, 767–783.

Arnett, J. J. (2001). Conceptions of the transition to adulthood: Perspectives from adolescence through midlife. *Journal of Adult Development, 8*, 133–143.

Baltes, M. M., & Horgas, A. L. (1997). Long-term care institutions and the maintenance of competence: A dialectic between compensation and overcompensation. In S. L. Willis, K. W. Schaie, & M. D. Hayward (Eds.), *Societal mechanisms for maintaining competence in old age* (pp. 142–181). New York: Springer.

Baltes, P. B. (1997). On the incomplete architecture of human ontogeny: Selection, optimization, and compensation as foundation of developmental theory. *American Psychologist, 52*, 366–380.

Barber, B. K., & Olsen, J. A. (2004). Assessing the transitions to middle and high school. *Journal of Adolescent Research, 19*, 3–30.

Birditt, K. S., & Fingerman, K. L. (2003). Age and gender differences in adults' descriptions of emotional reactions to interpersonal problems. *Journals of Gerontology B: Psychological Sciences and Social Sciences, 58*, P237–P245.

Birditt, K. S., Fingerman, K. L., & Almeida, D. M. (2005). Age differences in exposure and reactions to interpersonal tensions: A daily diary study. *Psychology and Aging, 20*, 330–340.

Blanchard-Fields, F., Mienaltowski, A., & Seay, R. B. (2007). Age differences in everyday problem-solving effectiveness: Older adults select more effective strategies for interpersonal problems. *Journals of Gerontology B: Psychological Sciences and Social Sciences, 62*, P61–P64.

Boduroglu, A., Yoon, C., Luo, T., & Park, D. C. (2006). Age-related stereotypes: A comparison of American and Chinese cultures. *Gerontology, 52*, 324–333.

Bugental, D. B., & Grusec, J. E. (2006). Socialization processes. In W. Damon, R. M. Lerner, & N. Eisenberg (Eds.), *Handbook of child psychology: Vol. 3. Social, emotional, and personality development* (6th ed., pp. 366–428). Hoboken, NJ: Wiley.

Cacioppo, J. T., Hawkley, L. C., & Thisted, R. A. (2010). Perceived social isolation makes me sad: 5-year cross-lagged analyses of loneliness and depressive symptomatology in the Chicago Health, Aging, and Social Relations Study. *Psychology and Aging, 25*, 453–463.

Carpenter, B. D. (2001). Attachment bonds between adult daughters and their older mothers: Associations with contemporary caregiving. *Journals of Gerontology B: Psychological Sciences and Social Sciences, 56*, 257–266.

Carrigan, M., & Szmigin, I. (1999). The representation of older people in advertisements. *International Journal of Market Research, 41*, 311–326.

Carstensen, L. L., Isaacowitz, D. M., & Charles, S. T. (1999). Taking time seriously: A theory of socioemotional selectivity. *American Psychologist, 54*, 165–181.

Chan, W., McCrae, R. R., De Fruyt, F., Jussim, L., Lockenhoff, C. E., De Bolle, M., et al. (2012). Stereotypes of age differences in personality traits: Universal and accurate? *Journal of Personality and Social Psychology, 103*, 1050–1066.

Charles, S. T. (2010). Strength and vulnerability integration: A model of emotional well-being across adulthood. *Psychological Bulletin, 136*, 1068–1091.

Charles, S. T., Piazza, J. R., Luong, G., & Almeida, D. M. (2009). Now you see it, now you don't: Age differences in affective reactivity to social tensions. *Psychology and Aging, 24*, 645–653.

Chasteen, A. L., Bhattacharyya, S., Horhota, M., Tam, R., & Hasher, L. (2005). How feelings of stereotype threat influence older adults' memory performance. *Experimental Aging Research, 31*, 235–260.

Chatters, L. M., Taylor, R. J., Lincoln, K. D., & Schroepfer, T. (2002). Patterns of informal support from family and church members among African Americans. *Journal of Black Studies, 33*, 66–85.

Cheng, S.-T., & Chan, A. C. (2006). Filial piety and psychological well-being in well older Chinese. *Journals of Gerontology B: Psychological Sciences and Social Sciences, 61*, P262–P269.

Cheung, C.-K., & Kwan, A. Y.-H. (2009). The erosion of filial piety by modernisation in Chinese cities. *Ageing and Society, 29*, 179–198.

Chou, R. J.-A. (2011). Filial piety by contract?: The emergence, implementation, and implications of the "Family Support Agreement" in China. *The Gerontologist, 51*, 3–16.

Codd, V., Nelson, C. P., Albrecht, E., Mangino, M., Deelen, J., Buxton, J. L., et al. (2013). Identification of seven loci affecting mean telomere length and their association with disease. *Nature Genetics, 45*, 422–427.

Connell, C. M., & Prinz, R. J. (2002). The impact of childcare and parent–child interactions on school readiness and social skills development for low-income African American children. *Journal of School Psychology, 40*, 177–193.

Coudin, G., & Alexopoulos, T. (2010). "Help me! I'm old!": How negative aging stereotypes create dependency among older adults. *Aging and Mental Health, 14*, 516–523.

DePaulo, B. M., & Morris, W. L. (2005). Target article: Singles in society and in science. *Psychological Inquiry, 16*, 57–83.

Depp, C. A., Schkade, D. A., Thompson, W. K., & Jeste, D. V. (2010). Age, affective experience, and television use. *American Journal of Preventive Medicine, 39*, 173–178.

DiMatteo, M. (2004). Social support and patient adherence to medical treatment: A meta-analysis. *Health Psychology, 23*, 207–218.

Dixon, R. A., Rust, T. B., Feltmate, S. E., & See, S. K. (2007). Memory and aging: Selected research directions and application issues. *Canadian Psychology, 48*, 67–76.

Duggan, M., & Brenner, J. (2013). The demographics of social media users—2012. Retrieved from *http://pewinternet.org/reports/2013/social-media-users.aspx*.

Dye, D., Goodman, M., Roth, M., Bley, N., & Jensen, K. (1973). The older adult volunteer compared to the nonvolunteer. *The Gerontologist, 13*, 215–218.

Ehlman, K., & Ligon, M. (2012). The application of a generativity model for older adults. *International Journal of Aging and Human Development, 74*, 331–344.

Elder, G. H., Jr. (1998). The life course as developmental theory. *Child Development, 69*, 1–12.

Elder, G. H., Jr., & Liker, J. K. (1982). Hard times in women's lives: Historical influences across forty years. *American Journal of Sociology, 88*, 241–269.

Ellis, S. R., & Morrison, T. G. (2005). Stereotypes of ageing: Messages promoted by age-specific paper birthday cards available in Canada. *International Journal of Aging and Human Development, 61*, 57–73.

Erber, J. T., Szuchman, L. T., & Prager, I. G. (2001). Ain't misbehavin': The effects of age and intentionality on judgments about misconduct. *Psychology and Aging, 16*, 85–95.

Erikson, E. (1950). *Childhood and society.* New York: Norton.

Erikson, E. H., Erikson, J. M., & Kivnick, H. Q. (1986). *Vital involvement in old age.* New York: Norton.

Feinberg, L. F., & Newman, S. L. (2004). A study of 10 states since passage of the National Family Caregiver support program: Policies, perceptions, and program development. *Gerontologist, 44,* 760–769.

Fiese, B. H., Tomcho, T. J., Douglas, M., Josephs, K., Poltrock, S., & Baker, T. (2002). A review of 50 years of research on naturally occurring family routines and rituals: Cause for celebration? *Journal of Family Psychology, 16,* 381–390.

Fingerman, K., Miller, L., Birditt, K., & Zarit, S. (2009). Giving to the good and the needy: Parental support of grown children. *Journal of Marriage and Family, 71,* 1220–1233.

Fingerman, K. L. (2001). *Aging mothers and their adult daughters: A study in mixed emotions.* New York: Springer.

Fingerman, K. L. (2003). *Mothers and their adult daughter: Mixed emotions, enduring bonds.* Amherst, NY: Prometheus Books.

Fingerman, K. L. (2004a). The consequential stranger: Peripheral relationships across the life span. In F. R. Lang & K. L. Fingerman (Eds.), *Growing together: Personal relationships across the lifespan* (pp. 183–209). New York: Cambridge University Press.

Fingerman, K. L. (2004b). The role of offspring and in-laws in grandparents' ties to their grandchildren. *Journal of Family Issues, 25,* 1026–1049.

Fingerman, K. L. (2009). Consequential strangers and peripheral ties: The importance of unimportant relationships. *Journal of Family Theory and Review, 1,* 69–86.

Fingerman, K. L., & Charles, S. T. (2010). It takes two to tango: Why older people have the best relationships. *Current Directions in Psychological Science, 19,* 172–176.

Fingerman, K. L., & Griffiths, P. C. (1999). Season's greetings: Adults' social contacts at the holiday season. *Psychology and Aging, 14,* 192–205.

Fingerman, K. L., Hay, E. L., Kamp Dush, C. M., Cichy, K., & Hosterman, S. (2007). Parents' and offspring's perceptions of change and continuity when parents experience the transition to old age. *Advances in Life Course Research, 12,* 275–306.

Fingerman, K. L., Miller, L., & Charles, S. (2008). Saving the best for last: How adults treat social partners of different ages. *Psychology and Aging, 23,* 399–409.

Fredrickson, B. L., & Carstensen, L. L. (1990). Choosing social partners: How old age and anticipated endings make people more selective. *Psychology and Aging, 5,* 335–347.

Friedman, H. S., & Martin, L. R. (2012). *The Longevity Project: Surprising discoveries for health and long life from the landmark eight-decade study.* New York: Plume.

Gardner, D., & Helmes, E. (2006). Interpersonal dependency in older adults and the risks of developing mood and mobility problems when receiving care at home. *Aging and Mental Health, 10,* 63–68.

Glass, J., Bengtson, V. L., & Dunham, C. C. (1986). Attitude similarity in three-generation families: Socialization, status inheritance, or reciprocal influence? *American Sociological Review, 51,* 685–698.

Hawkley, L. C., & Cacioppo, J. T. (2007). Aging and loneliness: Downhill quickly? *Current Directions in Psychological Science, 16,* 187–191.

Hazan, C., & Shaver, P. R. (1994). Attachment as an organizational framework for research on close relationships. *Psychological Inquiry, 5,* 1–22.

Heckhausen, J., Wrosch, C., & Schulz, R. (2010). A motivational theory of life-span development. *Psychological Review, 117,* 32–60.

Hertzog, C. (2008). Theoretical approaches to the study of cognitive aging: An individual-differences perspective. In S. M. Hofer & D. F. Alwin (Eds.), *Handbook of cognitive aging: Interdisciplinary perspectives* (pp. 34–49). Thousand Oaks, CA: Sage.

Hertzog, C., Kramer, A. F., Wilson, R. S., & Lindenberger, U. (2008). Enrichment effects on adult cognitive development: Can the functional capacity of older adults be preserved and enhanced? *Psychological Science in the Public Interest, 9,* 1–65.

Hess, T. M. (2006). Attitudes toward aging and their effects on behavior. In J. Birren & K. W. Schaie (Eds.), *Handbook of the psychology of aging* (6th ed., pp. 379–406). Amsterdam: Elsevier.

Hess, T. M., & Kotter-Grühn, D. (2011). Social knowledge and goal-based influences on social information processing in adulthood. *Psychology and Aging, 26*, 792–802.

Holt-Lunstad, J., Smith, T. B., & Layton, B. (2010). Social relationships and mortality risk: A meta-analytic review. *PLoS Medicine, 7*, 2–19.

Hong, S., & Morrow-Howell, N. (2010). Health outcomes of Experience Corps: A high-commitment volunteer program. *Social Science and Medicine, 71*, 414–420.

House, J. S. (2001). Social isolation kills, but how and why? *Psychosomatic Medicine, 63*, 273–274.

Hummert, M. L., Garstka, T. A., Shaner, J. L., & Strahm, S. (1994). Stereotypes of the elderly held by young, middle-aged, and elderly adults. *Journals of Gerontology B: Psychological Sciences and Social Sciences, 49*, 240–249.

Kern, M. L., & Friedman, H. S. (2011). Personality and differences in health and longevity. In T. Chamorro-Premuzic, S. von Stumm, & A. Furnham (Eds.), *The Wiley-Blackwell handbook of individual differences* (pp. 461–489). Oxford, UK: Wiley-Blackwell.

Kessler, E.-M., Schwender, C., & Bowen, C. E. (2010). The portrayal of older people's social participation on German prime-time TV advertisements. *Journals of Gerontology B: Psychological Sciences and Social Sciences, 65*, 97–106.

Kite, M. E., Stockdale, G. D., Whitley, B. E., Jr., & Johnson, B. T. (2005). Attitudes toward younger and older adults: An updated meta-analytic review. *Journal of Social Issues, 61*, 241–266.

Lang, F. R. (2000). Endings and continuity of social relationships: Maximizing intrinsic benefits within personal networks when feeling near to death. *Journal of Social and Personal Relationships, 17*, 155–182.

Lang, F. R. (2004). Social motivation across the life span. In F. R. Lang & K. L. Fingerman (Eds.), *Growing together: Personal relationships across the lifespan* (pp. 341–367). New York: Cambridge University Press.

Lee, M. M., Carpenter, B., & Meyers, L. S. (2007). Representations of older adults in television advertisements. *Journal of Aging Studies, 21*, 23–30.

Lefkowitz, E. S., Vukman, S. N., & Loken, E. (2012). Young adults in a wireless world. In A. Booth, S. L. Brown, N. S. Lansdale, W. D. Manning, & S. M. McHale (Eds.), *Early adulthood in a family context* (pp. 45–58). New York: Springer.

Lerner, R. M. (2002). *Concepts and theories of human development* (3rd ed.). Mahwah, NJ: Erlbaum.

Levy, B., Ashman, O., & Dror, I. (1999). To be or not to be: The effects of aging stereotypes on the will to live. *Omega: Journal of Death and Dying, 40*, 409–420.

Levy, B., & Langer, E. (1994). Aging free from negative stereotypes: Successful memory in China and among the American deaf. *Journal of Personality and Social Psychology, 66*, 989–997.

Levy, B. R. (1999). The inner self of the Japanese elderly: A defense against negative stereotypes of aging. *International Journal of Aging and Human Development, 48*, 131–144.

Levy, B. R. (2003). Mind matters: Cognitive and physical effects of aging self-stereotypes. *Journals of Gerontology B: Psychological Sciences and Social Sciences, 58*, 203–211.

Levy, B. R., Hausdorff, J. M., Hencke, R., & Wei, J. Y. (2000). Reducing cardiovascular stress with positive self-stereotypes of aging. *Journals of Gerontology B: Psychological Sciences and Social Sciences, 55*, P205–P213.

Levy, B. R., Slade, M. D., Kunkel, S. R., & Kasl, S. V. (2002). Longevity increased by positive self-perceptions of aging. *Journal of Personality and Social Psychology, 83*, 261–270.

Lewis, M. A., & Rook, K. S. (1999). Social control in personal relationships: Impact on health behaviors and psychological distress. *Health Psychology, 18*, 63–71.

Litwin, H., & Stoeckel, K. J. (in press). Social networks and subjective wellbeing among older Europeans: Does age make a difference? *Ageing and Society*.

Luong, G., Charles, S. T., & Fingerman, K. L. (2011). Better with age: Social relationships across adulthood. *Journal of Social and Personal Relationships, 28,* 9–23.

Magai, C., Consedine, N. S., Gillespie, M., O'Neal, C., & Vilker, R. (2004). The differential roles of early emotion socialization and adult attachment in adult emotional experience: Testing a mediator hypothesis. *Attachment and Human Development, 6,* 389–417.

Mallers, M. H., Charles, S. T., Neupert, S. D., & Almeida, D. M. (2010). Perceptions of childhood relationships with mother and father: Daily emotional and stressor experiences in adulthood. *Developmental Psychology, 46,* 1651–1661.

Markus, H. R., Ryff, C. D., Conner, A. L., Pudberry, E. K., & Barnett, K. L. (2001). Themes and variations in American understandings of responsibility. In A. S. Rossi (Ed.), *Caring and doing for others* (pp. 349–399). Chicago: University of Chicago Press.

Martin, M., & Wight, M. (2008). Dyadic cognition in old age: Paradigms, findings, and directions. In S. M. Hofer & D. F. Alwin (Eds.), *Handbook of cognitive aging: Interdisciplinary perspectives* (pp. 629–646). Thousand Oaks, CA: Sage.

McAdams, D. P. (2011). Life narratives. In K. L. Fingerman, C. Berg, J. Smith, & T. C. Antonucci (Eds.), *Handbook of life-span development* (pp. 589–610). New York: Springer.

McAdams, D. P., Diamond, A., de St. Aubin, E., & Mansfield, E. (1997). Stories of commitment: The psychosocial construction of generative lives. *Journal of Personality and Social Psychology, 72,* 678–694.

McLean, K. C., Pasupathi, M., & Pals, J. L. (2007). Selves creating stories creating selves: A process model of self-development. *Personality and Social Psychology Review, 11,* 262–278.

Miller, L. M., Charles, S. T., & Fingerman, K. L. (2009). Perceptions of social transgressions in adulthood. *Journals of Gerontology B: Psychological Sciences and Social Sciences, 64,* 551–559.

Monserud, M. A. (2011). Changes in grandchildren's adult role statuses and their relationships with grandparents. *Journal of Family Issues, 32,* 425–451.

Morrow-Howell, N., Hinterlong, J., Rozario, P. A., & Tang, F. (2003). Effects of volunteering on the well-being of older adults. *Journals of Gerontology B: Psychological Sciences and Social Sciences, 58,* S137–S145.

Mutchler, J. E., Burr, J. A., & Caro, F. G. (2003). From paid worker to volunteer: Leaving the paid workforce and volunteering in later life. *Social Forces, 81,* 1267–1293.

Okun, M. A., August, K. J., Rook, K. S., & Newsom, J. T. (2010). Does volunteering moderate the relation between functional limitations and mortality? *Social Science and Medicine, 71,* 1662–1668.

Ong, A. D., Rothstein, J. D., & Uchino, B. N. (2012). Loneliness accentuates age differences in cardiovascular responses to social evaluative threat *Psychology and Aging, 27,* 190–198.

Ory, M., Hoffman, M. K., Hawkins, M., Sanner, B., & Mockenhaupt, R. (2003). Challenging aging stereotypes: Strategies for creating a more active society. *American Journal of Preventive Medicine, 25,* 164–171.

Pasupathi, M. (2001). The social construction of the personal past and its implications for adult development. *Psychological Bulletin, 127,* 651–672.

Pasupathi, M., & Löckenhoff, C. E. (2002). Ageist behavior. In T. D. Nelson (Ed.), *Ageism: Stereotyping and prejudice against older persons* (pp. 201–246). Cambridge, MA: MIT Press.

Pfeil, U., Arjan, R., & Zaphiris, P. (2009). Age differences in online social networking: A study of user profiles and the social capital divide among teenagers and older users in MySpace. *Computers in Human Behavior, 25,* 643–654.

Rauers, A., Riediger, M., Schmiedek, F., & Lindenberger, U. (2011). With a little help from my spouse: Does spousal collaboration compensate for the effects of cognitive aging? *Gerontology, 57,* 161–166.

Roberto, K. A., & Stroes, J. (1992). Grandchildren and grandparents: Roles, influences, and relationships. *International Journal of Aging and Human Development, 34,* 227–239.

Roberts, D. F., & Foehr, U. G. (2008). Trends in media use. *Future of Children, 18,* 11–37.

Rook, K. S., Luong, G., Sorkin, D. H., Newsom, J. T., & Krause, N. (2012). Ambivalent versus problematic social ties: Implications for psychological health, functional health, and interpersonal coping. *Psychology and Aging, 27,* 912–923.

Rubin, K. H., Bukowski, W. M., & Parker, J. G. (2006). Peer interactions, relationships, and groups. In N. Eisenberg, W. Damon, & R. M. Lerner (Eds.), *Handbook of child psychology: Vol. 3. Social, emotional, and personality development* (6th ed., pp. 571–645). Hoboken, NJ: Wiley.

Russell, D., & Taylor, J. (2009). Living alone and depressive symptoms: The influence of gender, physical disability, and social support among Hispanic and non-Hispanic older adults. *Journals of Gerontology B: Psychological Sciences and Social Sciences, 64,* 95–104.

Sereny, M. (2011). Living arrangements of older adults in China: The interplay among preferences, realities, and health. *Research on Aging, 33,* 172–204.

Shaver, P. R., Belsky, J., & Brennan, K. A. (2000). The adult attachment interview and self-reports of romantic attachment: Associations across domains and methods. *Personal Relationships, 7,* 25–43.

Small, B. J., Dixon, R. A., McArdle, J. J., & Grimm, K. J. (2012). Do changes in lifestyle engagement moderate cognitive decline in normal aging?: Evidence from the Victoria Longitudinal Study. *Neuropsychology, 26,* 144–155.

Smetana, J. G. (2006). Social-cognitive domain theory: Consistencies and variations in children's moral and social judgments. In M. Killen & J. G. Smetana (Eds.), *Handbook of moral development* (pp. 119–153). Mahwah, NJ: Erlbaum.

Smetana, J. G., Campione-Barr, N., & Metzger, A. (2006). Adolescent development in interpersonal and societal contexts. *Annual Review of Psychology, 57,* 255–284.

Smith, J., Borchelt, M., Maier, H., & Jopp, D. (2002). Health and well-being in the young old and oldest old. *Journal of Social Issues, 58,* 715–732.

Thiele, D. M., & Whelan, T. A. (2006). The nature and dimensions of the grandparent role. *Marriage and Family Review, 40,* 93–108.

Thomas, P. A. (2012). Trajectories of social engagement and mortality in late life. *Journal of Aging and Health, 24,* 547–568.

Uchino, B. N. (2006). Social support and health: A review of physiological processes potentially underlying links to disease outcomes. *Journal of Behavioral Medicine, 29,* 377–387.

Uchino, B. N., Bowen, K., Carlisle, M., & Birmingham, W. (2012). Psychological pathways linking social support to health outcomes: A visit with the "ghosts" of research past, present, and future. *Social Science and Medicine, 74,* 949–957.

Uchino, B. N., Cawthon, R. M., Smith, T. W., Light, K. C., McKenzie, J., Carlisle, M., et al. (2012). Social relationships and health: Is feeling positive, negative, or both (ambivalent) about your social ties related to telomeres? *Health Psychology, 31,* 789–796.

Wrzus, C., Hänel, M., Wagner, J., & Neyer, F. J. (2013). Social network changes and life events across the life span: A meta-analysis. *Psychological Bulletin, 139,* 53–80.

Yoon, C., Hasher, L., Feinberg, F., Rahhal, T. A., & Winocur, G. (2000). Cross-cultural differences in memory: The role of culture-based stereotypes about aging. *Psychology and Aging, 15,* 694–704.

Yun, R. J., & Lachman, M. E. (2006). Perceptions of aging in two cultures: Korean and American views on old age. *Journal of Cross-Cultural Gerontology, 21,* 55–70.

Zickuhr, K., & Madden, M. (2012). Older adults and Internet use. Retrieved from *http://pewinternet.org/reports/2012/older-adults-and-internet-use.aspx.*

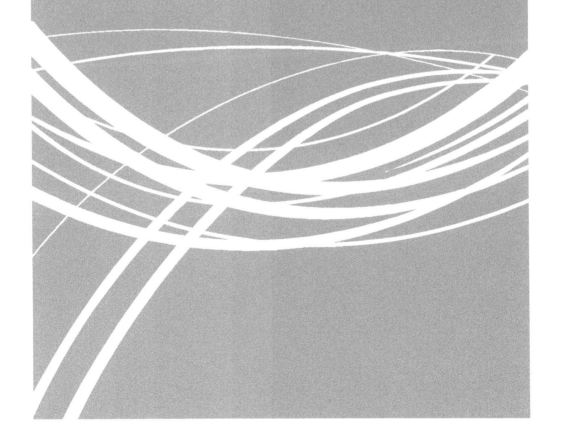

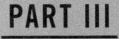

PART III

SOCIALIZATION IN THE CONTEXT OF DIFFERENT RELATIONSHIPS AND SETTINGS

CHAPTER 6

Socialization as Dynamic Process
A Dialectical, Transactional Perspective

Leon Kuczynski
C. Melanie Parkin
Robyn Pitman

During much of the past century, socialization theories have tended to be unidirectional and deterministic. Parents were portrayed as active in setting agendas, transmitting values, and controlling children's behavior, whereas children were considered as passive outcomes in the socialization process. The goal of research on socialization was to explain how intergenerational continuity or the conformity of the younger generation to the norms and expectations of the previous generation comes about.

Less emphasis has been placed on the possibility that socialization is a mechanism of intergenerational change. Vast macro-level social change has occurred since the 1960s in values concerning gender equality, racial, cultural and sexual diversity, family diversity, and the rights of children. The role of media and globalization of knowledge drives increasingly rapid change, such that decades rather than generations may soon become a more appropriate unit for measuring shifts in values. At the micro level, there is also lifelong change in the individual. Socialization does not end at young adulthood. Instead, socialization continues throughout the life span as individuals continue to change and develop the skills, behavior patterns, ideas, and values needed for competent functioning in a social context that is constantly changing. Parents also engage in a process of continuing resocialization as they adapt to the direct impact of having children (Palkovitz, Marks, Appleby, & Holmes, 2003); new social contexts, including the workplace; and life transitions, as well as social changes in the surrounding culture. Thus, from a developmental perspective, intergenerational change, not just intergenerational continuity, needs to be considered as an expected outcome of socialization.

Contemporary researchers have a much more dynamic conception of the process of socialization than was once the case. This revitalization of socialization theory can be traced to three important ideas. The first is that socialization is a bidirectional process incorporating the influence of both children and parents (Bell, 1968; Sameroff, 1975a, 1975b). The second is that children and parents are active interpretive agents who construct new meanings during transactions with each other (Grusec & Goodnow, 1994; Kuczynski, 2003). The third is a new focus on the neglected dialectical underpinnings of Sameroff's (1975a, 1975b, 2009) transactional model of human development, which emphasizes the nonlinear or qualitative change that emerges from interactions between human agents (Kuczynski & De Mol, in press).

Our purpose in this chapter is to explore dialectics as a conceptual metatheory for understanding causality in the parent–child relationships and the new directions that it offers for the study of socialization. In the first part of this chapter, we contrast mechanistic and dialectical conceptions of bidirectional influence in socialization. The argument is that mechanism and dialectics provide qualitatively different ways of thinking about the process of socialization. Next we explore the original dialectical foundation of Sameroff's (1975a, 1975b) transactional model of human development and how the concept of dialectics has been expanded within social relational theory (Kuczynski & De Mol, in press). We argue that social relational theory and dialectical transactional conceptions of bidirectionality add a focus on relational, not just interactional, processes in parent–child dynamics as well as new insights into the qualitative changes that occur in the process of socialization. Table 6.1 provides an overview of basic assumptions of mechanistic, dialectical, and social relational concepts that are the foci of this chapter.

Mechanistic versus Dialectical Models of Bidirectionality

There are two very different ways of thinking about the nature of bidirectional influence (Kuczynski & De Mol, in press; Overton & Reese, 1973). These correspond to mechanistic versus dialectical perspectives on the nature of phenomena (ontology).

The *mechanistic* model of bidirectionality considers parent–child social interactions as a reactive process that comprises immediate reciprocal exchanges of behaviors that

TABLE 6.1. Concepts of Mechanistic, Dialectical, and Social Relational Theories

	Mechanistic →	Dialectical ☉	Social relational ↔
Causality	Linear	Nonlinear	Transactional/systemic
Agency	Independent Inert elements	Interdependent Active components	Equal agency (construction, action, autonomy)
Context	N/A	Holism	Parent–child relationship
Source of change	Control strategies	Contradiction Uncertainty	Conflict, ambiguity Ambivalence, expectancy violations
Outcomes	Linear effects (e.g., compliance, intergenerational transmission)	Synthesis Novelty	Nonlinear outcomes (e.g., accommodation, negotiation, working models, nonlinear trajectories)

produce incremental or linear change. Research models that explicitly or implicitly follow a mechanistic ontology treat parents and children as separate inert elements and consider causality between the elements as operating in a direct, linear, and predictable manner. This is the ontology that underlies early unidirectional (parent → child) models of socialization. Mechanistic models of bidirectional causality added a child-to-parent (child → parent) direction of influence to the parent-to-child direction of influence, thus preserving an idea of direct cause and effect in a reciprocal sequence. For example, Sears (1951) conceptualized social interaction to be a series of stimulus → response sequences in which each person's behavior was simultaneously a reaction to the other's previous behavior and a stimulus for the partner's subsequent response. An underlying mechanistic idea of causal influence was also evident in the influential control process model of parent–child interaction (Bell & Harper, 1977). These authors proposed that parent–child interactions operated according to the properties of a homeostatic control process that keeps the child's behavior within upper and lower limits that are tolerated by the parent. The theoretical underpinning of the coercive family process model (see Patterson, 1982; Patterson, Reid, & Dishion, 1992) is also mechanistic. According to Patterson and colleagues, reciprocal exchanges of aversive behaviors among parents and children provide negative reinforcement for each other's behavior and escalate into habitual patterns of mutual coercion.

The mechanistic nature of these theories can be seen in the way agency, context, and causality are implicitly or explicitly conceptualized.

1. Parents and children are treated as if they are by nature relatively *inert, reactive,* or *passive* and do not change unless acted upon by an external force.
2. Parents and children are treated as if they are disconnected, interchangeable *elements*, with little consideration of the causal significance of the system or holistic relationship context in which they are embedded.
3. Causality is considered as direct and linear; this is evident in an emphasis on conformity, compliance, transmission of similarity, and continuity between the generations as the desired outcome of socialization.

Dialectical models of bidirectional influence consider parent–child social interactions to be a process of nonlinear transformation in which parents and children act as self-organizing agents, who are related as interdependent components of a larger system. Kuczynski and colleagues (Kuczynski & De Mol, in press; Kuczynski & Parkin, 2007) argue that dialectics implies a cognitive model of bidirectional influence in social transactions. In a dialectical perspective, bidirectional influence comes about as parents and children interpret or construct meanings out of each other's behaviors and resist, negotiate, and accommodate each other's perspectives within the constraints of the relationship.

Dialectics is a metatheory about the dynamic and contextualized nature of all phenomena. Dialectics has been conveyed by popular metaphors such as the *yin–yang* symbol of Chinese philosophy that captures the causal structure of dialectical systems, and the *thesis–antithesis–synthesis* process of Western Hegelian philosophy that captures the nonlinear model of dialectical causality. In dialectics, all phenomena and processes comprise a system (holistic context) of opposing forces that actively relate to produce continuous qualitative change (Kuczynski & Parkin, 2009; Kuczynski, Pitman, & Mitchell, 2009). Causality in dialectics is systemic rather than direct and emerges not only by the properties of the *active, self-organizing components* of the system but also by the properties of the *holistic* system of which they are a part. Valsiner and Connolly (2003) interpreted dialectics using contemporary dynamic systems theory:

> Development and the appearance of new emergent properties cannot arise in a single component or solely in the context; two or more components are always necessary. Hence, classical notions of linear causality (e.g., cause X leads to outcome Y) are inappropriate in the case of developing systems. Instead, developmental science operates with the notion of systemic causality (Valsiner, 2000). An outcome is a result of the systemic relationship between parts of a system: system $\{a–R–b\}$, where a and b are parts and R is their relation, leads to outcome Y. (p. xi)

Any system will have aspects that are harmonious, as well as aspects that are contradictory or dissonant. The potential for change exists in the tension of the interacting components of the system that has the potential for generating novel outcomes. In dialectics, *contradiction* is the source of change, just as a stimulus or a contingent punishment is the antecedent of change in mechanistic models. Riegel (1976) distinguished two types of contradiction. *Inner dialectics* are dialectical bidirectional $\leftrightarrow$ tensions within an individual, for example, competing thoughts or interpretations. *Outer dialectics* are dialectical bidirectional $\leftrightarrow$ tensions between an individual and some aspect of the social or physical environment that constitutes the relevant system. Examples include an opposing behavior in a relationship partner, or an unexpected event or change in the environment that clashes with an individual's current understanding (*thesis*). Contradictions are points of uncertainty that are experienced as tensions. In making sense of the contradiction (*antithesis*), each individual, or partner in a relationship, creates a new *synthesis* that sets the stage for new contradictions, new theses, and continuous qualitative change.

Dialectics has been a major source of ideas for psychology even if its foundations are not acknowledged or if its assumptions have not been fully implemented in particular theories. A dialectical conception of causality is the foundation of all organismic developmental theories (Goldhaber, 2000), as well as organismic/contextual or relational developmental systems metatheories (Overton, 2006). Approaches compatible with dialectics include social cognitive (Grusec & Goodnow, 1994) and constructionist (Smetana, 2011) theories of social development, as well as self-determination theory (Ryan & Deci, 2002), which all have a core assumption that parents and children are active agents who interpret and thereby reconstruct social messages. In this section, we review two theoretical frameworks for understanding dynamic bidirectional processes of influence in socialization that have an explicit dialectical orientation. The first is Sameroff's (1975a, 1975b, 2009) transactional model of human development, which is based in dialectics, and the second is social relational theory, which elaborates on the implications of a dialectical model of transaction for parent–child relationships and socialization.

The Transactional Model

Sameroff (1975a, 1975b) originally conceptualized bidirectional influence in his transactional model of human development as being dialectical in nature: Causes cannot be reduced to particular dispositions, cognitions, or behaviors of the parent or the child.

Parents and children are engaged in continual transformation as each partner responds to new emerging characteristics of the other (Sameroff, 1975a, 1975b, 2009). Sameroff proposed that contradiction is the mechanism for these qualitative transformations: "In every developing system, contradictions are generated and it is these contradictions which provide the motivation which lead the organisms to the higher level of organization found in developmental series" (Sameroff, 1975b, p. 74). Sameroff (2009) argued that changes in meaning systems occur whenever individuals are induced by a contradiction to think or act differently, or change their representation of a person or event.

Sameroff (2009) cited the social information-processing model of childhood aggression (Fontaine & Dodge, 2009) an example of the transactional approach. This model identifies a number of sites of changed representations including the encoding of cues, interpretation of cues, clarification of cues, construction of responses, and evaluation of responses that have been found to affect subsequent changes in behavior. Research on social cognitions and attributions in parent–child interactions also can be interpreted in a transactional way. For example, in studies on parent–child transactions, Bugental (2009) found that mothers who maltreat their children often respond on the basis of the threat that they perceive in their children's difficult behavior. The threat representation leads to mothers' negative affect, which affects the child's level of disregulation, which leads to subsequent withdrawal by the mother. Other examples include attributions of intentionality to children's behavior (Dix, Ruble, Grusec, & Nixon, 1986), as well as other cognitions or changed representations that parents or children individually or mutually form during interactions (e.g., Grusec, Rudy, & Martini, 1997). A well-researched example concerns the situational specificity of parental discipline strategies (Kuczynski, 1984). The most commonly used parental strategy during everyday interaction is mild power assertion, such as unexplained commands and prohibitions that are used to obtain immediate compliance. However, when parents interpret the child's behavior as requiring long-term change, for example, when the transgression involves a safety issue or a moral offense, parents qualitatively change their strategies to a more considered way of interacting and begin to use cognitive strategies such as reasoning (Kuczynski, 1984). A change in context evokes a changed representation (transaction) of the child's behavior, inducing the parent to send the interaction on a qualitatively new trajectory.

According to Sameroff (2009), there are methodological and conceptual barriers to implementing the original dialectical interpretation of transaction. Attempts to operationalize the transactional model often require a mechanistic measurement model that reduces dynamic processes into static scores that are isolated as independent variables when they are actually dependent interacting variables. In addition, dialectics involves many interconnected assumptions that have not been conceptually translated into empirical research models. Kuczynski and Parkin (2009) argued that the dialectical nature of Sameroff's transactional model, when originally proposed in 1975, was ahead of its time and required a framework of supportive research and theory about parent–child interactions and relationships.

Social Relational Theory

Social relational theory (Kuczynski & De Mol, in press; Kuczynski & Parkin, 2007) builds on the transactional model introduced by Sameroff (1975a, 1975b) by considering dialectics as a foundation for consolidating research on bidirectional processes in social-ization and bridging to the wider relational systems frameworks of contemporary devel-opmental science (Overton, 2006). In the next section, we consider how four aspects of the dialectical model—active components, holism, contradiction, and synthesis—can be used to reframe literature on socialization in the family and provide directions for future research. Although these aspects are presented separately for purposes of analysis, it is important to consider them as interrelated assumptions of a larger dialectical system of ideas.

The Components: Parent and Child Agents

Agency refers to parents and children as the active interacting causal components in a dialectical system. Agency is a multifaceted construct (Bandura, 2006; Cummings & Schermerhorn, 2003) that includes cognitive, behavioral, and motivational dimensions. In social relational theory, the dimensions of agency are the universal capacities for construction, action, and autonomy (Kuczynski, 2003; Kuczynski & De Mol, in press). *Construction* refers to the capacity of parents and children to reflect on their behavior and interpret messages communicated during social interactions. Parents interpret their children's behavior and the requirements of the situation and ideally tailor their mes-sages so that children can accurately understand and accept their perspective (Grusec & Goodnow, 1994). However, the constructive capacities of children means that they also interpret and evaluate parental communications, and thus determine how the messages are received or whether they are accepted (Kuczynski, 2003). *Action* refers to parents' and children's capacities to initiate purposeful behavior and strategically choose ways to achieve their goals. *Autonomy* refers to parents' and children's motives to feel that one's actions are undertaken with a sense of personal volition (Ryan & Deci, 2002) or to resist threats to their freedom to choose in situations that matter to them, block their goals (Kuczynski & Kochanska, 1990), or contravene their self-constructed understanding of social situations (Kuczynski & Knafo, 2014).

There are also individual aspects to agency (Kuczynski & De Mol, in press). Although parents and children are equally agents by virtue of being human, they are unequal in resources or power that supports their effectiveness as agents. In social relational theory, unequal power is conceptualized dialectically as a dynamic interdependent asymmetry. Parents have more individual resources (e.g., physical strength, assets, cognitive skills) to compel or persuade their children, especially early in childhood. However, children are never actually powerless with regard to such resources (Kuczynski, 2003). The asymmetry between parents and their children is constantly changing over time and varies depending on the context. Porta and Howe (2012) found that the relative power between parents and children and the specific power resources used by them change as they engage in dif-ferent personal, conventional, and prudential issues throughout the day. Moreover, as we elaborate in the section on holism, the dynamics of power inequality must be understood in the context of the long-term, interdependent parent–child relationship context. The interdependence of the parent and child means that parents are vulnerable and receptive to their children's influence despite differences in relative amounts of various resources.

A focus on human agency clarifies the contributions of parents and children to the socialization process. Correlational research is useful in identifying associations between child variables and parental variables, but does not illuminate the underlying processes of social interaction (Darling & Steinberg, 1993). The perspective of human agency guides researchers to be curious about what parents and children do in social interactions or how they interpret their experiences. One direction for future research implied by the concept that parents and children are equally human agents is to ask questions about their influence and agency in a parallel manner (Kuczynski, 2003). This would provide an enhanced perspective on what parents can accomplish as agents, as well as fill in knowledge about the neglected aspects of children's agency with regard to parents. A second direction is to extend the concept of equal agency to transactional models of social interaction. Such models would consider parents and children interacting "as if" they recognize each other's agency, thus anticipating and accommodating each other's interpretive capacities, autonomy motives, and different perspectives. A third direction, discussed in the next section, is to consider how the relationship context influences how parents and children experience and practice their agency; that is, a more comprehensive dialectical approach requires that parents and children be considered as interacting components of the holistic system of their shared relationship.

Holism: Relationship as Context for Agency

In social relational theory, the parent–child relationship corresponds to the dialectical idea of holism. Social development occurs within a system of close personal relationships (Reiss, Collins, & Berscheid, 2000). Different relationships, including relationships with parents, siblings, peers, teachers, and other adults (Piniata, 1999), come into prominence as contexts for socialization as children develop. With regard to the specific context of parent–child relationships, parents and children are considered to be embedded within a close, long-term, interdependent relationship that affects the nature of their influence and how they practice their agency as interacting partners (Kuczynski, 2003).

The assumption that relationships are holistic contexts, as well as dynamic processes, is a departure from socialization theories that consider parents and children as decontextualized individuals or use relationship variables such as "warmth" as a proxy for the relationship. Arguments for the causal role of relationship contexts and relational processes in socialization outcomes have been made in the past. Maccoby and Martin (1983) argued that the foundations for children's receptivity to parental influence are not parental discipline strategies but children's experiences of reciprocal cooperation developed in the early history of the relationship. Bretherton, Golby, and Cho's (1997) attachment perspective on socialization suggested that children's propensity to comply stems from the security of their relationships with parents. As well, Darling and Steinberg (1993) argued that authoritative, authoritarian, and permissive parenting styles (Baumrind, 1971a) reflect different relationship contexts rather than parenting practices. A relatively neglected finding from Baumrind's research program is also open to a relational interpretation. Baumrind (1971b) reported a harmonious parenting pattern (high warmth, moderate control, high tolerance), which she regarded as an anomaly that did not fit her more general conception of parenting styles. The harmonious pattern, in which children's cooperation is accomplished in the absence of parental firm control, can be viewed as consistent with research arguing for the causal role of mutually reciprocal or secure relationships. Taken together, such proposals point to a direction for future research. We know a great deal about parental practices and something about social interactional dynamics (Maccoby & Martin, 1983), but we know very little about relational practices and relational dynamics. In other words, we need to explore the transactional processes that underlie the variable known as "warmth."

Social relational theory draws from theory and research on personal relationships, as well as parent–child relationships (e.g., Bowlby, 1969; Hinde, 1979; Kelley et al., 1983; Maccoby, 2000) to understand dynamics associated with relationship contexts. Core ideas from this literature, including the interdependence of partners in a close relationship (Kelley et al. 1983), the significance of the past and future of the relationship, and the role of relationship expectancies formed during parent–child transactions (Hinde, 1979) have been consolidated into a transactional model of parent–child relationships (Kuczynski & De Mol, in press; Lollis & Kuczynski, 1997). These ideas provide the basis for a relational perspective on socialization that broadens the study of socialization processes beyond discipline and control strategies, and immediate contingencies between parent and child behaviors.

Interdependence

Interdependence is the degree to which the behaviors, emotions, and thoughts of two individuals are mutually and causally interconnected (Kelley et al., 1983). Interdependence has both a causal and an experiential meaning. The causal meaning of interdependence refers to the necessary bidirectional relation between the components of the whole in a close relationship. Indeed, bidirectional influence between partners must be present for the relationship to be considered a close relationship (Cook, 2001). The close coordination of parent and child actions in relationships has been represented in such constructs as intersubjectivity, scaffolding, coregulation, co-construction, and mutual responsiveness. Experientially, interdependence involves complex emotions and meanings that each partner constructs about the exchanges occurring in the relationship. The behavior of each person is dependent on and has consequences for the other. The child depends on the parent for love, security, care, and other resources for physical and psychological needs. Parents also depend on children to satisfy emotional needs for intimacy, companionship, joy, fun, pride, and meaning in their lives (Trommsdorff, Zheng, & Tardif, 2002). Parents and children both have a psychological and emotional investment in the relationship and create meanings about it. This mutual investment makes them more receptive to one another and also more vulnerable to being influenced by the other (Kuczynski, 2003). In other words, interdependence affects the way that children and parents respond to each other because they matter to each other (Marshall & Lambert, 2006).

Past and Future Dimensions of Relationships

Social relationships can be distinguished from social interactions using the concept of time. *Interactions* are discrete, moment-to-moment exchanges between individuals, whereas the relationship operates at a larger systemic level of analysis that considers the past and future time dimension of the relationship between the partners beyond the immediate interaction. According to Hinde (1979), as dyads accumulate a history of interactions, they form relationships, and the emergent relationship subsequently becomes the context for their future interactions. A single interaction between unfamiliar individuals does not constitute a relationship, but a relationship begins to be formed once individuals begin to form and act on expectations or predictions on the basis of their past experiences (Lollis & Kuczynski, 1997). Unlike interactions between unfamiliar individuals, the parent–child relationship has a rich history of transactions occurring over many years that contribute cognitive expectancies of the parent and child regarding the other's personality, preferences, and predictions of the others' responses to their actions (Kuczynski, Lollis, Parkin, & Oliphant, 2007). As well, the parent–child relationship has a long, anticipated future. The projected future of the relationship contributes future-oriented anticipations to interactions occurring in the present. An example is when parents act on the basis of future goals for children. Documented examples of parental goals include long-term socialization goals (Kuczynski, 1984), child-oriented goals that support the child's goals (Dix, 1992), and relationship goals (Hastings & Grusec, 1998) designed to promote and maintain the mutual relationship context. Dawber and Kuczynski's (1999) finding of a higher frequency of future goals in parents' interactions with their own children than with unfamiliar children lends support to the argument that the presence of future goals for the other is a relational phenomenon.

Acting on past expectancies and future anticipations are examples of transactions because they constitute cognitive representations of the relationship. The relationship itself is a cognitive construction that represents more than the sum of interactions that objectively occurred in the history of the relationship. Each partner interprets and makes sense of the other's behavior. These meanings become consolidated in representations of the relationship that then form the filter through which parent and child behaviors are experienced and predictions are made about how the other will respond in future interactions (Hinde, 1979; Kuczynski & De Mol, in press; Lollis, 2003; Lollis & Kuczynski, 1997).

Domain Complexity

The parent–child relationship has a complex structure incorporating not only a past and future but also various interrelated domains in which parents and children interact. It is now recognized that there are significant horizontal power dynamics in addition to long-standing conceptions of vertical power in parent–child relationships (Russell, Petitt, & Mize, 1998). This more complex view of power dynamics in parent–child relationships has been incorporated in relationship domain models (Bugental & Goodnow, 1998; Lollis & Kuczynski, 1997) and socialization domain models (Grusec & Davidov, 2010; Chapter 7, this volume) in which parents and children cycle through different domains within the relationship, and the goals, functions, and power dynamics underlying parent–child interactions change throughout the day. Three domains provide a starting point for understanding parent–child relationships in Western cultures: authority, attachment, and intimacy (Kuczynski & De Mol, in press). These can be conceptualized as having specific direct functions, unintended indirect transactional effects, and distinctive power dynamics that are also depicted to reflect Western patterns.

The *authority domain* has the specific direct function of socializing children and engages the parent in the role of legitimate authority and the child as active recipient of socialization messages (Grusec & Goodnow, 1994). Bidirectional dynamics in the authority domain occur in a context of interdependent power asymmetry, in which parents try to exercise their greater power in relation to a child who has resources to actively accommodate or resist their expectations. Transactions in the authority domain may have an indirect function in creating expectancies about the relationship. Examples of such expectancies include whether the parent's power will prevail during conflict (Cavell & Strand, 2003) or whether the relationship has democratic features and allows room for negotiation (Goodnow, 1997).

The *attachment domain* has the specific direct function of providing security and protection (Grusec & Davidov, 2010) and engages the parental role of caregiver and the child as seeker of care. Bidirectional dynamics occur in a complementary power relationship in which children provide cues about their needs and parents respond appropriately to those needs. Transactions in the attachment domain may indirectly contribute to the larger relationship, in addition to expectancies of security or insecurity. For example, Cummings and Schermerhorn (2003) argued that children's responses to mothers in the Strange Situation indicate that children develop a sense that they are able to influence the parent in the relationship from their experiences of parents' past responsiveness to their distress. In addition, Bretherton and colleagues (1997) speculated that representations that parents will meet children's needs in times of distress might generalize to trust that the parental demands or requests are in children's best interest.

The intimacy domain has the direct function of creating mutually pleasurable social interactions between parents and children. The *intimacy domain* (Harach & Kuczynski, 2005; Oliphant & Kuczynski, 2011) refers to a specific conception of interactions in the horizontal or reciprocal power domain of relationships that has been developed for middle childhood. Other conceptions of this domain focusing on infancy and early childhood include MacDonald's (1992) conception of the evolutionary significance of "warmth," which he proposed is based on pleasurable interactions, mutual attunement (Grusec & Davidov (2010), and shared positive affect or mutually responsive orientation (Aksan, Kochanska, & Ortmann, 2006; Kochanska, 2002).

Weingarten (1991) conceptualized parent–child intimacy as transient interactions in which parents and children share or co-create meaning. A coordination of actions is required to co-create meaning; whereas imposing meaning or withdrawing from meaning making is not experienced as intimacy. Intimacy conceptualized in this way has been explored in several qualitative studies. Harach and Kuczynski (2005) asked mothers and fathers of 4- to 7-year-old children what they do to strengthen relationships with their children. Parents reported ideas that corresponded more frequently to underlying concepts of intimacy and companionship (e.g., having fun together, treating each other with mutual respect), than to the ideas of attachment (e.g., security, trust), or authority (e.g., guidance teaching). Similarly, mothers and fathers (Oliphant & Kuczynski, 2011) were asked to identify recent interactions with their 7- to 11-year-old children in which they felt close to them. Oliphant and Kuczynski (2011) described these incidents as characterized by a close coordination of actions and positive affect. Examples of intimate interactions included shared thoughts, ideas, emotions, and activities that are experienced as moments of mutuality during routine activities such as mealtime, bedtime, car trips, or chores, as well as intentional, idiosyncratic rituals set up to create the opportunity for closeness or shared pleasure (Oliphant & Kuczynski, 2011). Bidirectional dynamics in the intimacy domain occur in the context of equal power that requires parents and children to coordinate their actions to achieve mutuality (Harach & Kuczynski, 2005; Oliphant & Kuczynski, 2011). Indirect outcomes of experiences in the intimacy domain may contribute to parents' or children's representations of the relationship as close and mutually cooperative, and perceptions that they can initiate or maintain such interactions.

Implications of Considering Relationships as Holistic Contexts

Considering the parent–child relationship as a holistic or systemic context suggests new phenomena in socialization, as well as directions for reinterpreting older ones. Kuczynski and De Mol (in press) discussed various directions for future research. Two that are highlighted here include the construction and maintenance of the relationship context, and relational dynamics.

Relationship Construction and Maintenance

A neglected aspect of the literature on parent–child relationships concerns how parents and children actively construct and maintain the relationship context that is crucial in determining the nature of their interactions. A key process is parental responsiveness and sensitivity (Laible, Thompson, & Froimson, Chapter 2, this volume), which plays a role in both constructing the relationship and mediating socialization processes. A domain perspective suggests that the construct of responsiveness may take different forms and have different outcomes depending on the domain in question. For example, Leerkes, Weaver, and O'Brien (2012) argue that the experiential origins of maternal sensitivity to distress cues and maternal sensitivity to nondistress cues in infants are different, and that the two forms of responsiveness make unique contributions to children's outcomes. In addition, receptiveness to parental influence (Maccoby & Martin, 1983; Parpal & Maccoby, 1985) or a mutually responsive orientation (Kochanska, 2002; Kochanska & Aksan, 1995) is viewed as growing out of parent–child relationships in which children and parents are engaged in cycles of positive affect and mutual cooperation. Grusec and Davidov (2010) argued that existing evidence suggests that positive mutual responsivity may have different associations with subsequent compliance and responsiveness to distress.

Studies on parents' perceptions of their efforts to maintain an intimate relationship with children (Harach & Kuczynski, 2005; Oliphant & Kuczynski, 2011) demonstrate a variety of relationship maintenance behaviors and include making time for mutually enjoyable interactions, managing their power in relationship to the child, communicating at the child's level, refraining from overpowering the child by imposing meaning, and making relational repairs through communication and apology. Parents report that children engage in analogous behaviors as their part in creating intimate interactions.

Relational Dynamics

An important direction for future research is to complement the extant body of interactional dynamics comprising immediate contingencies between behaviors such as control processes (Bell & Harper, 1977) and mutual negative reinforcement (Patterson, 1982) with a new exploration of relational dynamics that stem from the relationship context of social interactions. Kuczynski and De Mol (in press) discussed an initial list of relational principles that concern the causal nature of cognitions associated with the time dimension and interdependence of the relationship:

1. Parents and children act as if the relationship has a past (past expectancies).
2. Parents and children act as if the relationship has a future (future anticipations, goals).
3. Parents and children act as if their responses to each other's behavior matters to them (interdependence).

These dynamics can be considered as the effects of relational contexts that both *enable* and *constrain* how parents and children interact with each other as agents (Kuczynski & Parkin, 2007). For example, parents' effectiveness as agents is enabled by their knowledge of the child, developed in the history of the relationship (Dawber & Kuczynski, 1999), and a mutually responsive relationship that increases children's receptivity to their influence (e.g., Parpal & Maccoby, 1985), but their use of coercive power may be constrained by their desire to maintain an enjoyable and rewarding intimate relationship (Harach & Kuczynski, 2005). The enabling effects of the relationship for children are evident in adolescents' confidence in assertively resisting parents (Parkin & Kuczynski, 2012), but the constraining effects of the relationship are evident in situations in which children avoid aversive confrontational strategies in order not to damage their relationships with parents (Lundell, Grusec, McShane, & Davidov, 2008; Parkin & Kuczynski, 2012).

Another relational dynamic concerns how parents and children use the relationship that they have created to further their goals in interactions with each other. The idea of relationship-based control strategies was anticipated by Hoffman (1983), who described parents' use of contingent *love withdrawal* as well as *other-oriented induction*, as a form of reasoning that depends on affective relational resources such as guilt or empathy. These have been reinterpreted as having detrimental consequences in the construct of *psychological control* (Barber, 1996). However, there is evidence that parents may also use the relationship context in a constructive fashion. Researchers have found a positive association between parental knowledge and a number of relational variables, including parental responsiveness (Soenens, Vansteenkiste, Luyckx, & Goossens, 2006), warmth (Salafia, Gondoli, & Grundy, 2009), and trust (Smetana, Villalobos, Tasopoulos-Chan, Gettman, & Campione-Barr, 2009). In a recent qualitative study, Kuczynski, Wojciechowska, Dawczyk, and Pitman (2012) explored the processes of social interaction that may underlie the association between such relationship variables and parental knowledge. A majority of parents of 8- to 13-year-olds reported that they used relational strategies that included maintaining intimacy, solicitation during conversations, and ensuring trust/support in order to gain knowledge about their child. Essentially, parents created relationship contexts, such as routine intimate interactions, that enabled children to voluntarily disclose information about their activities, friendships, and internal states. In addition, parents attempted to foster trust in the relationship by assuring children that they could come to them when they were in trouble.

Cultural Embeddedness of Relationships

Hinde (1979) argued that relationships are systemically related to larger contexts, such as culture. Accordingly, it can be stated that there are cross-cultural differences, particularly in the dynamics of the domains comprising parent–child relationships. There are variations in the norms for appropriate power relations in parent–child relationships and the ways that functions such as authority, attachment, and intimacy are expressed

(Kuczynski, 2003; Trommsdorff & Kornadt, 2003). As well, there are cultural norms regarding the appropriate membership of the caregiving relationship, for instance, the extent to which fathers or grandparents are central in the day-to-day rearing of children (Goh & Kuczynski, 2010). Because parent–child relationships are embedded in culture, culture is important in understanding socialization processes and dynamics of bidirectionality, agency, and power in parent–child interactions.

Contradiction: The Source of Change

In social relational theory, the dialectical process of contradiction is considered to drive causal processes in socialization. Contradiction in dialectics, as in parent–child relationships, derives from considering the dynamic interplay between the whole and its components. Although parents and children have different perspectives, goals, and needs, they are nevertheless embedded in an interdependent mutual relationship. Socialization generates both external and internal contradictions (Riegel, 1976). External contradictions occur regularly during conflicts that pit the parent's needs against the child's needs, the parent's will against the child's will, the parent's interpretations of a behavior and the child's interpretations, and the parent's influence strategies and those of the child. In addition, parents and children continually interact with a larger ecological context of values, including those of peers, television, Internet, and school, that offer up contradictions and opportunities for change as parents and children adapt to each other's actions and choices (Kuczynski, Marshall, & Schell, 1997).

Internal contradictions for the parent occur during everyday interactions with children. For example, parents must allow exploration yet guard against danger, be responsive yet avoid spoiling the child, seek obedience and respect yet allow autonomy, be involved yet not overinvolved, and promote independence yet maintain dependence (Holden & Ritchie, 1988). The parental role itself involves diverse conflicting functions and roles such as authority, security provider, and intimacy that must be kept in balance (Harach & Kuczynski, 2005). In a recent qualitative study, Dawczyk and Kuczynski (2012) reported evidence of three aspects of the dialectical process that examined spontaneous occurrences of contradictions as parents described their recent interactions with children. First, contradictions could be classified according to the psychological processes of conflict, ambiguity, ambivalence, and violations of expectations, all of which have in common a state of uncertainty regarding what to do or think in specific situations (Kuczynski & Parkin, 2009; Kuczynski et al., 2009). Second, the majority of reports of contradiction were accompanied by affective reactions, conceptualized as dialectical tensions, ranging from mild dissonance to strong emotion. These included expressions of emotions indicative of anxiety, stress, surprise, anger, and sadness. Third, the contradictions were accompanied by evidence of problem solving (Holden & Hawk, 2003), which can be understood as attempts to resolve the contradiction.

Synthesis: Dialectical Models of Influence and Outcomes

A defining feature of a dialectical model of transaction is its focus on qualitative change or the emergence of novelty. Kuczynski and De Mol (in press) expanded Sameroff's (1975a, 1975b) transactional model using Lawrence and Valsiner's (1993, 2003) conception of the interpretive processes that take place as individuals engage in transactions with the social world. Lawrence and Valsiner (1993) argued that there are two internal processes to consider, internalization and externalization. *Internalization* refers to the cognitive processing that takes place as individuals make personal sense of messages from the environment. In the case of parent–child relations, this means that parents and children interpret events based on their personal understanding, evaluating the message along with competing messages from the environment, and reconstructing the message for their own use (Kuczynski et al., 1997). *Externalization* refers to the further processing that takes place as parents and children manifest or act on the internalized products of their interpretive processes. The concepts of internalization and externalization show how nonlinear qualitative change enters into processes of social guidance by parents. They also can be used to reframe deterministic concepts such as "control," "compliance," and "intergenerational transmission of values" in a way that captures the nonlinear or synthetic nature of socialization outcomes.

Reinterpreting Control

A key concept in socialization theory is *control*, which has been conceptualized as a parental practice, a process, and an outcome. Variations in firm control are the foundation of Baumrind's (1971a) parenting styles. As well, fostering parental control over child compliance is the focus of behavioral parent management interventions; children who are compliant are under control.

The word *control* may be valid if it is intended to mean no more than a pattern of parental behavior. However, the term is problematic from a dialectical-systems perspective if it implies a linear outcome such as the expectation of an exact match between what the parent demands and the child's response. For example, Baumrind (2012) recently described the control of authoritative parents as involving confrontive rather than coercive power assertion. Baumrind operationally defined confrontive power assertion as "confronts when child disobeys, cannot be coerced by the child, successfully exerts force or influence, enforces after initial noncompliance, exercises power unambivalently, uses negative sanctions freely, and discourages defiant stance" (p. 37). Although Baumrind's model of the authoritative parenting style acknowledges that parents may consider their children's opinions, the key feature of this style of parenting is that, in the end, the parents decide and exercise firm control.

Relational influence is proposed as a dialectical replacement for the construct of control (Kuczynski & De Mol, in press). Influence between human agents creates unpredictability or novelty during interpersonal transactions. In the process of relational influence, differences are created between the "control" attempt of one partner and the other's response as each partner interprets messages from the other in the transaction, then decides how to act on his or her understanding of messages. Conceptually, in the case of a disciplinary transaction, parents confronted with a child's transgression or a child's demand, first may interpret the situation (internalization), then decide how to act on their interpretation (externalization). Children similarly interpret the parents' message, then construct a response.

For example, the parent may make various attributions about the behavior such as intentionality (Dix et al. 1986) as well as the importance of the implied value for the parent (Grusec, Goodnow & Kuczynski 2000). In acting on this interpretation, the parent may select from various goals when deciding how to communicate with the child

(Hastings & Grusec 1998; Kuczynski, 1984). In response, the child may evaluate the legitimacy of the message or the parents' way of communicating it (Grusec & Goodnow, 1994) and then will decide whether to accept the message or to resist by confronting, negotiating, or complying behaviorally but rejecting the message cognitively (Kuczynski, Pitman, Parkin, & Rizk, 2011; Parkin & Kuczynski, 2012). These successive transactions interject creative elements into the interaction between the parent and the child and sever a direct link between the child's behavior and the parent's response, and between the parent's control attempt and the child's response. Thus, parents may sometimes *want* to control, but the best that they can realistically expect is relational influence.

Parents may develop a sense of *relational efficacy* through their experiences of relational influence (Kuczynski & De Mol, in press). Relational efficacy has two components. First, a sense of relational efficacy develops from the parents' awareness that their influence emerges from a history of interactions, and that they exert their own influence in a relationship context that includes the influence of their child. Second, a realistic sense of relational efficacy requires awareness that influence is dialectical in nature, and that the outcome has the potential for novelty. In other words, the relationship context may afford parents the expectation of a cooperative response from their child, even if its precise form is unintended. Parents may develop a sense of relational efficacy from their experiences of both cooperation and accommodative forms of resistance during the history of the relationship. A sense of relational efficacy may emerge, even in situations where parents may not be achieving behavioral compliance, from perceptions that they have been heard, that they matter, or that their influence has made a difference in the relationship (De Mol & Buysse, 2008).

Reinterpreting Compliance and Noncompliance

The transactional nature of relational influence implies that it is unrealistic to conceive of outcomes, such as conformity, as an exact match between the child's response and the parent's command, as is implied by standard operational definitions such as compliance in 6 seconds (McMahon & Forehand, 2003). Parental commands and children's responses to them occur in an interdependent relationship context that supports children's expression of autonomy. Within close relationships, the goal is less often to obtain exact compliance than it is to obtain conflict resolution, or some compromise of the original desires of the participants (Miller & Steinberg, 1975). *Accommodation* and *negotiation* are proposed as a dialectical replacement for the constructs of compliance and noncompliance. These terms convey the idea of synthesis. The outcomes of socialization interventions are coregulated and nondeterminate (Kuczynski & Hildebrandt, 1997). According to Dix and Branca (2003), "Because they are interdependent, parents and children must adjust to the needs and interests of the other if each is to succeed in promoting his or her concerns and if the interactions that do so are to be well coordinated and harmonious" (p. 170). Dix and Branca discuss various accommodation strategies that parents use to address their children's concerns on the way to achieving their goals. These include sequencing incompatible goals over time, compromising, replacing a less desirable activity with a somewhat more desirable activity, reframing, adapting, and convincing through explanation. Such accommodations may be a lengthy process that involves transformations of the parent's wishes in the short term. In their sample of preschool children, Crockenberg and Litman (1990) found that "obtaining compliance was quite extended; mothers reasoned, persuaded, suggested and adapted their request to what they thought the child would accept" (p. 970).

Children also play a role in the accommodation process. The argument is that socially competent children display a coregulated but inexact form of conformity and resistance that represents their expression of agency within the constraints of a close parent–child relationship (Kuczynski & Hildebrandt, 1997). Children who are inclined to cooperate with a parent's request may wish to do so in a different time frame than the parent had in mind, may indicate that they will attempt to coordinate their own plans with the parent's wishes, or that they are willing to negotiate a mutually acceptable course of action. Similarly, the construct of negotiation implies that children resist a request but simultaneously take the parent's wishes into account.

Fine-grained analyses of children's noncompliant behaviors during early childhood (Crockenberg & Litman, 1990; Kuczynski & Kochanska, 1990), middle childhood (Kuczynski, Pitman, Parkin, & Rizk, 2011) and adolescence (Parkin & Kuczynski, 2012) indicate that these responses can be interpreted as children's expressions of autonomy, reflecting variations in children's assertiveness and skill as agents. For example, Parkin and Kuczynski (2012) found that adolescents report that they express resistance both overtly by negotiating, asserting, delaying, ignoring or arguing, and covertly by complying in a minimal way or complying but not accepting the spirit of the parent's message. Kuczynski and De Mol (in press) speculated that in healthy parent–child relationships, children act as *connected agents* and express their agency in a way that takes the relationship into account. Resistance may be expressed in an adaptive way when children express their autonomy by pursuing their own goals in a way that accommodates the parents' point of view or avoids confrontations that are damaging to the relationship. An implication for future research is that such accommodations may not be present in unhealthy relationships in which children may act as *isolated agents* who are less constrained by a desire to protect the relationship.

Reinterpreting Intergenerational Transmission

In early models of socialization, values and ideas were considered to be "transmitted" between the generations (Strauss, 1992), and children were conceived as passive recipients and parents as passive conduits in the transmission process (Kuczynski et al., 1997). Building on Lawrence and Valsiner's (1993) conception of internalization as an individual's mental reconstruction of the world, Kuczynski and colleagues (1997) proposed that internalization is a process by which parents and children construct *personal working models* of the beliefs, attitudes, and values of their family and cultural contexts. The concept of working models of internalization (Kuczynski et al., 1997) and working models of culture (Kuczynski & Knafo, 2014) replaces the deterministic conception of internalization as a static transmission of similarity, with a conception that internalization is an ongoing process of synthesis in which beliefs, practices, and values are continuously being constructed and challenged throughout life. Because of different life experiences; different transactions with each other; and their different exposure and susceptibility to ideas of peers, media, or other institutions in their ecological contexts, each member of the family develops somewhat different personal working models as a product of his or her internalization processes (see Kuczynski & Knafo, 2014, for a review of relevant research).

Toward a Dialectical Model of Parenting

A question for future research is whether parents take an implicit dialectical perspective rather than a deterministic perspective in their role as socializing agents. Competent parents may well have a nonlinear view of their actions and may indeed approach socialization in a way that takes their children's agency into account. Parents do not always expect exact transmission of messages and exact conformity as outcomes (Grusec et al., 2000), and it is possible that when parents give commands or attempt to teach values, they have some expectation that their requests will be compromised or transformed through interpretation. A nondeterministic view of parenting would suggest that parents have a range of goals, from a rigid desire for exact transmission when the child's safety is at risk or when strongly held beliefs are at stake, to more indulgent attitudes regarding children's interpretations of their demands when less important personal and conventional issues are at stake (Kuczynski & Hildebrandt, 1997). Parents may therefore communicate a variety of positions with regard to acceptance of their child's behaviors, ranging from what is ideal to what is acceptable, tolerable, or "out of the question" (Goodnow, 1994). Children, in turn, discover how much stretch their parents' position affords and how much leeway there is for their own creative interpretation (Goodnow, 1997).

There is preliminary evidence that parents in families with typically developing children do have expectations and practices that are consistent with a dialectical perspective on influence. Parkin and Kuczynski (2012) found that adolescents perceived that, with the exception of issues concerning safety, parental expectations took the form of flexible, coregulated expectations rather than firm, and inflexible "rules." Robson and Kuczynski (2013) found that parents of 8- to 13-year-old children rarely conceived of or enforced their behavioral expectations of children in the sense of explicit, inflexible rules determined solely by the parent. Instead, flexibility was built into the nature of parental expectations. Flexibility was evident in that parents adjusted their expectations according to the child's emotional state and situational circumstances, and allowed leeway in the time frame for the child's cooperative response. Leeway was also inherent in the way parents perceived how they implemented their expectations. For instance, parents adjusted their rules based on the child's resistance and persuasive abilities. Resistance was anticipated and often interpreted as a legitimate sign of a child's autonomy, and parents granted greater leeway as the child demonstrated increasing capacity and strivings for autonomy. Thus, parents appeared to have an underlying dialectical conception of their influence both by incorporating leeway for the child's agency in their very conception of rules, and in anticipating and accepting novel outcomes during interactions with their child.

Parenting as Guiding Nonlinear Trajectories

Socialization is often conceived of as preparing the child for future success in society. The idea of a nonlinear trajectory that comprises a general orientation and decision points influenced by both the parent and the child along the way, with a wide range of possibilities for the final outcome, offers a dialectical conception of progress toward the future (Kuczynski & De Mol, in press; Sato, Hikada, & Fukuda, 2009).

Holden (2010) discussed the idea of trajectory from the perspective of the parents providing social guidance for children's progress toward the future. Holden argued that parents initiate trajectories by selecting environments that expose children to experiences and invest resources in particular activities. Parents may support trajectories through proactive and sustained efforts, including encouragement, time, helpful messages, and material assistance. Parents may mediate a child's chosen trajectories by helping the child to navigate roadblocks and avoid problematic trajectories. Finally, parents provide feedback by reacting positively or negatively to child-initiated trajectories. This includes supporting the child's choices of activities, education, and careers or using parental power to attempt to redirect the child or create barriers to the child's choices. However, the child is also active in negotiating parental guidance on the trajectory. Parents are not always perceived by adolescents as understanding what being a successful adult will entail in a given culture or point in time. Lightfoot (1997) described adolescents' reflections that adults have no idea about their experiences as adolescents. Thus, children's own efforts partially determine progress on the trajectory, and they may choose their own pathway, with or without the parents' support.

Conclusion

A dialectical perspective on parent–child relationships is an integrative framework that provides a conceptual home to research perspectives that involve constructs such as parent and child agency, goals, cognitions, and representations of relationships as critical factors in understanding socialization. Adopting a dialectical perspective is analogous to a change from a mechanistic lens that sees socialization as a means for intergenerational continuity to a dialectical lens that sees socialization as a dynamic process that also fosters differences between the generations. Perhaps a more apt metaphor is to consider dialectics to be a multifocal lens that allows researchers to have an integrated idea of the whole phenomenon, as well as its constituent features, by peering through the different aspects that the lens offers. The aspect that parents and children are equally active, interpretive, and self-organizing agents guides researchers to be curious about their concrete actions and experiences that feed into the causal processes that underlie empirical associations between abstract parent and child variables. The aspect of holism broadens the idea of what it means to parent a child beyond discipline and control strategies, and beyond a focus on immediate contingencies between behaviors exchanged by parents and children during social interactions. The aspect of contradiction provides a more complex view of the bidirectional processes involved, which include adapting to the conflict, expectancy violations, ambiguity, and ambivalence that are inherent in the relationship. This leads one to consider that parents do not always have a clear and certain idea of what to do, but they engage in problem solving when adapting to the uncertainty created by their rapidly developing child. The aspect of synthesis alerts researchers that parents do not have the sort of direct effect on their children that is assumed in unidirectional models. Parents' influence on children inherently occurs within a causal system that includes the influence and agency of children.

Working out the practical implications of such a complex perspective for parents is a challenge for the future. It is important to stress that parents do matter, and they do influence their children's socialization and development. Even if parents cannot directly determine final outcomes, they are still best placed to have considerable influence on the intervening processes of social interaction and relationship formation, as well as a role in the positive or negative trajectories on which children are initially launched. Moreover, contrary to the arguments of advocates of the extreme thesis that parents have little influence over child outcomes (Harris, 1998), parents do matter in that they can make the child's experience of parent–child relationships a happy or unhappy one. This is no small detail from a relational view of socialization!

Considerable empirical work is required to fill in the gaps in knowledge suggested by a dialectical perspective, as well as to determine the predictive utility for understanding children's outcomes or intervening in troubled families. It remains to be seen whether new users of the dialectical lens find it useful for understanding socialization as a dynamic phenomenon or whether they adapt the lens to create a different vision of synthesis.

REFERENCES

Aksan, N., Kochanska, G., & Ortmann, M. R. (2006). Mutually responsive orientation between parents and their young children: Toward methodological advances in the science of relationships. *Developmental Psychology, 42*, 833–848.

Bandura, A. (2006). Towards a psychology of human agency. *Perspectives on Psychological Science, 1*, 164–180.

Barber, B. K. (1996). Parental psychological control: Revisiting a neglected construct. *Child Development, 67*, 3296–3319.

Baumrind, D. (1971a). Current patterns of parental authority. *Developmental Psychology, 4*(1, Pt. 2), 1–103.

Baumrind, D. (1971b). Harmonious parents and their preschool children. *Developmental Psychology, 4*, 99–102.

Baumrind, D. (2012). Differentiating between confrontive and coercive kinds of parental power-assertive disciplinary practices. *Human Development, 55*, 35–51.

Bell, R. Q. (1968). A reinterpretation of the direction of effects in studies of socialization. *Psychological Review, 75*, 81–95.

Bell, R. Q., & Harper, L. V. (1977). *Child effects on adults*. Hillsdale, NJ: Erlbaum.

Bowlby, J. (1969). *Attachment and Loss: Vol. 1. Attachment*. New York: Basic Books.

Bretherton, I., Golby, B., & Cho, E. (1997). Attachment and the transmission of values. In J. Grusec & L. Kuczynski (Eds.), *Parenting and children's internalization of values* (pp. 103–134). New York: Wiley.

Bugental, D. B. (2009). Predicting and preventing child maltreatment: A biocognitive transactional approach. In A. Sameroff (Ed.), *Transactional processes in development: How children and contexts change each other* (pp. 97–116). Washington, DC: American Psychological Association.

Bugental, D. B., & Goodnow, J. J. (1998). Socialization processes. In W. Damon & N. Eisenberg (Eds.), *Handbook of child psychology: Vol. 3. Social, emotional, and personality development* (5th ed., pp. 389–462). New York: Wiley.

Cavell, T. A., & Strand, P. S. (2003). Parent-based interventions for aggressive, antisocial children: Adapting to a bilateral lens. In L. Kuczynski (Ed.), *Handbook of dynamics in parent–child relations* (pp. 395–419). Thousand Oaks, CA: Sage.

Cook, W. L. (2001). Interpersonal influence in family systems: A social relations model analysis. *Child Development, 72*, 1179–1197.

Crockenberg, S., & Litman, C. (1990). Autonomy as competence in 2-year-olds: Maternal correlates of child defiance, compliance, and self-assertion. *Developmental Psychology, 26*, 961–971.

Cummings, E. M., & Schermerhorn, A. C. (2003). A developmental perspective on children as agents in the family. In L. Kuczynski (Ed.), *Handbook of dynamics in parent–child relations* (pp. 91–108). Thousand Oaks, CA: Sage.

Darling, N., & Steinberg, L. (1993). Parenting style as context: An integrative model. *Psychological Bulletin, 113*(3), 487–497.

Dawber, T., & Kuczynski, L. (1999). The question of owness: Influence of relationship context on parental socialization strategies. *Journal of Social and Personal Relationships, 16*, 475–493.

Dawczyk, A., & Kuczynski, L. (2012, June). *Parents' experiences of contradictions while parenting in middle childhood.* Paper presented at the Jean Piaget Society Conference, Toronto, Ontario, Canada.

De Mol, J., & Buysse, A. (2008). The phenomenology of children's influence on parents. *Journal of Family Therapy, 30*, 163–193.

Dix, T. (1992). Parenting on behalf of the child: Empathic goals in the regulation of responsive parenting. In I. E. Sigel, A. V. McGillicuddy-DeLisi, & J. J. Goodnow (Eds.), *Parental belief system: The psychological consequences for children* (pp. 319–346). Mahwah, NJ: Erlbaum.

Dix, T., & Branca, S. H. (2003). Parenting as a goal-regulation process. In L. Kuczynski (Ed.), *Handbook of dynamics in parent–child relations* (pp. 167–188). Thousand Oaks, CA: Sage.

Dix, T. H., Ruble, D. N., Grusec, J., & Nixon, S. (1986). Social cognition in parents: Inferential and affective reactions to children of three age levels. *Child Development, 57*, 879–894.

Fontaine, R. G., & Dodge, K. A. (2009). Social information processing and aggressive behavior: a transactional perspective. In A. Sameroff (Ed.), *Transactional processes in development: How children and contexts change each other* (pp. 117–135). Washington, DC: American Psychological Association.

Goh, E., & Kuczynski, L. (2010). Only children and their coalition of parents: Considering grandparents and parents as joint caregivers in urban Xiamen, China. *Asian Journal of Social Psychology, 13*, 221–231.

Goldhaber, D. E. (2000). *Theories of human development: Integrative perspectives.* Mountain View, CA: Mayfield.

Goodnow, J. J. (1994). Acceptable disagreement across generations. *New Directions for Child Development, 66*, 51–63.

Goodnow, J. J. (1997). Parenting and the transmission and internalization of values: From social–cultural perspectives to within-family analyses. In J. E. Grusec & L. Kuczynski (Eds.), *Parenting and children's internalization of values: A handbook of contemporary theory* (pp. 333–361). New York: Wiley.

Grusec, J. E., & Davidov, M. (2010). Integrating different perspectives on socialization theory and research: A domain specific approach. *Child Development, 81*, 687–709.

Grusec, J. E., & Goodnow, J. J. (1994). Impact of parental discipline methods on the child's internalization of values: A reconceptualization of current points of view. *Developmental Psychology, 30*, 4–19.

Grusec, J. E., Goodnow, J. J., & Kuczynski, L. (2000). New directions in analyses of parenting contributions to children's acquisition of values. *Child Development, 71*, 205–211.

Grusec, J. E., Rudy, D., & Martini, T. (1997). Parenting cognitions and child outcomes: An overview and implications for children's internalization of values. In J. E. Grusec & L. Kuczynski (Eds.), *Parenting and children's internalization of values: A handbook of contemporary theory* (pp. 259–282). New York: Wiley.

Harach, L., & Kuczynski, L. (2005). Construction and maintenance of parent–child relationships: Bidirectional contributions from the perspective of parents. *Infant and Child Development, 14*, 327–343.

Harris, J. R. (1998). *The nurture assumption.* New York: Simon & Shuster.

Hastings, P. D., & Grusec, J. E. (1998). Parenting goals as organizers of responses to parent–child disagreement. *Developmental Psychology, 34*(3), 465–479.

Hinde, R. A. (1979). *Toward understanding relationships.* London: Academic Press.

Hoffman, M. L. (1983). Affective and cognitive processes in moral internalization: An information processing approach. In E. T. Higgins, D. Ruble, & W. Hartup (Eds.), *Social cognition and social development: A socio-cultural perspective* (pp. 236–274). New York: Cambridge University Press.

Holden, G. W. (2010). Childrearing and developmental trajectories: Positive pathways, off-ramps, and dynamic processes. *Child Development Perspectives, 4,* 197–204.

Holden, G. W., & Hawk, K. H. (2003). Meta-parenting in the journey of child rearing: A cognitive mechanism for change. In L. Kuczynski (Ed.), *Handbook of dynamics in parent–child relations* (pp. 189–210). Thousand Oaks, CA: Sage.

Holden, G. W., & Ritchie, K. L. (1988). Child rearing and the dialectics of parental intelligence. In J. Valsiner (Ed.), *Child development within socio-culturally structured environments: Parental cognition and adult–child interaction* (pp. 30–59). Norwood, NJ: Ablex.

Kelley, H. H., Berscheid, E., Christensen, A., Harvey, J. H., Huston, T. L., Levinger, G., et al. (1983). *Close relationships.* New York: Freeman.

Kochanska, G. (2002). Mutually responsive orientation between mothers and their young children: A context for the early development of conscience. *Current Directions in Psychological Science, 11,* 191–195.

Kochanska, G., & Aksan, N. (1995). Mother–child mutually positive affect, the quality of child compliance to requests and prohibitions, and maternal control as correlates of early internalization. *Child Development, 66*(1), 236–254.

Kuczynski, L. (1984). Socialization goals and mother–child interaction: Strategies for long-term and short-term compliance. *Developmental Psychology, 20,* 1061–1073.

Kuczynski, L. (2003). Beyond bidirectionality: bilateral conceptual frameworks for understanding dynamics in parent–child relations. In L. Kuczynski (Ed.), *Handbook of dynamics in parent–child relations* (pp. 1–24). Thousand Oaks, CA: Sage.

Kuczynski, L., & De Mol, J. (in press). Dialectical models of socialization. In R. M. Lerner (Editor-in-Chief) & W. F. Overton & P. C. Molenaar (Eds.), *Handbook of child psychology and developmental science: Vol. 1. Theory and method* (7th ed.). Hoboken, NJ: Wiley.

Kuczynski, L., & Hildebrandt, N. (1997). Models of conformity and resistance in socialization theory. In J. E. Grusec & L. Kuczynski (Eds.), *Parenting and the internalization of values: A handbook of contemporary theory* (pp. 227–256). New York: Wiley.

Kuczynski, L., & Knafo, A. (2014). Innovation and continuity in socialization, internalization and acculturation. In M. Killen & J. G. Smetana (Eds.), *Handbook of moral development* (2nd ed., pp. 93–112). New York: Psychology Press.

Kuczynski, L., & Kochanska, G. (1990). The development of children's noncompliance strategies from toddlerhood to age 5. *Developmental Psychology, 26,* 398–408.

Kuczynski, L., Lollis, S., Parkin, C. M., & Oliphant, A. (2007, March). *Children's choice of mothers and fathers as targets for influence: Using knowledge of distinct relationships.* Poster presented at the biennial meeting of the Society for Research on Child Development, Boston.

Kuczynski, L., Marshall, S., & Schell, K. (1997). Value socialization in a bidirectional context. In J. E. Grusec & L. Kuczynski (Eds.), *Parenting and the internalization of values: A handbook of contemporary theory* (pp. 23–50). New York: Wiley.

Kuczynski, L., & Parkin, C. M. (2007). Agency and bidirectionality in socialization: Interactions, transactions, and relational dialectics. In J. E. Grusec & P. D. Hastings (Eds.), *Handbook of socialization* (pp. 259–283). New York: Guilford Press.

Kuczynski, L., & Parkin, C. M. (2009). Pursuing a dialectical perspective on transaction: A social relational theory of micro family processes. In A. Sameroff (Ed.), *Transactional processes in development: How children and contexts change each other* (pp. 247–268). Washington, DC: American Psychological Association.

Kuczynski, L., Pitman, R., & Mitchell, M. B. (2009). Dialectics and transactional models: Conceptualizing antecedents, processes, and consequences of change in parent–child relationships. In J. A. Mancini & K. A. Roberto (Eds.), *Pathways of human development: Explorations of change* (pp. 151–170). Lanham, MD: Lexington Books.

Kuczynski, L., Pitman, R., Parkin, M., & Rizk, H. (2011, April). *Children's perspectives on resistance and noncompliance in middle childhood.* Paper presented at the biennial meeting of the Society for Research on Child Development, Montreal, Canada.

Kuczynski, L., Wojciechowska, I., Dawczyk, A., & Pitman, R. (2012, June). *Pathways to parental knowledge in middle childhood.* Paper presented at the annual conference of the Jean Piaget Society, Toronto, Ontario, Canada.

Lawrence, J. A., & Valsiner, J. (1993). Conceptual roots of internalization: From transmission to transformation. *Human Development, 36*(3), 150–167.

Lawrence, J. A., & Valsiner, J. (2003). Making personal sense: An account of basic internalization and externalization processes. *Theory and Psychology, 13*(6), 723–752.

Leerkes, E. M., Weaver, J. M., & O'Brien, M. (2012). Differentiating maternal sensitivity to infant distress and non-distress. *Parenting: Science and Practice, 12*, 175–184.

Lightfoot, C. (1997). *The culture of adolescent risk-taking.* New York: Guilford Press.

Lollis, S. (2003). Conceptualizing the influence of the past and the future in present parent–child relationships. In L. Kuczynski (Ed.), *Handbook of dynamics in parent–child relations* (pp. 67–89). Thousand Oaks, CA: Sage.

Lollis, S., & Kuczynski, L. (1997). Beyond one hand clapping: Seeing bidirectionality in parent–child relations. *Journal of Social and Personal Relationships, 14*, 441–461.

Lundell, L., Grusec, J. E., McShane, K., & Davidov, M. (2008). Mother–adolescent conflict: Adolescent goals, maternal perspective-taking, and conflict intensity. *Journal of Research on Adolescence, 18*, 555–571.

Maccoby, E. E. (2000). The uniqueness of the parent–child relationship. In W. A. Collins & B. Laursen (Eds.), *Relationships as developmental contexts* (pp. 157–175). Mahwah, NJ: Erlbaum.

Maccoby, E. E., & Martin, J. A. (1983). Socialization in the context of the family: Parent–child interaction. In P. H. Mussen (Ed.) & E. M. Hetherington (Vol. Ed.), *Handbook of child psychology: Vol. 4. Socialization, personality, and social development* (4th ed., pp. 1–101). New York: Wiley.

MacDonald, K. (1992). Warmth as a developmental construct: An evolutionary analysis. *Child Development, 63*, 753–773.

Marshall, S. K., & Lambert, J. D. (2006). Parental mattering: A qualitative inquiry into the tendency to evaluate the self as significant to one's children. *Journal of Family Issues, 27*, 1561–1582.

McMahon, R. J., & Forehand, R. L. (2003). *Helping the noncompliant child: Family-based treatment for oppositional behavior* (2nd ed.). New York: Guilford Press.

Miller, G., & Steinberg, M. (1975). *Between people: A new analysis of interpersonal communication.* Chicago: Science Research Associates.

Oliphant, A., & Kuczynski, L. (2011). Mothers' and fathers' perceptions of mutuality in middle childhood: The domain of intimacy. *Journal of Family Issues, 32*(8), 1104–1124.

Overton, W. F. (2006). Developmental psychology: Philosophy, concepts, methodology. In R. M. Lerner (Ed.), & W. Damon & R. M. Lerner (Editors-in-Chief), *Theoretical models of human development: The handbook of child psychology* (Vol. 1, pp. 18–88). New York: Wiley.

Overton, W. F., & Reese, H. W. (1973). Models of development: Methodological implications. In J. R. Nesselroade & H. W. Reese (Eds.), *Life-span developmental psychology: Methodological issues* (pp. 65–86). New York: Academic Press.

Palkovitz, R., Marks, L. D., Appleby, D. W., & Holmes, E. K. (2003). Processes and products of intergenerational relationships. In L. Kuczynski (Ed.), *Handbook of dynamics in parent–child relations* (pp. 307–324). Thousand Oaks, CA: Sage.

Parkin, C. M., & Kuczynski, L. (2012). Adolescent perspectives on rules and resistance within the parent–child relationship. *Journal of Adolescent Research, 27*, 555–580.

Parpal, M., & Maccoby, E. E. (1985). Material responsiveness and subsequent child compliance. *Child Development, 56*, 1326–1334.

Patterson, G., Reid, J., & Dishion, T. (1992). *Antisocial boys: Vol. 4. A social interactional approach.* Eugene, OR: Castalia.

Patterson, G. R. (1982). *Coercive family process.* Eugene, OR: Castalia.

Piniata, R. C. (1999). *Enhancing relationships between children and teachers.* Washington, DC: American Psychological Association.

Porta, S. D., & Howe, N. (2012). Assessing mothers' and children's perceptions of power through personal, conventional, and prudential conflict situations. *Merrill–Palmer Quarterly, 58,* 507–529.

Reiss, H. G. T., Collins, W. A., & Berscheid, E. (2000). The relationship context of human behavior and development. *Psychological Bulletin, 126,* 844–872.

Riegel, K. F. (1976). The dialectics of human development. *American Psychologist, 10,* 689–700.

Robson, J., & Kuczynski, L. (2013, November). *The construct of rules in middle childhood: How rules are negotiated.* Poster presented at the annual conference of the Society for the Study of Human Development, Fort Lauderdale, FL.

Russell, A., Petit, G., & Mize, J. (1998). Horizontal qualities in parent–child relationships: Parallels with and possible consequences for children's peer relationships. *Developmental Review, 18,* 313–352.

Ryan, R. M., & Deci, E. L. (2002). An overview of self-determination theory: An organismic-dialectical perspective. In E. L. Deci & R. M. Ryan (Eds.), *Handbook of self-determination research* (pp. 3–36). Rochester, NY: University of Rochester Press.

Salafia, E. H. B., Gondoli, D. M., & Grundy, A. M. (2009). The longitudinal interplay of maternal warmth and adolescents' self-disclosure in predicting maternal knowledge. *Research on Adolescence, 19*(4), 654–668.

Sameroff, A. (1975a). Early influences on development: Fact or fancy? *Merrill–Palmer Quarterly, 21,* 267–293.

Sameroff, A. (1975b). Transactional models of early social relations. *Human Development, 18,* 65–79.

Sameroff, A. (2009). The transactional model. In A. Sameroff (Ed.), *Transactional processes in development* (pp. 3–22). Washington, DC: American Psychological Association.

Sato, T., Hikada, T., & Fukuda, M. (2009). Depicting the dynamics of living the life: The trajectory equifinality model. In J. Valsiner, P. Molenaar, M. Lyra, & N. Chaudhary (Eds.), *Dynamic process methodology in the social and developmental sciences* (pp. 217–240). New York: Springer.

Sears, R. R. (1951). A theoretical framework for personality and social behavior. *American Psychologist, 6,* 476–482.

Smetana, J. G. (2011). *Adolescents, families, and social development: How adolescents construct their worlds.* West Sussex, UK: Wiley-Blackwell.

Smetana, J. G., Villalobos, M., Tasopoulos-Chan, M., Gettman, D. C., & Campione-Barr, N. (2009). Early and middle adolescents' disclosure to parents about activities in different domains. *Adolescence, 32*(3), 693–713.

Soenens, B., Vansteenkiste, M., Luyckx, K., & Goossens, L. (2006). Parenting and adolescent problem behavior: An integrated model with adolescent self-disclosure and perceived parental knowledge as intervening variables. *Developmental Psychology, 42*(2), 305–318.

Strauss, C. (1992). Models and motives. In R. G. D'Andrade & C. Strauss (Eds.), *Human motives and cultural models* (pp. 1–20). New York: Cambridge University Press.

Trommsdorff, G., & Kornadt, H. (2003). Parent–child relations in cross-cultural perspective. In L. Kuczynski (Ed.), *Handbook of dynamics in parent–child relations* (pp. 271–306). Thousand Oaks, CA: Sage.

Trommsdorff, G., Zheng, G., & Tardif, T. (2002). Value of children and intergenerational relations in cultural context. In P. Boski, F. J. R. van de Vijver, & A. M. Chodynicka (Eds.), *New directions in cross-cultural psychology* (pp. 581–601). Warsaw: Polish Psychological Association.

Valsiner, J., & Connolly, K. J. (2003). The nature of development: The continuing dialogue of processes and outcomes. In J. Valsiner & K. J. Connolly (Eds.), *Handbook of developmental psychology* (pp. xi–xviii). Thousand Oaks, CA: Sage.

Weingarten, K. (1991). The discourses of intimacy: Adding a social constructionist and feminist view. *Family Process, 30,* 285–305.

CHAPTER 7

Analyzing Socialization from a Domain-Specific Perspective

Joan E. Grusec
Maayan Davidov

Parents, peers, siblings, teachers, and the media all function as agents of socialization for children. By way of their interactions with these agents, children come to acquire a host of skills, standards, and values that are important for functioning well in their social world. We argue that socialization occurs in a variety of domains, with each of these domains marked by a different form of social interaction. We focus primarily on the roles played by parents in socialization because, as we suggest below, parents appear to be the most important in their impact on children's development and, indeed, this is the focus of most of the research literature. We note, however, that similar domains of interaction occur with other human agents of socialization as well, and toward the end of this chapter we briefly elaborate on this point.

In this chapter we focus predominantly on the emotional, cognitive, and behavioral processes associated with socialization and their antecedents in parenting actions. We also focus on parenting in a Western industrialized context, which is where most of the research has been done, referring the reader to other chapters in this handbook for reviews of parenting in other cultural contexts. Maccoby (Chapter 1, this volume) has provided a historical survey of parenting research that provides the background for what follows.

Socialization involves the acceptance of values, standards, and customs of society, as well as the ability to function in an adaptive way in the larger social context. These values, standards, and customs are not simply transmitted from one generation to the other; rather, they are, to some extent at least, constructed by each generation. Thus, parents are not so much purveyors of information as helpers in setting the stage for their children to become well-functioning members of the social group. Also, an important (but not the only) goal of socialization is that values and standards be internalized in the sense that members of the group behave in accord with them willingly rather than out of fear of external consequences or hope of reward. In this chapter, we briefly comment on parents as primary agents of socialization, as well as issues having to do with direction of effect in parent–child interactions. We then discuss socialization as situation- or domain-specific, expanding on this idea as a way of presenting what is known about the functions of parents and other agents in the socialization process.

The Primacy of Parents

Few contemporary researchers would argue with the proposition that parents are primary in socialization (Collins, Maccoby, Steinberg, Hetherington, & Bornstein, 2000). First, parents and children are part of a biosocial system that functions to protect offspring and to ensure that they are able to deal with the demands of social life. Thus, parents and children are biologically prepared to be attracted to and remain in close proximity to each other. Second, the strong human need for interrelatedness plays a substantial role in the socialization process, and opportunities for such interrelatedness abound in the parent–child relationship as parents protect, nurture, and express affection and warmth to their offspring. Moreover, the bonds of relatedness between parent and child can never be formally severed, unlike those between peers, teachers, and other biologically unrelated individuals. Third, in most societies, parents are formally assigned the role of primary agents of socialization. Fourth, practical reasons facilitate parents' motivation to socialize their children, given that they must live in close proximity to their children and that the lives of all are more comfortable when there is some agreement about the nature of appropriate behavior. Finally, parents are in a position to control resources available to their children, as well as manage their environments to ensure that they are either protected from or forewarned about undesirable influences.

Direction of Effect in Socialization

Researchers have long acknowledged that children also influence parents during the course of socialization and are currently making considerable strides in untangling the complexities of family interactions (Kuczynski, Parkin, & Pitman, Chapter 6, this volume). Behavior geneticists have argued that children affect their own outcomes by triggering particular responses (e.g., harshness) from their parents or by actively seeking out particular environments (e.g., Scarr & McCartney, 1983). Patterson (e.g., 1982) has documented how children can cause maternal loss of control through negative reinforcement, for example, by ceasing to whine when their mothers stop making aversive demands. Moreover, the mothers' repeated inability to gain compliance leads to feelings of incompetence that further interfere with attempts to control their children's actions. Others have described the parent–child interaction as transactional (e.g., Sameroff, 1975), with one member of the dyad changing the actions of the other, which in turn alters the actions of the first member. Thus, there is a constant process of reciprocal interchange that leads to constant transformation of interactions. What this all indicates is that children are highly involved in their own socialization.

Socialization as Situation-Specific

Traditionally, analyses of socialization assumed that there are general processes that operate across all settings. Increasingly, however, it has become evident that socialization involves different processes in different social contexts. Indeed, it has long been evident that many organisms are prepared to learn certain responses such as food aversion and fear of animals more easily than other responses (see Seligman, 1970). Bell and Ainsworth (1972) found that, contrary to the principles of reinforcement theory (which appeared to apply in many aspects of a child's development), maternal responding to infant cries in the first few months of life led to decreased crying toward the end of the first year. Distinctions have also been made between the child's need for protection and the need for warmth, with the argument that these two needs are biologically separate systems (MacDonald, 1992). Youniss, McLellan, and Strouse (1994) noted that peer relationships are governed by the principle of cooperation among equals as opposed to the asymmetrical power relationship that exists between parents and children. And Turiel (1998) has demonstrated that even very young children differentiate among moral (harm to others), social conventional (customs), prudential (harm to self), and personal issues, judging moral ones as obligatory and unalterable but seeing social conventional ones as capable of being changed by agreement or consensus.

Distinctions of context also appear in the actions of parents with respect to the goals that are activated in different socialization situations. Dix (1992) notes that parents on different occasions espouse personal goals relevant to obtaining obedience, empathic goals oriented toward satisfaction of their children's emotional needs, and socialization goals relevant to the acquisition of values. Similarly, Hastings and Grusec (1998) found that parents, in response to their children's misbehaviors, report a variety of goals that includes achieving obedience, teaching values, and maintaining harmony. In each case, they employ different strategies, ranging from power assertion (for obedience) through reasoning (for value acquisition) to negotiation and acceptance (for harmony). Finally, social domain theorists (e.g., Bugental, 2000; Fiske, 1992) talk about domains of social life in which there are different tasks to be solved and different rules or algorithms operate. This approach is applicable to socialization: Bugental (2000) identified and characterized different forms of interaction between children and agents of socialization, that is, different domains of socialization, and Grusec and Davidov (2007, 2010) built on this work.

Grusec and Davidov (2010) suggested that five domains involve different behavioral systems and are activated in different situations during the course of everyday life. Each system reflects a different state or motivation in the child. The *protection* domain involves the child's need for protection and security. The *control* domain has to do with not only the child's need to meet societal demands but also his or her developing sense of autonomy that can be threatened when parents attempt to impose too much control or intrusively direct the child's actions. The *guided learning* domain involves the child's need for instruction in order to master new skills, the *group participation* domain has to do with the child's need to identify with and be part of a social group, and the *reciprocity* domain involves the child's motivation and proclivity to reciprocate the behavior of others. These child needs and motivations come about in different situations, require different kinds of interventions in order to be satisfied, and ultimately lead to the acquisition of different skills.

We now elaborate on each domain, spending more time on the protection and control domains because these have been more extensively studied.

The Protection Domain

Humans at birth are far from able to care for themselves, so they have evolved to seek protection and nurturing from adults during infancy and beyond, and to provide protection and nurturing for their offspring during adulthood. Seeking the proximity of the caregiver in the face of threats to well-being is organized by the child's attachment behavioral system, whereas parental behavior aimed at ensuring the safety and well-being of the young is organized by the parent's caregiving system. These two behavioral systems are complementary and have likely evolved in parallel. Thus, when either the attachment or the caregiving system is activated, proximity between child and caregiver is increased and protection is thereby enhanced (Bowlby, 1969/1982; J. Cassidy, 1999).

The protection domain comes into play in situations involving real or potential threat, such as when the child is hurt, ill, in physical danger, or emotionally upset. Effective parenting in these situations engenders the child's confidence in the parent's protection (i.e., a secure attachment; Goldberg, Grusec, & Jenkins, 1999). Sensitive, protective caregiving involves the provision of help and emotional support in times of need in a manner suitable to the particular child. The specific actions taken by the parent to protect the child from harm vary depending (among other things) on the situation and the age of the child. With infants and toddlers, protection includes behaviors such as retrieving, maintaining proximity, calling, holding, soothing and comforting (soothing and comforting are important because they enable the parent to ascertain that the child is no longer in danger [J. Cassidy, 1999]). Because children differ in how much reassurance they need and what makes them feel secure, parents' knowledge of their children's reactions in stressful situations is important for effective protection. Thus, parents' knowledge of what children find distressing and comforting promotes their children's coping behavior (Sherman, Grusec, & Almas, 2013; Vinik, Almas, & Grusec, 2011). Moreover, effective parenting in the protection domain includes the provision of a safe environment for the child, even when the parent is not present. If children are exposed to environments outside the home in which their needs for protection and safety are not met (e.g., poor-quality day care, or the communal sleeping arrangements previously employed in some Israeli kibbutzim), then the child's sense of security in the parent's protection can be compromised (e.g., Sagi, Koren-Karie, Gini, Ziv, & Joels, 2002). Finally, we note that sensitive protection does not involve overprotective, restrictive practices, which can interfere with the development of competent self-regulatory abilities (e.g., Rubin, Burgess, & Hastings, 2002).

Responsiveness to Distress as Distinct

Our analysis of attachment relationships focuses on protective caregiving specifically, whereas much work in the area of attachment has assessed positive parenting more generally (Goldberg et al., 1999). Our more focused approach is based on theory and accumulating empirical evidence that suggests parenting in the protection domain (responsiveness to child distress) is distinct from other aspects of the parent–child relationship. For example, McElwain and Booth-LaForce (2006) reported that maternal sensitivity to a child's distress at 6 months predicted subsequent secure attachment, whereas sensitivity to nondistress did not (even though the two sensitivity measures were highly correlated). Furthermore, Davidov and Grusec (2006b) found that parental responsiveness to distress, but not parental warmth, predicted children's capacity to self-regulate their negative emotions and to respond with empathy and prosocial behavior to another's distress. Contrarily, maternal warmth, but not responsiveness to distress, was a significant predictor of children's competent regulation of positive affect and of boys' peer acceptance. Similarly, Leerkes, Blankson, and O'Brien (2009) showed that early responsiveness to distress contributed uniquely to children's subsequent positive social behavior, whereas early responsiveness to nondistress did not. Moreover, although maternal sensitivity to distress and nondistress are often positively associated, they have more unshared than shared variance, and are predicted by different antecedents (Leerkes, Weaver, & O'Brien, 2012). Thus, there is ample evidence that sensitive parenting in the protection domain (responsiveness to distress) differs from other aspects of responsive parenting.

Routes to Positive Socialization Outcomes in the Protection Domain

Sensitive, protective parenting can facilitate positive socialization outcomes in a number of ways. One way is by fostering children's ability to self-regulate negative affect competently. When children see that their distress signals reliably elicit parental assistance, negative events become less threatening: As a result, these events are less likely to trigger a frequent physiological stress response, with its attendant threat to the development and subsequent functioning of neurobiological systems responsible for the regulation of stress and negative emotion (Gunnar & Quevedo, 2007). Protective parents can also help their children gain control and understanding of negative emotions by allowing an outlet for their children's negative affect in a supportive context (Fabes, Leonard, Kupanoff, & Martin, 2001). Children's ability to regulate negative emotion, in turn, enables them to act more appropriately and maturely in everyday situations involving negative emotions (Chan, 2011; Gottman, Katz, & Hooven, 1996).

A second way that sensitive, protective parents facilitate socialization is through the fostering of children's empathy and concern for others. Sensitive parents model empathy and compassion, which children can then emulate when interacting with others (Denham, Bassett, & Wyatt, Chapter 25, this volume). Such parents also promote children's empathy by facilitating their ability to read others' emotions accurately (Fabes, Poulin, Eisenberg, & Madden-Derdich, 2002). Moreover, they promote children's competent regulation of negative affect, which in turn enables children to remain focused on distressed others and help them, instead of becoming self-distressed (e.g., Eisenberg, Wentzel, & Harris, 1998). Deficits in empathic capacity not only reduce prosocial responding but also may make antisocial behavior more likely: Individuals who cannot reflect on and identify with other persons' feelings and mental states do not experience guilt or discomfort as a consequence of hurting others (Bowlby, 1944; Malti & Krettanauer, 2012).

A third route to socialization in the protection domain involves facilitation of trust in the parent to act in the child's best interest. Children of supportive parents are more likely to perceive parental direction more as an expression of caring and goodwill than as intrusive or malevolent; such trust facilitates their willingness to share information with their parents and to listen to them (Bretherton, Golby, & Cho, 1997; Kerns, Aspelmeier,

Gentzler, & Grabill, 2001). Moreover, sensitive protection and trust promote children's ability to seek help openly when in need, and to accept and utilize such help once it is offered (e.g., Matas, Arend, & Sroufe, 1978; Newman, 2000). It also decreases the likelihood of engaging in health-threatening activities. Thus, controlling for earlier substance abuse, Branstetter, Furman, and Cottrell (2009) found that adolescents' secure attachment predicted reduced substance use 2 years later; this effect was mediated by mothers' greater knowledge of adolescents' whereabouts and social activities, at least some of which would come from children's voluntary disclosure of information to their parents. Similarly, Darling, Cumsille, and Martínez (2008) reported that Chilean adolescents who perceived their parents to be more supportive in times of need were more accepting of their parents' authority regarding both prudential (health and safety) and personal matters (e.g., choice of friends and activities).

The Control Domain

In the protection domain parents serve as "stronger and wiser" guardians who provide support, help, and reassurance in times of need. But the superior strength and resources of parents compared to children means that parents are not only providers of protection but also enforcers of rules. These rules are necessitated by the fact that humans live with others and must therefore be socialized to interact in predictable and peaceful ways. Thus, children must learn to abide by rules and to suppress desires to behave in an antisocial fashion. An important context for learning these lessons is interactions in the control domain, which occur when children break the rules or misbehave, and parents attempt to correct their behavior. Notably, this necessary setting of limits can threaten children's sense of autonomy. Children (and adults), regardless of culture, need to feel that their behavior is self-generated and that they are not impelled by external forces over which they have no power (e.g., Ryan & Deci, 2000), although too much autonomy is also problematic, as it may lead to indecisiveness and dissatisfaction (see Schwartz, 2000). What constitutes effective parenting in control interactions is therefore complex. We discuss three bodies of work that address these issues of parental control: self-determination theory and its emphasis on autonomy, the identification of different kinds of control, and evidence of the multiple moderators of the effects of control strategies.

Self-Determination Theory and Autonomy Support

Although children have a natural tendency to engage in many intrinsically rewarding behaviors, there are many socially expected behaviors that are not intrinsically rewarding, so conditions must be set in place to encourage their internalization. Self-determination theory (Grolnick, Deci, & Ryan, 1997) emphasizes three conditions that facilitate the internalization, or integration, of such behaviors with all aspects of the self: autonomy support (gentle control, provision of appropriate choice), which fosters the perception that behavior is self-generated rather than externally imposed; structure (setting clear expectations), which helps children understand what it is they are supposed to do; and interpersonal involvement or relatedness (being warm and caring, demonstrating interest in the child), which facilitates children's willingness to accept the structure. Self-determination theorists have provided considerable empirical evidence that these three conditions do in fact facilitate children's internalization of values (Grolnick, 2003; Ryan & Deci, 2000).

When autonomy is undermined, there are negative consequences for internalization and well-being. For example, frequent use of intrusive support (e.g., when parents check their children's homework or help them without being requested to do so) communicates caring but also undermines autonomy, and it can increase the risk of depression for some children (Pomerantz, 2001). As another example, when children are made to feel that their parents love them only if they behave or perform in specific ways, autonomy is sacrificed in order to maintain a sense of relatedness, with detrimental implications. Thus, college students who remember their parents responding with conditional positive regard report a more shallow and conflicted form of internalization, and short-lived satisfaction after success (Assor, Roth, & Deci, 2004). Adolescents' perception of their parents' conditional regard is associated with rigid behavior and feelings of internal compulsion, less adaptive regulation of negative emotions, resentment toward parents, and academic disengagement (Roth, Assor, Niemiec, Ryan, & Deci, 2009).

Varieties of Control

The exertion of parental control can take many specific forms, including persuasion, reasoning, and punishment or power assertion. In addition to studying specific discipline strategies, researchers have also identified different parenting styles or ways of imposing control. Baumrind's (1971) distinction between authoritarian and authoritative styles of control has guided thinking for many years. Recently, Baumrind (2012) has characterized these styles as involving coercive and confrontive use of power, respectively. The former is arbitrary, domineering, and focuses on making status distinctions; the latter is equally firm and demanding yet also negotiable, accompanied by reasoning, and focuses on teaching valuable skills.

Another distinction is that between behavioral and psychological control. Behavioral control involves the enforcement of clearly set rules and monitoring of children's behavior. Psychological control, which is not dissimilar to conditional positive regard discussed earlier (Soenens & Vansteenkiste, 2010), involves attempts to influence children's emotions by methods such as guilt induction, love withdrawal, and intrusiveness (Barber, 1996; Steinberg, 1990). Low levels of behavioral control are associated with externalizing problems, whereas high levels of psychological control are associated with internalizing ones, including anxiety, low self-esteem, and self-derogation (Barber & Harmon, 2002; Crouter & Head, 2002). Nevertheless, not every example of behavioral control is positive, nor is every instance of psychological control necessarily negative. High levels of behavioral control, if they involve perceived threats to autonomy, can be detrimental (e.g., Kerr & Stattin, 2000). And gentle tactics aimed at affecting children's emotional state, such as inducing empathy or feelings of responsibility, can have beneficial outcomes (e.g., Grusec & Goodnow, 1994).

Moderators of the Effects of Control Strategies

Further complexity with respect to control is added by the frequent observation of interactive effects involving parental control, which indicate that the effects of control depend on other variables. Thus, various characteristics of the child, parent, situation, and context can alter the outcomes of different forms of discipline (Collins et al., 2000; Grusec & Goodnow, 1994; Grusec, Goodnow, & Kuczynksi, 2000).

One very important moderator is temperament (see Bates & Pettit, Chapter 16, this volume, for a review). Although the general conclusion is that children with difficult temperaments are more adversely affected by negative forms of parenting, it has also been suggested that some children are especially sensitive to both positive and negative parenting (Belsky & Pluess, 2009).

Other interactions include age: Younger children, for example, are more likely than older children to see strong forms of intervention as fair and more issues as being under parental rather than personal jurisdiction (Smetana, Robinson, & Rote, Chapter 3, this volume). Thus, with adolescents, parents have to rely on more subtle interventions such as monitoring and guidance (Patterson, Crosby, & Vuchinich, 1992; Pettit, 1997). The nature of the misdeed in question matters as well: Punishment needs to fit the deed, a fit presumably mediated by children's perception of the fairness of a control strategy given the nature of the social rule that has been violated (Grusec & Goodnow, 1994). Thus, adolescents view maternal yelling as inappropriate in response to violation of conventional rules or personal issues, but not in response to moral transgressions (Padilla-Walker, 2008). Another important moderator is the affective context in which control occurs, with fewer negative effects when control is accompanied by warmth than when it is enacted with rejection and hostility (Brody & Flor, 1998; Kilgore, Snyder, & Lentz, 2000; Lansford et al., 2010). Moreover, the meaning and consequences of control strategies are also influenced by the family's cultural context (e.g., Chao, 2001; Rudy & Grusec, 2001, 2006).

Implications of Moderation Effects for Understanding Socialization in the Control Domain

The existence of so many variables that moderate the impact of parental control suggests that a focus on specific control strategies is insufficient. Accordingly, Grusec and Goodnow (1994) argued that internalization of values is better seen as a function of children's accurate perception of the parental message and acceptance of that message, with the latter determined by variables such as appropriateness of the strategy (e.g., fairness), the child's motivation (e.g., to please a warm parent), and the child's feeling that the message was self-generated and not threatening to autonomy. Grusec and colleagues (2000) argued that effective parenting in the control domain therefore involves parents' ability and willingness to select disciplinary responses that are suitable for the specific child in the current situation. Parents who are knowledgeable about their children's perceptions and reactions in control situations can tailor their interventions accordingly, thereby promoting positive socialization outcomes. For example, parents can accurately assess whether their children understand what they are supposed to do, whether their children feel they are being treated fairly or noncoercively, whether a particular strategy is seen as a manifestation of caring behavior or of hostility, or whether a power-assertive intervention is seen as an indication of the importance of the issue to the parent rather than an angry outburst.

Several studies support this position. Hastings and Grusec (1997) found that parents who were accurate in perceiving their adolescents' thoughts and feelings during conflict felt greater satisfaction with the outcomes of conflict (in the case of mothers) and had fewer conflicts (in the case of fathers). Lundell, Grusec, McShane, and Davidov (2008) reported that mothers who took the perspective of their adolescents were likely to have less intense conflicts with them, and that the link between perspective taking and reduced conflict intensity was through a reduction in the adolescents' desire to retaliate against the mother or alter her behavior. Davidov and Grusec (2006a) found that mothers who were more knowledgeable about their children's reactions to different discipline strategies were more likely to have children who complied, after initial resistance, with a request to tidy a playroom: It was the mothers' responsive reactions to their children's protests that mediated between maternal accuracy and children's ultimate compliance.

How is accurate knowledge acquired? It could be through careful observation of children's reactions, noncoercive questioning about their feelings, or modeling of the sharing of feelings and thoughts by the parent. Setting the conditions for a close and trusting relationship, which facilitates the child's sharing of information, is likely an important ingredient. A recent substantial literature on children's disclosure of information to their parents and the variety of conditions that facilitate such disclosure (e.g., Kerr & Stattin, 2000; Kerr, Stattin, & Burk, 2010; Smetana et al., Chapter 3, this volume) emphasizes the importance of such sharing of information in the socialization process. Authoritative parents may be more likely to use these various techniques: Davidov, Grusec and Wolfe (2012), for example, found that mothers who had greater knowledge of their children's views of discipline reported more authoritative parenting practices and were less likely to endorse permissive or authoritarian practices.

The Guided Learning Domain

Humans have needed to rely on teachable intellectual skills to survive in a world where they have limited physical prowess (see Gauvain & Perez, Chapter 24, this volume). The human capacity for language also enables the learning of complex skills through verbal communication. In interactions in the guided learning domain, the socialization agent assists the child's learning of a novel skill or piece of knowledge, working within the child's zone of proximal development; thus, the teacher helps the child master problems that he or she cannot yet solve independently, but can master with the help of a more knowledgeable other (Vygotsky, 1978). Guided learning must be scaffolded (Wood, Bruner, & Ross, 1976); that is, guidance and structuring are provided by the parent (e.g., in the form of leading questions, strategy suggestions, feedback), and this help needs to be continuously altered in order to match the child's changing skill level. In the course of this process, teacher and student arrive at a shared understanding of the task, which enables the child gradually to acquire a more advanced, deeper understanding of the task (Puntambekar & Hubscher, 2005; Vygotsky, 1978). In this way, children play an active role in guided learning interactions. For example, there is evidence that children's memory for an event and its importance is better when both mother and child discuss the event than when only the mother addresses it or there is no discussion (Haden, Ornstein, Eckerman, & Didow, 2001).

Guided learning is important not only for mastering cognitive tasks but also for learning socioemotional skills. For example, the children of parents who teach and coach them about the nature of emotions and how to express and manage them are better able to regulate their emotions physiologically and behaviorally (Denham, Bassett, & Wyatt,

Chapter 25, this volume; Gottman et al., 1996). And young children of mothers who talk coherently to them about emotion-provoking past events, and who scaffold the discussion by providing structure and feedback, are more advanced in their understanding of emotion (see Laible & Panfile, 2009, for a review).

Guided learning is important in moral development. Wright and Bartsch (2008), for example, report that even very young children engage in conversations about moral issues with their parents, often taking the lead in such conversations themselves. Parents who are high in *generativity*, that is, who see an important part of their role as the training of future generations, are more ready to engage in storytelling that focuses on the suffering, growth, and kindness of others (McAdams, 2004). Conversations in which parents elicit the child's opinion and check for understanding (the hallmarks of effective guided learning), and are supportive and not negative, are associated with increases in moral development (Walker, Hennig, & Krettenauer, 2000).

Guided Learning versus Reasoning in the Control Domain

A feature of effective parenting in the control domain is the use of reasoning to augment the impact of power assertion. Thus, parents who provide their child with reasons why his or her behavior is unacceptable are likely to be more successful in obtaining future compliance, even in situations in which the child is not being observed and is therefore not in danger of being punished (Grusec & Goodnow, 1994; Hoffman, 1970). One explanation for this outcome is that reasoning helps children understand why their behavior is unacceptable and therefore facilitates their attribution of compliance to internal reasons rather than external pressure (Grusec, 1983).

Reasoning in the control domain, then, has similarities to teaching in the guided learning domain. The difference, of course, is that when they have been caught misbehaving, children, as well as their parents, are likely to be in a state of high negative arousal, with parents struggling more or less successfully to contain their anger and to control their children's displays of negative affect, and children dealing with their own frustration and fear of parental punishment. Thus, parents might not be as efficient as teachers and children might not be as receptive to their teaching given that negative emotions lead to narrowing of attention (Fredrickson, 2003). Guided learning interactions, in contrast, are marked by children's motivation to learn the new skill, with parents facilitating that goal.

The Group Participation Domain

In the group participation domain, socialization occurs through a relatively implicit process as children observe others in their social group and adopt their behavior (see Bandura & Walters, 1963, who claimed that learning through observation is the fundamental learning process for humans). Many of the observed behaviors involve routinized or ritualized ways of doing things in the social milieu, which children are especially eager to emulate and often easily become part of their behavioral repertoires. Parents can therefore influence what their children learn in this domain by providing them with opportunities to observe and take part in valuable social activities, and by restricting their exposure to undesirable activities.

The adoption and valuing of group practices and symbols is important from an evolutionary perspective because it identifies the individual as a member of the ingroup, where good treatment is more likely (Brewer & Gardner, 1996). The powerful desire to emulate members of the ingroup is seen in young children's distress when an adult normative standard is violated, or when they are unable to imitate the actions of an adult model (Kagan, 1982). Rogoff, Moore, Correa-Chávez, and Dexter (Chapter 20, this volume) describe "learning by observing and pitching in," that is, learning through keen observation and listening in anticipation of engaging in a specific endeavor in the future. This form of learning occurs more frequently in cultural communities that are particularly inclined to involve children in adult activities as opposed to communities that segregate children in formal school settings. Nevertheless, learning through intent observation and participation does occur in these latter settings, too, as parents and children interact during the course of accomplishing everyday tasks together. Rheingold (1982), for example, describes the desire of young children to help with work around the house, even though they are not proficient at it and are even discouraged from doing so by their mothers. Young children also "play house," an indication of their motivation to engage in closely observed adult activity.

Children learn the customs and standards of their society by not only observing but also actively participating in relevant practices daily, at home and outside the home. Everyday ways of doing things include both *routines* (practices that are repeated to accomplish instrumental tasks) and *rituals* (practices that carry meaning, reflecting group membership and values); the same activities (e.g., family dinner) can combine aspects of both routine and ritual (e.g., Spagnola & Fiese, 2007). Notably, routines and rituals reflect myriad social expectations regarding how one should behave. This includes gender-based activities, work around the house, modes of dressing, what can be done in public and what is to be done in private, where to eat and sleep, how to play, and so on. As children take part in these everyday activities, they come to adopt these various social prescriptions because they are viewed as normal, typical behavior (the way things are done). Moreover, participation in these practices reflects group membership, and children are therefore motivated to adopt them in order to feel that they are part of the group. Finally, these behaviors and standards are also entrenched by frequent repetition, which makes them habitual and automatic (Davidov, 2013). Through group participation interactions, then, children are seamlessly induced to adopt many social practices and norms, without the need for discussion or conflict. (Only if these practices are questioned by the child will the interaction move into the area of conflict and autonomy preservation that forms the control domain [Bourdieu, 1977].)

Researchers have linked family rituals and routines to positive socialization outcomes such as psychosocial maturity (Eaker & Walters, 2002), school success (Spagnola & Fiese, 2007), and reduced family conflict (Dubas & Gerris (2002). The ability to maintain meaningful family rituals can protect children against some of the negative consequences of stressful experiences such as divorce or parental alcoholism (Spagnola & Fiese, 2007). Finally, Grusec, Goodnow, and Cohen (1997) demonstrated how routine performance of work around the house, done for the benefit of other family members, is linked with greater spontaneous prosocial behavior. In contrast, work done in response to a request or directive (that is, in the control domain), did not have a similar positive effect.

Managing the Child's Environment

Parents can take advantage of their children's desire to be like others by exposing them to favorable role models, limiting their access to negative ones, and managing their activities to encourage emulation of prosocial behavior and the acquisition of socially acceptable routines and rituals. They also need to know where their children are and to what they are being exposed, yet another indication of the importance of parental knowledge in the socialization process.

The Reciprocity Domain

Humans appear to have an inborn tendency to reciprocate what others have done for them (Trevarthen, Kokkinski, & Flamenghi, 1999), an evolutionarily adaptive response given the survival and reproductive benefits that arise from assisting others and receiving benefits from them in return. Humans are also alleged to be endowed with a "cheater mechanism" that makes them sensitive to times when they provide benefits to others but do not receive benefits in exchange (Cosmides & Tooby, 1992). Parent–child reciprocity interactions are marked by symmetry; that is, the parent and child operate temporarily as equal-status partners. In these interactions, parents and children are each attuned and responsive to the needs of the other, and they share common goals (in contrast to the conflicting goals that exist when parents actively attempt to alter undesirable behavior in the control domain). Parent–child play interactions provide an important opportunity for engaging in social reciprocity because these are situations in which parents can easily allow children to influence or determine the course of the interaction (although not all parents may do so). The sharing of pleasure and joy during play and other rewarding parent–child activities can also facilitate the establishment of mutual interests and goals, and therefore facilitate mutual reciprocity.

Forms of Reciprocity

Reciprocity in parent–child relationships has been defined and operationalized in several ways. Thus, some studies have focused on parents' willingness to be influenced by the child as a manifestation of reciprocity. Others have defined *reciprocity* as interactions that are symmetrical and mutual in nature, and still others have examined the more global concept of MRO—a mutually responsive orientation.

Reciprocity defined as parents' willingness to be influenced by their children is reflected in the classic study by Parpal and Maccoby (1985). They found that children of mothers who were instructed to follow their child's lead during a play interaction were more cooperative during a later cleanup period than children whose mothers received no instruction about how to play and who, in fact, were more directive and critical. The benefit of letting the child lead was especially pronounced for children who were viewed as difficult and noncompliant.

Parents may also reflect their willingness to be influenced by their children by cooperating with children's reasonable bids and requests, or by allowing children's input into family decisions. Davidov and Grusec (2006a) found that maternal willing compliance predicted children's compliance with a maternal request to clean up a playroom.

(Notably, this form of parental reciprocity no longer predicted compliance if children had protested the request, thereby moving the interaction into the control domain and illustrating the distinct effects of socialization processes in the reciprocity and the control domains.) Thus, by showing consideration of children's wishes (in the reciprocity domain), parents induce children into a system of mutual reciprocity, making it more likely that children will show goodwill in return. Moreover, children's responsiveness in the context of mutual reciprocity reflects a genuine willingness and interest in compliance that is not externally forced.

Other studies examining reciprocity have focused on the symmetrical, mutual quality of a given interaction (typically a play session or discussion), that is, the degree to which parent and child manage the interaction jointly and share positive affect. This form of mutual reciprocity predicts greater peer competence and prosocial behavior, and reduced externalizing behavior problems among children and adolescents (Criss, Shaw, & Ingoldsby, 2003; Deater-Deckard & Petrill, 2004; Lindsey, Cremeens, & Caldera, 2010).

Finally, Kochanska (2002) and her colleagues have identified the construct of MRO, which denotes a parent–child relationship that is mutually cooperative, harmonious, and affectively positive (e.g., Kochanska, Forman, Aksan, & Dunbar, 2005). They also include in this construct other aspects of the parent–child relationship, such as sensitive responses to distress signals, which we place in the protection domain, and responses to conflicting wishes, which we identify as part of the control domain. Parent–child MRO during the toddler and preschool years predicts the development of self-regulation and conscience in later childhood, as reflected by moral emotions, cognitions, and behavior, such as internalized conduct and guilt following perceived wrongdoing (Kochanska, 2002; Kochanska et al., 2005). Moreover, Kochanska and colleagues (2005) found that the link between early MRO and subsequent moral conduct was mediated by child responses indicative of reciprocity: enjoyment of the interaction with the mother and willing, committed compliance with her directions; in contrast, power assertion, a variable relevant to the control domain, was not an independent mediator.

Domains and Other Agents of Socialization: Peers, Siblings, and Teachers

We turn now to a discussion of peers, siblings, and teachers as they are implicated in the five domains of socialization. Peer interactions become increasingly important as children grow older. They differ from interactions with parents because they are more egalitarian and can be terminated. In contrast, sibling interactions can have a degree of asymmetry because of age differences, and they cannot be terminated. A feature of sibling interaction is its emotional intensity, with frequent negativity and conflict (see Dunn, Chapter 8, this volume). Such emotional intensity occurs less with peers because peer contact can be ended when it becomes unpleasant (Updegraff, McHale, & Crouter, 2001). Finally, teachers do not have enduring relationships with children in their classroom, but they do have control over resources, albeit somewhat less, of course, than parents. The influence they exert on children might differ at different school levels. For example, high school students perceive to a greater degree that teachers are less caring and more focused on academic achievement, competition, and maintaining control than do elementary school students (Harter, 1996).

Protection

In middle childhood and early adolescence, children view their parents and their friends as comparable in their ability to provide emotional support (Bokhorst, Sumter, & Westenberg, 2010). For example, by this age, a substantial portion of children who have been bullied report that they seek the comfort of a friend (Hunter, Boyle, & Warden, 2004). Moreover, having a friend who "sticks up" for them makes bullied children less prone to internalizing and externalizing problems (Hodges, Boivin, Vitaro, & Bukowski, 1999). Siblings also provide protection or comfort in the case of distress: Children who grow up in harsh or disharmonious homes have fewer problems when they have supportive relationships with their siblings (Jenkins, 1992). Finally, teachers are also important providers of comfort to children. For example, the receipt of emotional support from a teacher is one of the important experiences that helps parents who were themselves abused as children not to abuse their own offspring (Egeland, Jacobvitz, & Sroufe, 1988). Similarly, secure attachments to teachers have positive effects on the prosocial behavior of young children who are insecurely attached to their mothers (Mitchell-Copeland, Denham, & DeMulder, 1997).

Control

Social acceptance and rejection by peers are powerful features of peer pressure. This influence can be positive when it encourages prosocial behavior or sets limits on negative behavior (e.g., Komro, Perry, Veblen-Mortenson, & Williams, 1994); however, peer pressure can also encourage antisocial conduct such as bullying (e.g., Craig & Pepler, 1997). The influence of siblings in the control domain is revealed by the fact that the sibling relationship provides a context for learning conflict resolution strategies: Sibling relationship quality predicts how well children deal with conflicts and is a moderator of the relation between children's understanding of others and their positive conflict tactics (Recchia & Howe, 2009). And, in the school setting, teachers are responsible for enforcing the rules and limiting disruptive behavior. Teachers who convey high expectations of mature behavior yet avoid harsh feedback (thus striking a balance between authority and granting autonomy) promote students' responsibility, prosociality, and academic success (Wentzel, 2002). Furthermore, the emphasis that teachers often continue to place on discipline and control as children transition into junior high school is seen as problematic because it interferes with the adolescent need for autonomy (Eccles, Wigfield, & Schiefele, 1998).

Guided Learning

Most studies of peers and guided learning have addressed the role of peers in the acquisition of cognitive skills; for example, gains in ability are more likely to occur when more knowledgeable children provide explanations for their partners (Fawcett & Garton, 2005). Moreover, student-to-student conversations regarding moral issues can expose children to arguments that are somewhat above their current stage (but within their zone of proximal development) and are therefore effective for scaffolding the growth of their moral reasoning (Turner & Berkowitz, 2005). Interestingly, the features of moral discussions that are conducive to development differ for parents and peers. Thus, conversations with parents that are reflective, positive, and nonconfrontational are most effective in improving levels of moral reasoning. However, in the case of peers, negativity and challenge while discussing moral dilemmas facilitate moral development (Walker et al., 2000). These findings reflect a benefit of the more egalitarian nature of the peer relationship, which allows children greater freedom to express dissenting views.

Siblings also instruct each other and may on occasion be better at such instruction than parents because they are closer to the learner's zone of proximal development (K. W. Cassidy, Fineberg, Brown, & Perkins, 2005). The importance of guided learning in the classroom, beyond its central role in the acquisition of academic material, comes from studies of moral education. Simple exposure to moral stories, for example, does not lead to increased moral development. Rather, reflective discussion that takes into account the fact that students perceive the same story differently (that is, that students are working within different zones of proximal development) is essential (Narvaez, 2002). Class meetings, scaffolded by the teacher, in which social problems can be discussed and resolved, are another important method for promoting students' socioemotional competence and character development (Turner & Berkowitz, 2005).

Group Participation

Social acceptance and membership in groups of peers or cliques is very important in childhood and adolescence, and this is where children influence each other through modeling as they learn the practices and routines of the group. Comparison with friends and subsequent adjustments in behavior are also part of this process (Lubbers, Kuyper, & Van Der Werf, 2009). Exposure to various group activities through extracurricular participation is another important part of socialization in the group participation domain. For example, adolescents' participation in school clubs and sports groups is linked to better academic and psychological adjustment and reduced substance use, even after researchers control for prior self-selection variables (Fredricks & Eccles, 2006).

Not surprisingly, older siblings provide models for younger siblings and involve them in various group activities, both positive and negative (as indeed is the case with respect to peers). For example, joint delinquent behaviors are especially likely to occur with male siblings who are close in age and therefore spend more time together (Rowe, Rodgers, & Meseck-Bushey, 1992). Notably, however, some children may engage in behavior and activities that are the opposite of those modeled by their siblings (known as deidentification), which helps to set themselves apart as unique and to reduce sibling rivalry and competition (Whiteman, McHale, & Crouter, 2007).

Teachers and coaches also play an important role in exposing children to various routines and rituals in the classroom and on the playing field. Sociologists in the field of education talk about the "hidden curriculum" of the school—all the socialization messages that are conveyed implicitly through the everyday practices of classroom life, such as forms of address, waiting in line, working in groups, and so on (Brint, Contreras, & Matthews. 2001).

Mutual Reciprocity

There is considerable mutual reciprocity in the play activities of peers. Moreover, research suggests that children do better on academic tasks when cooperation rather than competition is emphasized (Johnson & Johnson, 1979). Younger siblings who report that they have more mutual and egalitarian exchanges with older siblings are more likely to have advanced social skills (Karos, Howe, & Aquan-Assee, 2007). Moreover, children who do not have siblings presumably do not have as much experience with the give-and-take of sibling interaction. Accordingly, they are less liked by their classmates and are more likely to be both aggressive toward and victimized by their peers (Kitzmann, Cohen, & Lockwood, 2002).

As for teachers, there is considerable evidence that this positive aspect of teacher–child relationships is influential in children's school adjustment. For example, a mutually positive teacher–child relationship (e.g., in which teacher and child enjoy each other's company) predicted greater school engagement and subsequent academic success, after researchers controlled for earlier achievement (Hughes & Kwok, 2007). Teacher–child mutual reciprocity is also reflected in teacher–child joint play at preschool (although this also depends on culture; see Farver, Kim, & Lee, 1995).

Conclusions

In this chapter we have argued that socialization happens in different domains or types of social interactions. These domains of interaction can be identified by a focus on different motives experienced by children, and different actions required by agents of socialization in response to those different motives. Children need to be protected, need to be reminded of limits yet also feel autonomous, need to be taught new knowledge and skills to be like other members of the group, and tend to reciprocate the behavior and goodwill of others. Socialization goes on in all these contexts. In the course of children's interactions with socialization agents, different domains become activated and deactivated, depending on features of the situation, as well as the characteristics, goals, and needs of both parent (or other socialization agent) and child.

This analysis suggests that what works effectively in one domain may be ineffective, or even counterproductive, when another domain is activated. Attention and comfort for a child who is crying because of distress will have a different impact than attention and comfort for a child who is crying in order to avoid an unpleasant task. Compliance with the request of a child who wants to play will have a different impact than compliance with the request of a child who wants to stay up too late. Discussion, reasoning, and praise in connection with the performance of household chores works well in the control domain but undermines the helpfulness of a child who sees such work as a badge of membership in the group. Belief that virtue should be its own reward and that reinforcement should not be given for positive action because it undermines intrinsic motivation, will be problematic unless the child views that positive action as part of a reciprocal exchange.

At the same time, however, some parental behaviors promote positive outcomes in more than one domain. Monitoring of a child's activities can aid both in effectively correcting that child's behavior through discipline and managing that child's environment. In the former case, the control domain is activated, whereas in the latter, it is the group participation domain. Similarly, parental expression of warmth and affection can make children more likely to go along with the demands of their parents in the control domain and can also foster the formation of shared goals and reciprocal positive exchanges in the mutual reciprocity domain. Moreover, parents who are reflective, and aware of their own strengths and weaknesses when interacting with their children, may be better able to steer interactions toward domains they prefer or in which they feel more comfortable. Finally, children's characteristics can, of course, influence the nature of parent–child interactions in the various domains. A particular child attribute might also have differential effects as a function of the interaction domain. For example, a child's strong need for autonomy might cause friction in the control domain yet facilitate the establishment of mutual reciprocity. The symmetry of power, parental openness to the child's influence, and pursuit of mutual goals characteristic of the latter domain should be particularly pleasing to children with a strong need to determine their own actions.

Notably, many real-life situations may include features of more than one domain. Thus, the domains of interaction noted here can be viewed as more basic units, which can be combined in various ways to create more complex amalgams. For example, the parent and child may be engaged in a mutually enjoyable conversation as part of a family dinner (reciprocity and group participation) or the child may be arguing with the parent but also seeking reassurance and emotional support (control and protection); the socialization agent may be supporting the child's learning (guided learning) of a skill that is relevant to another domain, for example, how to cope with stress (protection), how to partake in a cultural ritual (group participation), how to inhibit aggressive responses (control), and so on. Greater research-based knowledge regarding the features and consequences of each domain of socialization can promote better understanding of these more complex combinations as well.

Another important point is that interactions in one domain can affect processes in another domain. For example, when parents have been consistently supportive in the protection domain in the past, children may be less likely to become overly aroused in discipline situations in later control interactions (with parents, teachers, etc.). Similarly, Kochanska, Aksan, Knaack, and Rhines (2004) found that early secure attachment (protection) enhanced the subsequent positive effects of gentle discipline (control) on children's conscience development. In another study, early security augmented the effects of variables reflecting parent child mutual reciprocity on subsequent internalization of values and problem behavior (Kochanska et al., 2010). As another example, early mutual reciprocity may increase children's eagerness to adopt practices that are modeled by parents in the group participation domain (leisure activities, religious practices, etc.). Systematically uncovering the intricate connections and interplay between socialization processes in different domains is an important goal for future research.

In summary, then, we suggest that features of willing or well-socialized behavior differ. They may involve trust that a caregiver is making demands that are in the interests of the child, acceptance of rules and limits that is viewed as self-generated, mature behavior or skill that has been learned and internalized through coaching, adoption of the social customs and practices typical of one's group, or a feeling of shared goals and desire to cooperate and reciprocate. We do not mean to imply, however, that the nature of parent–child interaction is a fragmented one. Whereas it is helpful to outline different roles played by parents in different domains of socialization, in the end, these roles are embodied in the same persons and the same overall relationship. The implication is that parental responsivity or competence in one domain may well compensate for insensitivity or incompetence in another domain, and difficulties in one domain may well exacerbate problems in other domains. Moreover, interactions with parents in a given domain may influence and/or be affected by interactions with other socialization agents in that or other domains, and vice versa. We know relatively little about these complex processes and their implications. It is clear, however, that they provide important directions for future research on socialization.

REFERENCES

Assor, A., Roth, G., & Deci, E. L. (2004). The emotional costs of parents' conditional regard: A self-determination theory analysis. *Journal of Personality, 72,* 47–88.

Bandura, A., & Walters, R. H. (1963). *Social learning theory and personality development.* New York: Holt, Rinehart & Winston.

Barber, B. K. (1996). Parental psychological control: Revisiting a neglected construct. *Child Development, 67,* 3296–3319.

Barber, B. K., & Harmon, E. L. (2002). Violating the self: Parental psychological control of children and adolescents. In B. K. Barber (Ed.), *Intrusive parenting: How psychological control affects children and adolescents* (pp. 15–52). Washington, DC: American Psychological Association.

Baumrind, D. (1971). Current patterns of parental authority. *Developmental Psychology, 4,* 1–103.

Baumrind, D. (2012). Differentiating between confrontive and coercive kinds of parental power-assertive disciplinary practices. *Human Development, 55,* 35–51.

Bell, S. M., & Ainsworth, M. D. S. (1972). Infant crying and maternal responsiveness. *Child Development, 43,* 1171–1190.

Belsky, J., & Pluess, M. (2009). Beyond diathesis stress: Differential susceptibility to environmental influences. *Psychological Bulletin, 135,* 885–908.

Bokhorst, C. L., Sumter, S. R., & Westenberg, P. M. (2010). Social support from parents, friends, classmates, and teachers in children and adolescents aged 9 to 18 years: Who is perceived as most supportive? *Social Development, 19,* 417–426.

Bourdieu, P. (1977). *Outline of a theory of practice* (R. Nice, Trans.). Cambridge, UK: Cambridge University Press.

Bowlby, J. (1944). Forty-four juvenile thieves: Their characters and home life. *International Journal of Psycho-Analysis, 25,* 19–52, 107–127.

Bowlby, J. (1982). *Attachment and loss: Vol. 1. Attachment.* New York: Basic Books. (Original work published 1969)

Branstetter, S. A., Furman, W., & Cottrell, L. (2009). The influence of representations of attachment, maternal–adolescent relationship quality, and maternal monitoring on adolescent substance use: A 2-year longitudinal examination. *Child Development, 80,* 1448–1462.

Bretherton, I., Golby, B., & Cho, E. (1997). Attachment and the transmission of values. In J. E. Grusec & L. Kuczynski (Eds.), *Parenting and children's internalization of values* (pp. 103–134). New York: Wiley.

Brewer, J. B., & Gardner, W. (1996). Who is this "we"?: Levels of collective identity and self-representation. *Journal of Personality and Social Psychology, 71,* 83–93.

Brint, S., Contreras, M. F., & Matthews, M. T. (2001). Socialization messages in primary schools: An organizational analysis. *Sociology of Education, 74,* 157–180.

Brody, G. H., & Flor, D. L. (1998). Maternal resources, parenting practices, and child competence in rural, single-parent African American families. *Child Development, 69,* 803–816.

Bugental, D. B. (2000). Acquisition of the algorithms of social life: A domain-based approach. *Psychological Bulletin, 26,* 187–209.

Cassidy, J. (1999). The nature of the child's ties. In J. Cassidy & P. R. Shaver (Eds.), *Handbook of attachment: Theory, research, and clinical applications* (pp. 3–20). New York: Guilford Press.

Cassidy, K. W., Fineberg, D. S., Brown, K., & Perkins, A. (2005). Theory of mind may be contagious, but you don't catch it from your twin. *Child Development, 76,* 97–106.

Chan, S. M. (2011). Social competence of elementary-school children: Relationships to maternal authoritativeness, supportive maternal responses and children's coping strategies. *Child: Care, Health and Development, 37,* 524–532.

Chao, R. K. (2001). Extending research on the consequences of parenting style for Chinese Americans and European Americans. *Child Development, 72,* 1832–1843.

Collins, W. A., Maccoby, E. E., Steinberg, L., Hetherington, E. M., & Bornstein, M. H. (2000). Contemporary research on parenting: The case for nature and nurture. *American Psychologist, 55,* 218–232.

Cosmides, L., & Tooby, J. (1992). Cognitive adaptations for social exchange. In J. H. Barkow, L. Cosmides, & J. Tooby (Eds.), *The adapted mind: Evolutionary psychology and the generation of culture* (pp. 163–228). London: Oxford University Press.

Craig, W., & Pepler, D. (1997). Observations of bullying and victimization in the schoolyard. *Canadian Journal of School Psychology, 2,* 41–60.

Criss, M. M., Shaw, D. S., & Ingoldsby, E. M. (2003). Mother–son positive synchrony in middle childhood: Relation to antisocial behavior. *Social Development, 12,* 379–400.

Crouter, A. C., & Head, M. R. (2002). Parental monitoring and knowledge of children. In M. H. Bornstein (Ed.), *Handbook of parenting: Vol. 3. Being and becoming a parent* (2nd ed., pp. 461–483). Mahwah, NJ: Erlbaum.

Darling, N., Cumsille, P., & Martínez, M. L. (2008). Individual differences in adolescents' beliefs about the legitimacy of parental authority and their own obligation to obey: A longitudinal investigation. *Child Development, 79,* 1103–1118.

Davidov, M. (2013). The socialization of self-regulation from a domains perspective. In G. Seebass, M. Schmitz, & P. M. Gollwitzer (Eds.), *Acting intentionally and its limits: Individuals, groups, institutions* (pp. 223–244). Berlin: De Gruyter.

Davidov, M., & Grusec, J. E. (2006a). Multiple pathways to compliance: Mothers' willingness to cooperate and knowledge of their children's reactions to discipline. *Journal of Family Psychology, 20*(4), 705–708.

Davidov, M., & Grusec, J. E. (2006b). Untangling the links of parental responsiveness to distress and warmth to child outcomes. *Child Development, 77,* 44–58.

Davidov, M., Grusec, J. E., & Wolfe, J. L. (2012). Mothers' knowledge of their children's evaluations of discipline: The role of type of discipline and misdeed, and parenting practices. *Merrill–Palmer Quarterly, 58,* 314–340.

Deater-Deckard, K., & Petrill, S. A. (2004). Parent–child dyadic mutuality and child behavior problems: An investigation of gene–environment processes. *Journal of Child Psychology and Psychiatry, 45,* 1171–1179.

Dix, T. (1992). Parenting on behalf of the child: Empathic goals in the regulation of responsive parenting. In I. E. Sigel, A. V. McGillicuddy-DeLisi, & J. J. Goodnow (Eds.), *Parental belief systems: The psychological consequences for children* (2nd ed., pp. 319–346). Hillsdale, NJ: Erlbaum.

Dubas, J. S., & Gerris, J. R. M. (2002). Longitudinal changes in the time parents spend in activities with their adolescent children as a function of child age, pubertal status and gender. *Journal of Family Psychology, 16,* 415–462.

Eaker, D. G., & Walters, L. H. (2002). Adolescent satisfaction in family rituals and psychosocial development: A developmental systems theory perspective. *Journal of Family Psychology, 16,* 406–414.

Eccles, J. S., Wigfield, A., & Schiefele, U. (1998). Motivation to succeed. In W. Damon (Series Ed.) & N. Eisenberg (Volume Ed.), *Handbook of child psychology: Vol. 3. Social, emotional, and personality development* (5th ed., pp. 1017–1095). New York: Wiley.

Egeland, B., Jacobvitz, D., & Sroufe, L. A. (1988). Breaking the cycle of abuse. *Child Development, 59,* 1080–1088.

Eisenberg, N., Wentzel, M., & Harris, J. D. (1998). The role of emotionality and regulation in empathy-related responding. *School Psychology Review, 27,* 506–521.

Fabes, R. A., Leonard, S. A., Kupanoff, K., & Martin, C. L. (2001). Parental coping with children's negative emotions: Relations with children's emotional and social responding. *Child Development, 72,* 907–920.

Fabes, R. A., Poulin, R. E., Eisenberg, N., & Madden-Derdich, D. A. (2002). The Coping with

Children's Negative Emotions Scale (CCNES): Psychometric properties and relations with children's emotional competence. *Marriage and Family Review, 34*, 285–310.

Farver, J. A. M., Kim, Y. K., & Lee, Y. (1995). Cultural differences in Korean- and Anglo-American preschoolers' social interaction and play behaviors. *Child Development, 66*, 1088–1099.

Fawcett, L. M., & Garton, A. F. (2005). The effect of peer collaboration on children's problem-solving ability. *British Journal of Educational Psychology, 75*, 157–169.

Fiske, A. P. (1992). The four elementary forms of sociality: Framework for a unified theory of social relations. *Psychological Review, 99*, 689–723.

Fredricks, J. A., & Eccles, J. S. (2006). Is extracurricular participation associated with beneficial outcomes?: Concurrent and longitudinal relations. *Developmental Psychology, 42*, 698–713.

Fredrickson, B. L. (2003). The value of positive emotions: The emerging science of positive psychology is coming to understand why it's good to feel good. *American Scientist, 91*, 330–335.

Goldberg, S., Grusec, J. E., & Jenkins, J. (1999). Confidence in protection: Arguments for a narrow definition of attachment. *Journal of Family Psychology, 13*, 475–483.

Gottman, J. M., Katz, L. F., & Hooven, C. (1996). Parental meta-emotion philosophy and the emotional life of families: Theoretical models and preliminary data. *Journal of Family Psychology, 10*, 243–268.

Grolnick, W. (2003). *The psychology of parental control: How well-meant parenting backfires.* Mahwah, NJ: Erlbaum.

Grolnick, W. S., Deci, E. L., & Ryan, R. M. (1997). Internalization within the family: The self-determination theory perspective. In J. E. Grusec & L. Kuczynski (Eds.), *Parenting and children's internalization of values: A handbook of contemporary theory* (pp. 135–161). New York: Wiley.

Grusec, J. E. (1983). The internalization of altruistic dispositions: A cognitive analysis. In E. T. Higgins, D. N. Ruble, & W. W. Hartup (Eds.), *Social cognition and social development* (pp. 275–293). New York: Cambridge University Press.

Grusec, J. E., & Davidov, M. (2007). Socialization in the family: The roles of parents. In J. E. Grusec & P. D. Hastings (Eds.), *Handbook of socialization* (pp. 284–308). New York: Guilford Press.

Grusec, J. E., & Davidov, M. (2010). Integrating different perspectives on socialization theory and research: A domain-specific approach. *Child Development, 81*, 687–709.

Grusec, J. E., & Goodnow, J. J. (1994). The impact of parental discipline methods on the child's internalization of values: A reconceptualization of current points of view. *Developmental Psychology, 30*, 4–19.

Grusec, J. E., Goodnow, J. J., & Cohen, L. (1997) Household work and the development of children's concern for others. *Developmental Psychology, 32*, 999–1007.

Grusec, J. E., Goodnow, J. J., & Kuczynski, L. (2000). New directions in analyses of parenting contributions to children's acquisition of values. *Child Development, 71*, 205–211.

Gunnar, M., & Quevedo, K. (2007). The neurobiology of stress and development. *Annual Review of Psychology, 58*, 145–173.

Haden, C. A., Ornstein, P. A., Eckerman, C. O., & Didow, S. M. (2001). Mother–child conversational interactions as events unfold: Linkages to subsequent remembering. *Child Development, 72*, 1016–1031.

Harter, S. (1996). Teacher and classmate influences on scholastic motivation, self-esteem, and level of voice in adolescents. In J. Juvonen & K. Wentzel (Eds.), *Social motivation: Understanding children's school adjustment* (pp. 11–42). New York: Cambridge University Press.

Hastings, P., & Grusec, J. E. (1997). Conflict outcomes as a function of parental accuracy in perceiving child cognitions and affect. *Social Development, 6*, 76–90.

Hastings, P. D., & Grusec, J. E. (1998). Parenting goals as organizers of responses to parent–child disagreement. *Developmental Psychology, 34*, 465–479.

Hodges, E. V., Boivin, M., Vitaro, F., & Bukowski, W. M. (1999). The power of friendship: Protection against an escalating cycle of peer victimization. *Developmental Psychology, 35*, 94–101.

Hoffman, M. L. (1970). Moral development. In P. H. Mussen (Ed.), *Carmichael's manual of child psychology* (Vol. 2, pp. 261–360). New York: Wiley.

Hughes, J., & Kwok, O. M. (2007). Influence of student–teacher and parent–teacher relationships on lower achieving readers' engagement and achievement in the primary grades. *Journal of Educational Psychology, 99,* 39–51.

Hunter, S. C., Boyle, J. M., & Warden, D. (2004). Help seeking amongst child and adolescent victims of peer-aggression and bullying: The influence of school-stage, gender, victimisation, appraisal, and emotion. *British Journal of Educational Psychology, 74,* 375–390.

Jenkins, J. M. (1992). Sibling relationships in disharmonious homes. In F. Boer & J. Dunn (Eds.), *Children's sibling relationships: Developmental and clinical issues* (pp. 125–136). Hillsdale, NJ: Erlbaum.

Johnson, R. T., & Johnson, D. W. (1979). Type of task and student achievement and attitudes in interpersonal cooperation, competition, and individualization. *Journal of Social Psychology, 108,* 37–48.

Kagan, J. (1982). The emergence of self. *Journal of Child Psychology and Psychiatry, 23,* 363–381.

Karos, L., Howe, N., & Aquan-Assee, J. (2007). Reciprocal and complementary sibling interactions, relationship quality and socio-emotional problem solving. *Infant and Child Development, 16,* 577–596.

Kerns, K. A., Aspelmeier, J. E., Gentzler, A. L., & Grabill, C. M. (2001). Parent–child attachment and monitoring in middle childhood. *Journal of Family Psychology, 15,* 69–81.

Kerr, M., & Stattin, H. (2000). What parents know, how they know it, and several forms of adolescent adjustment: Further support for a reinterpretation of monitoring. *Developmental Psychology, 36,* 366–380.

Kerr, M., Stattin, H., & Burk, W. J. (2010). A reinterpretation of parental monitoring in longitudinal perspective. *Journal of Research on Adolescence, 20,* 39–64.

Kilgore, K., Snyder, J., & Lentz, C. (2000). The contribution of parental discipline, parental monitoring, and school risk to early-onset conduct problems in African American boys and girls. *Developmental Psychology, 36,* 835–845.

Kitzmann, K. M., Cohen, R., & Lockwood, R. L. (2002). Are only children missing out?: Comparison of the peer-related social competence of only children and siblings. *Journal of Social and Personal Relationships, 19,* 299–316.

Kochanska, G. (2002). Mutually responsive orientation between mothers and their young children: A context for the early development of conscience. *Current Directions in Psychological Science, 11,* 191–195.

Kochanska, G., Aksan, N., Knaack, A., & Rhines, H. M. (2004). Maternal parenting and children's conscience: Early security as moderator. *Child Development, 75,* 1229–1242.

Kochanska, G., Forman, D. R., Aksan, N., & Dunbar, S. B. (2005). Pathways to conscience: Early mother–child mutually responsive orientation and children's moral emotion, conduct, and cognition. *Journal of Child Psychology and Psychiatry, 46,* 19–34.

Kochanska, G., Woodard, J., Kim, S., Koenig, J. L., Yoon, J. E., & Barry, R. A. (2010). Positive socialization mechanisms in secure and insecure parent–child dyads: Two longitudinal studies. *Journal of Child Psychology and Psychiatry, 51,* 998–1009.

Komro, K. A., Perry, C. L., Veblen-Mortenson, S., & Williams, C. L. (1994). Peer participation in Project Northland: A community-wide alcohol use prevention project. *Journal of School Health, 64,* 318–322.

Laible, D., & Panfile, T. (2009). Mother–child reminiscing in the context of secure attachment relationships: Lessons in understanding and coping with negative emotion. In J. Quas & R. Fivush (Eds.), *Emotion and memory in development: Biological, cognitive, and social considerations* (pp. 166–195). Oxford, UK: Oxford University Press.

Lansford, J. E., Malone, P. S., Dodge, K. A., Chang, L., Chaudhary, N., Tapanya, S., et al. (2010). Children's perceptions of maternal hostility as a mediator of the link between discipline and children's adjustment in four countries. *International Journal of Behavioral Development, 34,* 452–461.

Leerkes, E. M., Blankson, A. N., & O'Brien, M. (2009). Differential effects of maternal sensitivity to infant distress and nondistress on social–emotional functioning. *Child Development, 80,* 762–775.

Leerkes, E. M., Weaver, J. M., & O'Brien, M. (2012). Differentiating maternal sensitivity to infant distress and non-distress. *Parenting: Science and Practice, 12,* 175–184.

Lindsey, E. W., Cremeens, P. R., & Caldera, Y. M. (2010). Mother–child and father–child mutuality in two contexts: Consequences for young children's peer relationships. *Infant and Child Development, 19,* 142–160.

Lubbers, M. J., Kuyper, H., & Van Der Werf, M. P. (2009). Social comparison with friends versus non-friends. *European Journal of Social Psychology, 39,* 52–68.

Lundell, L., Grusec, J. E., McShane, K., & Davidov, M. (2005). *Mother–adolescent conflict: Adolescent goals, maternal perspective-taking, and conflict intensity.* Unpublished manuscript, University of Toronto, Ontario, Canada.

MacDonald, K. (1992). Warmth as a developmental construct: An evolutionary analysis. *Child Development, 63,* 753–773.

Malti, T., & Krettenauer, T. (2012). The relation of moral emotion attributions to prosocial and antisocial behavior: A meta-analysis. *Child Development, 84,* 397–412.

Matas, L., Arend, R., & Sroufe, L. A. (1978). Continuity of adaptation in the second year: The relationship between quality of attachment and later competence. *Child Development, 49,* 547–556.

McAdams, D. P. (2004). Generativity and the narrative ecology of family life. In M. W. Pratt & B. H. Fiese (Eds.), *Family stories and the life course* (pp. 235–257). Mahwah, NJ: Erlbaum.

McElwain, N. L., & Booth-LaForce, C. (2006). Maternal sensitivity to infant distress and non-distress as predictors of infant–mother attachment security. *Journal of Family Psychology, 20,* 247–255.

Mitchell-Copeland, J., Denham, S. A., & DeMulder, E. K. (1997). Q-sort assessment of child–teacher attachment relationships and social competence in the preschool. *Early Education and Development, 8,* 27–39.

Narvaez, D. (2002). Does reading moral stories build character? *Educational Psychology Review, 14*(2), 155–171.

Newman, R. S. (2000). Social influences on the development of children's adaptive help seeking: The role of parents, teachers, and peers. *Developmental Review, 20,* 350–404.

Padilla-Walker, L. M. (2008). Domain-appropriateness of maternal discipline as a predictor of adolescents' positive and negative outcomes. *Journal of Family Psychology, 22,* 456–464.

Parpal, M., & Maccoby, E. E. (1985). Maternal responsiveness and subsequent child compliance. *Child Development, 56,* 1326–1334.

Patterson, G. R. (1982). *Coercive family process.* Eugene, OR: Castalia Press.

Patterson, G. R., Crosby, L., & Vuchinich, S. (1992). Predicting risk for early police arrest. *Journal of Quantitative Criminology, 8,* 335–355.

Pettit, G. S. (1997). The developmental course of violence and aggression: Mechanisms of family and peer influence. *Psychiatric Clinics of North America, 20,* 283–299.

Pomerantz, E. M. (2001). Parent × child socialization: Implications for the development of depressive symptoms. *Journal of Family Psychology, 15,* 510–525.

Puntambekar, S., & Hubscher, R. (2005). Tools for scaffolding students in a complex learning environment: What have we gained and what have we missed? *Educational Psychologist, 40,* 1–12.

Recchia, H. E., & Howe, N. (2009). Associations between social understanding, sibling relationship quality, and siblings' conflict strategies and outcomes. *Child Development, 80,* 1564–1578.

Rheingold, H. L. (1982). Little children's participation in the work of adults, a nascent prosocial behavior. *Child Development, 53,* 114–125.

Roth, G., Assor, A., Niemiec, C. P., Ryan, R. M., & Deci, E. L. (2009). The emotional and academic consequences of parental conditional regard: Comparing conditional positive regard, conditional negative regard, and autonomy support as parenting practices. *Developmental Psychology, 45,* 1119–1142.

Rowe, D. C., Rodgers, J. L., & Meseck-Bushey, S. (1992). Sibling delinquency and the family environment: Shared and unshared influences. *Child Development, 63,* 59–67.

Rubin, K. H., Burgess, K. B., & Hastings, P. D. (2002). Stability and social–behavioral consequences of toddlers' inhibited temperament and parenting behaviors. *Child Development, 73,* 483–495.

Rudy, D., & Grusec, J. E. (2001). Correlates of authoritarian parenting in individualist and collectivist cultures and implications for understanding the transmission of values. *Journal of Cross-Cultural Psychology, 32,* 202–212.

Rudy, D., & Grusec, J. E. (2006). Authoritarian parenting in individualist and collectivist groups: Associations with maternal emotion and cognition and children's self-esteem. *Journal of Family Psychology, 20,* 68–78.

Ryan, R. M., & Deci, E. L. (2000). Self-determination theory and the facilitation of intrinsic motivation, social development, and well-being. *American Psychologist, 55,* 68–78.

Sagi, A., Koren-Karie, N., Gini, M., Ziv, Y., & Joels, T. (2002). Shedding further light on the effects of various types and quality of early child care on infant–mother attachment relationship: The Haifa study of early child care. *Child Development, 73,* 1166–1186.

Sameroff, A. (1975). Transactional models of early social relations. *Human Development, 18,* 65–79.

Scarr, S., & McCartney, K. (1983). How people make their own environment: A theory of genotype–environment effects. *Child Development, 54,* 424–435.

Schwartz, B. (2000). Self-determination: The tyranny of freedom. *American Psychologist, 55,* 79–88.

Seligman, M. E. (1970). On the generality of the laws of learning. *Psychological Review, 77,* 406–418.

Sherman, A., Grusec, J. E., & Almas, A. N. (2013). *The role of maternal knowledge in the development of children's positive coping skills.* Unpublished manuscript, University of Toronto, Toronto, Ontario, Canada.

Soenens, B., & Vansteenkiste, M. (2010). A theoretical upgrade of the concept of parental psychological control: Proposing new insights on the basis of self-determination theory. *Developmental Review, 30,* 74–99.

Spagnola, M., & Fiese, B. H. (2007). Family routines and rituals: A context for development in the lives of young children. *Infants and Young Children, 20,* 284–299.

Steinberg, L. (1990). Autonomy, conflict, and harmony in the family relationship. In S. S. Feldman & G. R. Elliott, (Eds.), *At the threshold: The developing adolescent* (pp. 255–276). Cambridge, MA: Harvard University Press.

Trevarthen, C., Kokkinski, T., & Flamenghi, G. A., Jr. (1999). What infants' imitations communicate: With mothers, with fathers and with peers. In J. Nadel & G. Butterworth (Eds.), *Imitation in infancy: Cambridge studies in cognitive perceptual development* (pp. 127–185). New York: Cambridge University Press.

Turiel, C. (1998). Notes from the underground: Culture, conflict, and subversion. In J. Langer & M. Killen (Eds.), *Piaget, evolution, and development: The Jean Piaget symposium series* (pp. 271–296). Mahwah, NJ: Erlbaum.

Turner, V. D., & Berkowitz, M. W. (2005). Scaffolding morality: Positioning a socio-cultural construct. *New Ideas in Psychology, 23,* 174–184.

Updegraff, K. A., McHale, S. M., & Crouter, A. C. (2002). Adolescents' sibling relationship and friendship experiences: Developmental patterns and relationship linkages. *Social Development, 11,* 182–204.

Vinik, J., Almas, A. N., & Grusec, J. (2011). Mothers' knowledge of what distresses and what comforts their children predicts children's coping, empathy, and prosocial behavior. *Parenting: Science and Practice, 11,* 56–71.

Vygotsky, L. S. (1978). *Mind in society: The development of higher psychological processes.* Cambridge, MA: Harvard University Press.

Walker, L. J., Hennig, K. H., & Krettenauer, T. (2000). Parent and peer contexts for children's moral reasoning development. *Child Development, 71,* 1033–1048.

Wentzel, K. R. (2002). Are effective teachers like good parents?: Teaching styles and student adjustment in early adolescence. *Child Development, 73,* 287–301.

Whiteman, S. D., McHale, S. M., & Crouter, A. C. (2007). Competing processes of sibling influence: Observational learning and sibling deidentification. *Social Development, 16,* 642–661.

Wood, D., Bruner, J. S., & Ross, G. (1976). The role of tutoring in problem solving. *Journal of Child Psychology and Psychiatry, 17,* 89–100.

Wright, J. C., & Bartsch, K. (2008). Portraits of early moral sensibility in two children's everyday conversations. *Merrill–Palmer Quarterly, 54,* 56–85.

Youniss, J., McLellan, J. A., & Strouse, D. (1994). "We're popular, but we're not snobs": Adolescents describe their crowds. In R. Montemayor, G. R. Adams, & T. P. Gullotta (Eds.), *Advances in adolescent development: Vol. 6. Personal relationships during adolescence* (pp. 101–122). Thousand Oaks, CA: Sage.

CHAPTER 8

Siblings

Judy Dunn

The great majority of individuals grow up with siblings (around 80% in North America and in Europe). For many people, their relationships with their sisters and brothers are the longest lasting in their lives—longer than their relationships with parents, partners, or children. All over the world, siblings figure importantly in legends, history, and literature, yet the scientific study of the nature and influence of sibling relationships is relatively recent. From early in the 20th century, clinicians and family theorists have argued that siblings can influence individual adjustment and play a key role in family relationships (Adler, 1928). Ethnographic studies of siblings have shown how widespread and significant siblings' caregiving can be (Zukow-Goldring, 2002), yet systematic study of siblings was relatively rare until the 1970s and 1980s—an important exception being the classic research on siblings carried out by Koch (1954, 1960) in the 1950s and 1960s. Over the last three decades, the picture has changed markedly, and research interest in siblings has grown notably, focusing particularly on childhood and adolescence (Brody, 1998; Hetherington, Reiss, & Plomin, 1994; Howe, Ross, & Recchia, 2011). Siblings in adulthood remain relatively underresearched.

To consider sibling influences on socialization, I focus first on the nature of relationships between siblings, and on individual differences in those relationships, as well as associations with other family relationships. Second, I consider the evidence that these relationships influence individual socialization, with a focus on two domains: children's adjustment and the development of social understanding. Third, I compare the influence of siblings and of peers on socialization. Finally, I consider how research on siblings has challenged our understanding of family socialization more broadly considered—the issue of why siblings growing up within the same family differ from one another in personality and adjustment. Of particular importance, recent methodological advances in the use of multilevel modeling have been employed to study sibling differences in outcome (Pike, 2012; see also Jenkins et al., 2009; Jenkins, Rasbash, Leckie, Gass, & Dunn, 2012).

Sibling Relationships as Contexts for Socialization

Two striking characteristics of sibling relationships in childhood and adolescence stand out from systematic research—characteristics that make the relationships' potential for influence on socialization very high. These are, first, the emotional quality of the relationship between siblings, and, second, the familiarity and intimacy of siblings. On emotional quality, both intense positive and negative feelings are frequently and uninhibitedly expressed by siblings from infancy through adolescence. The translation of negative feelings into conflict and aggressive behavior between siblings is a persistent problem for many parents (frequently cited as a reason for attending family therapy), and sibling violence is the most common form of domestic abuse (Naylor, Petch, & Ali, 2011). Observational studies note that intense positive emotions are also frequent (Dunn, Creps, & Brown, 1996). And for many young siblings, the relationship is one in which mixed feelings are evident—with both positive and negative feelings freely expressed.

Studies of sibling conflict have continued over the past decade to illuminate a number of themes. For instance, detailed observational studies by Hildy Ross and her colleagues have shown the consistency of 2- and 4-year-olds in their patterns of sibling conflict (Perlman, Ross, & Garfinkel, 2009), while also documenting developmental changes. In general, more planning and less opposition were associated with siblings achieving resolutions: Information-sharing between siblings (ages 4–8 years) faced with a conflict of interest (Ram & Ross, 2008) was also reported to contribute to resolution of conflicts. Differences in resolution strategies of older and younger siblings have been described: When siblings ages 4–12 years were in conflict (Ross, Ross, Stein, & Trabasso, 2006), the older siblings provided leadership by suggesting, modifying, justifying, and requesting agreement to plans for resolution. Younger siblings countered and disagreed with these strategies, but they also contributed to planning and agreed to their siblings' plans. Mutually beneficial conflict resolution required that children shift focus from debating past wrongs to developing plans to meet their unrealized goals in future interaction.

An especially interesting study of antisocial behavior toward siblings, and its links with later behavior toward peers, was reported by Ensor, Marks, Jacobs, and Hughes (2010). Trajectories of antisocial behavior were studied for a socially diverse sample of 3- and 6-year-old children, and also with unfamiliar peers at age 6 years. Three indicators of antisocial behavior toward siblings (refusal to share/interact, bullying, and harming) were studied with latent growth models. The average trajectory of antisocial behavior toward siblings was stable and particularly high for boys with brothers and for children whose mothers had poor educational qualifications. Sustained and escalating antisocial behavior toward siblings predicted bullying and refusal to share with unfamiliar peers, and more subtle forms of antisocial behavior, such as social exclusion. The findings were independent of associations with concurrent antisocial behavior between young siblings. Earlier research on children's relations with siblings and peers indicated correlations between aggression with peers and with siblings (Vandell, Minnett, & Santrock, 1987), and similarities in behavior in disputes with siblings and with peers (Slomkowski & Dunn, 1992), but other studies of young children report no such links across the relationships (Abramovitch, Corter, Pepler, & Stanhope, 1986). Different methods, different samples, and different measures may have contributed to these inconsistencies across study findings.

The second feature of sibling relationships that heightens their potential for influence on socialization is the familiarity and intimacy of the relationship. From the preschool years through middle childhood, siblings spend more time together and in interaction with each other than they do with parents or peers (McHale & Crouter, 1996). They know each other very well, and this intimacy means that they can provide effective support or they can tease and undermine each other—as they do with great effectiveness from the second year onward (Dunn, 1988a). Either way, the impact of a sibling's behavior on each child's attitude toward conforming to the social rules of the family is likely to be high. In other words, in the face of conflict with a sibling, children exploit their understanding of social rules within the family to their own advantage, and to "do down" their sibling.

Individual Differences

Whereas the intimacy and emotional intensity of siblings' relationships make their potential for influence on socialization high, a third characteristic of siblings' relationships that mitigates against generalizing about sibling influence is the great range of individual differences between siblings. Some siblings describe their affection and interest in their siblings vividly in interviews and show cooperation, insight, and empathy in most of their interactions. Others describe their feelings of irritation, hostility and dislike, and show this hostility and aggression in interactions with their siblings. Still others show and describe their *ambivalent* feelings (for siblings' perceptions of their relationship, see, e.g., McGuire, Manke, Eftekhari, & Dunn, 2000). In assessing the developmental influence of the relationship on patterns of socialization, it is clearly crucial to take account of the quality of the sibling relationship and the factors that lead to these notable individual differences. The analytic tools that make possible the systematic analysis of the relationships between more than two siblings per family have now been developed (e.g., Jenkins et al., 2009, 2012). This allows differentiation of the aspects of a particular sibling dyad that are shared by all dyads within the family (between family effects) from those aspects that are unique to individual siblings in each sibling dyad within the family. The striking results reported in the Jenkins and colleagues articles indicate that the within-family variance between sibling dyads in the same family is both significant and greater in magnitude than the between family members (Pike, 2012).

Birth Order, Gender, and Age Gap

During the early years of childhood, there is some evidence that the quality of the relationship between siblings is more influenced by the affection, interest, or hostility of the firstborn than by the feelings of the second born. Longitudinal research shows that the reaction of firstborn children (their affection and interest, or hostility) to a new sibling is linked over time to the quality of both siblings' behavior toward each other (Dunn & Kendrick, 1982). However, the significance of the contribution of second-born siblings to the relationship quality increases during the preschool years (Dunn, 1988b).

Patterns of normative change in the quality of siblings' relationship depend on siblings' birth order; declines in emotional intimacy toward a sibling during the transition to adolescence are less characteristic of younger siblings than of older ones: Younger siblings tend to place greater value on the support they receive from older siblings than vice versa (Buhrmester, 1992). Research into the associations between sibling and friend relationships has highlighted differences between firstborn and second-born adolescents (Updegraff, McHale, & Crouter, 2002). In a study that took the "insider's perspective" by focusing on young adolescents' own reports of their sibling and friendship relationships, these researchers predicted that there would be stronger connections between the quality of sibling and peer relationships for second borns than firstborns, in terms of both dimensions of intimacy and control in the relationships. Support was found for the birth order effects: Second borns' reports of sibling intimacy were modestly associated with greater friendship intimacy, but this pattern was not found for firstborn adolescents. The authors concluded that these results support the notion that adolescents are most likely to learn from high-status models (McHale, Updegraff, Helms-Erikson, & Crouter, 2001; Tucker, Updegraff, McHale, & Crouter, 1999). The associations between the two relationships in this research were stronger for sibling and friendship *control*, for both firstborn and second-born siblings. Adolescents who reported high levels of controlling behavior with their siblings also reported high levels of control in their friendships. Patterns of longitudinal change in control also were similar in the two relationships. The researchers emphasize that the relationship connections may be more salient when the comparison involves same-sex sibling and friendship dyads, but they point out that it will be important in the future to consider the possibility that the extent to which siblings model behavior in accordance with masculine or feminine roles (e.g., how expressive or traditionally feminine they are) may be more important than sibling sex in the moderation of cross-relationship linkages.

Findings on how the quality of the sibling relationship is related to gender vary with the age and developmental stage of the siblings. In early childhood, the evidence on gender is inconsistent. During middle childhood, gender becomes more significant, with boys becoming less likely to describe intimacy and warmth in their sibling relationships (Dunn, Slomkowski, & Beardsall, 1994). It appears that the socialization influences of the wider world outside the family impact increasingly on siblings' relationships within the family in the teenage years.

Temperament and Personality

Associations between the temperamental or personality characteristics of siblings and the quality of their relationship have been described in preschoolers, in children in early and middle childhood, and in adolescents (e.g., Furman & Lanthier, 1996; Stocker, Dunn, & Plomin, 1989), But the results vary in the different studies, which tend to be based on different populations and to use various methods to study children of various ages. Furman and Lanthier (1996) noted, however, that a general pattern is evident across studies. Temperamental characteristics are more systematically related to conflict in the sibling relationship than to affection and warmth. This may be because although conflict between siblings is easy to measure (it shows up in a variety of settings and methods), the positive features of the relationship are less evident.

The frequencies of conflict and affection in siblings were found to be importantly linked to the *match* between siblings' temperaments, in studies in early and in middle childhood (Brody, 1996). Siblings who were more similar in temperament had more positive relationships—a finding that fits with the evidence on both adult and childhood friends that similarity makes for friendship: "Like me" attracts (Hartup, 1996; Hinde, 1979).

Associations with Other Family Relationships

A number of general developmental points have been established concerning links between sibling relationships and other relationships within the family. The first concerns parent–child relationships. Attachment research has shown that children who are secure in their attachments to their parents develop more positive sibling relationships than those who are insecure (Teti & Ablard, 1989; Volling & Belsky, 1992). And studies that investigate a broad range of dimensions of parent–child relationships consistently report that positive, prosocial sibling relationships are associated with warm positive parent–child relationships (e.g., Brody, 1998; Pike, Coldwell, & Dunn, 2005). Punitive, negative, and overcontrolled parent–child relations are associated with aggressive, hostile sibling relationships. The evidence for these associations is correlational, and this means that inferences about the direction of causal influence, or the family processes that are implicated, cannot be drawn. These associations may be due to parental influence or to child effects. Difficult children, for instance, may elicit negative behavior from both parents and siblings. Siblings who are very aggressive and hostile to each other are difficult to live with, and this hostility may in turn contribute to the difficulties in the relationship with their parents. It seems likely that all these family processes may be implicated in the links between relationships.

The second point, established in several research programs, is that the quality of the relationship between parents is associated with differences in the sibling relationship, with more positive marital/spousal relationships linked to more positive sibling relations (Dunn, Deater-Deckard, Pickering, Beveridge, & the ALSPAC Study Team, 1999; Stocker, Ahmed, & Stall, 1997). Both direct pathways from marital to sibling relationships and indirect pathways via the parent–child relationship are implicated. Interestingly, the pattern of associations between marital and sibling relationships differs in stepfamilies: Conflict between mother and stepfather was not related to conflict between siblings in a study in the United Kingdom, in contrast to the pattern found in families with two biological parents (Dunn et al., 1999; Hetherington & Clingempeel, 1992). Siblings' responses to marital conflict differ even within the same family, and these differences are linked to their adjustment (Jenkins, Dunn, Rasbash, O'Connor, & Simpson, 2005).

The third point also concerns parent–child and sibling relationships. There is some clinical evidence that in families in which parent–child relationships are extremely distant or uninvolved, the siblings can develop intensely supportive relationships with each other (Boer & Dunn, 1990). There is some evidence that this can be beneficial. For example, placing young adolescent siblings together in the same residential foster care versus separate residential care facilities has been associated with greater self-esteem, and siblings in the same residence reported more well-being when they had closer relationships and more time together (Davidson-Arad & Klein, 2011).

The fourth point is one that has received a great deal of research attention. Differential parent–child relationships within a family are associated with more conflicted, hostile sibling relationships and more adjustment problems in siblings. If parents show more affection, attention and warmth, or less discipline, control, or pressure for socialization in their relationship with one sibling than with another, the siblings are less likely to get along well than siblings in families in which parents and siblings do not describe such differential treatment (K. Conger & Conger, 1994; Reiss, Neiderhiser, Hetherington, & Plomin, 2000). Children's own perceptions of parental preferential treatment are key here, as shown in research by Meunier and colleagues (2012). Their findings confirm that the less favorable the parenting treatment received, the more externalizing behavior the children displayed.

Such differential patterns of treatment of siblings by parents are more evident when families are facing stress, for example, in families with disabled or sick children, those in which parents have recently separated, or stepfamilies (Bank, Patterson, & Reid, 1996). Differential parent–child relationships are associated with difficulties or distress in the parents' own relationship, and in turn with higher levels of sibling conflict both concurrently and longitudinally over time (Brody, Stoneman, & McCoy, 1992, 1994; Hetherington, Henderson, & Reiss, 1999). Differential paternal treatment has been included in some studies and also contributes to adjustment outcome. Volling and Elins (1998) found, for instance, that preschoolers had more symptoms of both an internalizing and externalizing nature when both parents disciplined them more than they disciplined their siblings. The evidence again is correlational, and the direction of causal influence is not clear. Children's interpretation of their parents' differential behavior is important here. If children interpret such behavior as evidence that their parents are less concerned about them than with their sibling, or that they are less worthy of love than their siblings, the sibling relationship is likely to be less positive (Kowal & Kramer, 1997). Note however, that children may perceive preferential treatment of one sibling as fair, and in these cases, lower levels of internalizing behavior problems and greater self-esteem have been reported than in families in which the children do not perceive such differential treatment as fair (Kowal, Kramer, Krull, & Crick, 2002).

These processes of monitoring and reflecting on the relations between other family members begin very early in development, before children's second birthday. This is seen in a study by Dunn, Brown, Slomkowski, Tesla, and Youngblade (1991), who found that the frequency of control and conflict between parents and older siblings contributed independent variance to the younger siblings' social understanding. Again, then, it is evident that the potential effects of one family relationship (between parent and sibling *A*) on the socialization of sibling *B* should be taken into account.

A final point on links between parent–child and sibling relationships is that the quality of the relationship that develops between young siblings is linked to the *changes* in the relationship between parent and firstborn that accompany the birth of a sibling. Both intensive, observational research (Dunn & Kendrick, 1982; Stewart, Mobley, Van Tuyl, & Salvador, 1987) and large-scale surveys (Baydar, Greek, & Brooks-Gunn, 1997) report that the birth of a sibling is accompanied by a decline in positive mother–child interactions, and increases in controlling negative interactions and behavioral problems in the child who has been "displaced" by a new sibling. In a recent comprehensive review, Volling (2012) notes that there are new socialization pressures on children when a new baby is born, and these may be reflected in increased conflict between parent and child. The large-scale studies show that these changes in family relationships with the birth of a sibling are accompanied by a decline in material resources for the family, and this decline may itself have sequelae for the children's adjustment and relationships. The general point to be emphasized by these findings is that such *indirect* links between parent–child and sibling relationships (via social or economic adversities or family stress) are implicated as influences on the quality of the siblings' relationships over time, as well as on children's socialization. This brings us to the issue of changes in siblings' relationships as both children grow up.

Developmental Changes in Sibling Relationships

Before considering sibling relationships as influences on children's socialization, it is important to recognize that there may be significant changes in the nature of the relationship as the siblings grow up, changes that affect the ways siblings influence one another. Longitudinal research has shown that as their powers of social understanding and communication develop in the preschool years, younger siblings within sibling dyads take an increasingly active role in the relationship. They begin to initiate more games, cooperate and participate in joint play more effectively (Dunn et al., 1996), and also use their powers of understanding to get their own way more effectively in sibling conflict (Tesla & Dunn, 1992). Both their presence and their increasingly powerful actions may be considered as potential influences on older siblings' socialization. To what degree is there continuity in the quality of sibling relationships from early to middle childhood?

Most of the studies of middle childhood and adolescence are cross-sectional, and these have mapped the normative changes in sibling relationships over these years—showing changes in the balance of power between siblings as the relationship becomes more egalitarian (Buhrmester, 1992; Buhrmester & Furman, 1990; Vandell et al., 1987). It is not clear to what degree this change in power relations reflects an increase in the ability of the younger sibling to influence the older one, and to be autonomous, or a decrease in the caregiving role of the older sibling, or indeed a decrease in dominance that both children attempt to exert on each other. In adolescence, there tends to be a decrease in the warmth and positivity that siblings express about each other (paralleling the changes in child–parent relationships over this period as adolescents become more involved with peers outside the family).

To what degree is there continuity in the marked individual differences in sibling relationships in early childhood as children grow up? The limited amount of longitudinal research that has addressed this question (e.g., Brody, 1998; Howe, Fiorentino, & Gariépy, 2003) suggests there is moderate to strong continuity in the quality of sibling relationships, but more studies are needed in this area. Beyond early childhood, sibling research has been chiefly cross-sectional. However, in two particular domains provide evidence from which to assess siblings' influence on each other from the early childhood years through adolescence. These are children's adjustment and their social understanding, which I consider next.

Sibling Relationships as Influences on Socialization

Influences on Children's Adjustment

Associations between the quality of sibling relationships and children's adjustment have been repeatedly demonstrated, with documentation of both concurrent links and associations over time. In seminal studies in the 1980s, through detailed observation of children and their families, Patterson and his colleagues in Oregon showed that siblings reinforce each other's aggressive behavior by fighting back, escalating conflict (e.g., Patterson, 1986). The evidence for direct socialization by siblings was clear. These patterns of coercive behavior were found both in community and clinical samples of children with conduct disorders. Snyder and Patterson (1995) made the important point that growing up in families in which children were thus "trained" to be coercive and aggressive had the doubly handicapping effect of not only reinforcing aggressive behavior but also failing to provide training in prosocial behavior.

In a longitudinal study following children from middle childhood to adolescence, Stocker, Burwell, and Briggs (2002) found that conflict between 7- and 10-year-olds accounted for unique variance in the children's anxiety, depression, and delinquent behavior 2 years later, beyond the variance explained by mothers' hostility, fathers' hostility, and marital conflict at the earlier time point. Such patterns begin early in siblings' lives: An observational study indicated that conflict between 5-year-old and preschool-age siblings was associated with internalizing problems both concurrently and 7 years later (Dunn, Slomkowski, Beardsall, & Rende, 1994), beyond the variance accounted for by mothers' current mental health. Such longitudinal patterns may extend beyond adolescence: Interactions with siblings during adolescence have been reported to predict the quality of couples' interactions in young adulthood (R. D. Conger, Cui, Bryant, & Elder, 2000).

Socialization Processes Implicated: Direct and Indirect

What mechanisms and socialization processes are implicated in these associations between sibling relationships and later adjustment outcome? Several possible explanations can be given. First, learning theorists would argue that children learn hostile behavior in conflict with their siblings that then generalizes to other relationship contexts. According to this model, sibling aggressive behavior has a direct shaping effect on a child's own conduct. The research of Patterson and colleagues supports such a view. Second, it may be plausibly argued that growing up with a sibling who continually behaves in a negative way toward one, and makes disparaging, diminishing comments, lowers children's self-esteem, increases their feelings of depression and anxiety, and also increases the likelihood that they will develop a negative attributional style—which, in itself, is a risk factor for later depression and anxiety. Third, as we saw earlier, Snyder and Patterson (1995) argued plausibly that children growing up with an aggressive, hostile sibling may be deprived of the social contexts in which their prosocial empathetic skills are developed. That is, they may have difficulties in developing powers of social understanding and of emotion regulation—limitations that in themselves may contribute both to internalizing and to externalizing problems—and may further contribute to the hostility in the sibling relationship.

It is also possible that a fourth, "common causal factor" underlies both the sibling conflict and the child's adjustment problems. An obvious candidate here is the relationship between parent and child, which as I indicated earlier, is implicated in patterns of family relationships and adjustment. Similarly, marital conflict or distress can lead to both adjustment problems in children and problems in the sibling relationship. To disentangle these pathways of influence, Stocker and her colleagues (2002) indicated that sibling conflict is associated with increases in children's adjustment problems over time even when they controlled for earlier parent–child hostility and marital conflict. Moreover, sibling adjustment at time 1 did not predict significant increases in sibling conflict at time 2; in contrast, sibling conflict at the first time point predicted increases in internalizing and externalizing problems at time 2. This study focused on the older sibling in each dyad. However, a substantial body of research indicates that *younger* siblings are influenced by their older siblings in the domain of adjustment (in some cases more than vice versa; see, e.g., Hetherington et al., 1999). In the key study noted earlier, the results of Ensor and colleagues (2010) indicated that the average trajectory of antisocial behavior toward the older sibling was stable or escalating, and was associated with bullying behavior toward unfamiliar peers, and other more subtle antisocial actions, such as social exclusion.

One process of sibling influence that has received serious attention—and some empirical support—is the notion of sibling deidentification (Whiteman, McHale, & Crouter, 2007). This was originally described by Adler (see Ansbacher & Ansbacher, 1956) as a psychological process by which siblings diverge in their development, finding different domains of interest in which to create separate and independent identities (see Schachter, Shore, Feldman-Rotman, Marquis, & Campbell, 1976). According to these theorists, deidentification will be most pronounced for siblings who are the same sex or more similar in age. Support for the idea of deidentification in the adjustment domain was reported by Feinberg and Hetherington (2001) in a study of adolescents: Siblings who were farther apart in age were more similar in adjustment than those who were close in age. Some evidence indicates that processes of deidentification become more pronounced as individuals reach adolescence (McHale et al., 2001).

While there is then evidence for sibling socialization effects that are independent of parent–child associations, it is also possible (indeed likely) that there are also interactive effects involving both parent–child and sibling relationships in the development of adjustment problems. Thus, Garcia, Shaw, Winslow, and Yaggi (2000) demonstrated, with a low-income sample of 5-year-old boys, that the interaction between sibling conflict and rejecting parent–child relationships predicted aggressive behavior problems over time. An increase in aggression was found for children who had both high scores on sibling conflict and experienced rejection in parent–child relationships.

In addition to these lines of evidence for direct socializing influence of siblings on one another's adjustment, several sources of evidence also suggest that siblings affect each other's adjustment through less direct processes. A particularly powerful process is the impact of *differential* parent–child relationships within the family, as outlined earlier. Several studies indicate that the sibling who is perceived or observed to be the least favored shows more adjustment problems than the favored sibling (K. Conger & Conger, 1994; Reiss et al., 2000). Differential paternal treatment has been included in some studies and also contributes to adjustment outcome (e.g., Brody, Stoneman, & McCoy, 1992; Stocker, 1995; Volling & Elins, 1998). Volling and Elins (1998) found, for instance, as noted earlier, that preschoolers showed more internalizing and externalizing symptoms when both mothers and fathers disciplined them more than they disciplined their siblings. Differential parental treatment has also been studied in a cross-ethnic framework. One study compared European American and Asian American families with late adolescents, and while in general the findings showed that perceptions of differential treatment predicted up to 13% of the variance in achievement and self-perceptions—a significant amount of variance beyond that predicted by absolute levels of affection and control (Barrett Singer & Weinstein, 2000), it is now clear that different cultural and ethnic groups can have very different attitudes toward differential treatment. The research of Mosier and Rogoff (2003) into Guatemalan and U.S. middle-class families with toddlers and preschoolers indicated that the Mayan toddlers were accorded a privileged position by both their mothers and their older siblings—and were allowed access to objects that their older siblings also wanted. In contrast, the U.S. toddlers were expected to follow the same rules for sharing as their older siblings. This pattern, the authors argue, fits the Guatemalan cultural model that prioritizes both responsibility and respect for others' freedom of choice.

A further source of evidence for indirect effects concerns the research on the family disruption caused by the birth of a second child, noted earlier. Home observations (Dunn & Kendrick, 1982; Stewart et al., 1987) and large-scale surveys (Baydar, Greek, et al., 1997; Baydar, Hyle, & Brooks-Gunn, 1997) have documented the disturbance in bodily functions, withdrawal, aggression, and anxiety that follows the birth of a sibling, correlated with changes in the older siblings' changed relationship with the parent. A variety of processes may be implicated here (see Dunn, 1988b); these differ in nature, ranging from general emotional disturbance as a mediating link to a series of processes of increasing specificity and cognitive complexity, such as children's monitoring of differential maternal behavior toward self and sibling, to processes involving maternal "attributional style" and communication about others. Even with children who are only preschoolers, it seems, maternal discourse about sibling differences can be linked to differences in children's outcome. It has been argued that individual differences in children and the developmental stage of the child influence which of these processes is developmentally significant (Dunn, 1988b).

Another indirect process of influence involves peer groups. Younger siblings are vulnerable to the influences of not only their older siblings but also their older siblings' friends (possibly deviant) (Rowe, Linver, & Rodgers, 1996; Slomkowski, Rende, Conger, Simons, & Conger, 2001).

Sources of Support

While much of the sibling research on adjustment has focused on the impact of hostility and negative interactions between siblings, there is also evidence that siblings can be an important source of support for children who are faced with stressful experiences. Early studies indicate that children growing up in disharmonious homes have fewer adjustment problems if they have a good sibling relationship (Jenkins, 1992; Jenkins & Smith, 1990). It seems that both offering comfort to a sibling and receiving support from a sibling are linked to benefits for children. Note that other studies of family transitions report that siblings relatively infrequently are sources of support through provision of a confiding relationship (Dunn & Deater-Deckard, 2001). However children faced with other negative life events, such as paternal unemployment or grandparental death, do report becoming more close and intimate following stressful life events (Dunn, Slomkowski, Beardsall, & Rende, 1994). Whether siblings function in this way to support each other depends crucially on the nature of their relationship—the extent to which they are affectionate and interested in each other. This issue of individual differences is crucial to the second domain of socialization influence considered here, the influence of siblings on the development of social understanding.

The Development of Social Understanding

Sibling research has importantly changed our understanding of the development of children's "discovery of the mind" (Astington, 1993). The growth of children's understanding of other people's emotions, thoughts, and beliefs, and their understanding of the links between such inner states and people's actions, is a topic that has dominated cognitive developmental psychology over the last two decades. It is a domain of development that is clearly implicated in children's socialization. In standard experimental settings designed to assess this ability to "mind-read," young preschool children show limited understanding of the connections between what someone thinks and his or her actions; not until children are 4 years of age can they reliably succeed in these standard assessments (Wellman, Cross, & Watson, 2001). However, in the context of interactions with their siblings—interactions of intense emotions and familiarity—much younger children show powers of anticipating the other's intentions and manipulating the other's emotions. Their ability to deceive, to tease, to manage conflict by anticipating the other's perspective, to share an imaginative world in joint pretend, and to engage in conversations about why people behave the way they do, referring to mental states and feelings as causes and consequences of action, all reflect a growing understanding of connections between inner states and behavior, and all are seen in the interactions between siblings from ages 2 to 4 years. Such observations of siblings have provided a new perspective on a central feature of social cognitive development (Dunn, 2002). The message of the sibling research is not only that these developments begin considerably earlier than suspected, but that the emotional context and familiarity of the sibling relationship also can play an important part in the growth of understanding.

Sibling research has been important in highlighting the development of *individual differences* in children's understanding of others, and sibling experiences are importantly linked to the development of such individual differences. Children who have engaged in frequent talk about mental states with family members or friends are particularly successful on assessments of understanding feelings and mental states (Dunn, 1999). Such conversations are particularly likely to take place in the context of joint pretend play with a sibling or a close friend, when both children have to plan narratives together about how the protagonists in the pretend play behave, and why. Children who have frequently engaged in shared pretend with an older sibling are likely to perform particularly successfully on the standard assessments of understanding of mind (Howe, Petrakos, & Rinaldi, 1998). Some studies indicate that children with older siblings in general perform better on such assessments than those without older siblings (Perner, Ruffman, & Leekam, 1994); other research indicates that family interaction with familiar kin, rather than siblings per se, is linked to this growth of understanding (Lewis, Freeman, Kyriakidou, Maridaki-Kassotaki, & Berridge, 1996). However, the connection with shared pretend play is well established, and this is particularly likely to occur between siblings *who like each other* and have a friendly relationship.

This research is chiefly correlational, so, again, one has to be cautious about inferring causal contributions from sibling interaction to growing understanding. Children who are precocious at understanding feelings and at mind reading are likely to be rewarding play companions; their abilities may contribute to the growth of shared imaginative experiences with sibling or friend, and these abilities in themselves may contribute to further growth in understanding other people's inner states (Howe et al., 1998). However, although the issue of direction of effects remains a difficult one, what researchers have learned from studying siblings is that certain social processes within the family are potentially of great significance in the development of such a central feature of human cognitive ability.

Siblings and Peers

How do the relationships that children develop with their siblings within the family relate to the kinds of relationship that they form with peers outside the family? If they are linked, then this has to be taken seriously as a "socialization" process, albeit an indirect one, since there is now a wealth of evidence that children's experiences with peers have an important role in their social development.

One might well expect that there are systematic links between the quality of sibling and peer relationships, either on the grounds of attachment theory, in terms of social learning theory (which would predict that what is learned within the sibling relationship will generalize to interactions with familiar peers), or because of evidence that individual characteristics elicit similar responses from different others. The processes underlying such links differ in these different theoretical frameworks, but each would predict positive connections between sibling and peer relationships.

There are however counterarguments that focus on the clear differences between sibling and peer relationships, and suggest that simple positive links should not be expected between them. Friendships involve commitment, trust, and support, and many siblings do not feel this way about each other. Friendships do not involve sharing parental love and attention, or resentment about preferential treatment by parents. Children select their friends, but they do not choose their siblings.

Given these differences, it is perhaps not surprising that evidence for positive associations between sibling and peer relationships is not consistent. Some research on young children indicates that the ways in which children behave during disputes is related to their behavior in conflict with peers (Slomkowski & Dunn, 1992), and correlations between aggression with peers and with siblings have been described (Vandell et al., 1987). Other studies of young children report only weak or nonsignificant links across the relationships (Abramovitch et al., 1986; McElwain & Volling, 2005). As for the positive dimensions of the relationships, some studies have pointed toward patterns of consistency. This has been observed in children's positive communication styles with siblings and peers (Slomkowski & Dunn, 1992), and in links between sibling relationship quality and popularity, positive peer behaviors, and friendship quality (Lockwood, Kitzmann, & Cohen, 2001; Modry-Mandell, Gamble, & Taylor, 2007; van Aken & Asendorpf, 1997). Findings have been inconsistent overall, though. Links between the sibling and peer relationships in controlling and positive behavior were reported by Stocker and Mantz-Simmons (1993), but they also noted that children who were especially cooperative with their siblings described lower levels of companionship with their friends. Other evidence that supports this suggestion of "compensatory" patterns across the two relationships has been reported (Mendelson, Aboud, & Lanthier, 1994; Stocker & Dunn, 1990). For instance, in a study of young adolescents, the individuals who were isolated from their peers described their sibling relationships as more supportive (East & Rook, 1992). And sometimes, even within the same study, evidence for both positive associations and negative links is found (e.g., Updegraff & Obeidallah, 1999; Volling, Youngblade, & Belsky, 1997).

Given the mixed findings for associations across these two important relationships, the conclusion of Parke and Buriel (1998), reviewing the field, remains appropriate: 'the challenge for future work is to discover the contexts under which strong, weak, or compensatory connections might be expected between (sibling and peer) relationship systems' (p. 485). As echoed by Howe and colleagues (2011), it is not yet clear when sibling relationships should be expected to have convergent versus divergent associations with the qualities of peer and friend relationships.

Siblings and Family Influence

The study of siblings has raised an important general issue for developmental psychologists concerning the ways in which family experiences affect individual development and influence socialization. Siblings who grow up in the same family nevertheless differ notably from one another in personality and adjustment (K. Conger & Conger, 1994; Dunn & Plomin, 1990; Reiss et al., 2000). These differences present a major challenge to those who study family influences on socialization. The various features of family life that have been investigated as important influences on children's and adolescents' development—such as parental education and occupation, marital relationship and parents' mental health, social adversities faced by the family, neighborhood effects—all are apparently shared by siblings within the same family. Why then do the siblings grow up to be so different from one another?

A range of answers to this question has been explored, including the notion that experiences within the family differ very much for siblings, and that these "within-family" or "nonshared" experiences are key to the development of individual differences. To clarify this issue, we need to study the experiences that are specific to each sibling rather than compare children growing up in different families—the "between-family" differences that have been the chief focus of research. The key message from this research is not that family influences are unimportant; rather, it is that families are experienced very differently by the siblings who are members of them (Hetherington et al., 1994).

This perspective on family processes is being systematically studied, with a focus on differential parent–child relationships, as described earlier, differential experiences within the sibling relationship itself (Dunn & Plomin, 1990), and analytic approaches such as multilevel modeling, which enable the researcher to separate out the variance in outcome that is attributable to *shared* family influence (affecting all the siblings within the family), and *nonshared* family influence, which affects specific children within the family and not others. Examples of such research include studies of the development of adjustment problems in siblings (O'Connor, Dunn, Jenkins, Pickering, & Rasbash, 2001), studies of the impact of marital conflict on siblings (Jenkins et al., 2005) and studies of parenting (O'Connor, Dunn, Jenkins, & Rasbash, 2006). It is clear that individual differences in sibling temperament, adjustment, and intelligence play a key part in eliciting different responses from other family members and from those outside the family, and in siblings' response to shared stresses, such as conflict between their parents. But to understand fully how families affect individual development, it is also clear that we need to include more than one child in each family.

Siblings in Cross-Cultural Perspective

We also need to broaden the range of communities studied. Research on siblings in minority communities is still relatively sparse, as are cross-cultural and non-Western studies. These lacunae are surprising given that from ethnographic studies we know that siblings play a key role as caregivers for very young children in many cultures (Weisner, 1989; Zukow, 1989; Zukow-Goldring, 2002). Weisner (1989) considers how experiences with siblings in many non-Western communities play an important role "in socialization for parenthood." Siblings can, anthropological research tells us, be central in adults' lives in many such communities (see, e.g., Nuckolls, 1993). Many of the issues discussed in this chapter would be illuminated by systematic cross-cultural comparisons, as demonstrated in the earlier example of the privileged treatment of toddlers in a Mayan community. In this study, Mosier and Rogoff (2003) argued convincingly that the pattern they observed in Guatemala, in which older siblings showed voluntary responsibility and the toddlers were privileged, "reflects early socialization in this model of individual freedom of choice in support of responsibility to the group" (p. 1056).

A second example is the evidence of the significance of siblings' teaching skills, highlighted in a study of Mayan children (Maynard, 2002). The Zinocantec older siblings were videotaped in caregiving interactions with their 2-year-old brothers and sisters. In the context of play, older siblings taught their younger siblings how to do everyday tasks, such as washing and cooking. Ethnographic observations and discourse analyses indicated that children's teaching skills increased over the course of middle childhood, and by age 8 years, children were highly skilled in using talk combined with demonstrations to guide their siblings, thus helping their younger siblings to increase their participation in culturally important tasks. This example illustrates a general point made by Zukow-Goldring (2002) in her review of sibling caregiving—that in agrarian societies, sibling caregivers do more than attend to immediate biological needs of their younger siblings: "Siblings are 'culture brokers,' introducing their sisters and brothers to ways of acting and knowing through unique styles of interaction" (p. 278).

We remain largely ignorant about the extent or significance of ethnic differences in sibling relationships, either in childhood or adulthood. A study in the United States compared adult sibling relationships in African American, Hispanic, non-Hispanic white, and Asian American adults, and concluded that the similarities across these groups in support and contact far outweighed the differences (Riedmann & White, 1996). Would the same be true for childhood and adolescence?

Summary: Socialization and Siblings

The study of siblings has provided a powerful perspective on both normative and individual differences in development and socialization. Research on the growth of social understanding, on social competence, on the links between emotional and cognitive development, on family influence on adjustment and socialization, and on peer relations has been illuminated by a focus on siblings. Recent research on siblings has given us the opportunity to learn more about not only their relationships and direct socialization influences but also key issues in developmental psychology. The relationships of step- and half-siblings, and individual differences in their development, is a growing area of research. Not only is this an important practical area, with the increasing numbers of families that include step-relationships, but also the comparison of full, half-, and step-siblings gives a useful approach to the study of the role of genetics in the development of individual differences (Deater-Deckard, Dunn, O'Connor, & Golding, 2002). In the clinical literature there has also been interest in siblings, as in the example of studies of children's response to illness, disability or injury, or death of their siblings (Dickens, 2014; Nabors et al., 2013; Stallard, Mastroyannopoulou, Lewis, & Lenton, 1997), of siblings as donors in organ or bone-marrow transplant surgery (Phipps, 2006; Vogel, 2011) and of traumatic experiences of siblings (Degeneffe, Gagne, & Tucker, 2013; Newman, Black, & Harris-Hendriks, 1997).

There are nevertheless some striking gaps in what we know about siblings and socialization. Although there is a welcome increase in studies of siblings in adolescence, there is still little longitudinal research into adulthood, or studies with an intergenerational perspective, despite the evidence for the importance of siblings in adulthood. The issue of how long term the significance of early experiences with siblings may be remains unclear. There is the notable gap in cross-cultural studies of siblings. However, sibling research is clarifying both normative developmental questions and key issues in socialization theory; the gaps in what is known provide opportunities for further research that is likely to be both illuminating in terms of developmental theory and important in terms of practical issues and our understanding of family processes and socialization.

REFERENCES

Abramovitch, R., Corter, C., Pepler, D. J., & Stanhope, L. (1986). Sibling and peer interaction: A final follow-up and a comparison. *Child Development, 57,* 217–229.

Adler, A. (1928). Characteristics of the first, second and third child. *Children, 3,* 14–52.

Ansbacher, H. L., & Ansbacher, R. R. (1956). *The individual psychology of Alfred Adler.* New York: Basic Books.

Astington, J. W. (1993). *The child's discovery of the mind.* Cambridge, MA: Harvard University Press.

Bank, L., Patterson, G. R., & Reid, J. B. (1996). Negative sibling interaction as predictors of later adjustment problems in adolescent and young adult males. In G. H. Brody (Ed.), *Sibling relationships: Their causes and consequences* (pp. 197–229). Norwood, NJ: Ablex.

Barrett Singer, A. T., & Weinstein, R. S. (2000). Differential parental treatment predicts achievement and self-perceptions in two cultural contexts. *Journal of Family Psychology, 14,* 491–509.

Baydar, N., Greek, A., & Brooks-Gunn, J. (1997). A longitudinal study of the effects of the birth of a sibling during the first 6 years of life. *Journal of Marriage and the Family, 59,* 939–956.

Baydar, N., Hyle, P., & Brooks-Gunn, J. (1997). A longitudinal study of the effects of the birth of a sibling during preschool and early grade school years. *Journal of Marriage and the Family, 59,* 957–965.

Boer, F., & Dunn, J. (1990). *Children's sibling relationships: Developmental and clinical issues.* Hillsdale, NJ: Erlbaum.

Brody, G., Stoneman, Z., & McCoy, J. (1992). Associations of maternal and paternal direct and differential behavior with sibling relationships: Contemporaneous and longitudinal analyses. *Child Development, 63,* 82–92.

Brody, G., Stoneman, Z., & McCoy, J. (1994). Forecasting sibling relationships in early adolescence from child temperaments and family processes in middle childhood. *Child Development, 65,* 771–784.

Brody, G. H. (1996). *Sibling relationships: Their causes and consequences.* Norwood, NJ: Ablex.

Brody, G. H. (1998). Sibling relationship quality: Its causes and consequences. *Annual Review of Psychology, 49,* 1–24.

Buhrmester, D. (1992). The developmental course of sibling and peer relationships. In F. Boer & J. Dunn (Eds.), *Children's sibling relationships: Developmental and clinical issues* (pp. 19–40). Hillsdale, NJ: Erlbaum.

Buhrmester, D., & Furman, W. (1990). Perceptions of sibling relationships during middle childhood and adolescence. *Child Development, 61,* 1387–1398.

Conger, K., & Conger, R. (1994). Differential parenting and change in sibling differences in delinquency. *Journal of Family Psychology, 8,* 287–302.

Conger, R. D., Cui, M. M., Bryant, C. M., & Elder, G. H., Jr. (2000). Competence in early adult relationships: A developmental perspective on family influences. *Journal of Personality and Social Psychology, 79,* 224–237.

Davidson-Arad, B., & Klein, A. (2011). Comparative well-being of Israeli youngsters in residential care with and without siblings. *Children and Youth Services Review, 33,* 2152–2159.

Deater-Deckard, K., Dunn, J., O'Connor, T. G., & Golding, J. (2002). Sibling relationships and social-emotional adjustment in different family contexts. *Social Development, 11,* 571–590.

Degeneffe, C. E., Gagne, L. M., & Tucker, M. (2013). Family systems changes following traumatic brain injury: Adult sibling perspectives. *Journal of Applied Rehabilitation Counseling, 44,* 32–41.

Dickens, N. (2014). Prevalence of complicated grief and posttraumatic stress disorder in children and adolescents following sibling death. *Family Journal, 22,* 119–126.

Dunn, J. (1988a). *The beginnings of social understanding.* Cambridge, MA: Harvard University Press.

Dunn, J. (1988b). Connections between relationships: Implications of research on mothers and siblings. In R. A. Hinde & J. Stevenson-Hinde (Eds.), *Relations between relationships* (pp. 168–180). Oxford, UK: Oxford University Press.

Dunn, J. (1999). Mindreading and social relationships. In M. Bennett (Ed.), *Developmental psychology: Achievements and prospects* (pp. 55–71). Philadelphia: Psychology Press.

Dunn, J. (2002). Mindreading, emotion understanding, and relationships. In R. Silbereisen & W. W. Hartup (Eds.), *Growing points in developmental science: An introduction* (pp. 55–71). Oxford, UK: Psychology Press.

Dunn, J., Brown, J., Slomkowski, C., Tesla, C., & Youngblade, L. (1991). Young children's understanding of other people's feelings and beliefs: Individual differences and their antecedents. *Child Development, 62,* 1352–1366.

Dunn, J., Creps, C., & Brown, J. (1996). Children's family relationships between two and five: Developmental changes and individual differences. *Social Development, 5,* 230–250.

Dunn, J., & Deater-Deckard, K. (2001). *Children's views of their changing families.* York, UK: York Publishing Services/Joseph Rowntree Foundation.

Dunn, J., Deater-Deckard, K., Pickering, K., Beveridge, M., & the ALSPAC Study Team. (1999). Siblings, parents and partners: Family relationships within a longitudinal community study. *Journal of Child Psychology and Psychiatry, 40,* 1025–1037.

Dunn, J., & Kendrick, C. (1982). *Siblings: Love, envy and understanding.* London: Grant McIntyre.

Dunn, J., & Plomin, R. (1990). *Separate lives: Why siblings are so different.* New York: Basic Books.

Dunn, J., Slomkowski, C., & Beardsall, L. (1994). Sibling relationships from the preschool period through middle school and adolescence. *Developmental Psychology, 30,* 315–324.

Dunn, J., Slomkowski, C., Beardsall, L., & Rende, R. (1994). Adjustment in middle childhood and early adolescence: Links with earlier and contemporary sibling relationships. *Journal of Child Psychology and Psychiatry, 35,* 491–504.

East, P. L., & Rook, K. S. (1992). Compensatory patterns of support among children's peer relationships: A test using school friends, nonschool friends, and siblings. *Developmental Psychology, 28,* 163–172.

Ensor, R., Marks, A., Jacobs, L., & Hughes, C. (2010). Trajectories of antisocial behavior toward siblings predict antisocial behavior toward peers. *Journal of Child Psychiatry and Psychology, 51*, 1208–1216.

Feinberg, M., & Hetherington, E. M. (2001). Differential parenting as a within-family variable. *Journal of Family Psychology, 15*, 22–37.

Furman, W., & Lanthier, R. P. (1996). Personality and sibling relationships. In G. H. Brody (Ed.), *Sibling relationships: Their causes and consequences* (pp. 127–146). Norwood, NJ: Ablex.

Garcia, M. M., Shaw, D. S., Winslow, E. B., & Yaggi, K. E. (2000). Destructive sibling conflict and the development of conduct problems in young boys. *Developmental Psychology, 36*, 44–53.

Hartup, W. W. (1996). The company they keep: Friendships and their developmental significance. *Child Development, 67*, 1–13.

Hetherington, E. M., & Clingempeel, W. G. (1992). Coping with marital transitions: A family systems approach. *Monographs of the Society for Research in Child Development, 57*, 2–3.

Hetherington, E. M., Henderson, S., & Reiss, D. (1999). Adolescent siblings in stepfamilies: Family functioning and adolescent adjustment. *Monographs of the Society for Research in Child Development, 64*, 1–222.

Hetherington, E. M., Reiss, D., & Plomin, R. (1994). *Separate social worlds of siblings: The impact of nonshared environment on development*. Hillsdale, NJ: Erlbaum.

Hinde, R. A. (1979). *Toward understanding relationships*. London: Academic Press.

Howe, N., Fiorentino, L. M., & Gariépy, N. (2003). Sibling conflict in middle childhood: Influence of maternal context and mother–sibling interaction over four years. *Merrill–Palmer Quarterly, 49*, 183–208.

Howe, N., Petrakos, H., & Rinaldi, C. (1998). "All the sheeps are dead. He murdered them": Sibling pretense, negotiation, internal state language and relationship quality. *Child Development, 69*, 182–191.

Howe, N., Ross, H. S., & Recchia, H. (2011). Sibling relations in early and middle childhood. In P. K. Smith & C. H. Hart (Eds.), The *Wiley-Blackwell handbook of childhood social development* (2nd ed., pp. 356–372). New York: Wiley-Blackwell.

Jenkins, J., & Smith, M. (1990). Factors protecting children living in disharmonious homes: Maternal reports. *Journal of the American Academy of Child and Adolescent Psychiatry, 29*, 60–69.

Jenkins, J. M. (1992). Sibling relationships in disharmonious homes: Potential difficulties and protective effects. In F. Boer & J. Dunn (Eds.), *Children's sibling relationships: Developmental and clinical issues* (pp. 125–138). Hillsdale, NJ: Erlbaum.

Jenkins, J. M., Cheung, C., Frampton, K., Rasbash, J., Boyle, M. H., & Georgiades, K. (2009). The use of multilevel modeling for the investigation of family process. *European Journal of Developmental Science, 3*, 131–149.

Jenkins, J. M., Dunn, J., Rasbash, J., O'Connor, T. G., & Simpson, A. (2005). The mutual influence of marital conflict and children's behavior problems: Shared and non-shared family risks. *Child Development, 76*, 24–39.

Jenkins, J. M., Rasbash, J., Leckie, G., Gass, K., & Dunn, J. (2012). The role of maternal factors in sibling relationship quality: A multilevel study of multiple dyads per family. *Journal of Child Psychology and Psychiatry, 53*, 622–629.

Koch, H. (1960). *The relation of certain formal attributes of siblings to attitudes held toward each other and toward their parents* (Vol. 25). Chicago: University of Chicago Press.

Koch, H. L. (1954). The relation of "primary mental abilities" in five- and six-year-olds to sex of child and characteristics of his sibling. *Child Development, 15*, 209–223.

Kowal, A., & Kramer, L. (1997). Children's understanding of parental differential treatment. *Child Development, 68*, 113–126.

Kowal, A., Kramer, L., Krull, J. L., & Crick, N. R. (2002). Children's perceptions of the fairness of parental preferential treatment and their socioemotional well-being. *Journal of Family Psychology, 16*, 297–306.

Lewis, C., Freeman, N. H., Kyriakidou, C., Maridaki-Kassotaki, K., & Berridge, D. M. (1996). Social influences on false belief access: Specific sibling influences or general apprenticeship? *Child Development, 67,* 2930–2947.

Lockwood, R. L., Kitzmann, K. M., & Cohen, R. (2001). The impact of sibling warmth and conflict on children's social competence with peers. *Child Study Journal, 31,* 47–69.

Maynard, A. E. (2002). Cultural teaching: The development of teaching skills in Maya sibling interactions. *Child Development, 73,* 969–982.

McElwain, N. L., & Volling, B. L. (2005). Preschool children's interactions with friends and older siblings: Relationship specificity and joint contributions to problem behavior. *Journal of Family Psychology, 19,* 486–496.

McGuire, S., Manke, B., Eftekhari, A., & Dunn, J. (2000). Children's perceptions of sibling conflict during middle childhood: Issues and sibling (dis)similarity. *Social Development, 9,* 173–190.

McHale, S. M., & Crouter, A. C. (1996). The family context of children's sibling relationships. In G. H. Brody (Ed.), *Sibling relationships: Their causes and consequences* (pp. 173–195). Norwood, NJ: Ablex.

McHale, S. M., Updegraff, K. A., Helms-Erikson, H., & Crouter, A. C. (2001). Sibling influences on gender development in middle childhood and early adolescence: A longitudinal study. *Developmental Psychology, 37,* 115–125.

Mendelson, M., Aboud, F., & Lanthier, R. (1994). Kindergartners' relationships with siblings, peers and friends. *Merrill–Palmer Quarterly, 40,* 416–427.

Meunier, J. C., Roskam, I., Stievenart, M., Van De Moortele, G. V., Browne, D. T., & Wade, M. (2012). Parental differential treatment, child's externalizing behavior and sibling relationships: Bridging links with child's perception of favoritism and personality, and parents' self-efficacy. *Journal of Social and Personal Relationships, 29,* 612–638.

Modry-Mandell, K. L., Gamble, W. C., & Taylor, A. R. (2007). Family emotional climate and sibling relationship quality: Influences on behavioral problems and adaptation in preschool-aged children. *Journal of Child and Family Studies, 16,* 61–73.

Mosier, C. E., & Rogoff, B. (2003). Privileged treatment of toddlers: Cultural aspects of individual choice and responsibility. *Developmental Psychology, 39,* 1047–1060.

Nabors, L., Bartz, J., Kichler, J., Sievers, R., Elkins, R., Pangallo, J., et al. (2013). Play as a mechanism of working through medical trauma for children with medical illnesses and their siblings. *Issues in Comprehensive Pediatric Nursing, 36,* 212–224.

Naylor, P. B., Petch, L., & Ali, P. A. (2011). Domestic violence: Bullying in the home. In C. P. Monks & L. Coye (Eds.). *Bullying in different contexts* (pp. 87–112). New York: Cambridge University Press.

Newman, M., Black, D., & Harris-Hendriks, J. (1997). Victims of disaster, war, violence or homicide: Psychological effects on siblings. *Child Psychology and Psychiatry Review, 2,* 140–149.

Nuckolls, C. (1993). *Siblings in South Asia.* New York: Guilford Press.

O'Connor, T., Dunn, J., Jenkins, J., Pickering, K., & Rasbash, J. (2001). Family settings and children's adjustment: Differential adjustment within and across families. *British Journal of Psychiatry, 179,* 110–115.

O'Connor, T. G., Dunn, J., Jenkins, J., & Rasbash, J. (2006). Predictors of between-family and within-family variation in parent–child relationships. *Journal of Child Psychology and Psychiatry, 47,* 498–510.

Parke, R. D., & Buriel, R. (1998). Socialization in the family: Ethnic and ecological perspectives. In W. Damon (Ed.), *Handbook of child psychology: Vol. 3. Social, emotional and personality development* (pp. 463–552). New York: Wiley.

Patterson, G. R. (1986). The contribution of siblings to training for fighting: A microsocial analysis. In D. Olweus, J. Block, & M. Radke-Yarrow (Eds.), *Development of antisocial and prosocial behavior* (pp. 235–261). New York: Academic Press.

Perlman, M., Ross, H. S., & Garfinkel, D. A. (2009). Consistent patterns of interaction in young children's conflicts with their siblings. *International Journal of Behavioral Development, 33,* 504–515.

Perner, J., Ruffman, T., & Leekam, S. R. (1994). Theory of mind is contagious: You catch it from your sibs. *Child Development, 65,* 1228–1238.

Phipps, S. (2006). Psychosocial and behavioral issues in stem cell transplantation. In R. T. Brown (Ed.), *Comprehensive handbook of childhood cancer and sickle cell disease: A biopsychosocial approach* (pp. 75–99). New York: Oxford University Press.

Pike, A. (2012). Commentary: Are siblings birds of a feather?: Reflections on Jenkins et al. (2012). *Journal of Child Psychology and Psychiatry, 53,* 630–631.

Pike, A., Coldwell, J., & Dunn, J. (2005). Sibling relationships in early/middle childhood: Children's perspectives and links with individual adjustment. *Journal of Family Psychology, 19,* 523–532.

Ram, A., & Ross, H. (2008). "We got to figure it out": Information-sharing and siblings' negotiations of conflicts of interests. *Social Development, 17,* 512–527.

Reiss, D., Neiderhiser, J. M., Hetherington, E. M., & Plomin, R. (2000). *The relationship code: Deciphering genetic and social patterns in adolescent development.* Cambridge, MA: Harvard University Press.

Riedmann, A., & White, L. (1996). Adult sibling relationships: Racial and ethnic comparisons. In G. H. Brody (Ed.), *Sibling relationships: Their causes and consequences* (pp. 105–126). Norwood, NJ: Ablex.

Ross, H., Ross, M., Stein, N., & Trabasso, T. (2006). How siblings resolve their conflicts: The importance of first offers, planning, and limited opposition. *Child Development, 77,* 1730–1745.

Rowe, D. C., Linver, M., & Rodgers, J. L. (1996). Delinquency and IQ: Using siblings to find source of variation. In G. H. Brody (Ed.), *Sibling relationships: Their causes and consequences* (pp. 147–171). Norwood, NJ: Ablex.

Schachter, F. F., Shore, E., Feldman-Rotman, S., Marquis, R. E., & Campbell, S. (1976). Sibling deidentification. *Developmental Psychology, 12,* 418–427.

Slomkowski, C., Rende, R., Conger, K., Simons, R., & Conger, R. (2001). Sisters, brothers, and delinquency: Evaluating social influence during early and middle adolescence. *Child Development, 72,* 271–283.

Slomkowski, C. L., & Dunn, J. (1992). Arguments and relationships within the family: Differences in young children's disputes with mother and sibling. *Developmental Psychology, 28,* 919–924.

Snyder, J., & Patterson, G. (1995). Individual differences in social aggression: A test of a reinforcement model of socialization in the natural environment. *Behavior Therapy, 26,* 371–391.

Stallard, P., Mastroyannopoulou, K., Lewis, M., & Lenton, S. (1997). The siblings of children with life-threatening conditions. *Child Psychology and Psychiatry Review, 2,* 26–33.

Stewart, R. B., Mobley, L., Van Tuyl, S., & Salvador, M. (1987). The firstborn's adjustment to the birth of a sibling. *Child Development, 58,* 341–355.

Stocker, C., Ahmed, K., & Stall, M. (1997). Marital satisfaction and maternal emotional expressiveness: Links with children's sibling relationships. *Social Development, 6,* 373–385.

Stocker, C., & Dunn, J. (1990). Sibling relationships in childhood: Links with friendships and peer relationships. *British Journal of Developmental Psychology, 8,* 227–244.

Stocker, C., Dunn, J., & Plomin, R. (1989). Sibling relationships: Links with child temperament, maternal behavior, and family structure. *Child Development, 60,* 715–727.

Stocker, C., & Mantz-Simmons, L. (1993). *Children's friendships and peer status: Links with family relationships, temperament and social skills.* Denver, CO: University of Denver.

Stocker, C. M. (1995). Differences in mothers' and fathers' relationships with siblings: Links with behavioral problems. *Development and Psychopathology, 7,* 499–513.

Stocker, C. M., Burwell, R. A., & Briggs, M. L. (2002). Sibling conflict in middle childhood predicts children's adjustment in early adolescence. *Journal of Family Psychology, 16,* 50–57.

Tesla, C., & Dunn, J. (1992). Getting along or getting your own way: The development of young children's use of argument in conflicts with mother and sibling. *Social Development, 1,* 107–121.

Teti, D. M., & Ablard, K. E. (1989). Security of attachment and infant-sibling relationships: A laboratory study. *Child Development, 60,* 1519–1528.

Tucker, C. J., Updegraff, K. A., McHale, S. M., & Crouter, A. C. (1999). Older siblings as socializers of younger siblings' empathy. *Journal of Early Adolescence, 19,* 176–198.

Updegraff, K. A., McHale, S. M., & Crouter, A. C. (2002). Adolescents' sibling relationship and friendship experiences: Developmental patterns and relationship linkages. *Social Development, 11,* 182–204.

Updegraff, K. A., & Obeidallah, D. A. (1999). Young adolescents' patterns of involvement with siblings and friends. *Social Development, 8,* 53–69.

van Aken, M. A., & Asendorpf, J. B. (1997). Support by parents, classmates, friends and siblings in preadolescence: Covariation and compensation across relationships. *Journal of Social and Personal Relationships, 14,* 79–93.

Vandell, D. L., Minnett, A. M., & Santrock, J. W. (1987). Age differences in sibling relationships during middle childhood. *Journal of Applied Developmental Psychology, 8,* 247–257.

Vogel, R. (2011). The management of the sibling hematopoietic stem cell donor. *Journal of Pediatric Oncology Nursing, 28,* 336–343.

Volling, B. L. (2012). Family transitions following the birth of a sibling: An empirical review of changes in the firstborn's adjustment. *Psychological Bulletin, 138,* 497–528.

Volling, B. L., & Belsky, J. (1992). The contribution of mother–child and father–child relationships to the quality of sibling interaction: A longitudinal study. *Child Development, 63,* 1209–1222.

Volling, B. L., & Elins, J. L. (1998). Family relationships and children's emotional adjustment as correlates of maternal and paternal differential treatment: A replication with toddler and preschool siblings. *Child Development, 69,* 1640–1656.

Volling, B. L., Youngblade, L. M., & Belsky, J. (1997). Young children's social relationships: An examination of the linkages between siblings, friends, and peers. *American Journal of Orthopsychiatry, 67,* 102–111.

Weisner, T. S. (1989). Comparing sibling relationships across cultures. In P. Zukow (Ed.), *Sibling interaction across cultures: Theoretical and methodological issues* (pp. 11–25). New York: Springer-Verlag.

Wellman, H. M., Cross, D., & Watson, J. (2001). Meta-analysis of theory of mind development: The truth about false belief. *Child Development, 72,* 655–684.

Whiteman, S. D., McHale, S. M., & Crouter, A. C. (2007). Competing processes of sibling influence: Observational learning and sibling deidentification. *Social Development, 16,* 642–661.

Zukow, P. (1989). *Sibling interaction across cultures.* New York: Springer-Verlag.

Zukow-Goldring, P. (2002). Sibling caregiving. In M. H. Bornstein (Ed.), *Handbook of parenting* (Vol. 3, pp. 253–286). Mahwah, NJ: Erlbaum.

CHAPTER 9

Socialization in the Context
of Family Diversity

Charlotte J. Patterson
Rachel H. Farr
Paul D. Hastings

The diversity of family structures in the Western world is arguably greater today than at any other point in history. Infants are being born into an array of different family types, some of which were not even recognized as existing as recently as 50 years ago. Babies conceived via reproductive technology may be biologically related to one, two, or none of the adults who intend to rear them. Adoption and remarriage add to the diversity of biologically related and unrelated parent–child relationships. Children today are being reared not only by married, mother–father couples but also by unmarried heterosexual couples, and by divorced or never-married single heterosexual men and women. Single lesbian women and single gay men, unmarried lesbian couples and unmarried gay couples, and, in a growing number of jurisdictions, married lesbian couples and married gay couples are also rearing children in an ever-growing number of nonheterosexual parent families. Substantial numbers of children are not being reared by parents at all but live instead with grandparents. What does all this mean for the socialization of infants and children?

This question has not always been of such central interest to scholars of human development. For many years, most researchers assumed that they knew the conditions that were most favorable for child development. Those conditions were generally considered to be provided most reliably by families that included two heterosexual parents, one male and one female, who were married to one another and biologically related to the child or children whom they were rearing. While fathers in such families were expected to be employed full time outside the home, mothers were expected to remain at home, where they were responsible for child care and household upkeep but did not earn money. Even though the existence of such so-called "traditional" families has not characterized much of human history, and even though many, if not most, families today—even in

Western countries—do not fit this pattern, it has nevertheless been widely considered the norm against which other family-rearing environments should be measured (Lamb, 1999b, 2012).

In this chapter, we consider the impact of family diversity on human development, with particular focus on processes of socialization. This topic has most often been studied in research that focused on family structure. For example, traditions of research have grown up around the study of single-parent families, stepfamilies, and dual-career two-parent families (Hetherington & Stanley-Hagan, 1999; Weinraub, Horvath, & Gringlas, 2002). Results of this research have consistently revealed that family resources, processes, and relationships are more important predictors of successful socialization than are assessments of family structure. As our examination of the literature reveals, when family processes and relationships are supportive, and when family resources are sufficient to meet children's needs, successful socialization of young children generally ensues, even when structural characteristics of the family may not conform to cultural norms.

We begin by considering some key aspects of family environments, interactions, and relationships. In light of these considerations, different nontraditional family structures and the evidence about their impact on human development are reviewed. Although many forms of diversity in family structure occur, space does not permit exploration of them all. In this chapter, nontraditional families—including one-parent families, unmarried heterosexual-parent families, families formed using reproductive technology, families with sexual minority parents (i.e., lesbian and gay parents), and grandparent-headed families—are discussed. In the final section, we summarize the overall findings and consider their possible implications.

Family Resources, Interactions, and Relationships

The possible impact of family structure on children's development is an important topic. Should there indeed be differences in children's behavior, characteristics, or abilities across family types, however, it is also important to understand *why* such differences exist. Differences in developmental outcomes that are observed across family types might be attributable to other factors that are confounded with family type. Families that share a given structure may also share similar socioeconomic conditions, for example, or similar ideas about family roles. Indeed, there is abundant evidence that single-parent families, on average, have lower incomes than do two-parent families. Identifying the variables and processes that contribute to similarities and differences in children's development across family structures is important for efforts to promote the well-being and positive development of all children.

Within and across different family types, there are fundamental resources, interactions, and relationships that are likely to be needed to support positive socialization (Lamb, 2012). First, it is clear that families need access to sufficient financial resources and to the satisfactory nutrition, adequate shelter, and health care that such financial resources make possible. Second, the qualities of parent–child interactions and relationships are important issues in any family. Third, the emotional climate and stability of families are important elements of environments they provide for the socialization of infants, children, and adolescents. In addition, the social embeddedness of the family and the availability of social support for parents facilitate appropriate socialization. In the sections that follow, we briefly outline the contributions of each of these resources to socialization.

Access to Resources

For socialization to proceed in positive directions, the basic needs of infants and children must be met. These include sufficient nutrition, adequate shelter, protection from dangers, and access to opportunities for socialization. In most parts of the Western world, basic needs such as food and shelter are generally purchased using a family's economic resources. Inasmuch as family financial resources play a central role in providing for the needs of infants, children, and adolescents, wealth and poverty are central issues for research on socialization. When families are impoverished, the difficulties in socialization of infants and children are multiple (Lamb, 2012). Infants from low-income families are less likely than those from more affluent families to receive adequate nutrition and appropriate health care (Brooks-Gunn & Duncan, 1997a, 1997b). Low birthweights, poor nutrition, and poor childhood health are all more common in impoverished than in affluent families (Alaimo, Olson, Frongillo, & Breifel, 2001). Similarly, low-income families are less likely than others to have adequate housing (Bradley, 2002). They have greater exposure to toxins, such as lead-based paint (Nordin et al., 1998), and to environmental harms, such as exposure to air pollution, experience of community or family violence, and direct victimization via physical abuse or neglect (Bolger & Patterson, 2003; Bradley, 2002).

Research has consistently shown that parents with low incomes and less access to resources show poorer socialization practices and less authoritative parenting styles compared to more financially well-off parents (Magnuson & Duncan, 2002). Across racial groups (Bradley, Corwyn, McAdoo, & Garcia Coll, 2001; Brody, Flor, & Gibson, 1999), parents with fewer economic resources have been found to be less confident in their parenting, less warm and engaged with their children, and more verbally and physically punitive than parents with greater financial resources. This seems to be true for both mothers and fathers (Burbach, Fox, & Nicholson, 2004),

Children from low-income families are less likely than those from more affluent homes to have access to enriching opportunities (Bradley et al., 2001; Conger, Conger, & Martin, 2010). They are less likely to live in homes that contain many books, to have access to music or to works of art, and to visit libraries and museums (Bradley, 2002). They are less likely to have the opportunity to take music or dance lessons, to participate in clubs, or to play on sports teams (Fields, Smith, Bass, & Lugalia, 2001).

Children in socioeconomically disadvantaged families also fare less well than their more advantaged counterparts, showing more adjustment difficulties and problematic behaviors (Conger et al., 2010; Offord, Boyle, & Jones, 1987). The effects of socioeconomic stress on children are likely to be at least partially mediated by effects on parents (Hoff, Laursen, & Tardif, 2002; Ross, Roberts, & Scott, 1998). One study showed that socioeconomic status (SES) is positively correlated with better parenting practices among divorced mothers; in turn, better parenting practices predict children's adaptive and pro-social behavior at school (DeGarmo, Forgatch, & Martinez, 1999). Job loss, income loss, and persistent economic hardship undermine parents' ability to respond in nurturing ways to their children. Indeed, Evans and Kim (2013) identified chronic stress and coping as a pathway through which childhood poverty has ramifications throughout the life course.

Quality of Parenting

The consensus of many years of research on infant and child socialization clearly reveals the importance of quality of parenting. Attachment theory emphasizes the influence of sensitive and responsive parenting on the qualities of parent–infant, parent–child, and parent–adolescent relationships (Cassidy & Shaver, 1999). Baumrind (1967, 1971, 1973) and others have emphasized the importance of a parenting style that combines high parental warmth, communication, and control (Parke & Buriel, 1998). Others have suggested the importance of parental ability to monitor child and adolescent activities (G. R. Patterson & Fisher, 2002). In all these ways and more, children whose parents exhibit more favorable parenting strategies are more likely to develop well (as discussed in several chapters in this volume). Should these aspects of parenting be found to vary across family types, socialization might be expected to confer relative advantages or disadvantages to children living in different family structures.

Family Climate and Stability

Over and above the qualities of parenting by individual parents, the larger family climate is also an important factor in the socialization of infants, children, and adolescents. The role of marital relations—whether harmonious or conflictual—is an important factor here; children exposed to a great deal of conflict between their parents are less likely to show positive developmental outcomes (Cummings & Davies, 1994). In addition, the extent to which families are characterized by mutuality, support, and emotional harmony is an important influence on socialization (McHale et al., 2002).

Another factor that appears to be important to socialization efforts is the stability of children's environments (Adam, 2004). Those who have greater numbers of separations from primary caregivers or greater numbers of residential moves are more likely to have problems in adjustment (Adam & Chase-Lansdale, 2002). Multiple residential moves are often associated with school transfers, and these are important stressors for children and adolescents. Residential moves may often be associated with family disruptions, such as separation or divorce of parents, so they may be markers for other stresses. In all, children and adolescents whose families provide stable, supportive environments seem to be at an advantage over those in more chaotic home situations (Wood, Halfon, Scarlata, Newacheck, & Nessim, 1993).

Social Networks

Positive social relationships outside the family are another element of supportive environments for children. The other family members, adult friends, and community members with whom parents have regular contact may support parental socialization efforts (Cochran & Niego, 2002). Support can be *emotional*, bolstering a parent's confidence and providing an outlet for stress; *informational*, giving useful advice about childrearing; or *instrumental*, offering practical assistance (Crockenberg, 1988). Other adults may also act as additional socialization agents for children, through their involvement in child care, provision of social or material resources to children, or status as models of healthy adult social functioning (Cochran & Brassard, 1979).

Supportive social networks benefit both parents and children. Parents with greater social support are less stressed, more authoritative, and have warmer interactions with their children (Cochran & Niego, 2002). Children of parents who maintain more frequent and satisfying contacts with their social networks themselves have more friends and are more socially competent (Homel, Burns, & Goodnow, 1987; Markiewicz, Doyle, & Brendgen, 2001). Access to supportive adults through parents' social networks has also been found to protect children from the adverse effects of economic hardship (Stanton-Salazar & Spina, 2003; Zimmerman, Bingenheimer, & Notaro, 2002).

Summary

Overall, then, physical resources, high-quality parenting, favorable family climate, reasonable stability, and supportive extrafamilial social networks are important resources for socialization (Lamb, 2012). These resources are not necessarily independent factors. Many vary with family income, so that children growing up in poverty receive less of everything. On the other hand, not all children or adolescents from affluent families are well adjusted, and important resources (e.g., parental attention) may be in short supply for some children from wealthy homes (Luthar & Latendresse, 2005).

To address the question of why children typically fare better in some family structures (e.g., married, two-parent households) as compared to others (e.g., cohabiting couple and single-mother families), Waldfogel, Craigie, and Brooks-Gunn (2010) reviewed research based on data from the Fragile Families and Child Wellbeing Study. They identified five key factors that might affect child adjustment: (1) parental resources, (2) parental mental health, (3) parental relationship quality, (4) parenting quality, and (5) father involvement. Waldfogel and colleagues also noted the importance of family stability, as well as the possible role of selection by individual women and men into different family types. Even so, such factors did not shape all of children's outcomes in the same ways. For instance, family instability was an important determinant of children's cognitive outcomes, whereas family structure (e.g., having a single mother) was a more important influence on child behavior problems. Taken together, these results do, however, parallel other findings that children in stable families with single or cohabiting parents are less at risk than those in unstable families with single or cohabiting parents. What may matter most, then, for parents' socialization of positive development for children is access to sufficient physical, psychological, and social resources to offset whatever ill effects are incurred through deficiencies in some resources or occurrences of other risk factors.

Diverse Family Structures and the Socialization of Children

We now consider research on socialization in various nontraditional families from the standpoint of the family resources and processes outlined previously. We begin by examining never-married one-parent families, then explore research on unmarried two-parent heterosexual parent families, families formed with assisted reproductive technologies, sexual minority–parented families, and custodial grandparent families. In each case, we assess research findings to determine how the family structure in question fares in terms of both the resources and processes outlined earlier, and socialization outcomes. We acknowledge a variety of other "nontraditional" family systems, such as adoptive families, interracial and multicultural families, and blended and reconstituted families following divorce and remarriage. Given length constraints, however, discussion of these families remains outside the scope of this chapter.

Never-Married, Mother-Headed, One-Parent Families

Single-parent families are a sizable and diverse group in the United States today (Weinraub et al., 2002). In addition to those who become single parents after divorce, many single parents have never been married. More than one-third of births in the United States were to unmarried women in 2003—more than 1 million babies (Martin, Kochanek, Strobino, Guyer, & MacDornan, 2005). Some never-married mothers are single professional women who decided to have children in their 30s, but the largest number is unmarried adolescent mothers (Martin et al., 2005). These figures vary widely across countries, though. For example, approximately 25% of live births in Canada in 2003 were to unmarried mothers, and less than 20% of these were to teenage mothers (Statistics Canada, 2005). Internationally, it is likely that differences in sex education, access to methods of contraception and pregnancy termination (e.g., "morning-after" pill; abortion), and attitudes about premarital sex all affect the relative proportions of single women who give birth. Regardless of such percentages, though, the experiences of children born to single adolescent mothers compared to single adult mothers can be very different.

Young single mothers face many challenges. Coming, as they most often do, from backgrounds that are educationally and economically disadvantaged, these young mothers face tasks of establishing personal identities, preparing for adulthood, and becoming parents all at the same time (Weinraub et al., 2002). This pattern is especially common among African American adolescents; as we discuss later, these young women often establish residence with their own mothers, who may help in the rearing of children (Smith & Drew, 2002).

Because these families often have limited economic resources, they are likely to have access only to less desirable housing, in neighborhoods that may be characterized by violence and other environmental hazards. Parents facing economic hardship also have been found to be more likely than others to act in punitive ways with their children (Hanson, McLanahan, & Thomson, 1997). Given the multiple disadvantages of these families, it is not surprising that their children often experience many problems (McLanahan & Sandefur, 1994; Weinraub et al., 2002).

The fastest growing group of unmarried mothers is employed, college-educated women in their 30s who have become parents without marriage (Bachu, 1998; Smock & Greenland, 2010). Due to greater educational and employment opportunities for women, declining stigma associated with single parenthood, and delayed childbearing, single parenthood has increased dramatically among women in managerial and professional occupations (Weinraub et al., 2002). Research on this group is still somewhat limited, but available results paint a very different picture for children than the one just outlined for younger single mothers.

In one study of children reared by older unmarried mothers versus same-age married couples, Weinraub and her colleagues (2002) reported that the women had middle-class incomes and were able to provide food, shelter, and many opportunities for their children. They reported that when levels of stress were relatively low, 8- to 13-year-olds from single-parent and matched two-parent families were equally well adjusted (Gringlas & Weinraub, 1995). When families had experienced many stressful life events, however, children of single parents showed more behavior problems than did those from low-stress one-parent or two-parent homes (Weinraub et al., 2002). Thus, under difficult circumstances, children of single mothers—even single mothers with many resources—were more vulnerable. Whether this was due to less positive parenting among stressed mothers or to other factors is not known. Most of the time, however, when life went smoothly, children of older unmarried mothers were well adjusted.

Social support may help single mothers meet the challenges of parenting. Single mothers with young children exhibited more optimal parenting when they felt that they had more social support (Weinraub & Wolf, 1983, 1987). However, they also felt that they received less social support than mothers in two-parent families. A program designed to strengthen the social networks of low-income mothers with preschool-age children revealed that as European American single mothers built larger and closer networks of non-kin friends, the mothers felt greater confidence in their parenting and were more active in preparing their children for school (Cochran, 1991). African American single mothers with strong social connections with relatives and non-kin adults were more engaged with their children. More recently, Kalil and Ryan (2010) studied sources of practical support for single-mother families and found that the economic burdens of single mothers are significantly lessened by a variety of public programs. These mothers also turn to private sources of support, such as their friends, boyfriends, or family members for cash or other types of assistance. Overall, these studies indicate that social support is associated with better quality parenting at least as strongly for single parents as for other family types (Cochran & Niego, 2002; Weinraub et al., 2002).

Resource issues are therefore crucial to the parenting issues of single-mother families. For families with few economic resources and little social support, many difficulties arise. For single mothers whose economic resources allow them to provide for children's needs and to offer stimulating opportunities as well, outcomes may be very different. Even in these affluent families, however, parental resources may be overwhelmed in stressful circumstances; when this happens, children of single parents are likely to have adjustment problems. Although the research findings are still somewhat limited, the most important explanatory factors appear to be available resources and qualities of family interactions rather than the nature of the family structure itself (Hanson et al., 1997; McLanahan & Sandefur, 1994).

Single-Father Families

Although there are far fewer single fathers than single mothers, and fewer studies of single-father families, the number of single-father families is growing (Weinraub et al., 2002). Higher rates of adoption by single men and custody awards to men following divorce and family dissolution are contributing to this social change. Some studies suggest that the socialization by single fathers and single mothers is similar. For example, they have both been found to be more permissive than mothers and fathers in two-parent families (Dornbusch & Gray, 1988).

Compared to single mothers, single fathers have more economic resources, feel more confident, have more authority over their children, and are more positively engaged with children (Hilton & Devall, 1998). Some studies indicate no difference in the well-being of elementary school-age children living in single-father, single-mother, and two-parent families (Hilton, Desrochers, & Devall, 2001; Schnayer & Orr, 1989).

The results of other studies, however, suggest differences among these family types. Song, Benin, and Glick (2012) reported that after they controlled for SES, children were faring better in single-mother families than in single-father or stepparent families. Bronte-Tinkew, Scott, and Lilja (2010) argued that single-father families should be seen as distinct from single-mother families and two-parent, biological-parent families in terms of not only sociodemographic characteristics but also parenting styles and parental involvement. Other research has indicated that daughters of single fathers showed more adjustment difficulties than girls in other family types, including decreased sociability and increased neediness, whereas sons of single fathers did not differ in social competence from their peers (Santrock, Warshak, & Elliott, 1982), suggesting the possibility of gender differences in children's responses to being raised by single fathers. Similarly, using data from the National Longitudinal Study of Adolescent Health, Benson and Johnson (2009) found that the quality of parent–child relationships, as well as the experience of living in single-parent families (including single-father families), appeared to be more consequential for adolescent daughters than for sons. Benson and Johnson also noted that parental control seemed particularly influential for adolescents in single-father families compared to other family structures.

Like single-mother families, single-father families tend to have fewer economic resources than two-parent families (Meyer & Garasky, 1993). Single fathers who obtain custody after divorce receive more offers of informational and instrumental support from their social networks than do newly divorced single mothers (Weinraub et al., 2002), although they may not use the support that is offered. Overall, the limited amount of research available suggests that many of the socialization processes and experiences affecting single-mother families also pertain to single-father families, although, clearly, more work in this area is needed.

Unmarried Heterosexual, Two-Parent Families

Increasing numbers of cohabiting heterosexual couples are choosing to conceive, bear, and rear children within the context of unmarried two-parent families (Cancian & Reed, 2001; Ermisch, 2001; Smock & Greenland, 2010). Until recently, little empirical attention had been devoted to child development or parenting practices within this family structure. Even now, there have been only a few studies.

A number of factors associated with problematic socialization have been found to characterize unmarried, two-parent families more often than married families. Cohabitating parents, on average, have fewer economic resources than do married couples (McLanahan & Teitler, 1999). Satisfaction with the couple relationship tends to be lower (Nock, 1995), and the stability of unmarried relationships is also lower. Thus, it is not surprising that cohabiting couples separate earlier and more often than do married couples (DeMaris & Rao, 1992; Lillard, Brien, & Waite, 1995). Having a child is associated with greater stability of unmarried couple relationships (Wu, 1995), especially if the child is conceived within the relationship (Manning, 2004), although this may also mean that more committed cohabiting couples are likely to choose parenthood.

A few recent studies indicate that, compared to married heterosexual two-parent families, children and parents in unmarried heterosexual two-parent families are more likely to manifest difficulties. Examining data from the National Institute of Child Health and Human Development (NICHD) Study of Early Child Care, Aronson and Huston (2004) found that infants and mothers in cohabitating relationships were more similar to their counterparts in single-mother families than to those in married, two-parent families. Cohabitating mothers were less attentive and positive toward their infants and provided less structured and stimulating home environments than did married mothers. Infants of cohabitating mothers showed less warmth and were less securely attached to their mothers. Mothers in unmarried families were younger, had fewer economic resources, and were less well educated than mothers in married families. These contextual factors did not account for differences in parenting or infant measures, however. The quality of the partner relationship did, however, mediate the relation of family structure with parenting: The less optimal parenting of unmarried mothers was attributable to lower intimacy and support they felt with their partners.

Studies with older children and adolescents have shown that compared to children of married heterosexual parents, children of unmarried but cohabitating heterosexual parents experience more academic problems, achieve lower grades, and have more behavioral problems (Brown, 2004; Dunifon & Kowaleski-Jones, 2002; Thompson, Hanson, & McLanahan, 1994). Although unmarried parents tend to use less optimal socialization practices than married parents, researchers have not found that differences in warmth, control, and punishment across family structures account for differences in children's well-being (Dunifon & Kowaleski-Jones, 2002; Thompson et al., 1994). Thus, associations between children's functioning and living in unmarried, two-parent families may be explained by access to resources, quality of parent relationship, social networks, or other factors.

It is important to note that most of the research on socialization in unmarried, two-parent families has been conducted in the United States, where attitudes about unmarried cohabitation have historically been negative. Associations between cohabitation and development may be very different in nations and cultures in which childrearing by unmarried couples is more common and accepted. For example, heterosexual couples in Québec, Canada, are now more likely to cohabitate than to marry, and for over a decade there have been more children born to unmarried heterosexual couples than to married heterosexual couples (Institut de la Statistic Québec, 2005). It would be informative to pursue cross-cultural research on variations in the relations between parental marriage versus cohabitation and children's development, depending on changing attitudes and on the relative prevalence of these two family types within societies.

Families Formed Using Reproductive Technologies

With the advent of alternative reproductive technologies (ARTs), many new options have become available to couples and other adults who would otherwise experience infertility. Since the birth of Louise Brown, the first "test-tube baby," in 1978, many new choices have emerged (Golombok, 2002, 2013; Golombok, MacCallum, & Goodman, 2001). *Donor insemination* (DI) involves the insemination of a woman with sperm from a male donor. The donor may be the husband, another man known to the woman, or a man who remains anonymous. *In vitro* fertilization (IVF) involves the fertilization of egg by sperm in the laboratory, with the resulting embryo transferred to the mother's womb for gestation. *Egg donation* (ED) involves the removal of fertile eggs from the body of a female donor (who may either be known or anonymous) and fertilization via IVF, with the resulting embryo transferred to the womb of a gestational mother. These techniques are sometimes combined with *surrogacy*, in which a woman (called a *surrogate*) carries to term a baby she agrees to give up at birth to be raised by others. Thus, ARTs make possible the birth of children who are genetically linked to one, two, or none of the adults who expect to rear them. Considerable controversy has surrounded medical, legal, and ethical questions about these new practices, but here we focus on issues related to parenting and the development of children who have been conceived using the new reproductive technologies (Golombok, 2013).

How might children conceived via ART be expected to fare? The expenses involved in pursuing ART can be high, and those who become parents in this way are likely to have economic resources. These people are highly motivated to become parents and are willing to undergo arduous medical procedures in order to do so. Given that they have probably undergone diagnosis and treatment for infertility, these people are also likely to be older than other parents of same-age children. All these factors may contribute to favorable predictions about the parenting circumstances and skills of those who have formed families using ART.

On the other hand, additional factors seem to suggest that children conceived via ART might have difficulties (Golombok, 2002). For instance, the lack of a genetic link between the child and at least one of the parents might be seen as a cause for concern, especially if it is thought to be related to reduced interest in parenting by the parent who is not biologically linked with the child. Consistent with this idea, Dunn, Davies, O'Connor, and Sturgess (2000) reported that in natural conception heterosexual-parent families, stepparents were less affectionate toward and less supportive of stepchildren than of biological children. If the lack of genetic links between some ART parents and their children results in less warmth and less supportive parenting, then this might result in negative outcomes for children conceived via ART. Of course, stepparents also differ from biologically linked parents in other ways, such as the length of time they have known the child.

Research addressing these issues has been extensive in recent years, and normal patterns of socialization among children conceived using ART have been reported (Golombok, 2002, 2013). For instance, Golombok and her colleagues (1996; Golombok, Cook, Bish, & Murray, 1995) examined the quality of parenting, as well as outcomes for children among IVF and DI heterosexual parent families, as well as among heterosexual natural conception families, when their children were between 4 and 8 years of age. This original group of families was recruited in the United Kingdom, but observations from more families were later added to the study from Spain, Italy, and the Netherlands (Golombok et al., 1995, 1996); because the results revealed no national differences, only the overall results are described here. Measures of the quality of parenting included assessments of maternal warmth, emotional involvement in parenting, and qualities of mother–child and father–child interaction. In addition, parents completed assessments of marital adjustment, parenting stress, anxiety and depression. Assessments of child development included social competence, as well as behavior problems.

Results revealed positive patterns of parenting, as well as favorable outcomes for children (Golombok, 2013; Golombok et al., 1995, 1996). Child adjustment, parenting, and marital quality among IVF and DI mothers were similar in most respects to those in mothers who had conceived naturally. Mothers who had used ART reported greater warmth toward and higher emotional involvement with their children than did those who had conceived naturally, and they also reported less parenting stress. ART fathers were described as interacting more with their children than did natural conception fathers. Children were found to have few cognitive or behavior problems and to be functioning well. The qualities of ART children's attachment relationships with parents were no different than those of naturally conceived children. No differences between DI and IVF families were reported. Similar findings come from a study in Taiwan, in which teachers described IVF mothers as more affectionate with their children than natural conception mothers but otherwise similar (Hahn & DiPietro, 2001). Related studies have also indicated few if any reasons for concern; most differences between ART and other families have favored the ART offspring (Golombok & MacCallum, 2003).

The authors also conducted a follow-up study of these families when the children were 12 years of age (Golombok et al., 2001; Golombok, MacCallum, Goodman, & Rutter, 2002), when possible problems with children's self-esteem and sense of positive identity might be expected to emerge. Golombok and colleagues (2001, 2002) reported that both ART parents and their youngsters showed good adjustment. Parents who had conceived children via ART were similar to those who had conceived naturally on measures of psychological adjustment, parenting, and marital relations. Children conceived via ART had scholastic records, peer relations, and emotional development that did not differ significantly from those of other children (Golombok et al., 2002). Another follow-up study examined parent–child relationships in these families when the children were in late adolescence (Owen & Golombok, 2009). The results indicated that levels of mother–adolescent warmth were higher in ART families than in adoptive families, and in DI families compared with IVF and natural conception families. Mothers in IVF families demonstrated more disciplinary aggression than did DI mothers, but there were no differences among fathers across family types with regard to warmth and conflict. Interestingly, only two of the 26 DI children were aware that they were conceived via DI, even by late adolescence. Overall, even with some differences observed across different family structures, the extant data suggest that socialization of children conceived via DI and IVF proceeds in a typical fashion (Golombok, 2013; Golombok & MacCallum, 2003; Owen & Golombok, 2009; Wagenaar, Huisman, Cohen-Kettenis, & van de Wall, 2008).

Somewhat less information is available about the development of children conceived using ED, though available data are similar to those for children conceived using other forms of ART. Both in early studies (e.g., Raoul-Duvan, Bertrand-Servais, Letur-Konirsch, & Frydman, 1994) and in more recent ones (Golombok, Murray, Brinsden, & Abdalla, 1999), results of assessments of parenting were similar to those for natural conception families, except that ED mothers reported less parenting stress. The self-esteem and behavioral adjustment of young children in ED families was similar to that in natural conception families (Golombok et al., 1999).

A pair of recent studies comparing infants and toddlers conceived via ED, and those who were naturally conceived, confirmed the earlier finding of positive parenting profiles in ED and DI families (Golombok, Jadva, Lycett, Murray, & MacCallum, 2005; Golombok, Lycett, et al., 2004). MacCallum, Golombok, and Brinsden (2007) investigated parenting and child development among ED, IVF, and adoptive families with children ages 2–5 years and discovered higher emotional overinvolvement, as well as greater defensiveness and secrecy about the child's origins, in ED families compared to the other family groups. No differences were observed among children with respect to psychological problems (MacCallum et al., 2007).

Mothers who used ART to conceive infants showed greater emotional involvement with them than did mothers who had conceived naturally, but the groups did not differ on personal or marital adjustment (Golombok, Lycett, et al., 2004). When children were 2 years of age, follow-up assessments revealed that there were still no differences in parents' personal or marital adjustment as a function of mode of conception. Mothers who had conceived using ART described feeling greater pleasure in their children and saw their children as more vulnerable than did those who had conceived naturally. No developmental differences among the children were noted (Golombok et al., 2005). A similar study of ED-conceived children up to 8 years of age (Golombok et al., 1999) revealed that their adjustment was also similar to that of naturally conceived children. In a study of ED families, Applegarth and Riddle (2007) reported that parents indicated that the lack of genetic tie between mother and child felt less important over time, but mothers did report continued thoughts about the donor.

Little is known about the childhood development of children born through surrogacy (Golombok & MacCallum, 2003), but there are a few studies of such families in the first years of the children's lives. In one study (Golombok, Murray, Jadva, MacCallum, & Lycett, 2004), surrogacy, ED, and natural conception families were compared over the infant's first year. Results indicated more favorable psychological adjustment and better adjustment to parenthood among surrogacy than among natural conception families (Golombok, Murray, et al., 2004). No differences in infant temperament were observed, but qualities of parent–infant relationships were more favorable among ART than among natural conception parents. In a follow-up to this study when children were 2 years old, Golombok, MacCallum, Murray, Lycett, and Jadva (2006) found that mothers in families formed through surrogacy demonstrated more positive parent–child relationships, and that fathers in these families demonstrated less parenting stress than did the mothers and fathers in natural conception families. Furthermore, children in each family type did not differ in terms of their cognitive or socioemotional development. Finally, this sample of families was also studied when children were 7 years old (Golombok et al., 2011). Interestingly, at age 7, mother–child interaction was less positive among both surrogacy and ED families than in natural conception families. However, there were no differences across family types with regard to maternal positivity and negativity, or with regard to child adjustment. Overall, the available evidence suggests that children of surrogacy are developing in typical ways (Golombok, 2002; Golombok, Murray, et al., 2004).

Successful outcomes among offspring conceived via ART suggest that, at least among the families that have been studied, the desire and ability to parent are not related to biological linkages. The greater resources of the older, financially secure ART parents, as well as their greater than average desire for parenthood, appear to be important elements in their ability to parent, as well as to create harmonious family environments. Thus, it appears that the financial and psychological resources of these parents have been important elements in their success (Golombok, 2002, 2013; Golombok & MacCallum, 2003). Indeed, results of research on families created through ARTs have shown that concerns about detrimental outcomes for children and parents in these families are generally unfounded.

Sexual-Minority-Parent Families

Most of the literature on sexual-minority families has focused on lesbian- and gay-parent families rather than on bisexual- (or transgender-) parent families. Whether through the use of ART, adoption, or by means of earlier heterosexual marriages, many nonhetero-sexual individuals have become parents (C. J. Patterson, 2000, 2002, 2005; C. J. Patterson & Riskind, 2010). For instance, of the same-sex couples who identified themselves on the U.S. Census, 33% of women and 22% of men reported that they were rearing at least one child in their home (Simmons & O'Connell, 2003). Children growing up in gay- and lesbian-parented homes may live with one parent or two, and they may or may not be biologically linked to the adults who are their parents. These children are genetically related to both parents only in rare cases (e.g., in ART conceptions, when one partner is a genetic parent, and the egg or sperm donor is a biological relative of the other parent; see C. J. Patterson & Riskind, 2010). Although laws have changed recently in some countries and states, in much of the world, same-sex partners still do not have access to the legal institution of marriage, so most children growing up in lesbian- and gay-parented households live with unmarried—and many with never-married—parents (C. J. Patterson, 2007; C. J. Patterson, Riskind, & Tornello, 2014). In addition, of course, children with same-sex parents do not have the male and female parents prescribed by cultural norms. Thus, lesbian- and gay-parented families differ from cultural expectations in a number of ways.

What is the impact on children of growing up with lesbian or gay parents? More than two decades of research on children's self-esteem, academic achievement, behavior, and emotional development has revealed that, for the most part, children with lesbian or gay parents develop in much the same ways that other children do (Hastings et al., 2006; C. J. Patterson, 2000, 2002, 2005; Perrin & the Committee on Psychosocial Aspects of Child and Family Health, 2002; Stacey & Biblarz, 2001). For instance, in a study in England, Golombok and colleagues (2003) compared psychological development of 7-year-old children with lesbian mothers to that of same-age children with heterosexual parents from the same communities. Only two differences in parenting emerged as a function of sexual orientation. Lesbian mothers were more likely to report engaging in imaginative play with their children and less likely to report "smacking" (i.e., using corporal punishment with) their children—both differences that might be seen as favoring children in the lesbian mother families. On measures of self-concept, peer relations, conduct, and gender development, however, no significant differences emerged between children with lesbian and heterosexual parents (Golombok et al., 2003).

Particularly notable was Golombok and colleagues' (2003) finding of no differences in gender development. They employed an activities inventory designed specifically to identify variations in children's gendered behavior and characteristics (e.g., interest in playing with jewelry) that had been extensively validated against behavioral observations, and that had good reliability (Golombok & Rust, 1993). Especially given the strengths of this instrument, the fact that gender development scores of children with lesbian and heterosexual parents did not differ was of particular interest. The results are, however, consistent with those from a substantial body of research on children of lesbian mothers (Farr, Forssell, & Patterson, 2010; C. J. Patterson, 2000, 2005; Perrin & the Committee on Psychosocial Aspects of Child and Family Health, 2002).

The Golombok and colleagues (2003) study included single-lesbian-, coupled-lesbian-, single-heterosexual-, and coupled-heterosexual-parent families in a fully crossed design. Thus, the study allowed comparisons based on not only parental sexual orientation but also the number of parents in the home. These latter comparisons provided an instructive contrast to those based on sexual orientation. Regardless of sexual orientation, single mothers reported significantly more dysfunctional interactions with their children, more severe disputes with them, less enjoyment of motherhood, lower overall quality of parenting, and greater parenting stress than did mothers with partners. Parenting stress was a significant predictor of children's behavioral and socioemotional problems, such that greater stress was associated with more problems. Single mothers did not see their children as experiencing more problems than other children, but teachers identified children of single parents as having more emotional and conduct problems than children with two parents (Golombok et al., 2003). Thus, while parental sexual orientation was unrelated to children's outcomes, increased parenting stress and lower-quality parenting in single-parent families were related to difficulties. Contrasting results were, however, reported by others; for example, Chan, Raboy, and Patterson (1998) reported no differences in child adjustment in single-parent versus two-parent-lesbian- versus heterosexual-parent families.

Studies with older children and adolescents have also reported generally positive development among children of lesbian mothers (e.g., Gartrell, Deck, Rodas, Peyser, & Banks, 2005; Gershon, Tschann, & Jemerin, 1999; Huggins, 1989; O'Connor, 1993; Tasker & Golombok, 1997; Wainright, Russell, & Patterson, 2004; for a review, see Hastings et al., 2006). For example, in their longitudinal study of children born to lesbian mothers, Gartrell and colleagues (2005) interviewed children and their mothers when the children were 10 years of age. Standardized scores for children's social competence and behavior problems on a maternal interview measure were compared to those for the norming group of same-age schoolchildren in the United States. Results showed that both social competence and conduct of children with lesbian mothers were comparable to those of the children in the norming sample. Although a substantial minority of the children acknowledged having experienced antigay incidents (e.g., other children expressing dislike for nonheterosexual people or activities), most reported speaking up in response to them (Gartrell et al., 2005).

Actual experiences or concerns of children and youth about discrimination due to the sexual orientation of their gay and lesbian parents have been reported by a number of investigators (Crosbie-Burnett & Helmbrecht, 1993; Gartrell et al., 2000; Javaid, 1993; Ray & Gregory, 2001; van Dam, 2004). Adolescents with gay and lesbian parents may feel more concern than younger children do about negative peer reactions to their family structure. There appears, however, to be little, if any, impact of discrimination on the overall well-being of the children of lesbian and gay parents.

A study by Wainright and colleagues (2004) explored personal, social, and academic development among adolescents (12–18 years of age) living with same-sex and opposite-sex parents. The two samples were matched on demographic characteristics and drawn from a national sample (the National Longitudinal Study of Adolescent Health). Adolescents living with same-sex parents were at least as well adjusted as their peers living with opposite-sex parents in terms of psychological well-being (e.g., depression, anxiety, and self-esteem), school outcomes (e.g., grades, trouble in school, and connectedness at school), and family and relationship processes (e.g., perceived care from adults and peers, perceived parental warmth, feelings of neighborhood integration, and perceived autonomy). Among both adolescents living with same-sex and those living with opposite-sex parents, the best predictors of overall adjustment were parent reports of warm, close relationships with their teenage offspring. Thus, not only were adolescents with same-sex parents well adjusted, but familial predictors of adolescent adjustment remained the same regardless of family structure (see also Wainright & Patterson, 2006, 2008).

Another finding of interest from the Wainright and colleagues (2004) study is that there were no differences in adolescents' reports of romantic attractions and behaviors as a function of family structure. Few adolescents reported same-sex attractions, so only opposite-sex romantic relationships were examined. When asked whether they had been involved in a romantic relationship within the past 18 months, 68% of adolescents with same-sex parents and 59% of adolescents with opposite-sex parents reported that they had; the difference was not statistically significant. Results also revealed that equal proportions of adolescents with same- and opposite-sex parents reported having ever engaged in sexual intercourse (34% of each group). Thus, romantic and sexual development of adolescents in the two groups appeared to be comparable.

Tasker and Golombok (1997) interviewed the offspring of divorced lesbian and divorced heterosexual mothers when they were young adults. They found no differences in anxiety or depression, employment histories, age at first intercourse, number of sexual relationships, current relationship status, or happiness in current romantic relationship (if any). The young adults with lesbian mothers were no more likely than those with heterosexual mothers to describe themselves as attracted to same-sex romantic or sexual partners. If they were attracted to same-sex partners, the offspring of lesbian mothers were more likely to say that they would consider acting on their attraction, or that they already done so. In the end, however, the young adult offspring of lesbian mothers were not more likely than those of heterosexual mothers to describe themselves as lesbian, gay, or bisexual (Tasker & Golombok, 1997). This last result is consistent with a substantial body of research showing that a large majority of children with lesbian and gay parents themselves grow up to be heterosexual (C. J. Patterson, 1992, 2000, 2005; C. J. Patterson & Chan, 1999; Perrin & the Committee on Psychosocial Aspects of Child and Family Health, 2002). Thus, for better or worse, parental sexual orientation seems to have little impact on sexual development.

The similarities between children reared by heterosexual parents and those reared by gay and lesbian parents are striking and may be seen as being at odds with some predictions based on risk models of developmental psychopathology. Some children of gay and lesbian parents experience discrimination, and they are at increased risk of living in conditions of economic hardship. Gay men earn less than heterosexual men with the same education, experience, and occupation who live in the same region (Badgett, 1995), although differences between lesbian and heterosexual women are less dramatic. Lesbian and gay couples who become parents after coming out have generally been relatively affluent, but divorced lesbian and gay parents may have fewer economic resources (C. J. Patterson, 2000; van Dam, 2004). The economic disadvantages of lesbian and gay couples (e.g., lack of access to health insurance through the partner's job) might be expected to result in disadvantages for families.

However, gay and lesbian parents also appear to be, on average, effective socialization agents. A number of studies have noted few differences in the socialization attitudes and behaviors of heterosexual parents compared to gay and lesbian parents (Bos, van Balen, & van den Boom, 2004; Wainright et al., 2004). When researchers have noted differences, these have generally favored gay and lesbian parents. For instance, when compared to heterosexual parents, lesbian mothers in two-parent households were able to identify more potential child care problems and generate more solutions to those problems (Flaks, Ficher, Masterpasqua, & Joseph, 1995), and they reported more positive relationships with their children (Brewaeys, Ponjeart, Van Hall, & Golombok, 1997). Lesbian mothers and gay fathers are less likely than heterosexual parents to report the use of physical punishment (Golombok et al., 2003; Johnson & O'Connor, 2001). Gay fathers put more emphasis than heterosexual fathers on the importance of tradition and security in their decision to have children, and they were more likely to report using an authoritative parenting style with their children (Bigner & Jacobsen, 1989a, 1989b).

Family relationships and social support networks also play a role in the positive development of children of gay and lesbian parents. Studies indicate that lesbian couples report sharing household tasks and parenting duties more equally than do heterosexual couples, and that they report high satisfaction with the quality of their couple relationships (Bos et al., 2004; Brewaeys et al., 1997; C. J. Patterson, 2002). Similar to results of the research on single-mother versus two-parent families, gay fathers who share their home with another supportive adult, including a partner, roommate, or parent, report fewer difficulties with parenting than do single gay fathers (Barrett & Tasker, 2001).

Support from social networks appears to be an important part of the lives of gay and lesbian parents. In a Dutch study, younger lesbian mothers were especially likely to use informal social support, such as talking to friends, which could protect the young mothers and their children from some of the risks associated with early parenthood (Bos et al., 2004). Children of lesbian mothers may also benefit from their mothers' social networks. In a U.S. study, children who had more frequent contacts with their grandparents or with their lesbian mothers' friends reported less anxiety and greater well-being than did children who were less involved in their mothers' social networks (C. J. Patterson, Hurt, & Mason, 1998). Thus, as has been observed in families with heterosexual parents, well-functioning family systems and supportive social networks are associated with the adjustment and effective socialization of gay and lesbian parents and to their children's overall positive development even in the presence of social and economic risks.

Favorable development among offspring of lesbian mothers and gay fathers suggests that the desire and ability to parent effectively are not related to parental sexual orientation. Because the achievement of parenthood often requires significant efforts on their part, lesbian and gay parents as a group may have greater than average desire for parenthood (C. J. Patterson & Riskind, 2010). Lesbians and gay men are less likely to become parents unintentionally than are heterosexual women and men; thus, it is possible that lesbian and gay parents are a more self-selected group of individuals with better-than-average potential for parenthood. Many lesbian and gay parents who choose to become parents through ART or adoption are able to draw on considerable personal, financial, or social resources that serve to support their ability to exhibit favorable patterns of parenting. Regardless of parental sexual orientation, single parents may have fewer resources, feel more stressed, and have more problematic interactions with their children. Evidence about whether children of single-lesbian or gay parents have more emotional or behavioral problems than do those with two lesbian or gay parents is, however, mixed (Chan et al., 1998; Golombok et al., 2003). Overall, these findings suggest that while two parents may often be better than one, access to resources and to social support is a more important determinant of socialization outcomes than is parental sexual orientation.

Custodial-Grandparent Families

Almost 10% of children in the United States—at least 5–6 million children—live in a household in which a grandparent is present, and a wide range of experiences is represented in this group (Pinazo-Hernandis & Tompkins, 2009; Smith & Drew, 2002). In some families, a grandparent needing help lives with parents and children in the parents' household; in this case, parents are generally offering assistance to a grandparent. In other families, parent and child live in the grandparent's home; in this case, a young or unemployed parent (usually, a mother) and child accept help from a grandparent (usually, a grandmother). Finally, due to issues such as parental death, drug addiction, or incarceration, grandparents may be the sole custodial guardians of their grandchildren (Dunifon, 2013).

These diverse types of homes are likely to provide very different environments for children (Smith & Drew, 2002). As an example, custodial grandparents in the United States are more likely than any other grandparents to be living below the official poverty line, to have no health insurance, and to be receiving public assistance. Younger African American grandmothers who have not graduated from high school are most likely to take custodial roles with grandchildren. Considering the lack of economic power of these women, the fact that they experience financial problems when required to care for grandchildren cannot be viewed as surprising (Minkler & Fuller-Thompson, 2000). Custodial grandparents are also more likely than other grandparents to feel depressed and to report poor health (Baker & Silverstein, 2008; Minkler & Fuller-Thompson, 1999, 2001; Minkler, Fuller-Thompson, & Driver, 1997). Grandparents raising grandchildren with special needs are particularly likely to feel distressed (Emick & Hayslip, 1999), probably because the task of caring for such children can easily overwhelm the resources of any family. Both formal and informal social support have been found to at least partially mitigate such stress (Landry-Meyer, Gerard, & Guzell, 2005).

From the sparse research on parenting among grandparents, especially those with few financial or other resources, it appears that stress and difficulties abound among these families. Thus, even though they share genetic links with the grandparents who rear them, children living in these households face many challenges and are likely to experience many problems of adjustment (Smith & Drew, 2002).

Summary and Conclusions

Although cultural norms in the Western world describe only a narrow range of family structures as optimal for childrearing, substantial numbers of children are in fact growing up in other kinds of families. The norms prescribe that children should be reared by heterosexual, married couples who are their genetic parents. In reality, however, many children are being reared by never-married couples, by lesbian and gay couples, by parents to whom they are not genetically linked, by single parents, or by their grandparents (Lamb, 1999a, 2012).

What are the socialization outcomes for childrearing in these varied family environments? To address this question, we reviewed research on socialization in families that differ from the cultural norm in one or more ways. In this section, we consider each assumption of the cultural norm in turn and examine the evidence regarding its significance. First, however, we discuss the issue of economic resources as it relates to family structure and to socialization processes.

Clearly, children growing up in economically impoverished families are at greater risk of encountering problems in development. These range from poor nutrition and housing to inadequate access to health care, to coercive parenting and family instability. Family economic circumstances are related to children's health, behavior, and educational opportunities, and those whose families have fewer economic resources are likely to suffer on all these counts (Brooks-Gunn & Duncan, 1997a, 1997b).

Economic resources are, of course, unevenly distributed across family structures. Because of long-standing patterns of discrimination (e.g., on gender or racial grounds), some family types generally have fewer resources than others. Thus, it can be difficult to avoid attribution of the problems associated with economic issues to various family structures. There have been well-known efforts to separate economic from family structure issues (e.g., McLanahan & Sandefur, 1994), and these have served to underline the importance of economic resources. Overall, though, economic inequalities are not always acknowledged fully in research on family structure.

Of all the cultural prescriptions for the "traditional" family, the one that receives the most powerful support from the available research literature is that children are better off when they have two parents rather than only one. First, two parents together generally have access to greater economic resources than either one alone. They may also have more extensive social support networks together than does either one alone, and they may provide important support and encouragement for one another. It is clear that some single parents—especially those with considerable economic resources—arrange family life in ways that support positive socialization, but this is more difficult for a lone parent than for two parents working closely together. Other things being equal, two parents are usually better than one.

Does it benefit children if their parents are married? Looking first at heterosexual couples who have access to civil marriage, the evidence suggests that children of married parents show better adjustment. Even though there is an association between marriage and children's adjustment, the reasons or mechanisms for this link are far from clear. Does marriage favor children because of the differences between parents who do or do not marry? Because of the economic and social benefits that flow from marriage? Because of the added family stability that comes with marriage? Or are the benefits of marriage for children due to some combination of these and other factors? We know that those who choose to marry differ in some ways from those who do not (see Arnett, Chapter 4, this volume), and we know that many economic, social, and health benefits are associated with marriage (General Accounting Office, 1997; Horwitz & White, 1998; Horwitz, White, & Howell-White, 1996; Schoenborn, 2004). How important each of these elements may be for children's socialization, however, is not yet known.

For same-sex couples rearing children, the issues regarding marriage have been, and in many jurisdictions continue to be, different. Until recently, no same-sex couples had access to the institution of civil marriage. Thus, the selection factors that apply to married versus unmarried heterosexual couples might not be similarly evident among lesbian or gay couples. As same-sex couples have begun to gain access to civil marriage around the world, the situation in this regard is in flux. It seems likely that the economic and social rewards of marriage will benefit same-sex couples, just as they seem to have benefited opposite-sex couples. For example, both parents would share legal decision-making capacities for their children, and in the event of the death of one parent, the other parent's inheritance and custody rights would not be challenged. Furthermore, to the degree that civil marriage might encourage family stability, it should be expected to benefit children in same-sex parent families.

Although some of the prescriptions of cultural norms have received support from the research on nontraditional families, others clearly have not. First, it is clear from research on ART that genetic links between parents and children are not necessary for favorable socialization outcomes to occur. Studies of families whose children were conceived via DI, ED, IVF, and surrogacy show that positive parenting and favorable child outcomes can occur in the absence of genetic links between parents and children. Although difficulties in socialization may yet be uncovered, results of research to date are not consistent with the idea that genetic linkages are necessary for favorable parenting and socialization.

Similarly, the research findings to date do not support the view that parental sexual orientation is an important factor in the socialization of children. Other things being equal, the offspring of lesbian and gay parents appear to develop in ways that are very similar to the development of those with heterosexual parents. Although some of these children acknowledge encounters with antigay sentiments, these do not seem, on average, to have an appreciable impact on their overall development at home or at school. In all, the childrearing behaviors, parenting styles, and family management practices of a parent are much more important than parental sexual orientation for children's psychosocial development.

Finally, we come to the issue of gender in parenting and socialization. Our reading of the socialization literature does not support the traditional view that children need both male and female parents in order to develop in positive ways (Biblarz & Stacey, 2010; Lamb, 2012). Even if two parents are often better than one, this is not relevant to the issues of gender in parenting. When families are headed by heterosexual parents, number and gender of parents are confounded because parents of each gender are required if there are to be two parents. In gay-father and lesbian-mother families, in contrast, number and gender of parents are not confounded. As of this writing, data on children reared by gay couples are still sparse, so arguments in this area cannot be advanced with great confidence. In general, however, the successful socialization of children by lesbian couples suggests that parental gender, like parental sexual orientation, may not be as important for socialization as cultural norms tend to suggest.

Overall, then, the theoretical yield of research on nontraditional families has already been substantial and holds promise of further contributions. While the results of research uphold the importance of some prescriptions, others receive little or no support. The research has revealed fairly robust support for the importance of having two parents and tentative support for the importance of the two parents being married. Traditional expectations about the importance of genetic linkages, parental sexual orientation, and parental gender have not, however, borne up under close scrutiny. Thus, research on nontraditional families has been valuable in evaluating the significance of widely held views about factors that are most important in socialization.

REFERENCES

Adam, E. K. (2004). Beyond quality: Parental and residential stability and children's adjustment. *Current Directions in Psychological Science, 13*, 210–213.

Adam, E. K., & Chase-Lansdale, P. L. (2002). Home sweet home(s): Parental separations, residential moves, and adjustment problems in low-income adolescent girls. *Developmental Psychology, 38,* 792–805.

Alaimo, K., Olson, C. M., Frongillo, E. A., Jr., & Breifel, R. R. (2001). Food insufficiency, family income, and health in U. S. preschool and school-aged children. *American Journal of Public Health, 91,* 781–786.

Applegarth, L. D., & Riddle, M. R. (2007). What do we know and what can we learn from families created through egg donation? *Journal of Infant, Child, and Adolescent Psychotherapy, 6*(2), 90–96.

Aronson, S. R., & Huston, A. C. (2004). The mother–infant relationship in single, cohabiting, and married families: A case for marriage? *Journal of Family Psychology, 18,* 5–18.

Bachu, A. (1998). *Trends in marital status of U.S. women at first birth* (Population Division Working Paper No. 20). Washington, DC: U.S. Government Printing Office.

Badgett, M. V. (1995). The wage effects of sexual orientation discrimination. *Industrial and Labor Relations Review, 48,* 726–739.

Baker, L. A., & Silverstein, M. (2008). Depressive symptoms among grandparents raising grandchildren: The impact of participation in multiple roles. *Journal of Intergenerational Relationships, 6*(3), 285–304.

Barrett, H., & Tasker, F. (2001). Growing up with a gay parent: Views of 101 gay fathers on their sons' and daughters' experiences. *Education and Child Psychology, 18,* 62–77.

Baumrind, D. (1967). Childcare practices anteceding three patterns of preschool behavior. *Genetic Psychology Monographs, 75,* 43–88.

Baumrind, D. (1971). Current patterns of parental authority. *Developmental Psychology Monographs, 4*(1, Pt. 2), 1–103.

Baumrind, D. (1973). The development of instrumental competence through socialization. *Minnesota Symposium on Child Psychology, 7,* 3–46.

Benson, J. E., & Johnson, M. K. (2009). Adolescent family context and adult identity formation. *Journal of Family Issues, 30*(9), 1265–1286.

Biblarz, T. J., & Stacey, J. (2010). How does the gender of parents matter? *Journal of Marriage and Family, 72,* 3–22.

Bigner, J. J., & Jacobsen, R. B. (1989a). Parenting behaviors of homosexual and heterosexual fathers. In F. W. Bozett (Ed.), *Homosexuality and the family* (pp. 173–186). New York: Haworth Press.

Bigner, J. J., & Jacobsen, R. B. (1989b). The value of children to gay and heterosexual fathers. In F. W. Bozett (Ed.), *Homosexuality and the family* (pp. 163–172). New York: Haworth Press.

Bolger, K. E., & Patterson, C. J. (2003). Sequelae of child maltreatment: Vulnerability and resilience. In S. S. Luthar (Ed.), *Resilience and vulnerability: Adaptation in the context of childhood adversities* (pp. 156–181). New York: Cambridge University Press.

Bos, H. M. W., van Balen, F., & van den Boom, D. C. (2004). Experiences of parenthood, couple relationship, social support, and child-rearing goals of lesbian mothers families. *Journal of Child Psychology and Psychiatry, 45,* 755–764.

Bradley, R. H. (2002). Environment and parenting. In M. H. Bornstein (Ed.), *Handbook of parenting: Vol. 2. Biology and ecology of parenting* (pp. 281–314). Mahwah, NJ: Erlbaum.

Bradley, R. H., Corwyn, R. F., McAdoo, H. P., & Garcia Coll, C. (2001). The home environments of children in the United States, Part I: Variations by age, ethnicity, and poverty status. *Child Development, 72,* 1844–1867.

Brewaeys, A., Ponjeart, I., Van Hall, E. V., & Golombok, S. (1997). Donor insemination: Child development and family functioning in lesbian mother families. *Human Reproduction, 12,* 1349–1359.

Brody, G. H., Flor, D. L., & Gibson, N. M. (1999). Linking maternal efficacy beliefs, developmental goals, parenting practices, and child competence in rural single-parent African American families. *Child Development, 70,* 1197–1208.

Bronte-Tinkew, J., Scott, M. E., & Lilja, E. (2010). Single custodial fathers' involvement and parenting: Implications for outcomes in emerging adulthood. *Journal of Marriage and Family, 72*(5), 1107–1127.

Brooks-Gunn, J., & Duncan, G. J. (Eds.). (1997a). *Consequences of growing up poor.* New York: Russell Sage Foundation.

Brooks-Gunn, J., & Duncan, G. J. (1997b). The effects of poverty on children. *The Future of Children, 7,* 58–69.

Brown, S. L. (2004). Family structure and child well-being: The significance of parental cohabitation. *Journal of Marriage and Family, 66,* 351–367.

Burbach, A. D., Fox, R. A., & Nicholson, B. C. (2004). Challenging behaviors in young children: The father's role. *Journal of Genetic Psychology, 165,* 169–183.

Cancian, M., & Reed, D. (2001). Changes in family structure: Implications for poverty and related policy. In S. Danziger & R. Haveman (Eds.), *Understanding poverty in America: Progress and problems* (pp. 69–97). New York: Harvard University Press.

Cassidy, J., & Shaver, P. R. (Eds.). (1999). *Handbook of attachment: Theory, research, and clinical applications.* New York: Guilford Press.

Chan, R. C., Raboy, B., & Patterson, C. J. (1998). Psychosocial adjustment among children conceived via donor insemination by lesbian and heterosexual mothers. *Child Development, 69,* 443–457.

Cochran, M. (1991). Personal social networks as a focus of support. In D. Unger & D. Powell (Eds.), *Families as nurturing systems* (pp. 45–68). New York: Haworth Press.

Cochran, M., & Brassard, J. (1979). Child development and personal social networks. *Child Development, 50,* 609–615.

Cochran, M., & Niego, S. (2002). Parenting and social networks. In M. H. Bornstein (Ed.), *Handbook of parenting: Vol. 4. Social conditions and applied parenting* (2nd ed., pp. 123–148). Mahwah, NJ: Erlbaum.

Conger, R., Conger, K., & Martin, M. (2010). Socioeconomic status, family processes, and individual development. *Journal of Marriage and Family, 72,* 685–704.

Crockenberg, S. (1988). Social support and parenting. In W. Fitzgerald, B. Lester, & M. Yogman (Eds.), *Research on support for parents and infants in the postnatal period* (pp. 67–92). New York: Ablex.

Crosbie-Burnett, M., & Helmbrecht, L. (1993). A descriptive empirical study of gay male stepfamilies. *Family Relations, 42,* 256–262.

Cummings, E. M., & Davies, P. (1994). *Children and marital conflict: The impact of family dispute and resolution.* New York: Guilford Press.

DeGarmo, D. S., Forgatch, M. S., & Martinez, C. R. (1999). Parenting of divorced mothers as a link between social status and boys academic outcomes: Unpacking the effects of socioeconomic status. *Child Development, 70,* 1231–1245.

DeMaris, A., & Rao, V. (1992). Premarital cohabitation and subsequent marital stability in the United States: A reassessment. *Journal of Marriage and the Family, 54,* 178–190.

Dornbusch, S. M., & Gray, K. D. (1988). Single-parent families: Perspectives on marriage and the family. In M. H. Strober & S. M. Dornbusch (Eds.), *Feminism, children, and the new families* (pp. 274–296). New York: Guilford Press.

Dunifon, R. (2013). The influence of grandparents on the lives of children and adolescents. *Child Development Perspectives, 7*(1), 55–60.

Dunifon, R., & Kowaleski-Jones, L. (2002). Who's in the house?: Race differences in cohabitation, single parenthood, and child development. *Child Development, 73*(4), 1249–1264.

Dunn, J., Davies, L. C., O'Connor, T. G., & Sturgess, W. (2000). Parents' and partners' life course and family experiences: Links with parent–child relationships in different family settings. *Journal of Child Psychology and Psychiatry, 41,* 955–968.

Emick, M. A., & Hayslip, B. (1999). Custodial grandparenting: Stresses, coping skills, and relationships with grandchildren. *International Journal of Aging and Human Development, 48,* 35–61.

Ermisch, J. (2001). Cohabitation and childbearing outside of marriage in Britain. In B. Wolfe &

L. L. Wu (Eds.), *Out of wedlock: Causes and consequences of nonmarital fertility* (pp. 109–139). New York: Russell Sage Foundation.

Evans, G. W., & Kim, P. (2013). Childhood poverty, chronic stress, self-regulation, and coping. *Child Development Perspectives, 7*(1), 43–48.

Farr, R. H., Forssell, S. L., & Patterson, C. J. (2010). Parenting and child development in adoptive families: Does parental sexual orientation matter? *Applied Developmental Science, 14*, 164–178.

Fields, J. M., Smith, K., Bass, L. E., & Lugalia, T. (2001). *A child's day: Home, school and play (selected indicators of child well-being)* (Current Population Reports P70–68). Washington, DC: U.S. Census Bureau.

Flaks, D. K., Ficher, I., Masterpasqua, F., & Joseph, G. (1995). Lesbians choosing motherhood: A comparative study of lesbian and heterosexual parents and their children. *Developmental Psychology, 31*, 105–114.

Gartrell, N., Banks., A., Reeds, N., Hamilton, J., Rodas, C., & Deck, A. (2000). The National Lesbian Family Study: 3. Interviews with mothers of five-year-olds. *American Journal of Orthopsychiatry, 70*, 542–548.

Gartrell, N., Deck, A., Rodas, C., Peyser, H., & Banks, A. (2005). The National Lesbian Family Study: 4. Interviews with the 10-year-old children. *American Journal of Orthopsychiatry, 75*, 518–524.

General Accounting Office. (1997). Tables of laws in the United States Code involving marital status, by category. Retrieved from *www.gao.gov/archive/1997/og97016.pdf*.

Gershon, T. D., Tschann, J. M., & Jemerin, J. M. (1999). Stigmatization, self-esteem, and coping among the adolescent children of lesbian mothers. *Journal of Adolescent Health, 24*, 437–445.

Golombok, S. (2002). Parenting and contemporary reproductive technologies. In M. H. Bornstein (Ed.), *Handbook of parenting: Vol. 3. Being and becoming a parent* (pp. 339–360). Mahwah, NJ: Erlbaum.

Golombok, S. (2013). Families created by reproductive donation: Issues and research. *Child Development Perspectives, 7*(1), 61–65.

Golombok, S., Brewaeys, A., Cook, R., Giavazzi, M. T., Guerra, D., Mantovanni, A., et al. (1996). The European study of assisted reproduction families. *Human Reproduction, 11*, 2324–2331.

Golombok, S., Cook, R., Bish, A., & Murray, C. (1995). Families created by the new reproductive technologies: Quality of parenting and social and emotional development of the children. *Child Development, 66*, 285–298.

Golombok, S., Jadva, V., Lycett, E., Murray, C., & MacCallum, F. (2005). Families created by gamete donation: Follow-up at age 2. *Human Reproduction, 20*, 286–293.

Golombok, S., Lycett, E., MacCallum, F., Jadva, V., Murray, C., Rust, J., et al. (2004). Parenting infants conceived by gamete donation. *Journal of Family Psychology, 18*, 443–452.

Golombok, S., & MacCallum, F. (2003). Outcomes for parents and children following nontraditional conception: What do clinicians need to know? *Journal of Child Psychology and Psychiatry, 44*, 303–315.

Golombok, S., MacCallum, F., & Goodman, E. (2001). The "test-tube" generation: Parent–child relationships and the psychological well-being of *in vitro* fertilization children at adolescence. *Child Development, 72*, 599–608.

Golombok, S., MacCallum, F., Goodman, E., & Rutter, M. (2002). Families with children conceived by donor insemination: A follow-up at age twelve. *Child Development, 73*, 952–968.

Golombok, S., MacCallum, F., Murray, C., Lycett, E., & Jadva, V. (2006). Surrogacy families: Parental functioning, parent–child relationships and children's psychological development at age 2. *Journal of Child Psychology and Psychiatry, 47*(2), 213–222.

Golombok, S., Murray, C., Brinsden, P., & Abdalla, H. (1999). Social versus biological parenting: Family functioning and the socioemotional development of children conceived by egg or sperm donation. *Journal of Child Psychology and Psychiatry, 40*, 519–527.

Golombok, S., Murray, C., Jadva, V., MacCallum, F., & Lycett, E. (2004). Families created through surrogacy arrangements: Parent–child relationships in the first year of life. *Developmental Psychology, 40*, 400–411.

Golombok, S., Perry, B., Burston, A., Murray, C., Mooney-Somers, J., Stevens, M., et al. (2003). Children with lesbian parents: A community study. *Developmental Psychology, 39*, 20–33.

Golombok, S., Readings, J., Blake, L., Casey, P., Marks, A., & Jadva, V. (2011). Families created through surrogacy: Mother–child relationships and children's psychological adjustment at age 7. *Developmental Psychology, 47*(6), 1579–1588.

Golombok, S., & Rust, J. (1993). The Pre-School Activities Inventory: A standardized assessment of gender role in children. *Psychological Assessment, 5*, 131–136.

Gringlas, M., & Weinraub, M. (1995). The more things change: Single parenting revisited. *Journal of Family Issues, 16*, 29–52.

Hahn, C., & DiPietro, J. A. (2001). *In vitro* fertilization and the family: Quality of parenting, family functioning, and child psychosocial adjustment. *Developmental Psychology, 37*, 37–48.

Hanson, T. L., McLanahan, S., & Thomson, E. (1997). Economic resources, parental practices, and children's well-being. In G. J. Duncan & J. Brooks-Gunn (Eds.), *Consequences of growing up poor* (pp. 190–238). New York: Russell Sage Foundation.

Hastings, P. D., Vyncke, J., Sullivan, C., McShane, K. E., Benibgui, M., & Utendale, W. (2006). *Children's development of social competence across family types.* Ottawa, Ontario, Canada: Department of Justice, Family, Children and Youth Section.

Hetherington, E. M., & Stanley-Hagan, M. M. (1999). Stepfamilies. In M. E. Lamb (Ed.), *Parenting and child development in "nontraditional" families* (pp. 137–159). Mahwah, NJ: Erlbaum.

Hilton, J. M., Desrochers, S., & Devall, E. L. (2001). Comparison of role demands, relationships, and child functioning in single-mother, single-father, and intact families. *Journal of Divorce and Remarriage, 35*(1/2), 29–56.

Hilton, J. M., & Devall, E. L. (1998). Comparison of parenting and children's behavior in single-mother, single-father, and intact families. *Journal of Divorce and Remarriage, 29*, 23–54.

Hoff, E., Laursen, B., & Tardif, T. (2002). Socioeconomic status and parenting. In M. H. Bornstein (Ed.), *Handbook of parenting: Vol. 4. Social conditions and applied parenting* (pp. 231–251). Mahwah, NJ: Erlbaum.

Homel, R., Burns, A., & Goodnow, J. (1987). Parental social networks and child development. *Journal of Social and Personal Relationships, 4*, 159–177.

Horwitz, A. V., & White, H. R. (1998). The relationship of cohabitation and mental health: A study of a young adult cohort. *Journal of Marriage and the Family, 60*, 505–514.

Horwitz, A. V., White, H. R., & Howell-White, S. (1996). Becoming married and mental health: A longitudinal study of a cohort of young adults. *Journal of Marriage and the Family, 58*, 895–907.

Huggins, S. L. (1989). A comparative study of self-esteem of adolescent children of divorced lesbian mothers and divorced heterosexual mothers. In F. W. Bozett (Ed.), *Homosexuality and the family* (pp. 123–135). New York: Harrington Park Press.

Institut de la Statistic Québec. (2005). Conjugal life of the parents. Gouvernement du Québec, Canada. Retrieved from *www.stat.gouv.qc.ca/donstat/societe/demographie/naisn_deces/naissance/410.htm.*

Javaid, G. A. (1993). The children of homosexual and heterosexual single mothers. *Child Psychiatry and Human Development, 23*, 235–249.

Johnson, S. M., & O'Connor, E. (2001). *Lesbian and gay parents: The National Gay and Lesbian Family Study* (APA Workshop 2). San Francisco: American Psychiatric Association Press.

Kalil, A., & Ryan, R. M. (2010). Mother's economic conditions and sources of support in fragile families. *Future of Children, 20*(2), 39–61.

Lamb, M. E. (1999a). Parental behavior, family processes, and child development in nontraditional and traditionally understudied families. In M. E. Lamb (Ed.), *Parenting and child development in "nontraditional" families* (pp. 1–14). Mahwah, NJ: Erlbaum.

Lamb, M. E. (Ed.). (1999b). *Parenting and child development in "nontraditional" families.* Mahwah, NJ: Erlbaum.

Lamb, M. E. (2012). Mothers, fathers, families, and circumstances: Factors affecting children's adjustment. *Applied Developmental Science, 16*, 98–111.

Landry-Meyer, H., Gerard, J. M., & Guzell, J. R. (2005). Caregiver stress among grandparents raising grandchildren: The functional role of social support. *Marriage and Family Review, 37*(1–2), 171–190.

Lillard, L. A., Brien, M. J., & Waite, L. J. (1995). Premarital cohabitation and subsequent marital dissolution: A matter of self-selection? *Demography, 32*, 437–457.

Luthar, S. S., & Latendresse, S. J. (2005). Children of the affluent: Challenges to well-being. *Current Directions in Psychological Science, 14*, 49–53.

MacCallum, F., Golombok, S., & Brinsden, P. (2007). Parenting and child development in families with a child conceived through embryo donation. *Journal of Family Psychology, 21*(2), 278–287.

Magnuson, K. A., & Duncan, G. J. (2002). Parents in poverty. In M. H. Bornstein (Ed.), *Handbook of parenting: Vol. 4. Social conditions and applied parenting* (2nd ed., pp. 95–121). Mahwah, NJ: Erlbaum.

Manning, W. D. (2004). Children and the stability of cohabiting couples. *Journal of Marriage and Family, 66*, 674–689.

Markiewicz, D., Doyle, A. B., & Brendgen, M. (2001). The quality of adolescents' friendships: Associations with mothers' interpersonal relationships, attachment to parents and friends, and prosocial behaviours. *Journal of Adolescence, 24*, 429–445.

Martin, J., Kochanek, K. D., Strobino, D. M., Guyer, B., & MacDornan, M. F. (2005). Annual summary of vital statistics—2003. *Pediatrics, 115*, 619–634.

McHale, J., Khazan, I., Erera, P., Rotman, T., De Courcey, W., & McConnell, M. (2002). Coparenting in diverse family systems. In M. H. Bornstein (Ed.), *Handbook of parenting: Vol. 3. Being and becoming a parent* (pp. 75–107). Mahwah, NJ: Erlbaum.

McLanahan, S., & Sandefur, G. (1994). *Growing up with a single parent: What hurts, what helps?* Cambridge, MA: Harvard University Press.

McLanahan, S., & Teitler, J. (1999). The consequences of father absence. In M. E. Lamb (Ed.), *Parenting and child development in "nontraditional" families* (pp. 83–102). Mahwah, NJ: Erlbaum.

Meyer, D. R., & Garasky, S. (1993). Custodial fathers: Myths, realities and child support policies. *Journal of Marriage and the Family, 55*, 73–89.

Minkler, M., & Fuller-Thompson, E. (1999). The health of grandparents raising grandchildren: Results of a national study. *American Journal of Public Health, 89*, 1384–1389.

Minkler, M., & Fuller-Thompson, E. (2000). Second time around parenting: Factors predictive of grandparents becoming caregivers for their grandchildren. *International Journal of Aging and Human Development, 50*, 185–200.

Minkler, M., & Fuller-Thompson, E. (2001). Physical and mental health status of American grandparents providing extensive child care to their grandchildren. *Journal of the American Medical Women's Association, 56*, 199–205.

Minkler, M., Fuller-Thompson, E., & Driver, D. (1997). Depression in grandparents raising grandchildren: Results of a national longitudinal study. *Archives of Family Medicine, 6*, 445–452.

Nock, S. L. (1995). A comparison of marriages and cohabiting relationships. *Journal of Family Issues, 16*(1), 53–76.

Nordin, J., Rolnick, S., Ehlinger, E., Nelson, A., Arneson, T., Cherney-Stafford, L., et al. (1998). Lead levels in high-risk and low-risk young children in the Minneapolis–St. Paul metropolitan area. *Pediatrics, 101*, 72–76.

O'Connor, A. (1993). Voices from the heart: The developmental impact of a mother's lesbianism on her adolescent children. *Smith College Studies in Social Work, 63*, 281–299.

Offord, D. R., Boyle, M. H., & Jones, B. R. (1987). Psychiatric disorder and poor school performance among welfare children in Ontario. *Canadian Journal of Psychiatry, 32*, 518–525.

Owen, L., & Golombok, S. (2009). Families created by assisted reproduction: Parent–child relationships in late adolescence. *Journal of Adolescence, 32*(4), 835–848.

Parke, R. D., & Buriel, R. (1998). Socialization in the family: Ethnic and ecological perspectives. In N. Eisenberg (Vol. Ed.) & W. Damon (Series Ed.), *Handbook of child psychology: Vol. 3. Social, emotional, and personality development* (pp. 463–552). New York: Wiley.

Patterson, C. J. (1992). Children of lesbian and gay parents. *Child Development, 63,* 1025–1042.

Patterson, C. J. (2000). Family relationships of lesbians and gay men. *Journal of Marriage and the Family, 62,* 1052–1069.

Patterson, C. J. (2002). Lesbian and gay parenthood. In M. H. Bornstein (Ed.), *Handbook of parenting: Vol. 3. Being and becoming a parent* (2nd ed., pp. 317–338). Hillsdale, NJ: Erlbaum.

Patterson, C. J. (2005). *Lesbian and gay parents and their children: Summary of research findings.* Washington, DC: American Psychological Association.

Patterson, C. J. (2007). Lesbian and gay family issues in the context of changing legal and social policy environments. In K. J. Bieschke, R. M. Perez, & K. A. DeBord (Eds.), *Handbook of counseling and psychotherapy with lesbian, gay, bisexual, and transgender clients* (2nd ed., pp. 359–377). Washington, DC: American Psychological Association.

Patterson, C. J., & Chan, R. W. (1999). Families headed by lesbian and gay parents. In M. E. Lamb (Ed.), *Parenting and child development in "nontraditional" families* (pp. 191–219). Mahwah, NJ: Erlbaum.

Patterson, C. J., Hurt, S., & Mason, C. (1998). Families of the lesbian baby-boom: Children's contact with grandparents and other adults. *American Journal of Orthopsychiatry, 68,* 390–399.

Patterson, C. J., & Riskind, R. G. (2010). To be a parent: Issues in family formation among gay and lesbian adults. *Journal of GLBT Family Studies, 6,* 326–340.

Patterson, C. J., Riskind, R. G., & Tornello, S. L. (2014). Sexual orientation and parenting: A global perspective. In A. Abela & J. Walker (Eds.), *Contemporary issues in family studies: Global perspectives on partnerships, parenting, and support in a changing world* (pp. 189–202). New York: Wiley-Blackwell.

Patterson, G. R., & Fisher, P. A. (2002). Recent developments in our understanding of parenting: Bidirectional effects, causal models, and the search for parsimony. In M. H. Bornstein (Ed.), *Handbook of parenting: Vol. 5. Practical issues in parenting* (pp. 59–88). Mahwah, NJ: Erlbaum.

Perrin, E. C., & the Committee on Psychosocial Aspects of Child and Family Health. (2002). Technical report: Coparent or second-parent adoption by same-sex parents. *Pediatrics, 109,* 341–344.

Pinazo-Hernandis, S., & Tompkins, C. J. (2009). Custodial grandparents: The state of the art and the many faces of this contribution. *Journal of Intergenerational Relationships, 7(2–3),* 137–143.

Raoul-Duvan, A., Bertrand-Servais, M., Letur-Konirsch, H., & Frydman, R. (1994). Psychological follow-up of children born after *in-vitro* fertilization. *Human Reproduction, 9,* 1097–1101.

Ray, V., & Gregory, R. (2001). School experiences of the children of lesbian and gay parents. *Family Matters, 59,* 28–34.

Ross, D. P., Roberts, P. A., & Scott, K. (1998). *Mediating factors in child development outcomes: Children in lone-parent families.* Hull, Québec, Canada: Applied Research Branch Strategic Policy, Human Resources Development.

Santrock, J. W., Warshak, R. A., & Elliott, G. L. (1982). Social development and parent–child interaction in father custody and stepmother families. In M. L. Lamb (Ed.), *Nontraditional families* (pp. 289–314). Hillsdale, NJ: Erlbaum.

Schnayer, R., & Orr, R. (1989). A comparison of children living in single-mother and single-father families. *Journal of Divorce, 12,* 171–184.

Schoenborn, C. A. (2004, December 15). *Marital status and health: United States, 1999–2002* (Advance Data from Vital and Health Statistics, No. 351). Washington, DC: National Center for Health Statistics.

Simmons, T., & O'Connell, M. (2003). *Married-couple and unmarried-partner households: 2000.* Washington, DC: U.S. Bureau of the Census.

Smith, P. K., & Drew, L. M. (2002). Grandparenthood. In M. H. Bornstein (Ed.), *Handbook of parenting: Vol. 3. Being and becoming a parent* (pp. 141–172). Mahwah, NJ: Erlbaum.

Smock, P. J., & Greenland, F. R. (2010). Diversity in pathways to parenthood: Patterns, implications, and emerging research directions. *Journal of Marriage and Family, 72,* 576–593.

Song, C., Benin, M., & Glick, J. (2012). Dropping out of high school: The effects of family structure and family transitions. *Journal of Divorce and Remarriage, 53*(1), 18–33.

Stacey, J., & Biblarz, T. J. (2001). (How) does the sexual orientation of parents matter? *American Sociological Review, 66,* 159–183.

Stanton-Salazar, R. D., & Spina, S. U. (2003). Informal mentors and role models in the lives of urban Mexican-origin adolescents. *Anthropology and Education Quarterly, 34,* 231–254.

Statistics Canada. (2005). *Births 2003* (Catalogue No. 84F0210XIE). Ottawa, Ontario, Canada: Author.

Tasker, F. L., & Golombok, S. (1997). *Growing up in a lesbian family: Effects on child development.* New York: Guilford Press.

Thompson, E., Hanson, T., & McLanahan, S. (1994). Family structure and child well-being: Economic resources vs. parental behaviors. *Social Forces, 73,* 221–242.

van Dam, M. A. (2004). Mothers in two types of lesbian families: Stigma experiences, supports and burdens. *Journal of Family Nursing, 10,* 450–494.

Wagenaar, K., Huisman, J., Cohen-Kettenis, P. T., & van de Wall, H. A. (2008). "An overview of studies on early development, cognition and psychosocial well-being in children born after in vitro fertilization": Erratum. *Journal of Developmental and Behavioral Pediatrics, 29*(5), 410.

Wainright, J. L., & Patterson, C. J. (2006). Delinquency, victimization, and substance use among adolescents with female same-sex parents. *Journal of Family Psychology, 20,* 526–530.

Wainright, J. L., & Patterson, C. J. (2008). Peer relations among adolescents with female same-sex parents. *Developmental Psychology, 44,* 117–126.

Wainright, J. L., Russell, S. T., & Patterson, C. J. (2004). Psychosocial adjustment, school outcomes, and romantic relationships of adolescents with same-sex parents. *Child Development, 75,* 1886–1898.

Waldfogel, J., Craigie, T., & Brooks-Gunn, J. (2010). Fragile families and child wellbeing. *Future of Children, 20*(2), 87–112.

Weinraub, M., Horvath, D. L., & Gringlas, M. B. (2002). Single parenthood. In M. H. Bornstein (Ed.), *Handbook of parenting: Vol. 3. Being and becoming a parent* (pp. 109–140). Mahwah, NJ: Erlbaum.

Weinraub, M., & Wolf, B. M. (1983). Effects of stress and social supports on mother–child interactions in single- and two-parent families. *Child Development, 54,* 1297–1311.

Weinraub, M., & Wolf, B. M. (1987). Stressful life events, social supports, and parent–child interactions: Similarities and differences in single-parent and two-parent families. In C. Boukydis (Ed.), *Research on support for parents and infants in the postnatal period* (pp. 114–135). Westport, CT: Ablex.

Wood, D., Halfon, N., Scarlata, D., Newacheck, P., & Nessim, S. (1993). Impact of family relocation on children's growth, development, school function, and behavior. *Journal of the American Medical Association, 270,* 1334–1338.

Wu, Z. (1995). The stability of cohabitation relationships: The role of children. *Journal of Marriage and the Family, 57,* 231–236.

Zimmerman, M. A., Bingenheimer, J. B., & Notaro, P. C. (2002). Natural mentors and adolescent resiliency: A study with urban youth. *American Journal of Community Psychology, 30,* 221–243.

CHAPTER 10

Socialization and Experiences with Peers

William M. Bukowski
Melisa Castellanos
Frank Vitaro
Mara Brendgen

Consider the daily life of many children in multiple areas of the contemporary world. Just after waking up they head off to school to join their peers. Even before arriving at school, they may have had the company of their peers as they walked, rode their bikes, or took the same transportation together. Even before leaving the house, they may have checked for news from peers in their favored social media sites. Once in school they first hang out with their peers in the schoolyard, the hallways, or the school cafeteria. They then spend the formal instructional part of the school day in their classrooms with their peers. These within-classroom peer experiences comprise many forms of interaction. Peers help each other, observe each other, talk to each other or engage in other forms of communication, and, at times, may get into verbal or even physical tussles. More interactions occur during breaks in the classroom routine such as "recess" and the time set aside for lunch. At the end of the school day, these interactions continue during afterschool activities, such as participation in team sports, afterschool care, and in play with peers in one's neighborhood. Even after face-to-face interactions have come to an end, peers can maintain their contact with each other through 20th- and 21st-century forms of media.

Starting during the preschool years, when many children spend their days in day care centers, experiences with peers can make up a large part of a child's daily life. These experiences can be sources of companionship, stimulation, information, help, rewards, security, joy, and, at times, frustration and harm. They can be as important as they are extensive. For at least seven decades, researchers have been testing hypotheses about the effects that peers have on each other. In this chapter we review and comment on the theory and the empirical data base related to the premise that experiences with peers constitute an important socialization domain for children and adolescents. According to this view, peers serve an important function in children's lives that goes beyond opportunities for companionship. We demonstrate that there is increasing evidence that experiences with peers affect the emotions that children and adolescents experience, how they think about themselves, and how they behave. We also demonstrate that some basic hypotheses about peer relations require more empirical scrutiny than they have received already.

There have been several large reviews of the literature on peer relations. These reviews, written by Hartup (1970, 1983) and others (e.g., Parker & Asher, 1987; Rubin, Bukowski, & Parker, 1998, 2006 , in press), have covered a broad set of domains in which peers appear to function, however unwittingly, as socialization agents. These domains include prosocial behavior, school performance, affect, aggression, the self-concept, and other areas of development. This chapter is organized in the following way. We first describe a model of the structure of the peer group, then discuss the major theoretical perspectives regarding the effects of peer experience. Finally, we present findings from the empirical literature that shows how peer relations affect children's development.

Organizing the Features of Peer Relations

For at least a century, social developmental psychologists have shown an interest in understanding the experiences that children have with their agemates (Monroe, 1986). Influenced by ethology and by social psychologists interested in the social mechanisms underlying behavior change, the study of peers was initially steeped in observational traditions that emphasized the influence that children had on each other. In parallel to this interest in influence was a concern with the antecedents and consequences of how much a child was liked and disliked by peers (Northway, 1944). During the past 30 years, the study of peers has increased, especially as investigators have recognized the extent to which measures of functioning with peers are related to subsequent measures of well-being and adjustment (Parker & Asher, 1987).

Levels of Social Complexity

Children's experiences with peers can be organized according to a multilevel model in which aspects of peer relations may occur at the level of the individual, the dyad, or the group (Rubin et al., 2006). According to this organizational scheme, based largely on the work of Hinde (1995), phenomena from different levels of experience are conceptually distinct from but functionally and experientially *interdependent* with phenomena at other levels. According to this model, the *level* of the individual refers to the characteristics that children bring with them to their experiences with peers. *Interactions* refer to what children do with each other. They are a form of experience that occurs at the level of the dyad, and are believed to be influenced by these individual characteristics, as well as by features of the social situation, such as the partner's characteristics, overtures, and responses. Interactions, in turn, form the basis of relationships. *Relationships* refer to the internal representations that members of the dyad build up, based on interactional experiences. Important examples of relationship variables are security and closeness (Bukowski, Hoza, & Boivin, 1993; Furman & Buhrmester, 1985). Finally, relationships are embedded within *groups*, or networks of relationships with more or less clearly defined boundaries (e.g., cliques, teams, school classes). Groups are defined by the affective and behavioral links between their members and by the types of behavioral tendencies and attitudes shared by the group members. Groups are not the same as a mere aggregate of relationships; through properties such as norms or shared cultural conventions, groups help define the type and range of relationships and interactions that are likely or permissible. Furthermore, groups have properties and processes, such as hierarchical organization and cohesiveness, that affect the extent to which children have opportunities for connection with and influence over others. A critical feature of this approach is the premise that although experiences and characteristics from the levels of the individual, the dyad, and the group are very different forms of social complexity, they are nevertheless interrelated.

The heuristic value of the three-level model comes from its apparent utility. It provides an intuitive and well-structured organizational scheme for categorizing the constructs and variables that are used in research on peer relations. It is important to recognize, however, that in spite of these benefits, the application of the model to some crucial variables can be more challenging than the model's apparent conceptual clarity would suggest. Ironically, the difficulty of applying the multilevel model in an unambiguous manner can be demonstrated when one uses it to categorize one of the most widely used constructs in the peer literature, specifically, *peer acceptance* (i.e., the extent to which a child is liked by members of the peer group). Insofar as acceptance refers to how much a person is liked by others, it can be seen as the result of an intersection between characteristics and processes at the level of the person, and characteristics and processes at the level of the group. For this reason, acceptance exists at the interface between the person and the group rather than clearly belonging to one or the other. These concerns can be applied to three other widely studied constructs, specifically, *rejection* (i.e., the degree to which a child is disliked by peers), *popularity* (i.e., the extent to which a child is *perceived* to be well liked or to have a position of status within a group; Bukowski, 2011), and *victimization* (i.e., the extent to which a child is treated badly by peers). Whereas acceptance and rejection are measured directly via the use of *sociometric measures* (i.e., techniques that measure the attractions and repulsions between persons; see Bukowski, Cillessen, & Velasquez, 2012), popularity is typically measured with peer assessments (i.e., techniques that measure how a child is perceived by others) that assign a "popularity" score to children according to how often they are chosen for items such as "someone who is popular" or "someone who is liked by everyone" (see Cillessen & Marks, 2011, for a full discussion of how popularity is measured). Victimization also is typically measured with peer assessment techniques.

This lack of clarity about where some constructs fit within the multilevel model does not invalidate the model but instead points to the critical interdependencies that exist between levels. This interdependency poses two interrelated challenges for research on peer relations. One is conceptual, whereas the other is methodological. The conceptual challenge concerns the development and application of theory about not only the constructs and processes at each level but also the ways that constructs from different levels intersect to affect outcome. The methodological challenge concerns the techniques needed to bring multiple levels of social complexity together in the same model. Each of these challenges is discussed in the next section.

Theory

Starting with the Dyad

Broad conceptual approaches to understanding peer relations were developed in the mid-20th century, more than 50 years ago. Typically, the models developed at that time emphasized dyadic-level variables and processes. They did so in an implied rather than an explicit way. Specifically, these perspectives emphasized aspects of interaction that were derived from the basic processes implicated in social learning theory. Two forms of interaction, specifically, reinforcement and imitation, were given the most attention. Research by Hartup and his colleagues, using laboratory-based analogue studies, provided compelling evidence that children imitate their peers, and that children's behavior can be shaped by reinforcements received from peers (see Hartup, 1964; Hartup & Coates, 1967; Hartup, Glazer, & Charlesworth, 1967). These laboratory-based studies were important in that they showed clearly that peers could affect each other and that these patterns of influence could occur via well-established behavioral mechanisms. They led to the widespread adoption of a traditional learning theory perspective that peers function as agents of behavioral control and behavioral change via the application of rewards for the behaviors considered appropriate and competent, and the use of punishments or the absence of rewards for behaviors that are seen to impede individual or group functioning. Moreover, findings from studies of the effects of imitation indicated that children use each other as sources of information about the forms of behavior that are most appropriate for functioning with peers.

Theory at the level of the dyad has also taken a relationships perspective. The best-known theory about the effects of peer relationships can be found in the writings of Sullivan (1953). Sullivan proposed that as children enter early adolescence, they begin to develop "chumships" or close, intimate mutual relationships with same-sex peers. As a relationship between "co-equals," chumship differs from the hierarchical relationships that children experience with their parents and the play-based interactions of childhood. Accordingly, Sullivan argued that this close relationship was a child's first true interpersonal experience of reciprocity and exchange. He proposed that it was within chumships that children had their first opportunities to experience a sense of self-validation. This validation would result from the internalization of the positive regard and care that their chums provided to them. Sullivan went so far as to propose that the positive experiences of having a "chum" in adolescence would be powerful enough to enable adolescents to overcome trauma that may have resulted from prior family experiences. Conversely, Sullivan believed that the experience of being isolated from the group, during the juvenile period, would lead a child to have concerns about his or her own competencies and acceptability as a desirable peer. Consequently, Sullivan suggested that children who are unable to establish a position within the peer group would develop feelings of inferiority that could contribute to a sense of psychological distress. One posited outcome of the lack of supportive chumship was the development of loneliness, or "the exceedingly unpleasant and driving experience connected with the inadequate discharge of the need for human intimacy" (Sullivan, 1953, p. 290).

Although the studies of the processes drawn from social learning theory were largely concerned with interactional mechanisms, they also revealed evidence of the power of relationships. Hartup (1964) showed that children were more likely to be reinforced by friends than by nonfriends, and that the reinforcement received from friends had stronger effects than reinforcement from nonfriends. Similar conclusions can be reached about the effects of imitation (see Hartup, 1970, for a summary). Specifically, it has been shown that children are more likely to imitate friends than nonfriends.

To some extent, the role of the dyad is apparent also in the work of Piaget (1932). In parallel with the ideas of Sullivan, Piaget claimed that the critical feature of peer relationships is the degree of balance in power between peers. He argued that, in contrast to relationships with parents, experiences with peers would be more egalitarian, and along a more or less horizontal plane of dominance and power assertion. Thus, it was in the peer context that children could experience opportunities to examine conflicting ideas and explanations, to negotiate and discuss multiple perspectives, and to decide to compromise with or to reject the ideas and perspectives held by peers. In these ways, interactions with peers were an ideal context for the development of social constructs such as those related to moral judgment.

The influence of Piaget is seen in the work of co-constructivist thinkers such as Azmitia, Lippman, and Ittel (1999). These writers introduced the notion that the quality of the relationship between the peers who are interacting with each other may contribute to cognitive and social cognitive growth and development. Given that friends are more sensitive to each other's needs, and more supportive of each other's thoughts and well-being than nonfriends, it may be that children are more likely to talk openly and challenge each other's thoughts and deeds in the company of friends than nonfriends. Accordingly, these relationships are likely to have unique effects on a child's thoughts and behaviors.

Peers also play a role in the theory of Vygotsky (1978). Whereas Piaget emphasized the effects of conflict between peers (i.e., that conflicts would led to disequilibrium that would, in turn, lead to accommodation), Vygotsky proposed that it was *cooperation* and the discussion of ideas that would promote change. According to Vygotsky, the cooperative co-construction of social events led to the formation of social constructs. Researchers such as Rogoff (1997) have argued that the child's peers can play the role of co-constructivist, and that the pairing of a less mature child with a more competent "expert" peer may facilitate a child's development.

Aside from its positive effects on affect and the self-concept, friendship has been ascribed two important protective effects. We alluded to one already, specifically, Sullivan's claim that friendship has the capacity to minimize the negative effects of being from a nonoptimal family. The second form of protection is related to negative peer experiences, specifically, victimization and rejection. Two theorists (Davies, 1982; Rizzo, 1989) ascribed a particular protective function to friendship, specifically, the ability to protect at-risk children from victimization by peers. Both theorists claimed that children who were at risk for victimization due to their own individual characteristics, such as aggression and withdrawal, would be spared from victimization by having a friend. Like Blatz (1966) and Sullivan (1953), they adopted the view that relationships (i.e., friendships) function so as to maximize security. In an extension of these views, it has been argued that, beyond their capacity to protect at-risk children from negative experiences, friendships can protect children from the affective consequences that typically result from being victimized or rejected by peers (see Hodges, Boivin, Vitaro, & Bukowski, 1999; Parker & Asher, 1993).

One of the weaknesses of most theories about friendship is the lack of a clear identification of the basic features of friendship. It has been pointed out already that some theories have emphasized particular aspects of the friendship. An example would be Sullivan's emphasis on security and validation. A more comprehensive approach can be found in the provision model proposed by Furman and his colleagues (Furman & Buhrmester, 1985; Furman & Robbins, 1985). Building on Sullivan's (1953) implicit claim that it is the features or provisions of friendship that matter, they proposed that children seek specific opportunities or affordances in their friendships. Whereas some provisions are forms of interaction (e.g., companionship, disclosure, and help), others refer to aspects of relationships (e.g., intimacy, security). A very strong claim appears to be central to Furman and colleagues' ideas about friendship and its provisions. It is that children and adolescents whose friendships offer these provisions show higher levels of well-being than children whose friendships lack them.

In summary, theory at the level of the dyad has emphasized interactions and relationships. Understandably, interaction-oriented perspectives have emphasized peer effects on behavior, whereas relationship-oriented perspectives have emphasized peer effect on affect and self-perceptions. A limitation to interaction-oriented models is the lack of clear ideas about how the effects of interactions would vary across relationship partners. In contrast, relationships models provide inspiring ideas about the importance of friendship for well-being, but they never specify the exact processes by which these experiences produce their effects.

Theory at the Level of the Group

Peer research has seen an increase of interest in group processes. *Groups* are collections of peers who interact and have relationships with each other. Although groups are the context for many dyadic experiences, they are not a mere collection of dyads (Kindermann & Gest, 2009). Instead, they present their own dynamics and need to be understood according to their own constructs and processes.

The peer group can be conceptualized according to constructs representing content and structure. Measures of *content*, such as group norms, refer to the behaviors, activities, values, and attitudes that characterize a group and distinguish it from other groups. *Norms* have been defined as the acceptable and expected behavior of the members of a social group (Shaw, 1981). Levine and Moreland (1998) added to this concept the idea that all members of the group should to a large extent share such expectations. It has been proposed that norms serve four functions: (1) to integrate people into the group; (2) to establish a frame of reference for interactions within the group; (3) to provide an implicit justification for group activities; and (4) to facilitate ingroup identification by providing a point of distinction from other groups (Shaw, 1981). In summary, norms act as the social regulators of any given group. Their essential form is quantitative in the sense that measures of content refer to how much or how little of a particular variable is seen in a particular group.

Structure refers to the strength and pattern of association between the persons in a group (Kelly, Ryan, Altman, & Stelzner, 2000). Measures of structure are indices of the interconnections between group members. Well-known structural aspects of the peer group are cohesion, collectivism and individualism, and dominance or hierarchy. *Cohesion* has been defined as the set of forces that keep group members together (Dion, 2000). It may also be defined as the organization of the links between group members (Vacha, McDonald, Coburn, & Black, 1979). This organization can be indexed according to the strength of the direct and indirect links between persons, which can be measured with sociometric procedures (see Cillessen, 2009). It can also be conceptualized according to the relative emphasis in the group on collectivism and individualism (Triandis, 2001). Whereas *collectivism* refers to an emphasis on the connections between people and respect for and sensitivity to the needs and emotions of others, *individualism* refers to the emphasis placed on individual achievement, self-reliance, and autonomy. These two dimensions refer to different conceptualizations of how the members of a group are interrelated.

Dominance, or *hierarchy*, another important structural feature of groups, refers to the degree to which there are imbalances or heterogeneity in power and influence among group members. Whereas some groups have an egalitarian structure, in which all members have the same effect on the direction and activity of the group, others are structured along lines of power, in which some members have more influence than others. The concept of dominance can be used not only to distinguish groups from each other and to describe the position of individuals within groups, but they can also identify smaller groups within the larger peer structure. For example, groups include core and marginal members (Hogg & Reid, 2006). Within a group, core members are highly visible, popular, and socially powerful. Thus, core members have the power to persuade other group members to think like them and agree with them (Berscheid & Reis, 1998). In some cases, status as a core member spans a number of groups. For example, Sussman, Pokhrel, Ashmore, and Brown (2007) have identified a core group of "populars" who dominate the school setting. In contrast, marginal group members have relatively little status and power, and their membership status within the group is more likely to fluctuate than that of a core member.

Although the content and the structure of groups can be seen as distinct concepts, it is likely that their effects derive from an interaction between them. That is, the effects of content are likely to vary as a function of structure. When structural components such as cohesion or collectivism are higher, the impact of the group's content (e.g., positive attitudes about academic achievement) may be stronger than when they are lower. In this regard, the interactive combination of structure and content may be a more effective way of understanding and measuring the group climate than use of either of these phenomena alone.

There appear to be two conceptual points of departure to recent efforts to put the "group" back into peer group research. One is the perspective that the human urge to belong to social groups motivates children and adolescents to conform to group expectations and norms (Baumeister & Leary, 1995). As noted earlier, the "glue" or cohesive forces that hold groups together are drawn from the shared values, attitudes, and behaviors of its constituent members (Brown, McNeil, & Glenberg, 2009; Bukowski & Sippola, 2001; Kindermann & Gest, 2009). Group members are interconnected via patterns of dyadic associations and the sharing of common interests and social conventions. These shared values and norms enforce appropriate within-group interactions between members. Presumably it is the motivation to fit in and the effect of within-group pressures to conform that account for the effect of group experience on children's and adolescents' behavior. According to another view, recently summarized by Gazelle (2013), group structures can offer affective provisions that are similar to those available in friendship relations. Gazelle has argued that via processes such as inclusion and exclusion, groups create an affective climate that can either support or minimize individual-level characteristics such as anxiety beyond the level of the child's own sense of exclusion.

In summary, there has been a renewed interest in the features and functions of the peer group. Peer researchers have developed new constructs to measures the "content" of the group and to assess aspects of group structure. Content-based group characteristics (e.g., norms), structural features of groups (e.g., cohesion and hierarchy strength), and cultural dimensions (e.g., individualism and collectivism) have been identified as factors that account for the effects of group experience in individual-level behavior.

Theory at the Level of the Individual

Typically, the individual is seen as the most basic level of the multilevel approach. In this discussion, theory related to the individual is presented last, since most of the ideas regarding individual-level constructs are intertwined with either dyadic or group functioning. This intersection between levels is implied in the conceptualization of individual-level variables as the person-centered characteristics that children bring to and take away from their dyadic and group experiences with peers. Individual-level variables are diverse. They can be demographic (e.g., age, sex, and race), aspects of personality (e.g., temperament and patterns of physiological response to arousal such as inhibition, exuberance, sociability, and emotion reactivity and regulation), ontogenetic (i.e., developmental history), reputational (i.e., how a person is seen by peers), social cognitive skills and forms of social competence (e.g., social problem-solving and social information-processing skills), self-perceptions (e.g., perceptions of one's competence and self-esteem), and social goals and motivation (e.g., needs for dominance or affiliation). The key feature of variables at the level of the individual is that they are characteristics of the person per se.

The individual-level variables that have been studied most extensively are aggression, sociability, and withdrawal. These broadband constructs reflect the fundamental behavioral orientations of moving against others, moving toward others, and moving away from others. These dimensions of peer-related social behavior have been a mainstay of peer research (see reviews in Bukowski & Véronneau, 2014; Rubin et al., in press). Individual-level variables can function as the antecedents, or even the causes, of individual differences in peer experience at the level of the dyad or group, and they can be the result or consequences of experiences at other levels of complexity. For example, aggression has been known to be a cause of rejection by peers (Bukowski & Newcomb, 1984) presumably due to the disruptive effects that this behavior has on interactions with peers, whereas the stability of anxious withdrawal is known to be exacerbated by features of the group, such as the degree to which some group members are excluded from group activities (Gazelle, 2013). The basic point of theory regarding the level of the individual is that insofar as children bring specific characteristics, such as behavioral tendencies, competencies, and needs, to their interactions with peers at the dyadic and group levels, there will be corresponding differences between children in dyadic and group experiences and differences in the effects of these experiences. It is well known that, in general, withdrawal and aggression put children at risk for rejection (Newcomb, Bukowski, & Pattee, 1993) and that individual-level characteristics are implicated in friendship formation (Hawley, Little, & Card, 2007).

In the past decade, peer researchers have focused on several new individual-level constructs and variables. Three new and important directions in the assessment of individual characteristics related to peer relations are especially noteworthy. They are behavior genetics, the assessment of behavioral activation and inhibition, and developmental variations in neural functioning. Quantitative genetic models, described by Brendgen, Vitaro, and Girard (2012), have allowed researchers to assess the extent to which a particular outcome or phenotype derives from genetic factors, which is an individual-level variable, and environmental factors that are unique to a person and that are shared between people. Well-structured statistical analyses of data taken from monozygotic and dizygotic twins provide powerful methods for assessing the effects of a basic individual-level feature. More complex models that include measures of the environment can provide estimates of the degree to which genetic factors are correlated with environmental factors and, more importantly, the extent to which genetic effects are moderated by environmental conditions (Brendgen et al., 2012).

Another new direction concerns individual differences in the degree to which persons prefer to approach or to avoid social situations. Initially outlined by Gray and McNaughton (2000), this perspective was restated to include an emphasis on peer interaction and social anxiety by Wardell, O'Connor, Read, and Colder (2011). Whereas the *behavioral activation system* (BAS) was conceived as a neural-based mechanism that increases approach behaviors via sensitivity to reward, the *behavioral inhibition system* (BIS) was conceived as a system that inhibits social behavior in response to conditioned aversive stimuli. There is already evidence that children who score high on measures of BIS are more likely than other children to have negative views of their peer relations and to have elevated levels of internalizing problems such as depression, anxiety, and behavioral avoidance (e.g., Coplan, Wilson, Frohlick, & Zelenski, 2006; Kingsbury, Coplan, Weeks, & Rose-Krasnor, 2013; Muris, Meesters, de Kanter, & Timmerman, 2005). There is also evidence that the combination of low levels of BIS and high levels of BAS predicts socioemotional competence (Kingsbury et al., 2013).

Another neural-based individual-level approach is seen in research showing that during early adolescence, reward-sensitive aspects of neural functioning develop earlier than neural mechanisms related to control (Paus, 2005), and that this age-related difference in neural development moderates the effects of peer experience. Specifically, there is evidence that the effects of peer influence are stronger during early adolescence, when reward-sensitive areas of the limbic system have matured, than they are in late adolescence, after the control mechanisms based in the prefrontal cortex have developed (Albert, Chein, & Steinberg, 2013; Albert & Steinberg, 2011; Chein, Albert, O'Brien, Uckert, & Steinberg, 2011; Paus et al., 2008).

In summary, children bring multiple personal characteristics with them to their peer relations. These include behavioral tendencies, skills, needs, forms of temperament, developmental history, competencies, and predispositions that derive from neural or genetic processes. It is probably not an exaggeration to say that nearly every study of peer relations includes at least one individual-level variable as either an antecedent or consequence of dyadic or group experiences.

The Interface between Individual, Dyad, and Group

Theory about peer relations needs to address three challenges related to the intersection or interdependency between different levels of social complexity. The first challenge is to explain how phenomena at one level are associated with phenomena at another level. Nearly every theory deals with this challenge to at least a minimal degree in the sense that particular processes are typically identified relative to the associations between measures from different levels. Theories vary, however, in the degree to which they deal with the second challenge, which concerns the degree to which the measures identified at the two levels are given the same level of attention and detailed description and explanation. In many theories there is an imbalance in the description of the measures from different levels. For example, Sullivan (1953) and others (Furman & Robbins, 1985) provide a rich conceptualization of friendship, but do not provide an equally rich conceptualization or description of the specific outcomes to which aspects of friendship are expected to be associated. This issue is a challenge for researchers because of its critical importance for the understanding of the particular effects that a form of experience is expected to have. This lack of clarity impedes our understanding of the processes and effects related to peers relations, and it hinders the development of clear hypotheses. To some extent, the third challenge is parallel to the second. It concerns the degree of variation in the effects of peer experiences. Theories differ in the degree to which they claim that effects of particular processes are general or specific. Whereas general effects are roughly the same across individuals (i.e., they are invariant), specific effects are those that are stronger for some persons than for others. These specific effects can either be "person effects" that vary as a function of individual-level characteristics (Magnusson & Stattin, 1998) or contextual effects that vary as a function of group or cultural characteristics (Spencer, 2006). Some theories appear to make claims about both generality and specificity. A good example of this focus on the intersection between multiple levels of complexity is the hypothesis proposed by Davies (1982) and Rizzo (1989) that friendship protects at-risk children from victimization by peers. Central to this hypothesis is the claim that the effects of an experience at the level of the dyad (i.e., friendship) will have stronger effects on children whose individual-level characteristics (i.e., aggression and withdrawal) put them at risk for a negative experience within the peer group. In this way, friendship may have some general positive effects, but its effects will be stronger for some children than for others.

Summary

Theory about peer relations has emphasized constructs and processes at the level of the dyad, the group, and the individual. According to these perspectives, experiences with peers can affect behavior, cognition, self-perceptions, and emotional well-being. There are differences in the degree to which various theories emphasize forms of experience or processes. Whereas Sullivan (1953), Piaget (1932), and Vygotsky (1978) emphasized the dyad, more recent theorists have emphasized group constructs. Other theories, especially social learning theory, did not explicitly focus on a particular level of experience but instead emphasized processes that would account for the effects of experiences, particularly those that occurred within peer interactions. Although theory about the dyad is rich in constructs and outcomes, it has not been as effective in promoting the development of well-defined measures and in demonstrating the processes underlying dyadic effects. The strength of current theory about the group is the specification of a set of well-defined constructs and variables that can be used to measure content- and structure-oriented aspects of group characteristics. In contrast, theory about the group has been weak in its specification of the processes by which its rich constructs affect behavioral and affective outcomes. The next wave of theoretical advances in the area of peer relations needs to focus on the intersection between phenomena from different levels of social complexity.

In spite of these limitations in theory, empirical research on peer relations has produced an extensive data base demonstrating the effects that experiences with peers have on behavior and well-being. In the second half of this chapter we provide a selective review of this literature. In the version of this chapter (Bukowski, Brendgen, & Vitaro, 2007) in the previous edition of this volume, our discussion of the effects of peer relations centered largely on internalizing and eternalizing problems. In this chapter, we provide a summary and update of the literature and expand our discussion to cover a broader set of topics, including the socialization of emotions.

Effects of Peer Relations on Externalizing Problems

An important theme of research on peer relations and aggression is that to understand how aggression develops, one needs to look beyond factors at the level of the individual (Brechwald & Prinstein, 2011; Cohen, Hsueh, Russell, & Ray, 2006). Cohen and colleagues (2006) emphasized the need to recognize that aggression can result, at least indirectly, from group and dyadic experiences. At the level of the group, researchers have shown that negative experiences with peers can lead to subsequent aggression. Much of this research has emphasized rejection. Dyad-oriented research has emphasized the effects of associating with deviant peers.

A methodological challenge to demonstrating the effects of peer experience is the need to control for selection effects. Specifically, an observed association between a child's behavior and the characteristics of friends may be due to multiple factors, such as the homophilic tendency of children to associate with peers to whom they are similar. Accordingly, the observation of a correlation between a child's behavior and the behavior of the peers with whom the child affiliates is not sufficient evidence of a socialization effect. Instead, one needs to use procedures to control for initial values either statistically, as in a longitudinal design, or via random assignment, as in an experimental approach.

Negative Experiences with Peers

Studies of peer rejection, exclusion, and victimization provide evidence of a causal effect of peer experience on externalizing problems. The findings are strongest for rejection. Typically, these studies show that earlier peer rejection uniquely predicts later externalizing problems, even after researchers control for initial levels of problems, particularly when accumulative peer rejection (i.e., rejection by peers for more than 1 year) is considered (Brendgen, Vitaro, & Bukowski, 2000; Deater-Deckard, Dodge, Bates, & Pettit, 1998; Ladd & Troop-Gordon, 2003; Lansford, Malone, Dodge, Pettit, & Bates, 2010). For example, Ladd and Troop-Gordon (2003) showed that the number of years children were rejected by their peers during the first 3 years of primary school predicted later externalizing problems (i.e., teacher-rated aggression and delinquency), above and beyond previous aggressive behaviors (which predicted chronic rejection), concurrent peer victimization, and involvement in mutual friendships. Moreover, as argued by Nelson and Dishion (2004), peer rejection during childhood may predict later delinquent–criminal problems at periods even when these problems are declining in most individuals, such as young adulthood. The predictive power of peer rejection with respect to early adulthood outcomes, however, may not be independent of the presence or the absence of friendships. For example, Bagwell, Newcomb, and Bukowski (1998) showed that the presence of externalizing problems (i.e., trouble with the law) during early adulthood was predicted only by a combination of peer rejection and absence of mutual friends over two consecutive years. Indeed, there is evidence that other forms of negative peer experience that may co-occur with rejection (e.g., victimization and exclusion) can lead to aggression (Cohen et al., 2006).

Lansford and colleagues (2010) took a process-oriented approach to understand how rejection leads to aggression. They reported that the association between rejection and aggression can be explained by the mediating effects of decreased problem-solving skills. Specifically, their findings supported a mediational model in which peer rejection led to a decrease in social problem-solving skills, which in turn led to higher levels of aggression. As importantly, they showed that rejection and aggression were associated in a transactional manner, with each functioning as an antecedent of the other. Similar findings have been reported by Prinstein, Rancourt, Guerry, and Browne (2009). Consistent with this pattern of results, other studies have shown that the link between personal dispositions (i.e., aggression) and later externalizing problems was exacerbated for individuals who were also rejected by their peers (Bierman & Wargo, 1995). For example, Dodge and colleagues (2003) found that peer rejection in kindergarten interacted with early aggression in predicting later aggression. More specifically, children who were initially aggressive and also rejected by their peers were more likely to show an increase in their aggressive behavior than were rejected classmates who were not initially aggressive. This effect was particularly true for children who scored high on reactive but not on proactive aggression, and for girls.

However, some studies that did not find support for peer rejection as a moderator of the link between childhood aggression and later externalizing problems. For example, Miller-Johnson, Coie, Maumary-Gremaud, Bierman, and the Conduct Problems Prevention Research Group (2002) showed that peer rejection in grade 1 predicted conduct problems 4 years later, independently of children's initial levels of aggression and hyperactivity–inattention. More recent research has replicated and extended these findings. An experimental study has shown that the effects of being rejected relative to aggression are especially strong for children who are isolated from peers (i.e., not included in activities), and that the subsequent aggressive behavior shown by an isolated and rejected child is typically aimed at the peers who have rejected him or her (Reijntjes et al., 2010).

With respect to potential moderators of the link between early peer rejection and subsequent antisocial behavior, some researchers have concluded that the link appears to be stronger and more consistent across studies for boys than for girls (McDougall, Hymel, Vaillancourt, & Mercier, 2001). As noted by Deater-Deckard (2001), however, this conclusion may very well be an artifact of the number of studies including only males and of the use of measures that apply more to males than to females. The picture may change as girls are more frequently included in studies of externalizing problems.

It is likely that several processes account for the effect of peer rejection on aggression. One may be that peer rejection alters self-perceptions and self-capabilities for achieving positive outcomes (McDougall et al., 2001). Moreover, peer rejection can also decrease school motivation and increase school difficulties, which in turn may exacerbate or trigger externalizing behaviors (Hymel, Comfort, Schonert-Reichl, & McDougall, 1996). Rejection reduces a child's opportunities to interact with and learn normative values from conventional peers. As proposed by Furman and Robbins (1985), a unique function of peer acceptance is to provide a sense of inclusion and a source of motivation to participate in activities involving peers. The absence of such feelings may very well drive rejected children away from their normative but rejecting peers and the contexts in which they interact with them, including the school. As they become more extensively associated with non-normative peers, they may be more susceptible to more deviant influences, including those that support externalizing problems.

Effects at the Level of the Dyad

There is substantial empirical evidence supporting the negative influence of deviant peers. Several researchers have shown that association with deviant peers at the dyadic level (i.e., on a one-to-one basis) is related to externalizing problems (Kim, Hetherington, & Reiss, 1999; Scaramella, Conger, Spoth, & Simons, 2002; Simons, Chao, Conger, & Elder, 2001). Consistent with social learning principles, both behaviors and attitudes favorable to aggression can be learned from association with a deviant friend (Brendgen, Bowen, Rondeau, & Vitaro, 1999). According to this model, affiliation with a deviant friend may mediate the link between aggression and peer rejection on the one hand, and the emergence or increases in externalizing problems on the other. It can also mediate the link between family dysfunction and antisocial behavior in adolescence (Kim et al., 1999). Finally, affiliation with a deviant peer can have a unique additive effect, above and beyond other factors. As suggested by Fergusson, Swain-Campbell, and Horwood (2002), the weight of the contribution of having a deviant peer to criminal activity and substance use may depend on when it is assessed (i.e., adolescence vs. early adulthood).

More recent studies provide ample evidence for the role of aggression in dyadic processes. Sijtsema and colleagues (2010) showed that during early adolescence, instrumentally and relationally aggressive peers became mutual friends with similar peers, and that evidence of the influence of friends as leading to either higher or lower levels of aggression could be observed for all types of aggression except physical aggression. These findings suggest that the more socially oriented forms of aggression (e.g., instrumental, reactive, and relational aggression) may be the most susceptible to social influence. Similarly, Laursen Hafen, Kerr, and Stattin (2012) used a two-wave social relations model to demonstrate friendship effects on delinquent behavior. Their findings are especially informative in their demonstration that the effects of a friend are stronger when the friend is well liked by other peers.

Effects of dyadic experiences on aggression have been attributed to reward-based mechanisms, sometimes referred to as *deviancy training* (Dishion & Piehler, 2009). Deviancy training comprises several forms of interaction, such as encouragement, praise, and expression of expectations, that function to increase a peer's overall level of aggressive behavior. Deviancy training takes place when a child rewards or models aggression for a friend or partner. There is evidence that deviancy training occurs in children as young as 5 years old, and that its effects can be seen across childhood and adolescence (e.g., Snyder, Schrepferman, Bullard, McEachern, & Patterson, 2012). It is important to recognize that the concept of deviancy training is the intellectual descendant of Hartup's (1964) studies of peer reinforcement from five decades ago.

Effects at the Level of the Group

There are two forms of evidence showing that group-level experience leads to changes in levels of aggression. One form of evidence was reported by Espelage, Holt, and Henkel (2003). They used a longitudinal design to examine the effect of group context on children's aggressive behavior. Data regarding friendship choice patterns at the first of two assessments were used to create peer groups. An aggression score was computed for each child and for each group. Using a multilevel approach, Espelage and colleagues showed that being in an aggressive group led either to stability or to an increased level of aggression, whereas being in a group low in aggression led to a decrease.

Another form of evidence comes from studies of popularity and aggression. Since the 1980s, it has been known that measures of aggression are often positively associated with measures of popularity and acceptance in the peer group (Cairns, Cairns, Neckerman, Gest, & Gariépy, 1988). This association has been observed to be stronger for girls than for boys, and stronger for measures of relational aggression than for measures of physical aggression (Rose, Swenson, & Waller, 2004). There is also evidence from two well-known longitudinal studies that measures of status predict subsequent levels of aggression, even after researchers accounted for the original level of aggression (Cillessen & Mayeux, 2004; Rose, Swenson, et al., 2004). Cillessen and Mayeux (2004) reported that a measure of popularity predicted physical and relational aggression for both genders across multiple 6-month intervals. Using a similar design, Rose, Swenson, and colleagues (2004) found that for early adolescent girls and boys, a measure of popularity predicted increased relational aggression also across a 6-month interval. These findings are consistent with experimental results (Keltner, Gruenfeld, & Anderson, 2003) indicating that individuals who were assigned higher status within a group context showed an increase in uninhibited negative social assertion relative to other group members. Interpretations of these findings typically invoke the idea that the power inherent in status has the insidious effect of providing a form of *license* that permits high-status persons to function outside of usual social constraints, such as the sanctions against aggressive behavior and other types of proscribed risk. These findings might appear to contradict the previously discussed evidence that rejection can lead to aggression. To understand what might appear to be a contradiction, one needs to remember that measures of popularity typically are only weakly associated with measures of acceptance. Most importantly, these findings indicate that there are many pathways by which experiences with peers can lead to aggression.

Summary

Four kinds of experience—peer rejection, associations with aggressive friends, being in aggressive groups, and being popular—have been shown to contribute to changes in aggressive behaviors in peers. Each of these experiences has resulted in higher levels of externalizing behaviors. With the exception of the research on rejection, research in the area has been more concerned with "content" than with "structure." Specifically, the current data base points to the importance of group norms and friend characteristics as the factors that account for behavioral change. Attention to structural features of groups should be included in the next wave of studies in this area, including the degree to which factors such as cohesion may minimize within-group antagonism. Also, aspects of friendship and interactional processes, such as reward mechanisms and imitation, which were the focus of studies five decades ago, need to be included in research on dyads.

Peer Relations and Internalizing Issues/Emotional Well-Being

A major point of peer research is that experiences with peers influence affective well-being (Parker & Asher, 1987). The study of effects of peer relations on affective well-being has typically targeted three variables, specifically, rejection by the peer group, peer victimization, and friendships. The overriding conclusion of the literatures on rejection and victimization is that these negative experiences with peers subsequently lead to higher levels of affective distress (see Prinstein et al., 2009, for a review). Several well-controlled studies have shown that being victimized by peers predicts internalizing problems such as anxiety, depression, and loneliness (e.g., Reijntjes, Kamphuis, Prinzie, & Telch, 2010). As with the effect of rejection on aggression, however, the relation between victimization and negative outcomes appears to be best understood as following a transactional course (Ostrov, 2010; van Lier et al., 2012). Insofar as victimized children often attribute these negative experiences to their own characteristics, they put themselves at risk for problems of an internalizing nature (Graham & Juvonen, 1998; Perren, Ettekal, & Ladd, 2013; Prinstein, Cheah, & Guyer, 2005; Singh & Bussey, 2011) and they heighten their subsequent risk for victimization. Recently, Boivin, Petitclerc, Feng, and Barker (2010) reported that children who experienced increased victimization between grades 3 and 6 could best be described as becoming less aggressive and more withdrawn and emotionally vulnerable over time; in short, children viewed by peers (and possibly by themselves) as "easy marks" become increasingly victimized. These results complement the findings that both social withdrawal and victimization predict subsequent difficulties of an internalizing nature.

Difficulties in friendship relations have also been linked to internalizing problems. Specifically, the absence of a mutual friend, as indicated by a lack of reciprocal friendship nominations, is significantly correlated with concurrent feelings of loneliness and depression (Brendgen et al., 2000; Bukowski, Hoza, & Boivin, 1993; Parker & Asher, 1993; Windle, 1994). Two recent longitudinal studies have shown that the effects of friendlessness are especially strong for withdrawn children. In a two wave longitudinal study, Laursen, Bukowski, Aunola, and Nurmi (2007) showed that the effect of being friendless on internalizing problems was more pronounced for withdrawn children (i.e., those who were seen by peers as being isolated from the group) than for their peers who were not withdrawn. They interpreted these findings as evidence of not only Sullivan's (1953) ideas about the importance of friendship but also in terms of the broader individual level characteristics of withdrawn children (e.g., heightened emotional sensitivity) that may account for their risk.

The second study was a multiwave longitudinal study that used a cascade model (Bukowski, Laursen, & Hoza, 2010). The purpose of the study was to assess whether friendlessness over time would lead to substantial increases in internalizing problems (i.e., a cascade) in comparison with being friendless at just one time point. Two important findings regarding the effects of being friendless were observed in this project. The first was that the effects of friendlessness were especially strong for children who showed both forms of withdrawn behavior, specifically, children who were self-isolating (i.e., they preferred to be by themselves) and those who were excluded from the group, rather than either form of withdrawal alone. The second finding was that the effects of chronic friendlessness led to particularly steep increases in internalizing problems over time (i.e., to a cascade). These studies point to the specificity, rather than to the generality, of the effects of friendship, in the sense that these effects are seen only in those children who show the highest level of risk. More importantly, consistent with the concept of the cascade, the effects of friendship were not observed to be linear and additive but instead demonstrated a curvilinear increase in internalizing problems.

These findings beg the question of what accounts for the effects of friendlessness on internalizing problems. A possible explanation of these results may be taken from a study of the association between friendship and the functioning of the hypothalamic–pituitary–adrenal (HPA) axis (Adams, Santo, & Bukowski, 2011). This study examined the extent to which the arousal of the HPA axis in response to a negative experience is moderated by the presence of a best friend. Using an experience-sampling procedure in a school-based study, early adolescent boys and girls were assessed 16 times across a 4-day period. Three forms of data were available for each child at each assessment: a self-report of the degree to which the child's experience at that time was positive or negative, an index of whether the child was with a friend, and an index of salivary cortisol as an indicator of HPA activity. The findings showed that there was less arousal of the HPA axis following a negative experience when a child was with a friend than when exposed to similar negative moments when he or she was not with a friend. An implication of these findings is that prolonged friendlessness may have especially negative effects on an individual's capacity to deal with stressful events.

Together these studies show the negative effects of a lack of positive dyadic experiences. Although one can interpret these findings as providing support for ideas about friendship expressed by theorists such as Sullivan (1953), it is important to recognize their limitations. Sullivan made particular claims about the aspects of friendship that would account for the positive effects of having a best friend. He referred specifically to constructs and processes such as security and validation. Typically, peer researchers have not assessed the constructs emphasized by Sullivan directly and have been content to rely on "proxy" measures of friendship, such a reciprocated liking. Although it is well known that the use of reciprocated liking as an operational definition of friendship has its advantages (see Bukowski & Hoza, 1989), this index is extremely limited by its lacks of emphasis on the specific features that are hypothesized to account for the effects that friendship has on well-being.

Peers and Emotion Socialization

Aside from efforts to more carefully assess how the features of friendship affect well-being, there may be value also in trying to understand how experiences with friends contribute to the socialization of emotion. There is reason to expect that peers, like parents (see Denham, Bassett, & Wyatt, Chapter 25, this volume), may affect the experience and expression of emotions. Although direct evidence about friends' socialization of emotions is currently weak, findings from the peer relations and coping literatures provide evidence suggesting that children turn to friends when in emotional distress and that, in turn, friends act as important emotion regulation "coaches." As of early adolescence, friends are sought out as emotional guides. While mothers and fathers have been found to be the most frequent providers of support in childhood, as children enter into adolescence, they begin perceiving friends to be just as supportive as parents and, more importantly, friends become the most frequent providers of support (e.g., Furman & Buhrmester, 1992). Findings from studies on coping suggest that both boys and girls seek out social support from friends following stressful social situations, but girls may do so more often (e.g., Eschenbeck, Kohlmann, & Lohaus, 2007). Indeed, Rose and colleagues (2012) found that both boys and girls told their friends about negative experiences (e.g., being treated badly by another child). It has also been demonstrated that friends are not only aware of but they are responsive to their chum's emotional displays. Friends have been found to be much more sensitive to the emotional cues and states of their friends than nonfriends (e.g., Foot, Chapman, & Smith, 1977).

In an effort to capture children's perceptions of their friends' responses to emotional displays, Klimes-Dougan, Klingbeil, and Meller (2013) adapted the concepts developed by Malatesta-Magai, Jonas, Shepard, and Culver (1992) to understand parental social-ization of emotion. Their goal was to show how adolescent peers may directly socialize emotion. In this adaptation, four strategies described by Malatesta-Magai and colleagues were used: reward (i.e., providing comfort and acceptance), override (i.e., providing com-ments that dismiss or minimize the value of an emotion), neglect (i.e., ignoring or failing to notice an emotional expression), and magnify (i.e., engaging in emotional contagion by mirroring back the emotion that is expressed). They then added two more strate-gies that were specific to friends: overt and relational aggression. Using this framework, Klimes-Dougan and colleagues discovered that friends were perceived as being more likely to respond to negative emotions (i.e., aggregated mean score of friends' responses to sadness, anxiety, and anger) with supportive (reward and override) rather than puni-tive reactions. Their findings demonstrated that boys and girls differed in their percep-tions of how best friends responded. Across two time points, girls reported that their friends used higher levels of reward, override, and magnify responses compared with boys, whereas boys reported that their friends used overt and relational aggression, as well as neglect, more often than girls. This set of findings shows that whereas girls may be more welcoming of emotional talk, boys may respond in more punitive or dismissive ways. Indeed, such perceptions may also account for girls' increased tendency to disclose their thoughts and feelings to friends and boys' perceptions of feeling odd or wasting their time when doing so (Rose et al., 2012). Overall, this work points to importance of best friends as emotion socializers who influence the management of emotion in both boys and girls. Understanding how emotions are experienced within early adolescent friendships appears critical given that these relationships are both deeply meaningful and increasingly less controlled by adults, making them particularly important and strong extrinsic influences on strategies youth learn to rely on in regulating strong negative emo-tions (Underwood, Mayeux, & Galperin, 2006).

Summary

The study of peer relationships has been an area of interest to developmental psycholo-gists for more than a century, and it has been especially intense during the past 25 years as researchers have developed and tested several models of peer influence. In contrast with the study of other socialization domains, the study of the effects of peers poses several unique challenges. Insofar as peers are not "assigned" to a child in the way that parents are, either through biology or adoption, the peer domain is fluid and dynamic in ways that the family system cannot be. Research on the socializing effects of peer experiences has emphasized how much a child is liked and disliked, the characteristics of the peers with whom the child associates, and the features of children's interactions and relationships. As we have indicated in this discussion, these factors affect develop-ment via several pathways and processes that involve both mediation and moderation. Moreover, the current data show that different aspects of experiences with peers can affect internalizing and externalizing problems. Whereas being rejected by peers and the characteristics of the peers with whom a child associates appear to affect externalizing behavior, the properties of a child's relationship with peers, especially friends, appear to affect internalizing tendencies. Currently, the results of the studies we have discussed do not always provide clear support for any particular underlying process. Nevertheless, there is no doubt that children's behavior, thoughts, and emotions are highly associated with and likely influenced by their experiences with peers. These effects derive from a set of processes rather than from any particular mechanism. Ongoing longitudinal studies under way around the world will shed further light on the importance of the various facets of the peer system.

ACKNOWLEDGMENTS

Work on this project was supported by grants to William M. Bukowski, Frank Vitaro, and Mara Brendgen from the Social Sciences and Humanities Research Council of Canada and the Fonds de Recherche de Québec: La Société et la Culture.

REFERENCES

Adams, R. E., Santo, J., & Bukowski, W. M. (2011). The presence of a best friend buffers the effects of negative experiences. *Developmental Psychology, 47*, 1786–1791.

Albert, D., Chein, J., & Steinberg, L. (2013). The teenage brain peer influences on adolescent decision making. *Current Directions in Psychological Science, 22*(2), 114–120.

Albert, D., & Steinberg, L. (2011). Judgment and decision making in adolescence. *Journal of Research on Adolescence, 21*(1), 211–224.

Azmitia, M., Lippman, D. N., & Ittel, A. (1999). On the relation of personal experience to early adolescents' reasoning about best friendship deterioration. *Social Development, 8*(2), 275–291.

Bagwell, C. L., Newcomb, A. F., & Bukowski, W. M. (1998). Preadolescent friendship and peer rejection as predictors of adult adjustment. *Child Development, 69*(1), 140–153.

Baumeister, R. F., & Leary, M. R. (1995). The need to belong: desire for interpersonal attachments as a fundamental human motivation. *Psychological Bulletin, 117*(3), 497.

Berscheid, E., & Reis, H. T. (1998). Attraction and close relationships. In L. Gardner, D. Gilbert, & S. T. Fiske (Eds.), *The handbook of social psychology* (pp. 193–281). New York: McGraw-Hill.

Bierman, K. L., & Wargo, J. B. (1995). Predicting the longitudinal course associated with aggressive-rejected, aggressive (nonrejected), and rejected (nonaggressive) status. *Development and Psychopathology, 7*(4), 669–682.

Blatz, W. (1966). *Human security: Some reflections.* Toronto: University of Toronto Press.

Boivin, M., Petitclerc, A., Feng, B., & Barker, E. D. (2010). The developmental trajectories of peer victimization in middle to late childhood and the changing nature of their behavioral correlates. *Merrill–Palmer Quarterly, 56*(3), 231–260.

Brechwald, W. A., & Prinstein, M. J. (2011). Beyond homophily: A decade of advances in understanding peer influence processes. *Journal of Research on Adolescence, 21*(1), 166–179.

Brendgen, M., Bowen, F., Rondeau, N., & Vitaro, F. (1999). Effects of friends' characteristics on children's social cognitions. *Social Development, 8*(1), 41–51.

Brendgen, M., Vitaro, F., & Bukowski, W. (2000). Deviant friends and early adolescents' emotional and behavioral adjustment. *Journal of Research on Adolescence, 10*, 173–189.

Brendgen, M., Vitaro, F., & Girard, A. (2012). Evaluating gene–environment interplay. In B.

Laursen, T. D. Little, & N. A. Card (Eds.), *Handbook of developmental research methods* (pp. 687–705). New York: Guilford Press.

Brown, M. C., McNeil, N. M., & Glenberg, A. M. (2009). Using concreteness in education: Real problems, potential solutions. *Child Development Perspectives, 3*(3), 160–164.

Bukowski, W. M. (2011). Popularity as a social concept: Meanings and significance. In A. H. N. Cillessen, D. Schwartz, & L. Mayeux (Eds.), *Popularity in the peer system* (pp. 3–24). New York: Guilford Press.

Bukowski, W. M., Brendgen, M., & Vitaro, F. (2007). Peers and socialization: Effects on externalizing and internalizing problems. In J. E. Grusec & P. D. Hastings (Eds.), *Handbook of socialization: Theory and research* (pp. 355–381). New York: Guilford Press.

Bukowski, W. M., Cillessen, A. H. N., & Velasquez, A. M. (2012). Peer ratings. In B. Laursen, T. D. Little, & N. A. Card (Eds.), *Handbook of developmental research methods* (pp. 211–230). New York: Guilford Press.

Bukowski, W. M., & Hoza, B. (1989). Popularity and friendship: Issues in theory, measurement, and outcomes. In T. Berndt & G. Ladd (Eds.), *Peer relations in child development* (pp. 15–45). New York: Wiley.

Bukowski, W. M., Hoza, B., & Boivin, M. (1993). Popularity, friendship, and emotional adjustment during early adolescence. In B. Laursen (Ed.), *Close friendships in adolescence* (pp. 23–37). San Francisco: Jossey-Bass.

Bukowski, W. M., Laursen, B., & Hoza, B. (2010). The snowball effect: Friendship moderates escalations in depressed affect among avoidant and excluded children. *Development and Psychopathology, 22*(4), 749–757.

Bukowski, W. M., & Newcomb, A. F. (1984). The stability and determinants of sociometric status and friendship choice: A longitudinal perspective. *Developmental Psychology, 20*, 941–952.

Bukowski, W. M., & Sippola, L. K. (2001). Groups, individuals, and victimization: A view of the peer system. In J. Juvonen & S. Graham (Eds.), *Peer harassment in school: The plight of the vulnerable and victimized* (pp. 355–377). New York: Guilford Press.

Bukowski, W. M., & Véronneau, M. H. (2014). Studying withdrawal and isolation in the peer group. In R. J. Coplan & J. C. Bowker (Eds.), *The handbook of solitude: Psychological perspectives on social isolation, social withdrawal, and being alone* (pp. 14–28). New York: Wiley.

Cairns, R. B., Cairns, B. D., Neckerman, H. J., Gest, S. D., & Gariépy, J. L. (1988). Social networks and aggressive behavior: Peer support or peer rejection? *Developmental Psychology, 24*(6), 815.

Chein, J., Albert, D., O'Brien, L., Uckert, K., & Steinberg, L. (2011). Peers increase adolescent risk taking by enhancing activity in the brain's reward circuitry. *Developmental Science, 14*(2), F1–F10.

Cillessen, A. H. N. (2009). Sociometric methods. In K. H. Rubin, W. M. Bukowski, & B. Laursen (Eds.), *Handbook of peer interactions, relationships, and groups* (pp. 82–99). New York: Guilford Press.

Cillessen, A. H., & Marks, P. E. (2011). Conceptualizing and measuring popularity. In A. H. N. Cillessen, D. Schwartz, & L. Mayeux (Eds.), *Popularity in the peer system* (pp. 25–56). New York: Guilford Press.

Cillessen, A. H. N., & Mayeux, L. (2004). From censure to reinforcement: Developmental changes in the association between aggression and social status. *Child Development, 75*, 147–163.

Cohen, R., Hsueh, Y., Russell, K. M., & Ray, G. E. (2006). Beyond the individual: A consideration of context for the development of aggression. *Aggression and Violent Behavior, 11*(4), 341–351.

Coplan, R. J., Wilson, J., Frohlick, S. L., & Zelenski, J. (2006). A person-oriented analysis of behavioral inhibition and behavioral activation in children. *Personality and Individual Differences, 41*(5), 917–927.

Davies, B. (1982). *Life in the classroom and playground*. London: Routledge & Kegan Paul.

Deater-Deckard, K. (2001). Annotation: Recent research examining the role of peer relations in the development of psychopathology. *Journal of Child Psychology and Psychiatry, 42*, 565–579.

Deater-Deckard, K., Dodge, K. A., Bates, J. E., & Pettit, G. S. (1998). Multiple risk factors in the development of externalizing behavior problems: Group and individual differences. *Development and Psychopathology, 10*(3), 469–493.

Dion, K. L. (2000). Group cohesion: From "field of forces" to multidimensional construct. *Group Dynamics: Theory, Research, and Practice, 4*, 7–26.

Dishion, T. J., & Piehler, T. F. (2009). Deviant by design: Peer contagion in development, interventions, and schools. In K. H. Rubin, W. M. Bukowski, & B. Laursen (Eds.), *Handbook of peer interactions, relationships, and groups* (pp. 589–602). New York: Guilford Press.

Dodge, K. A., Lansford, J. E., Burks, V. S., Bates, J. E., Pettit, G. S., Fontaine, R., et al. (2003). Peer rejection and social information-processing factors in the development of aggressive behavior problems in children. *Child Development, 74*(2), 374–393.

Eschenbeck, H., Kohlmann, C. W., & Lohaus, A. (2007). Gender differences in coping strategies in children and adolescents. *Journal of Individual Differences, 28*(1), 18.

Espelage, D., Holt, M., & Henkel, R. (2003) Examination of peer-group contextual effects on aggression during early adolescence. *Child Development, 74*, 205–220.

Fergusson, D. M., Swain-Campbell, N. R., & Horwood, L. J. (2002). Deviant peer affiliations, crime and substance use: A fixed effects regression analysis. *Journal of Abnormal Child Psychology, 30*(4), 419–430.

Foot, H. C., Chapman, A. J., & Smith, J. R. (1977). Friendship and social responsiveness in boys and girls. *Journal of Personality and Social Psychology, 35*(6), 401.

Furman, W., & Buhrmester, D. (1985). Children's perceptions of the personal relationships in their social networks. *Developmental Psychology, 21*(6), 1016–1024.

Furman, W., & Buhrmester, D. (1992). Age and sex differences in perceptions of networks and personal relationships. *Child Development, 63*, 103–115.

Furman, W., & Robbins, P. (1985). What's the point?: Issues in the selection of treatment objectives. In B. H. Schneider, K. H. Rubin, & J. E. Ledingham (Eds.), *Children's peer relations: Issues in assessment and intervention* (pp. 41–54). New York: Springer.

Gazelle, H. (2013). Is social anxiety "in the child" or in the anxiety-provoking nature of the child's environment? *Child Development Perspectives, 4*, 221–226.

Graham, S., & Juvonen, J. (1998). Self-blame and peer victimization in middle school: An attributional analysis. *Developmental Psychology, 34*(3), 587.

Gray, J. A., & McNaughton, N. (2000). *The neuropsychology of anxiety.* Oxford, UK: Oxford University Press.

Hartup, W. W. (1964). Friendship status and the effectiveness of peers as reinforcing agents. *Journal of Experimental Child Psychology, 1*(2), 154–162.

Hartup, W. W. (1970). Peer interaction and social organization. In P. H. Mussen (Ed.), *Carmichael's manual of child psychology* (Vol. 2, pp. 361–456). New York: Wiley.

Hartup, W. W. (1983). Peer relations. In P. H. Mussen (Ed.), *Handbook of child psychology: Vol. 4. Socialization, personality, and social development* (pp. 103–196). New York: Wiley.

Hartup, W. W., & Coates, B. (1967). Imitation of a peer as a function of reinforcement from the peer group and rewardingness of the model. *Child Development, 38*, 1003–1016.

Hartup, W. W., Glazer, J. A., & Charlesworth, R. (1967). Peer reinforcement and sociometric status. *Child Development, 38*, 1017–1024.

Hawley, P. H., Little, T. D., & Card, N. A. (2007). The allure of a mean friend: Relationship quality and processes of aggressive adolescents with prosocial skills. *International Journal of Behavioral Development, 31*(2), 170–180.

Hinde, R. A. (1995). A suggested structure for a science of relationships. *Personal Relationships, 2*, 1–15.

Hodges, E. V. E., Boivin, M., Vitaro, F., & Bukowski, W. M. (1999). The power of friendship: Protection against an escalating cycle of peer victimization. *Developmental Psychology, 35*(1), 94–101.

Hogg, M. A., & Reid, S. A. (2006). Social identity, self-categorization, and the communication of group norms. *Communication Theory, 16*(1), 7–30.

Hymel, S., Comfort, C., Schonert-Reichl, K., & McDougall, P. (1996). Academic failure and school dropout: The influence of peers. In J. Juvonen & K. R. Wentzel (Eds.), *Social motivation: Understanding children's school adjustment* (pp. 313–345). Cambridge, UK: Cambridge University Press.

Kelly, J. G., Ryan, A. M., Altman, B. E., & Stelzner, S. P. (2000). Understanding and changing social systems. In J. Rappaport & E. Seidman (Eds.), *Handbook of community psychology* (pp. 133–159). New York: Springer.

Keltner, D., Gruenfeld, D. H., & Anderson, C. (2003). Power, approach, and inhibition. *Psychological Review, 110*(2), 265.

Kim, J. E., Hetherington, E. M., & Reiss, D. (1999). Associations among family relationships, antisocial peers, and adolescents' externalizing behaviors: Gender and family type differences. *Child Development, 70*(5), 1209–1230.

Kindermann, T. A., & Gest, S. D. (2009). Assessment of the peer group: Identifying naturally occurring social networks and capturing their effects. In K. H. Rubin, W. Bukowski, & B. Laursen (Eds.), *Handbook of peer interactions, relationships, and groups* (pp. 100–117). New York: Guilford Press.

Kingsbury, A., Coplan, R. J., Weeks, M., & Rose-Krasnor, L. (2013). Covering all the BAS's: A closer look at the links between BIS, BAS, and socio-emotional functioning in childhood. *Personality and Individual Differences, 55*, 521–526.

Klimes-Dougan, B., Klingbeil, D. A., & Meller, S. J. (2013). The impact of universal suicide-prevention programs on the help-seeking attitudes and behaviors of youths. *Crisis: The Journal of Crisis Intervention and Suicide Prevention, 34*(2), 82.

Ladd, G. W., & Troop-Gordon, W. (2003). The role of chronic peer difficulties in the development of children's psychological adjustment problems. *Child Development, 74*, 1344–1367.

Lansford, J. E., Malone, P. S., Dodge, K. A., Pettit, G. S., & Bates, J. E. (2010). Developmental cascades of peer rejection, social information processing biases, and aggression during middle childhood. *Development and Psychopathology, 22*(03), 593–602

Laursen, B., Bukowski, W. M., Aunola, K., & Nurmi, J. E. (2007). Friendship moderates prospective associations between social isolation and adjustment problems in young children. *Child Development, 78*, 1395–1404.

Laursen, B., Hafen, C. A., Kerr, M., & Stattin, H. (2012). Friend influence over adolescent problem behaviors as a function of relative peer acceptance: To be liked is to be emulated. *Journal of Abnormal Psychology, 121*, 88–94.

Levine, J. M., & Moreland, R. L. (1998). Small groups. In D. Gilbert, S. Fiske, & G. Lindzey (Eds.), *The handbook of social psychology* (4th ed., Vol. 2, pp. 415–469). Boston: McGraw-Hill.

Magnusson, L., & Stattin, H. (1998). Person–context interaction theories. In W. Damon & R. Lerner (Eds.), *Handbook of child psychology: Vol. 1: Theoretical models of human development* (5th ed., pp. 685–759). Hoboken, NJ: Wiley.

Malatesta-Magai, C., Jonas, R., Shepard, B., & Culver, L. C. (1992). Type A behavior pattern and emotion expression in younger and older adults. *Psychology and Aging, 7*(4), 551.

McDougall, P., Hymel, S., Vaillancourt, T., & Mercer, L. (2001). The consequences of childhood peer rejection. In M. Leary (Ed.) *Interpersonal rejection* (pp. 213–247). New York: Oxford University Press.

McNaughton, N., & Gray, J. A. (2000). Anxiolytic action on the behavioural inhibition system implies multiple types of arousal contribute to anxiety. *Journal of Affective Disorders, 61*(3), 161–176.

Miller-Johnson, S., Coie, J. D., Maumary-Gremaud, A., Bierman, K., & Conduct Problems Prevention Research Group. (2002). Peer rejection and aggression and early starter models of conduct disorder. *Journal of Abnormal Child Psychology, 30*, 217–230.

Monroe, W. S. (1986). Social consciousness in children. *Psychological Review, 5*, 68–70.

Muris, P., Meesters, C., de Kanter, E., & Timmerman, P. E. (2005). Behavioural inhibition and behavioural activation system scales for children: Relationships with Eysenck's personality traits and psychopathological symptoms. *Personality and Individual Differences, 38,* 831–841.

Nelson, S. E., & Dishion, T. J. (2004). From boys to men: Predicting adult adaptation from middle childhood sociometric status. *Development and Psychopathology, 16*(2), 441–459.

Newcomb, A. F., Bukowski, W. M., & Pattee, L. (1993). Children's peer relations: A meta-analytic review of popular, rejected, neglected, controversial, and average sociometric status. *Psychological Bulletin, 113,* 99–128.

Northway, M. L. (1944). Outsiders: A study of the personality patterns of children least acceptable to their age mates. *Sociometry, 7,* 10–25.

Ostrov, J. M. (2010). Prospective associations between peer victimization and aggression. *Child Development, 81,* 1670–1677.

Parker, J. G., & Asher, S. R. (1987). Peer relations and later personal adjustment: Are low-accepted children at risk? *Psychological Bulletin, 102*(3), 357–389.

Parker, J. G., & Asher, S. R. (1993). Friendship and friendship quality in middle childhood: Links with peer group acceptance and feelings of loneliness and social dissatisfaction. *Developmental Psychology, 29*(4), 611–621.

Paus, T. (2005). Mapping brain maturation and cognitive development during adolescence. *Trends in Cognitive Sciences, 9*(2), 60–68.

Paus, T., Toro, R., Leonard, G., Lerner, J. V., Lerner, R. M., Perron, M., et al. (2008). Morphological properties of the action-observation cortical network in adolescents with low and high resistance to peer influence. *Social Neuroscience, 3*(3-4), 303–316.

Perren, S., Ettekal, I., & Ladd, G. (2013). The impact of peer victimization on later maladjustment: Mediating and moderating effects of hostile and self-blaming attributions. *Journal of Child Psychology and Psychiatry, 54*(1), 46–55.

Piaget, J. (1932). *The moral judgment of the child.* London: Kegan Paul, Trench, Trübner.

Prinstein, M. J., Cheah, C. S., & Guyer, A. E. (2005). Peer victimization, cue interpretation, and internalizing symptoms: Preliminary concurrent and longitudinal findings for children and adolescents. *Journal of Clinical Child and Adolescent Psychology, 34*(1), 11–24.

Prinstein, M. J., Rancourt, D., Guerry, J. D., & Browne, C. B. (2009). Peer reputations and psychological adjustment. In K. H. Rubin, W. M. Bukowski, & B. Laursen (Eds.), *Handbook of peer interactions, relationships, and groups* (pp. 548–567). New York: Guilford Press.

Reijntjes, A., Kamphuis, J. H., Prinzie, P., & Telch, M. J. (2010). Peer victimization and internalizing problems in children: A meta-analysis of longitudinal studies. *Child Abuse and Neglect, 34*(4), 244–252.

Rizzo, T. A. (1989). *Friendship development among children in school.* Norwood, NJ: Ablex.

Rogoff, B. (1997). Evaluating development in the process of participation: Theory, methods and practice building on each other. In E. Amsel & K. A. Renninger (Eds.), *Change and development: Issues of theory, method, and application* (pp. 265–285). Hillsdale, NJ: Erlbaum.

Rose, A. J., Schwartz-Mette, R. A., Smith, R. L., Asher, S. R., Swenson, L. P., Carlson, W., et al. (2012). How girls and boys expect disclosure about problems will make them feel: Implications for friendships. *Child Development, 83*(3), 844–863.

Rose, A. J., Swenson, L. P., & Waller, E. M. (2004). Overt and relational aggression and perceived popularity: developmental differences in concurrent and prospective relations. *Developmental Psychology, 40*(3), 378–387.

Rubin, K. H., Bukowski, W. M., & Parker, J. G. (1998). Peer interactions, relationships and groups. In W. Damon (Series Ed.) & N. Eisenberg (Vol. Ed.), *The handbook of child psychology* (5th ed., pp. 619–700). New York: Wiley.

Rubin, K. H., Bukowski, W., & Parker, J. G. (2006). Peer interactions, relationships, and groups. In W. Damon (Series Ed.) & N. Eisenberg (Vol. Ed.), *Handbook of child psychology: Vol. 3. Social, emotional, and personality development* (6th ed., pp. 571–645). New York: Wiley.

Rubin, K. H., Bukowski, W. M., & Parker, J. G. (in press). Peer interactions, relationships and groups. In W. Damon (Series Ed.) & N. Eisenberg (Vol. Ed.), *The Handbook of Child Psychology* (6th ed.). New York: Wiley.

Scaramella, L. V., Conger, R. D., Spoth, R., & Simons, R. L. (2002). Evaluation of a social contextual model of delinquency: A cross-study replication. *Child Development, 73*(1), 175–195.

Shaw, M. (1981). *Group dynamics* (3rd ed.). New York: McGraw-Hill.

Sijtsema, J. J., Ojanen, T., Veenstra, R., Lindenberg, S., Hawley, P. H., & Little, T. D. (2010). Forms and functions of aggression in adolescent friendship selection and influence: A longitudinal social network analysis. *Social Development, 19*(3), 515–534.

Simons, R. L., Chao, W., Conger, R. D., & Elder, G. H. (2001). Quality of parenting as mediator of the effect of childhood defiance on adolescent friendship choices and delinquency: A growth curve analysis. *Journal of Marriage and the Family, 63*(1), 63–79.

Singh, P., & Bussey, K. (2011). Peer victimization and psychological maladjustment: The mediating role of coping self-efficacy. *Journal of Research on Adolescence, 21*(2), 420–433.

Snyder, J. J., Schrepferman, L. P., Bullard, L., McEachern, A. D., & Patterson, G. R. (2012). Covert antisocial behavior, peer deviancy training, parenting processes, and sex differences in the development of antisocial behavior during childhood. *Development and Psychopathology, 24*(3), 1117–1138.

Spencer, M. B. (2006). Revisiting the 1990 Special Issue on Minority Children: An editorial perspective 15 years later. *Child Development, 77*, 1149–1154

Sullivan, H. S. (1953). *The interpersonal theory of psychiatry*. New York: Norton.

Sussman, S., Pokhrel, P., Ashmore, R. D., & Brown, B. B. (2007). Adolescent peer group identification and characteristics: A review of the literature. *Addictive Behaviors, 32*(8), 1602–1627.

Triandis, H. C. (2001). Individualism–collectivism and personality. *Journal of Personality, 69*(6), 907–924.

Underwood, M. K., Mayeux, L., & Galperin, M. (2006). Peer relations during middle childhood: Gender, emotions, and aggression. In L. Balter & C. S. Tamis-LeMonda (Eds.), *Child psychology: A handbook of contemporary issues* (2nd ed., pp. 241–261). New York: Psychology Press.

Vacha, E. F., McDonald, W. A., Coburn, J. M., & Black, H. E. (1979). *Improving classroom climate*. New York: Holt, Rinehart & Winston.

van Lier, P. A., Vitaro, F., Barker, E. D., Brendgen, M., Tremblay, R. E., & Boivin, M. (2012). Peer victimization, poor academic achievement, and the link between childhood externalizing and internalizing problems. *Child Development, 83*(5), 1775–1788.

Vygotsky, L. S. (1978). *Mind in society: The development of higher psychological processes*. Cambridge, MA: Harvard University Press.

Wardell, J. D., O'Connor, R. M., Read, J. P., & Colder, C. R. (2011). Behavioral approach system moderates the prospective association between the behavioral inhibition system and alcohol outcomes in college students. *Journal of Studies on Alcohol and Drugs, 72*(6), 1028–1036.

Windle, M. (1994). A study of friendship characteristics and problem behaviors among middle adolescents. *Child Development, 65*(6), 1764–1777.

CHAPTER 11

Socialization in School Settings

Kathryn R. Wentzel

Most American children over the age of 6 spend a minimum of 108 days each year in formal educational settings. Many younger children also spend significant portions of their lives in day care or preschool settings. Although these settings are designed primarily to engage children in academic and intellectual activities, they also create social worlds of major importance and significance to children. In many respects, schools provide social experiences that are highly similar to, and overlap with, those provided by families, the broader community, and the peer group. However, school settings are relatively unique in their focus on specific skills that are central to children's future roles as citizens and workers. These include skills related to being socially responsible and responsive to group goals, and to behaving in prosocial, cooperative ways with peers. For instance, schoolchildren spend significant amounts of time in large groups, engaged in activities that require the coordination of personal goals and behavior with those of others. In addition, children's relationships with teachers are less personal and intimate than their relationships with parents. While accomplishing these socially integrative tasks, children also are expected to assert themselves academically by competing successfully with others or by developing mastery in specific areas of interest.

If these outcomes reflect the primary objectives of educators and nonfamilial caregivers, how might their achievement be accomplished? Rarely have scholars attempted to align school-based objectives with specific socialization processes to identify what might promote the development and achievement of such objectives (see Pianta, Hamre, & Downer, 2011). The goal of this chapter, therefore, is to describe what is known about the process of socialization within school settings and to offer suggestions for future theory development and research in this area. In this chapter, *socialization* is defined with reference to contextual affordances, that is, supports and opportunities that facilitate the development of children's school-based competencies. In this regard, schools are viewed as complex systems that can provide students with multiple affordances as a function of the school itself (e.g., size, heterogeneity of student body, teacher:child ratios), as well as through social interactions and interpersonal relationships that are embedded in the educational process.

This chapter begins with a consideration of how to define *competence* within the context of school settings. Then, the literature on the processes of socialization is reviewed, including those associated with structural characteristics of schools, as well as more proximal social and interpersonal processes that might support competence development. Children's experiences in preschool and child care as well as in K–12 schools are considered. Finally, the chapter ends with a discussion of remaining issues and challenges to the field.

Defining Competence at School

In the developmental literature, competence has been described from a variety of perspectives ranging from children's development of individual skills, such as effective behavioral repertoires, problem-solving skills, positive beliefs about the self, and achievement of socially valued goals, to more general adaptation within a particular setting, as reflected in the gaining of social approval and acceptance. In this manner, competence reflects the achievement of personal goals and positive developmental outcomes for the individual, as well as the achievement of goals that are situationally relevant, using appropriate means to achieve these goals (Ford, 1992).

In addition, central to many definitions of competence is the notion that contextual affordances and constraints contribute to and mold the development of competencies in ways that enable these competencies to support the social good (Bronfenbrenner & Morris, 2006). More specifically, social contexts are believed to play an integral role in competence development by not only providing opportunities for the development of intrapersonal outcomes (e.g., achieving goals to make friends or to learn algebra) but also defining the appropriate parameters of accomplishments, such that individual skills and attributes can contribute to the social cohesion and smooth functioning of the group (e.g., establishing friendship groups that are socially inclusive rather than exclusive; engaging in learning activities during math class).

Together, these definitions suggest that competence can be understood in terms of context-specific effectiveness, being a product of personal attributes such as goals, values, self-regulatory skills, and cognitive abilities, and of ways in which these attributes contribute to meeting situational requirements. The application of this perspective to the realm of schooling results in a multifaceted description of children who are competent. First, competent students achieve goals that are personally valued, as well as those that are sanctioned by others. Second, the goals they pursue result in both social integration and positive developmental outcomes for themselves. Socially integrative outcomes are those that promote the smooth functioning of social groups at school (e.g., cooperative behavior) and are reflected in levels of social approval and social acceptance. Self-enhancing outcomes reflect healthy development of the self (e.g., mastery of skills, positive feelings of competence and self-determination, emotional well-being).

Achieving these outcomes is accomplished not just by one student's efforts but often as the result of compromise or conflict resolution with classmates and teachers. Indeed, an ecological perspective reminds us that the ability to be competent at school is contingent on opportunities and affordances that support students in their efforts to achieve a balance between accomplishing personal goals and behaving in ways that lead to social acceptance and approval (see Wentzel, 2004, 2013). This chapter reviews work on several aspects of school contexts that have the potential to provide such supports: structural characteristics, social interactions with teachers and classmates, and interpersonal relationships with teachers and classmates. First, however, I describe the goals that teachers, peers, and students themselves value within school contexts. This section is followed by a discussion of socialization processes by which individuals in school contexts promote the achievement of these goals.

Goals for Students at School

The notion that schools provide children with unique socialization experiences has been acknowledged since the beginning of public schooling. For example, in the United States, public schools were initially developed with an explicit function of educating children to become healthy, moral, and economically productive citizens. Since then, social behavior in the form of moral character, conformity to social rules and norms, cooperation, and positive styles of social interaction has been promoted consistently as a goal for students to achieve (see Wentzel, 1991, for a review). Given these overarching social goals for education, are there specific goals that are valued more than others in school settings? Do teachers and peers have goals for students concerning what they value and believe should be accomplished within the classroom? In the following sections, research on teachers', peers', and students' goals for themselves is reviewed.

Teachers' Goals for Students

Researchers rarely have asked teachers about their specific educational or behavioral goals for students. In preschool and child care settings, researchers typically identify desirable outcomes of care, often with an implicit assumption that these settings might in fact be detrimental to children's social development in comparison to parental care (e.g., Belsky, 2001). As a result, the focus of empirical investigations has been on outcomes that reflect developmentally appropriate milestones for young children, such as secure attachments to mothers and cooperative interactions with peers (Shonkoff & Phillips, 2000), rather than on specific outcomes that teachers would like children to achieve. As an indirect measure of their goals for students, K–12 teachers have been asked to characterize their ideal students (e.g., Meisgeier & Kellow, 2007; Verasalo, Tuomivaara, & Lindeman, 1996). Elementary school teachers (typically first through fifth grade) report preferences for students who are cooperative, conforming, cautious, and responsible rather than independent, assertive, argumentative, or disruptive. Similarly, in the middle school grades (sixth through eighth graders ranging in age from 11 to 14 years), teachers describe their "ideal" students as sharing, helpful, and responsive to rules, persistent, intrinsically interested, and as earning high grades (see Wentzel, 2013, for a review).

Researchers also have documented social values and expectations that teachers communicate to their students, including appropriate ways to respond to requests, appropriate contexts for different types of behavior, and expectations for impulse control, mature problem solving, and involvement in class activities. Teachers also communicate expectations for students' interactions with each other. Preschool teachers tend to focus on the development of prosocial behavior by modeling and encouraging prosocial interactions, discouraging social exclusion, and creating cooperative activities (e.g., Hagens, 1997). Elementary and secondary teachers focus on establishing norms for sharing, working well with others, and adherence to rules concerning aggression, manners, stealing, and loyalty (Wentzel, 2013).

Students' Goals for Each Other

The classroom goals that students would like each other to achieve are not well documented. However, it is reasonable to assume that students also communicate to each other expectations concerning valued forms of behavior. For example, Wentzel, Battle, Russell, and Looney (2010) reported that young adolescents indicate that their classmates expect them to perform well academically at school; approximately 80% of students from three predominantly middle-class middle schools reported that their peers strongly valued academic learning. However, in samples of high school students, only 40% of adolescents report similar levels of peer academic expectations (Wentzel, Monzo, Williams, & Tomback, 2007). This suggests that, at least in some schools, peers actively promote the pursuit of positive social and academic outcomes. However, these data also suggest that as students advance through their middle school and high school years, the degree to which their goals and values support positive academic accomplishments might become fairly attenuated (see also Wentzel, Baker, & Russell, 2012).

Insights concerning peer expectations and values also can be gleaned from research on personal characteristics and outcomes related to peer approval and acceptance at school. Researchers typically have defined children's involvement in peer relationships in three ways: degree of peer acceptance or rejection by the larger peer group, peer group membership, and dyadic friendships. Positive correlates of each of these types of relationships, however, are similar with respect to school-related outcomes. For example, socially accepted students also tend to be highly cooperative, helpful, sociable, and self-assertive compared to their socially rejected peers (Rubin, Bukowski, & Parker, 1998). Similarly, children with friends at school tend to be more sociable, cooperative, prosocial, and emotionally supportive when compared to their classmates without friends (e.g., Barry & Wentzel, 2006; Crosnoc & Needham, 2004). With regard to pursuit of specific goals, peer acceptance in middle school has been associated positively with pursuit of goals to behave prosocially and responsibly (e.g., Wentzel, Filisetti, & Looney, 2007).

Of additional interest is the finding that being socially accepted and enjoying popular sociometric status (as opposed to popularity, see Cillessen & van den Berg, 2012) are related to successful academic performance, and being unpopular and having rejected sociometric status are related to academic difficulties. Results are most consistent with respect to classroom grades, although peer acceptance has been related positively to standardized test scores as well as to IQ (see Wentzel, 2005). These findings are robust for elementary school-age children, as well as adolescents, and longitudinal studies document the stability of relations between peer acceptance and academic accomplishments over time (e.g., Schwartz, Gorman, Nakamoto, & McKay, 2006; Wentzel & Caldwell, 1997). Other indices of social acceptance such as the ability to establish close friendships also have been related positively to grades and test scores in elementary and middle school (Wentzel, Barry, & Caldwell, 2004).

Finally, students who perceive relatively high expectations for academic learning and engagement from their peers report that they pursue goals to learn for internalized reasons (or because it is important) rather than because they believe they will get in trouble or lose social approval if they do not (Wentzel, 2004). Therefore, peers who communicate a sense of importance or enjoyment with regard to engagement in academic tasks are likely to lead others to form similar attitudes toward the task. Although this literature suggests that peer acceptance is related positively to academic pursuits and accomplishments, it is likely that the mechanisms that explain these relations are complex. For example, it is likely that socially competent students are likely to have social skills that support both peer-related and academically related competencies, such as the ability to elicit help and resources from others, to recognize and conform to social rules and norms, and to work collaboratively with others toward common goals (see Wentzel, 2005, 2013).

Students' Goals for Themselves

Research on students' school-related goals has focused most often on academic outcomes; students actively pursue goals to learn and to perform well academically on a daily basis (Wentzel & Wigfield, 2009). However, students also consistently express interest in social goals such as to have fun and make friends (e.g., Ryan & Shim, 2008; Wentzel, 1989). Of particular interest from a school socialization perspective is that establishment of rewarding relationships with peers becomes increasingly important for students in middle school and high school. One likely reason for this growing interest in peers is that many young adolescents enter new middle school structures that necessitate interacting with larger numbers of peers on a daily basis. In contrast to elementary school classrooms, the relative uncertainty and ambiguity of having multiple teachers and different sets of classmates for each class, new instructional styles, and more complex class schedules often result in middle school students turning to each other for information, social support, and ways to cope.

Establishing positive relationships with teachers is also of concern to most students. However, clear developmental trends are evident. Whereas elementary school-age children often describe teachers as being important sources of social and academic support (Reid, Landesman, Treder, & Jaccard, 1989), adolescents rarely mention relationships with teachers as being important in their lives except as academic instructors (Lempers & Clark-Lempers, 1992). Finally, when given a list of possible social and academic goals to pursue at school, high school students indicate frequent attempts to achieve a range of social goals and rank having fun, making friends, being dependable and responsible, and being helpful as the most frequently pursued goals (Wentzel, 1989; also see Dowson & McInerney, 2003).

Summary

Although teachers' and students' goals for education have not been studied extensively, it is clear that a core set of competencies is valued by teachers as well as students. In addition to academic accomplishments, positive forms of behavior that are reflected in compliance to classroom rules and norms, and that demonstrate cooperation and caring for classmates, also are related to social approval and acceptance by others. Students themselves also mention trying to achieve these same outcomes, although they also mention more personal goals such as having fun. Given these multiple goals, how might a student learn which goals are valued by others and decide which goals to pursue at school? Although little is known about how students coordinate multiple, competing goals, it is clear that schools can play a powerful role in defining socially valued outcomes for students to achieve, and that teachers and students actively promote these outcomes in their day-to-day interactions with each other. In the following section, I discuss processes by which schools, as well as teachers and peers, might influence students to pursue these outcomes.

Processes of Socialization within School Settings

Although children try to achieve multiple goals for many reasons, the question of what leads them to engage willingly in the pursuit of goals that are valued by others lies at the heart of research on socialization (e.g., Grusec & Goodnow, 1994). If schools promote the adoption and pursuit of socially valued goals, how then does this influence occur? Models of socialization at school are not well developed. However, models of family socialization suggest at least three general mechanisms whereby social resources and experiences might influence competent functioning. First, the structure and general features of social contexts afford opportunities and resources that can directly support or hinder competence development. Second, ongoing social interactions and communications teach children about themselves and what they need to do to become accepted and competent members of their social worlds. Within the context of these interactions, children learn which goals and standards for behavior they should strive to achieve (Grusec & Goodnow, 1994). Third, the qualities of children's social relationships are likely to have motivational significance. Children are more likely to adopt and internalize expectations and goals that are valued by others if their interpersonal relationships are responsive and nurturant than if their relationships are harsh and critical (e.g., Ryan, 1993).

When considered with respect to educational settings, these mechanisms reflect the nested quality of children's experiences at school. Structural features of schools, such as school and class size, teacher:student ratios, and funding, can influence the amount and quality of resources and opportunities available to students. Social interactions and dyadic relationships with teachers and peers describe the more proximal contexts that can influence student adjustment, by way of communicating goals and expectations and creating emotionally supportive contexts that promote their adoption. In the following sections, I review research on each of these mechanisms.

Structural Characteristics of Schooling

Numerous studies have documented significant differences in student outcomes as a function of the structural features of the schools attended. These differences have been documented at the preschool level and in elementary and secondary school settings.

Preschool and Child Care Settings

Out-of-family care of preschool children takes place in a diversity of arrangements and settings. However, there is general agreement that structural aspects of quality care are reflected in specific characteristics of staff and settings (e.g., Brooks-Gunn, Fuligni, & Berlin, 2003; Fitzgerald, Mann, Cabrera, & Wong, 2003). Staff characteristics include staff:child ratios, amount and type of staff education and training, years of experience, turnover, and wages. Setting features include type and availability of developmentally appropriate curricular materials, cleanliness, safety, and group size. Researchers also have examined the amount of time children spend in child care settings in relation to child outcomes (National Institute of Child Health and Human Development [NICHD] Early Child Care Research Network, 2006).

In general, research has documented significant relations of staff characteristics with a range of social and cognitive outcomes in children across a variety of child care settings (e.g., Burchinal, Kainz, & Cai, 2011). Few studies have examined these features while taking into account other important predictors of child outcomes, such as family characteristics or the quality of parent–child relationships (cf. Fitzgerald et al., 2003; NICHD Early Child Care Network, 2002, 2006). However, the NICHD Early Child Care Study, in which a range of child care, home and family (structural, quality, and parent characteristics), and child characteristics have been assessed (see Brooks-Gunn et al., 2003) are beginning to shed light on the combined impact of these multiple factors on child outcomes over time.

A sampling of these findings indicates that child care factors by themselves do not predict young children's social adjustment (as indexed by attachment classifications with mothers), unless mothers' characteristics also are taken into account; time spent in child care is related to young children's increased risk for insecure attachment to mothers at 12 and 36 months only if maternal sensitivity also is low (NICHD Early Child Care Network, 1997, 2001). The more time young children spend in nonmaternal care also predicts externalizing problems and conflict with adults at 54 months and in kindergarten, but not in first grade (McCartney et al., 2010; NICHD Early Child Care Network, 2003a, 2003c). Finally, quality of early care has been related positively to academic outcomes 15 years later, due in part to its positive effects on cognitive development early on (Vandell, Belsky, Burchinal, Steinberg, & Vandergrift, 2010).

In general, these findings are robust, even when taking into account quality of parent–child interactions, type of setting (e.g., center and home-based), instability of child care arrangements, and maternal sensitivity, level of education, and depression. However, levels of problem behavior (e.g., disobedience and aggression) exhibited by children who spend the most time in child care are not at clinical levels, and the effect sizes are relatively small (NICHD Early Child Care Network, 2006). In addition, significant effects often differ depending on who is rating child behavior (mothers or caregivers), making it difficult to draw definitive conclusions (see, e.g., NICHD Early Child Care Network, 2003a).

More systematic intervention studies have documented the effects of preschool programs such as Head Start on young children. These studies have shown that in the short term, participation in high-quality preschool programs can have significant, positive effects on cognitive and school readiness outcomes, especially for children living in poverty (e.g., Resnick, 2010). These programs also appear to have short-term and long-term effects on social outcomes such as aggression, although only when interventions also focus on changing parent behavior (Schweinhart, Barne, Weikart, Barnett, & Epstein, 1993). Conclusions concerning preschool effects also must be tempered given that researchers typically cannot randomly assign children to control and intervention groups; comparison groups that are comparable with respect to subject and program characteristics are rare.

Formal Schooling

In contrast to research on day care and preschool settings, research on structural effects of elementary and secondary schooling has been guided by specific goals for enhancing the academic and social skills that form the basis of public education policy. For example, policy-driven work in the 1960s (e.g., Coleman et al., 1966) led to conclusions that physical features and administrative structures of schools, such as school size, funding, space, class size, teacher:child ratio, and curricular resources, explained minimal variance in student outcomes relative to nonschool variables, such as family and demographic factors. Much subsequent research has confirmed these findings, in that the strength of school effects relative to nonschool factors is typically small, except when comparing schools at the two extremes of quality continua (Scheerens & Bosker, 1997).

However, other research has documented the positive effects of one aspect of school context—school climate—on students' motivational and academic outcomes, underscoring the importance of the academic, behavioral, social, and moral climate and school authority structures for understanding student success (Roeser, Urdan, & Stephens, 2009). Much of this work has focused on *school climate*, as defined by students' sense of school community and school belonging. School climate has been related positively (albeit modestly) to social behavioral and academic outcomes (Anderman, 2002; Klein, Cornell, & Konold, 2012), with effects that are often moderated by students' sex, race (e.g., Kuperminc, Leadbetter, Emmons, & Blatt, 1997), school size (Anderman, 2002), and poverty level of the school's community (Hopson & Lee, 2011). To illustrate, beliefs that their schools are cohesive, responsive, and caring communities predict young adolescents' decreased drug use and delinquency, even when accounting for within-school differences and the poverty level of the school's community (Battistich & Hom, 1997). Significant negative relations between school climate and young adolescents' externalizing behavior also have been documented, even when controlling for race, socioeconomic status, stress levels, and self-concept, with the greatest effects of positive climate shown for African American and single-parent students (Kuperminc et al., 1997). Similar findings have been reported for Latino students making the transition to middle school (Espinoza & Juvonen, 2010). Finally, intervention studies designed to enhance the quality of school climate also have demonstrated that when students begin to experience a greater sense of school community, they also display more positive social skills (e.g., Limber, 2012).

The effects of school structures on student outcomes also can be gleaned from school transition studies in which students move from one school level to another, with each level marked by somewhat unique characteristics. Research on transitions of preschool children entering into kindergarten, and then into elementary school is rare, but studies of later transitions are more frequent. The transition from elementary school to middle school entails attending larger schools and requires students to interact with greater numbers of peers and establish new peer groups, and to adjust to new instructional styles (see Eccles & Roeser, 2013, for a review). Predictable changes associated with transitions to middle school are student perceptions that teachers are less caring and that they become more focused on students earning high grades, promoting competition between students, and maintaining control than teachers in elementary school.

The transition into high school is associated with changes similar to those associated with the middle school transition; the focus on academic accomplishments becomes even more demanding, peer groups must once again be reestablished, and the school environment becomes more impersonal. The transition to high school also is associated with declines in academic performance, attendance, participation in extracurricular activities, and in a perceived loss of teacher and school social support for many adolescents (Eccles & Roeser, 2013).

School-level norms also can have a negative impact on ways in which students interact with each other and on subsequent academic motivation and achievement. This occurs most often when schools establish competitive academic standards and norm-referenced criteria for evaluating achievements that heighten social comparison among students. In turn, high levels of social comparison tend to result in students adopting orientations toward learning that focus on performance rather than mastery of subject matter, and in lowered levels of academic efficacy and aspirations for achievement, especially among students with low ability (Butler, 2005).

On a positive note, schools that employ universal, schoolwide policies and programs that accentuate the importance of students' prosocial development also can create environments in which more positive relationships are likely to be formed. In this regard, social skills training programs can increase the prevalence of students' prosocial behaviors (e.g., sharing, cooperating) by teaching them skills such as how to recognize emotions more effectively, negotiate conflict resolutions, and control impulsive behaviors (Gresham, Van, & Cook, 2006; Raver, 2012). Researchers have documented that in elementary school-age samples, the acquisition of these skills facilitates a reduction in children's maladaptive social skills and strategies, thus enabling the formation of more functional relationships with peers (e.g., Bierman & Powers, 2009).

Other structured efforts to enhance prosocial behavior and corresponding peer interactions are exemplified by the Child Development Project (CDP), which provides cooperative learning activities and class meetings designed to communicate and reinforce positive behavioral and social norms of the classroom, foster cognitive and social problem solving, and build a sense of community. CDP schools outperform comparison schools on factors such as conflict resolution skills, increased levels of positive behavioral outcomes, and lower levels of negative behaviors (What Works Clearinghouse, 2007). Similarly, the Fast Track Program (Conduct Problems Prevention Research Group, 2010), designed in part to promote friendship building skills and social problem solving strategies, has documented improvements in the quality of elementary school–age students' peer relationships and social interactions (Lavallee, Bierman, & Nix, 2005).

Finally, although the literature implies that peers might be the primary source of threats to students' physical safety and well-being, teachers and school administrators can play a central role in creating schools that are free of peer harassment and in alleviating the negative effects of harassment once it has occurred. For example, antibullying programs focus on improving peer relationships by creating and fostering a safe and positive school environment and the development of prosocial skills in children (e.g., Salmivalli, Garandeau, & Veenstra, 2012). There also is evidence that when schools stress intergenerational bonding (i.e., between students and teachers), they support the development of teacher–student relationships that can act as buffers against the negative effects of aggressive peers on behavior (Crosnoe & Needham, 2004).

In summary, a number of features that characterize school settings at the preschool and K–12 level appear to be related to children's overall social and academic adjustment to school. For the most part, however, the effects are small; this is especially true for preschool and child care settings when family characteristics are taken into account. Moreover, specific processes that might explain these relations are rarely examined. However, several researchers have demonstrated that classroom-level processes can explain associations between school-level features and student outcomes (e.g., Finn, Pannozzo, & Achilles, 2003). As proposed by several scholars (Connell & Wellborn, 1991; Hamre & Pianta, 2007; Wentzel, 2004), these processes entail teacher and peer communications of goals and expectations for specific behavioral outcomes and creation of interpersonal contexts that motivate students to achieve them. These processes are discussed in the following sections.

Social Interactions: Transmitting Values and Providing Help, Advice, and Instruction

How might students learn what is valued by their teachers and peers? One approach to addressing this question has been to focus on teachers and peers as socialization agents who create interpersonal contexts that influence levels and quality of student motivation and engagement. Although the affective tone of teacher–student interactions is a central focus of discussion (see Connell & Wellborn, 1991; Wentzel, 2004), these perspectives propose that the contribution of teachers' and peers' relationships with students should be defined in terms of multiple dimensions that combine with emotional support to motivate students to engage in classroom activities.

Similar to those described in models of effective parenting and parenting styles (e.g., Baumrind, 1971; Darling & Steinberg, 1993), these dimensions reflect levels of concern with a student's emotional and physical well-being, predictability and structure, and instrumental resources. These dimensions are believed to reflect necessary interpersonal resources that support a child's pursuit of social and academic goals that are valued by others. When applied to the social world of the classroom, these dimensions are reflected in opportunities for learning, as reflected in communications of rules and expectations for behavior and performance, provisions of instrumental help, and opportunities for emotional support and interpersonal connectedness. Here I review research on ways in which teachers and peers communicate specific values concerning what it means to be competent, and on interactions with teachers and peers that provide help, advice, and instruction with respect to socially valued outcomes.

Social Interactions with Teachers

In the classroom, teachers' central pedagogical function is to transmit knowledge and train students in academic subject areas, primarily through direct instruction. Teachers also can be effective in teaching students social skills (Durlak, Weissberg, & Dymnicki, 2011). During the course of instruction, teachers also promote the development of student competencies by organizing and structuring learning environments in ways that make expectations and goals for behavioral and learning outcomes more salient to students. For example, cooperative learning activities can be designed to promote students' pursuit of social goals to cooperate and help each other, to be responsible to the group, and to achieve common objectives (Slavin, 2011). Providing clear expectations for behavior, monitoring student activities, and maximizing instructional times has also been associated with positive student outcomes in social and academic domains (see Pianta, Hamre, & Allen, 2012). It is reasonable to assume that the degree to which students pursue goals valued by teachers is dependent on whether teachers communicate clearly and consistently their values and expectations concerning classroom behavior and performance. As with parents, these practices promote a climate of interpersonal trust and fairness that promotes students' willingness to listen to teachers' communications and adopt their behavioral and learning goals and values.

The potential power of teachers' expectations for students is also demonstrated in findings that many teachers hold negative stereotypes of minority and low-achieving students, and expect less competent behavior and lower levels of academic performance from them than from other students (Weinstein, 2002). These expectations can then become self-fulfilling prophecies, with student performance changing to conform to teachers' expectations. However, teachers who communicate high expectations can bring about positive changes in performance: Teachers' overestimations of ability seem to have a somewhat stronger effect in raising levels of achievement than teachers' underestimations have on lowering achievement, especially for low-performing students (see Jussim, Robustelli, & Cain, 2009).

Social Interactions with Peers

Interactions with peers also can lead directly to resources and information that help students to be socially competent. In preschool settings, playing with peers who differ in terms of their self-regulatory skills can create beneficial (as well as risky) contexts for the development of childrens' own self-regulatory skills (Fabes, Hanish, & Martin, 2003). At older ages, peers provide information and advice, model behavior, or provide specific experiences that facilitate learning social expectations for behavior. Students frequently clarify and interpret their teacher's instructions concerning what they should be doing and how they should do it, and provide mutual assistance in the form of volunteering substantive information and answering questions (Cooper, Ayers-Lopez, & Marquis, 1982). Classmates also provide each other with important information about themselves; information concerning social self-efficacy and skills can be gleaned by observing social competencies and skills demonstrated by peers (McCullagh, Law, & Ste-Marie, 2012; Schunk & Zimmerman, 1997).

Help giving is perhaps the most explicit and obvious way in which peers have a direct influence on students' academic and social competence. Indeed, students who enjoy positive relationships with their peers also have greater access to resources and information to help them accomplish academic and social tasks than those who do not. These resources are viewed as adaptive forms of help when they take the form of information and advice, modeled behavior, or specific experiences that facilitate learning specific skills (e.g., Newman, 2000). Recent research indicates that students' perceptions of their teachers influence their propensity to seek adaptive help from peers (e.g., perceptions of competitive classroom structures are associated with lower levels of adaptive peer help seeking; Ryan & Shim, 2008).

Peers also can have an impact on students' goals and expectations for performance by influencing perceptions of ability. This is important for understanding academic competence because students' efficacy beliefs are powerful predictors of academic performance (Schunk & Pajares, 2009). Children utilize their peers for comparative purposes as early as 4 years of age (Butler, 2005). As children work on academic tasks that require fairly specific skills and are evaluated with respect to clearly defined standards, they use each other to monitor and evaluate their own abilities. Experimental work also has shown that peers serve as powerful models that influence the development of academic self-efficacy (Schunk & Pajares, 2009), especially when children observe similar peers who demonstrate successful ways to cope with failure. These modeling effects are especially likely to occur when students are friends (Crockett, Losoff, & Petersen, 1984).

Interpersonal Relationships: Providing Responsive and Emotionally Supportive Contexts

Feelings of emotional security and being socially connected also are believed to facilitate the adoption of goals and interests valued by others, and desires to contribute in positive ways to the overall functioning of the social group. Similar to parent–child relationships, the affective quality of interpersonal relationships at school is believed to provide children with responsive and nurturing environments that promote personal growth, as well as adaptive social functioning. Feelings of relatedness and belongingness at school are expected to contribute directly to feelings of self-worth and self-esteem (Pianta, Hamre, & Stuhlman, 2003). In turn, levels of emotional well-being are believed to contribute to both social and academic competence (e.g., Harter, 2012).

Perspectives on children's interpersonal relationships at school tend to differ according to the age of the child. Using a developmental systems approach, Pianta and his colleagues (2003) argue for the centrality of teacher–student attachments in the lives of preschool and elementary students. They describe qualities of the teacher–child relationship in terms of three features: closeness (e.g., warmth and open communication), conflict, and dependency. Research on middle childhood and adolescence has focused more often on specific qualities or dimensions of teacher–student interactions, and expressions of warmth and approval are central to most descriptions (see Wentzel, 2009). Although the affective quality of teacher–student relationships has been the focus of most research in this area, relationships with peers also appear to play an important role in creating emotionally supportive contexts at school.

Responsive and Warm Relationships with Teachers

During the preschool years, changes in the quality of child–teacher attachments as children move to new child-care settings are related to changes in various aspects of their social functioning (Howes & Hamilton, 1993). Although there is a significant amount of concordance between parent–child and teacher–child attachment quality (Ahnert, Pinquart, & Lamb, 2006), secure attachments to teachers appear to have some positive compensatory effects on the prosocial behavior of preschool children who are insecurely attached to their mothers (see Sabol & Pianta, 2013). Findings from the NICHD Early Child Care Study have demonstrated that close relationships with teachers (as perceived by teachers) are related positively to children's social behavior concurrently in kindergarten and 2 years later, with stronger effects for children with less-well-educated mothers (Peisner-Feinberg et al., 2001). However, in observational studies of quality of teacher–child relationships, emotionally supportive interactions with teachers are not related significantly to child outcomes when family and child characteristics (e.g., child sex and maternal sensitivity) are taken into account (NICHD Early Child Care Research Network, 2003b, 2003c).

Longitudinal studies indicate that young children who enjoy emotionally secure relationships with their teachers also are more likely to demonstrate more socially competent behavior and positive relationships with peers than those who do not have positive relationships (e.g., Curby et al., 2009; Mashburn et al., 2008). The quality of teachers' emotional interactions with young children also has been related to children's positive attitudes about school (Valeski & Stipek, 2001), and to academic outcomes over time (Pianta, Belsky, Vandergrift, Houts, & Morrison, 2008).

In the elementary school years, student reports of close and supportive teacher–student relationships predict low levels of aggression, especially for African American and Hispanic students (Meehan, Hughes, & Cavell, 2003). This latter finding is especially important in that African American students at this age tend to enjoy less positive relationships with teachers than do European American children (e.g., Hamre & Pianta, 2001; Meehan et al., 2003). In late elementary school, students' reports of negative relationships with teachers also are related to externalizing behavior problems, anxiety, and depression (Murray & Greenberg, 2000), and positive relationships are related to identification with teachers' values and positive social self-concept (Davis, 2001).

Adolescents' perceptions that teachers are emotionally supportive and caring have been related most often to positive motivational outcomes, including the pursuit of goals to learn and to behave prosocially and responsibly; academic interest; educational aspirations and values; and positive self-concept (see Wentzel, 2009, for a review). Having supportive relationships with teachers also appears to predict, in part, whether students at this age drop out of school (Rumberger, 1995). In studies of perceived support from teachers, parents, and peers (e.g., Wentzel et al., 2012), perceived support from teachers was unique in its relation to students' pursuit of goals to learn. Of additional interest is that Wentzel and colleagues (2012) found that teachers' communication of specific expectations for social and academic outcomes was more predictive of adolescents' academic motivation and engagement if communicated within the context of an emotionally caring relationship.

In summary, many correlational studies have demonstrated significant associations between teacher–student relationships and students' social and academic outcomes at school. However, it is important to note that the causal mechanisms that might explain these associations have not been examined in systematic fashion. Therefore, it might be that a student's behavioral style determines the nature of relationships with teachers over time, or that the quality of these relationships is able to influence student outcomes in positive or negative ways as children advance through school. It is also likely that these associations between relationship quality and outcomes become reciprocal over time, representing complex interrelated systems of social interactions (see Sabol & Pianta, 2013).

Responsive and Warm Relationships with Peers

Researchers have not adapted parenting models to the study of peer relationships (see Wentzel, 2004). However, it is reasonable to assume that when peers create responsive and emotionally supportive interpersonal contexts, students benefit in positive ways. In young children, high levels of peer acceptance and positive friendships have been linked to academic and socioemotional adjustment in school, including positive affect, academic and social engagement, and positive attitudes toward school (e.g., Buhs & Ladd, 2001; Ladd, Kochenderfer, & Coleman, 1996). In addition, young children who have friends who display prosocial behavior are less likely to respond in a hostile or impulsive manner in response to peer provocation or bullying behaviors than are children without highly prosocial friends (Lamarche et al., 2006). Presumably, this is because prosocial friends are able to provide instrumental help and to model effective ways to decrease and defuse threats from peers. Furthermore, having highly prosocial friends was found to protect against the negative relation between peer victimization and academic competence in a sample of middle school students (Tu, Erath, & Flanagan, 2012).

During adolescence, students also report that their peer groups and crowds provide them with a sense of emotional security and a sense of belonging (Brown, Eicher, & Petrie, 1986), whereas adolescents without friends or those who are socially rejected often are lonely, emotionally distressed, and depressed, and suffer from poor self-concepts (Prinstein, Rancourt, Guerry, & Browne, 2009). As with younger children, students in middle childhood and adolescence who are accepted by their peers and have established friendships with classmates also are more likely to enjoy a relatively safe school environment and less likely to be the targets of peer-directed violence and harassment than their peers who do not have friends (see Vitaro, Boivin, & Bukowski, 2009). In contrast, children who are rejected by their peers or do not have friends tend to be bullied and victimized more frequently than others.

In addition, adolescents who perceive that their peers support and care about them tend to be interested and engaged in academic pursuits, whereas students who do not perceive their relationships with peers as positive and supportive tend to be at risk for motivational and academic problems (Wentzel, 2005; Wentzel et al., 2010). Similarly, perceived social support also has been related to positive social outcomes. In particular, perceived social and emotional support from peers has been associated positively with prosocial outcomes in the classroom, such as helping, sharing, and cooperating, and negatively with antisocial forms of behavior (e.g., Wentzel et al., 2007).

Summary

The extant literature supports the notion that structural features, social interactions with teachers and peers, and the provisions of responsiveness and warmth by teachers and peers have the potential to provide tangible resources, opportunities, and experiences that support competence development at school. In this regard, children's experiences at school, whether in preschool or K–12 settings, appear to support the pursuit and achievement of goals that are espoused by teachers and peers, as well as the development of positive outcomes for students themselves. In the following section, I offer remaining questions and challenges for continued work in this area.

Conclusions and Future Directions

In this chapter, I have described social competence at school as the achievement of personal goals that include healthy developmental outcomes, in balance with the achievement of socially valued goals, such as displays of prosocial forms of behavior and high levels of academic performance. Furthermore, I have argued that the socialization of these competencies within school settings can be understood as a function of the amount and quality of structural-level resources of schools, as well as interpersonal contacts with teachers and peers that support students' efforts to achieve both personal and socially valued goals. Social interactions are likely to teach students what they are expected to accomplish and how to achieve it. In turn, the transmission of values and knowledge is more likely to occur if students enjoy supportive and caring relationships with teachers and peers. In conclusion, I raise several general issues that require additional consideration and empirical investigation if the field is to make progress in understanding the socialization functions of schools. These issues concern the nature of social competence at school and how it is socialized, the unique role of schools in promoting the development of competent outcomes, and the need for more sophisticated research methods and designs that can test theoretical models relevant for school settings.

Social Competence at School

Although we are beginning to understand the basic outcomes that most teachers and students value at school, we know little about how and why students come to learn about and to adopt these goals as their own. For instance, it is clear that teachers communicate their expectations and goals to students on a daily basis. However, less is known about factors that predispose students to accept or reject these communications. The family socialization literature suggests that parental messages are more likely to be perceived accurately by children if they are clear and consistent, are framed in ways that are relevant and meaningful to them, require decoding and processing by the child, and are perceived by the child to be of clear importance to the parent and as being conveyed with positive intentions (Grusec & Goodnow, 1994). Adapting this work to the realm of the classroom might provide important insights into effective forms of teacher and peer communication that lead to the adoption of socially valued goals.

Similarly, a greater focus on understanding student characteristics that facilitate acceptance of teachers' and peers' communications is needed. Factors such as students' beliefs regarding the fairness, relevance, and developmental appropriateness of others' goals and expectations (e.g., Smetana & Bitz, 1996) and aspects of social cognitive processing, such as selective attention, attributions, and social biases and stereotypes (Price & Dodge, 1989), are likely to influence students' interpretations and acceptance of social communications. Other individual characteristics, such as attachment security and family functioning (e.g., Fuligni, Eccles, Barber, & Clements, 2001), racial identity (Graham, Taylor, & Hudley, 1998), and the extent that students are oriented toward gaining social approval, also are likely to affect the degree to which they are influenced by teacher and peer expectations.

Consideration of student characteristics also must take into account age-related capabilities. For example, primary developmental tasks of young children under age 6 involve basic self-regulatory skills (managing physiological arousal, emotions, and attention), executive functions (e.g., the ability to monitor and plan behavior, language, and communication skills), and peer interaction skills (Shonkoff & Phillips, 2000). As they make their way through school, children are challenged with school transitions requiring skills related to social integration, flexible coping, and adaptation to new environments. In part, these successful adaptations require the development of positive self-perceptions of autonomy, competence, and personal identity (Grolnick, Friendly, & Bellas, 2009). Mastery of these developmental tasks as they relate to children's understanding and adoption of socially valued goals and objectives of teachers and peers needs to be incorporated into models of school success.

A developmental focus also is necessary for understanding the demands of teachers on students of different ages. A few researchers (e.g., Eccles & Midgley, 1989) have observed that teachers treat students differently and focus on different tasks and goals depending on the age of their students. For example, teachers of early elementary (i.e., first grade) and junior high school students tend to spend more of their time on issues related to social conduct than do teachers at other grade levels. However, little else is known about these differences. Therefore, a critical look at the normative requirements for competent classroom functioning also is necessary to advance knowledge of school socialization processes.

An additional issue concerns what it is that develops or is changed on the part of students as a result of exposure to supportive teacher and peer contexts. In part, responsive and warm relationships are likely to promote a sense of emotional well-being and corresponding desires to contribute to the smooth functioning of classroom activities (see Wentzel, 2012). Continued research that focuses on additional psychological mediators and moderators might be particularly fruitful in determining specific ways in which students' social interactions and interpersonal relationships at school ultimately influence the development of school-based competencies. For example, an additional area for consideration is the influence of social relationships on self-regulatory processes that promote goal pursuit, such as positive beliefs about ability, personal values, and attributions for success and failure (see Wentzel, 2004). The role of these intrapersonal processes in mediating relations between aspects of socialization and competent functioning has not been studied extensively. The differential impact of teachers and peers in contributing to these outcomes also deserves further study (e.g., Wentzel et al., 2012).

Schools as Unique Socializing Contexts

One of the enduring issues with respect to school-related influence concerns the possibility that school experiences mainly afford the practice, refinement, and reinforcement of skills and values learned at home. If so, continuity across home and school settings might explain children's competence at school more than experiences unique to schools (see Ahnert et al., 2006). This notion also is supported by findings that family socialization models are useful for describing socialization processes at school (Wentzel, 2002), and evidence that family factors are typically strong predictors of school outcomes (e.g., Rumberger, 1995) and often completely explain variance predicted by school variables when they are taken into account (e.g., Jimerson, Egeland, Sroufe, & Carlson, 2000). Research that examines core socialization processes that are common across multiple settings and domains of functioning is a natural extension of this work.

Another intriguing issue concerns the role of peers in the school socialization process. As I noted at the beginning of this chapter, a fairly unique aspect of schooling is the requirement that students learn to cooperate and get along with same-age nonfamilial peers. Although this implies that socializing children to function well in formalized peer groups might be a central function of schools, the development of cooperative, prosocial behavior is often attributed to interactions with peers rather than with adults (Youniss, 1994). As noted earlier, researchers are beginning to document ways in which teachers and school settings might influence the development and quality of peer interactions independently of the influence that students exert on each other (also see Ladd, Kochenderfer-Ladd, Visconti, & Ettekal, 2012). Therefore, it is reasonable to assume that the development of positive forms of behavior might be due in large part to systematic regulation of peer interactions in formal school settings. This is an important area of inquiry for both developmental and educational psychologists to pursue.

Theory, Methods, and Designs

Most conclusions concerning socialization in school settings are based on findings from nonexperimental correlational studies. These correlational strategies have resulted in a wealth of data that can serve as a strong foundation for further theory building and research. Descriptive designs also are useful for developing profiles of behavior that characterize competent students. However, more extensive research that can identify variations in these characterizations across classrooms and schools requires in-depth conversations with and extensive observations of students and teachers as they carry out their day-to-day lives at school. In addition, correlational designs typically have focused on a limited number of variables at one point in time. As a result, it is rare that process-oriented variables such as teacher–student interactions are included in studies of structural effects, or familial and nonschool predictors in studies of classroom processes. It also is likely that schools can have effects on children by way of their positive impact on the economic (Sederberg, 1987) and political (Reynolds, 1995) life of communities; school-to-work and service learning programs are good examples of school-based resources that have the potential to provide positive benefits to communities and families. The notion that community and family effects might mediate the impact of schools on children is intriguing but rarely studied in a systematic fashion. Therefore, a necessary next step is the development of conceptual models that consider ways in which children, and the various social systems in which they develop, including home, peer groups, communities, and schools, interact to support the development of school-related competence.

In addition, correlational research cannot advance understanding of causal influence or direction of effects. Indeed, is it that responsive and supportive teachers and peers have the potential to influence the development of competencies and skills they value, or is it that competent students influence teachers and peers to interact with them in specific ways? Although the likely answer is that both are true, identifying ways in which teachers and peers actively promote the development of social competencies at school requires systematic longitudinal and experimental research. Large-scale longitudinal studies have begun to document school-based predictors of young children's competence over time (e.g., Vandell et al., 2010). Others have begun to document correlates of change related to qualities of older students' relationships with teachers and peers (e.g., Hamre & Pianta, 2001; Wentzel & Caldwell, 1997).

A welcome change to this area of research is that intervention and experimental studies designed to examine processes that support competence development at schools have become more common over the past 10 years. Studies designed to test the effects of school-based interventions are beginning to shed light on the efficacy of training teachers and peers to interact with each other in positive ways in order to facilitate the development of social and academic skills (Durlak et al., 2011; Vazsonyi, Belliston, & Flannery, 2004). Training teachers to facilitate the development of young children's social competencies and self-regulatory skills that in turn promote academic competence also has shown promising results (e.g., Raver, 2012).

Our current understanding of school socialization also is based primarily on studies of white middle-class children from the United States. Therefore, more diverse samples with respect to race and socioeconomic status (SES) also are needed in this area of research. For instance, in response to findings reported by the NICHD Child Care Study, researchers have argued that when child-care variables are assessed in more diverse samples that include a broader range of SES and ethnicity, different results are obtained (e.g., Fouts, Roopnarine, Lamb, & Evans, 2012; Sagi, Koren-Karie, Gini, Ziv, & Joels, 2002). Researchers of older children also have found that race moderates relations between dropping out of school and features of schools and families, such that the SES of families and schools predicts dropping out for European American and Hispanic adolescents but not for African American students (Rumberger, 1995). Some studies also have demonstrated differential teacher treatment of students as a function of student gender, race (Jussim et al., 2009), and behavioral styles (Chang, 2003), with these differences sometimes attributed in part to teachers' own race and gender (Saft & Pianta, 2001). Although it is likely that the underlying psychological processes that contribute to school adjustment (e.g., self-regulation, values, competence beliefs) are similar for all students regardless of race, ethnicity, gender, or other contextual and demographic variables, the degree to which these latter factors moderate the effects of these psychological processes on adjustment outcomes is not well known (e.g., Blair, Berry, & Friedman, 2012). Achieving a better understanding of such interactions deserves our full attention. Similarly, beliefs about how to characterize a competent student are likely to vary as a function of race, gender, neighborhood, or family background (e.g., Harkness et al., 2008). The fact that many results concerning child outcomes and schooling differ as a function of who provides the assessments of behavior (e.g., parents, teachers, or students themselves) attests to this possibility (e.g., NICHD Early Child Care Research Network, 2003a; Toro et al., 1985). Expanding our data base to include the voices of underrepresented populations both as research participants and as researchers can only enrich our understanding of how and why children make successful adaptations to school.

In conclusion, I have argued that being a competent student requires children to achieve positive developmental outcomes and personal goals while meeting social objectives that are imposed externally by teachers and peers. Identifying the precise socialization experiences that lead to a healthy balance between personal growth and social integration remains a significant challenge to the field. However, we have gained some important insights into students' experiences within school settings as they relate to social approval and acceptance, as well as to the development of personal competencies and interests. Socialization of these outcomes within school settings can be understood, in part, as a function of the amount and quality of structural-level resources of schools, as well as interpersonal contacts with teachers and peers. Ideally, these insights can serve as a foundation for continued research on the social antecedents of children's competent functioning at school.

REFERENCES

Ahnert, L., Pinquart, M., & Lamb, M. E. (2006). Security of children's relationships with nonparental care providers: A meta-analysis. *Child Development, 77,* 664–679.

Anderman, E. M. (2002). School effects on psychological outcomes during adolescence. *Journal of Educational Psychology, 94,* 795–809.

Barry, C., & Wentzel, K. R. (2006). The influence of middle school friendships on prosocial behavior: A longitudinal study. *Developmental Psychology, 42,* 153–163.

Battistich, V., & Hom, A. (1997). The relationship between students' sense of their school as a community and their involvement in problem behaviors. *American Journal of Public Health, 87,* 1997–2001.

Baumrind, D. (1971). Current patterns of parental authority. *Developmental Psychology Monograph, 4*(1, Pt. 2), 1–103.

Belsky, J. (2001). Emanuel Miller lecture: Developmental risks (still) associated with early child care. *Journal of Child Psychology and Psychiatry and Allied Disciplines, 42,* 845–859.

Bierman, K. L., & Powers, C. J. (2009). Social skills training to improve peer relations. In K. H. Rubin, W. M. Bukowski, & B. Laursen (Eds.), *Handbook on peer interactions, relationships, and groups* (pp. 603–621). New York: Guilford Press.

Blair, C., Berry, D. J., & Friedman, A. H. (2012). The development of self-regulation in infancy and early childhood: An organizing framework for the design and evaluation of early care and education programs for children in poverty. In S. L. Odom, E. P. Pungello, & N. Gardner-Neblett (Eds.), *Infants, toddlers, and families in poverty: Research implications for early child care* (pp. 127–152). New York: Guilford Press.

Bronfenbrenner, U., & Morris, P. A. (2006). The bioecological model of human development. In W. Damon (Series Ed.) & R. Lerner (Vol. Ed.), *Handbook of child psychology: Vol. 1. Theoretical models of human development* (6th ed., pp. 793–828). Hoboken, NJ: Wiley.

Brooks-Gunn, J., Fuligni, A. S., & Berlin, L. J. (2003). *Early childhood development in the 21st century.* New York: Teachers College Press.

Brown, B. B., Eicher, S. A., & Petrie, S. (1986). The importance of peer group ("crowd") affiliation in adolescence. *Journal of Adolescence, 9,* 73–96.

Buhs, E. S., & Ladd, G. W. (2001). Peer rejection as an antecedent of young children's school adjustment: An examination of mediating processes. *Developmental Psychology, 37,* 550–560.

Burchinal, M., Kainz, K., & Cai, Y. (2011). How well do our measures of quality predict child outcomes?: A meta-analysis and coordinated analysis of data from large-scale studies of early childhood settings. In M. Zaslow, I. Martinez-Beck, K. Tout, & T. Halle (Eds.), *Quality measurement in early childhood settings* (pp. 11–31). Baltimore: Brookes.

Butler, R. (2005). Competence assessment, competence, and motivation between early and middle childhood. In A. J. Elliot & C. S. Dweck (Eds.), *Handbook of competence and motivation* (pp. 202–221). New York: Guilford Press.

Chang, L. (2003). Variable effects of children's aggression, social withdrawal, and prosocial leadership as functions of teacher beliefs and behaviors. *Child Development, 74,* 535–548.

Cillessen, A., & van den Berg, Y. (2012). Popularity and school adjustment. In A. M. Ryan & G. W. Ladd (Eds.), *Peer relationships and adjustment at school* (pp. 135–164). Charlotte, NC: Information Age.

Coleman, J. S., Campbell, E. Q., Hobson, C. J., McPartland, J., Mood, A. M., Weinfeld, F. D., et al. (1966). *Equality of educational opportunity.* Washington, DC: U.S. Government Printing Office.

Conduct Problems Prevention Research Group. (2010). The effects of a multiyear universal social–emotional learning program: The role of student and school characteristics. *Journal of Consulting and Clinical Psychology 78*, 156–168.

Connell, J. P., & Wellborn, J. G. (1991). Competence, autonomy, and relatedness: A motivational analysis of self-system processes. In M. R. Gunnar & L. A. Sroufe (Eds.), *Self processes and development: The Minnesota Symposia on Child Development* (Vol. 23, pp. 43–78). Hillsdale, NJ: Erlbaum.

Cooper, C. R., Ayers-Lopez, S., & Marquis, A. (1982). Children's discourse during peer learning in experimental and naturalistic situations. *Discourse Processes, 5*, 177–191.

Crockett, L., Losoff, M., & Petersen, A. C. (1984). Perceptions of the peer group and friendship in early adolescence. *Journal of Early Adolescence, 4*, 155–181.

Crosnoe, R., & Needham, B. (2004). Holism, contextual variability, and the study of friendships in adolescent development. *Child Development, 75*, 264–279.

Curby, T. W., LoCasale-Crouch, J., Konold, T. R., Pianta, R. C., Howes, C., Burchinal, M., et al. (2009). The relations of observed pre-K classroom quality profiles to children's achievement and social competence. *Early Education and Development, 20*, 346–372.

Darling, N., & Steinberg, L. (1993). Parenting style as context—an integrative model, *Psychological Bulletin, 113*, 487–496.

Davis, H. A. (2001). The quality and impact of relationships between elementary school students and teachers. *Contemporary Educational Psychology, 26*, 431–453.

Dowson, M., & McInerney, D. M. (2003). What do students say about their motivational goals?: Towards a more complex and dynamic perspective on student motivation. *Contemporary Educational Psychology, 28*, 91–113.

Durlak, J. A., Weissberg, R. P., & Dymnicki, A. B. (2011). The impact of enhancing students' social and emotional learning: A meta-analysis of school-based universal interventions. *Child Development, 82*, 405–432.

Eccles, J. S., & Midgley, C. (1989). Stage–environment fit: Developmentally appropriate classrooms for young adolescents. In C. Ames & R. Ames (Eds.), *Research on motivation in education: Vol. 3* (pp. 139–186). New York: Academic Press.

Eccles, J., & Roeser, R. (2013). Schools as developmental contexts during adolescence. In R. Lerner, M. Easterbrooks, J. Mistry, & I. Weiner, (Eds.), *Handbook of psychology: Vol. 6. Developmental psychology* (2nd ed., pp. 321–337). Hoboken, NJ: Wiley.

Espinoza, G., & Juvonen, J. (2011). Perceptions of the school social context across the transition to middle school: Heightened sensitivity among Latino students? *Journal of Educational Psychology, 103*, 749–758.

Fabes, R. A., Hanish, L. D., & Martin, C. (2003). Children at play: The role of peers in understanding the effects of child care. *Child Development, 74*, 1039–1043.

Finn, J. D., Pannozzo, G. M., & Achilles, C. M. (2003). The "why's" of class size: Student behavior in small classes. *Review of Educational Research, 73*, 321–368.

Fitzgerald, H., Mann, T., Cabrera, N., & Wong, M. (2003). Diversity in caregiving contexts. In R. Lerner, A. Easterbrooks, & J. Mistry (Ed.), *Handbook of psychology: Vol. 6. Developmental psychology* (pp. 135–167). Mahwah, NJ: Erlbaum.

Ford, M. E. (1992). *Motivating humans: Goals, emotions, and personal agency beliefs.* Newbury Park, CA: Sage.

Fouts, H., Roopnarine, J., Lamb, M., & Evans, M. (2012). Infant social interactions with multiple caregivers: The importance of ethnicity and socioeconomic status. *Journal of Cross-Cultural Psychology, 43*, 328–348.

Fuligni, A. J., Eccles, J. S., Barber, B. L., & Clements, P. (2001). Early adolescent peer orientation and adjustment during high school. *Developmental Psychology, 37*, 28–36.

Graham, S., Taylor, A., & Hudley, C. (1998). Exploring achievement values among ethnic minority early adolescents. *Journal of Educational Psychology, 90*, 606–620.

Gresham, F., Van, M., & Cook, C. (2006). Social-skills training for teaching replacement behaviors: Remediating acquisition in at-risk students. *Behavioral Disorders, 31*, 363–377.

Grolnick, W., Friendly, R., & Bellas, V. (2009). Parenting and children's motivation at school. In K. Wentzel & A. Wigfield (Eds.), *Handbook of motivation at school* (pp. 279–300). New York: Routledge/Taylor & Francis.

Grusec, J. E., & Goodnow, J. J. (1994). Impact of parental discipline methods on the child's internalization of values: A reconceptualization of current points of view. *Developmental Psychology, 30,* 4–19.

Hagens, H. E. (1997). Strategies for encouraging peer interactions in infant/toddler programs. *Early Childhood Education Journal, 25,* 147–149.

Hamre, B. K., & Pianta, R. C. (2001). Early teacher–child relationships and the trajectory of children's school outcomes through eighth grade. *Child Development, 72,* 625–628.

Harkness, S., Blom, M., Oliva, A., Moscardino, U., Zylicz, P., Bermudez, M., et al. (2008). Teachers' ethnotheories of the "ideal student" in five Western cultures. In J. Elliott & E. Grigorenko (Eds.), *Western psychological and educational theory in diverse contexts* (pp. 113–135). New York: Routledge.

Harter, S. (2012). *The construction of the self: Developmental and sociocultural foundations* (2nd ed.). New York: Guilford Press.

Hopson, L. M., & Lee, E. (2011). Mitigating the effect of family poverty on academic and behavioral outcomes: The role of school climate in middle and high school. *Children and Youth Services Review, 33,* 2221–2229.

Howes, C., & Hamilton, C. E. (1993). The changing experience of child care: Changes in teachers and in teacher–child relationships and children's social competence with peers. *Early Childhood Research Quarterly, 8,* 15–32.

Jimerson, S., Egeland, B., Sroufe, L. A., & Carlson, B. (2000). A prospective longitudinal study of high school dropouts: Examining multiple predictors across development. *Journal of School Psychology, 38,* 525–549.

Jussim, L., Robustelli, S., & Cain, T. (2009). Teacher expectations and self-fulfilling prophecies. In K. R. Wentzel & A. Wigfield (Eds.), *Handbook of motivation at school* (pp. 349–380). New York: Taylor & Francis.

Klein, J., Cornell, D., & Konold, T. (2012). Relationships between bullying, school climate, and student risk behaviors. *School Psychology Quarterly, 27,* 154–169.

Kuperminc, G. P., Leadbetter, B. J., Emmons, C., & Blatt, S. J. (1997). Perceived school climate and difficulties in the social adjustment of middle school students. *Applied Developmental Psychology, 1,* 76–88.

Ladd, G. W., Kochenderfer, B. J., & Coleman, C. C. (1996). Friendship quality as a predictor of young children's early school adjustment. *Child Development, 67,* 1103–1118.

Ladd, G. W., Kochenderfer-Ladd, B., Visconti, K. J., & Ettekal, I. (2012). Classroom peer relations and children's social and scholastic development: Risk factors and resources. In A. M. Ryan & G. W. Ladd (Eds.), *Peer relationships and adjustment at school* (pp. 11–50). Charlotte, NC: Information Age.

Lamarche, V., Brendgen, M., Boivin, M., Vitaro, F., Perusse, D., & Dionne, G. (2006). Do friendships and sibling relationships provide protection against peer victimization in a similar way? *Social Development, 15,* 373–393.

Lamb, M. E. (1998). Nonparental child care: Context, quality, correlates. In W. Damon, I. E. Sigel, & K. A. Renninger (Eds.), *Handbook of child psychology: Vol. 4. Child psychology in practice* (pp. 73–134). New York: Wiley.

Lavallee, K. L., Bierman, K. L., & Nix, R. L. (2005). The impact of first-grade "friendship group" experiences on child social outcomes in the Fast Track Program. *Journal of Abnormal Child Psychology, 33,* 307–324.

Lempers, J. D., & Clark-Lempers, D. S. (1992). Young, middle, and late adolescents' comparisons of the functional importance of five significant relationships. *Journal of Youth and Adolescence, 21,* 53–96.

Limber, S. (2012). The Olweus Bullying Prevention Program: An overview of its implementation and research basis. In S. Jimerson, A. Nickerson, M. Mayer, & M. Furlong (Eds.), *Handbook of school violence and school safety: International research and practice* (pp. 369–381). New York: Routledge.

Mashburn, A. J., Pianta, R. C., Downer, J. T., Barbarin, O. A., Bryant, D., Burchinal, M., et al. (2008). Measures of classroom quality in prekindergarten and children's development of academic, language, and social skills. *Child Development, 79,* 732–749.

McCartney, K., Burchinal, M., Clarke-Stewart, A., Bub, K., Owen, M., Belsky, J., et al. (2010). Testing a series of causal propositions relating time in child care to children's externalizing behavior. *Developmental Psychology, 46,* 1–17.

McCullagh, P., Law, B., & Ste-Marie, D. (2012). Modeling and performance. In S. Murphy (Ed.), *The Oxford handbook of sport and performance psychology* (pp. 250–272). New York: Oxford University Press.

Meehan, B. T., Hughes, J. N., & Cavell, T. A. (2003). Teacher–student relationships as compensatory resources for aggressive children. *Child Development, 74,* 1145–1157.

Meisgeier, C., & Kellow, T. (2007). Type, temperament and teacher perceptions of ideal and problem students. *Journal of Psychological Type, 67,* 39–49.

Murray, C., & Greenberg, M. T. (2000). Children's relationships with teachers and bonds with school: An investigation of patterns and correlates in middle childhood. *Journal of School Psychology, 38,* 423–445.

Newman, R. S. (2000). Social influences on the development of children's adaptive help seeking: The role of parents, teachers, and peers. *Developmental Review, 20,* 350–404.

NICHD Early Child Care Research Network. (1997). The effects of infant child care on infant–mother attachment security: Results of the NICHD Study of Early Child Care. *Child Development, 68,* 860–879.

NICHD Early Child Care Research Network. (2001). Child-care and family predictors of preschool attachment and stability from infancy. *Developmental Psychology, 37,* 847–862.

NICHD Early Child Care Research Network. (2002). Parenting and family influences when children are in child care: Results from the NICHD Study of Early Child Care. In J. Borkowski, S. Ramey, & M. Bristol-Power (Eds.), *Parenting and the child's world: Influences on academic, intellectual, and social–emotional development* (pp. 99–123). Mahwah, NJ: Erlbaum.

NICHD Early Child Care Research Network. (2003a). Does amount of time spent in child care predict socioemotional adjustment during the transition to kindergarten? *Child Development, 74,* 976–1005.

NICHD Early Child Care Research Network. (2003b). Does quality of child care affect child outcomes at age 4½? *Developmental Psychology, 39,* 451–469.

NICHD Early Child Care Research Network. (2003c). Social functioning in first grade: Associations with earlier home and child care predictors and with current classroom experiences. *Child Development, 74,* 1639–1662.

NICHD Early Child Care Research Network. (2006). Child-care effect sizes for the NICHD Study of Early Child Care and Youth Development. *American Psychologist, 61,* 99–116.

Peisner-Feinberg, E. S., Burchinal, M. R., Clifford, R. M., Culkin, M. L., Howes, C., Kagan, S. L., et al. (2001). The relation of preschool child-care quality to children's cognitive and social development trajectories through second grade. *Child Development, 72,* 1534–1553.

Pianta, R. C., Belsky, J., Vandergrift, N., Houts, R., & Morrison, F. J. (2008). Classroom effects on children's achievement trajectories in elementary school. *American Educational Research Journal, 45,* 365–397.

Pianta, R. C., Hamre, B. K., & Allen, J. P. (2012). Teacher–student relationships and engagement: Conceptualizing, measuring, and improving the capacity of classroom interaction. In S. L. Christenson, A. L. Reschly, & C. Wylie (Eds.), *Handbook on student engagement* (pp. 365–386). New York: Springer.

Pianta, R. C., Hamre, B., & Downer, J. (2011). Aligning measures of quality with professional development goals and goals for children's development. In M. Zaslow, I. Martinez-Beck,

K. Tout, & T. Halle (Eds.), *Quality measurement in early childhood settings* (pp. 297–315). Baltimore: Brookes.

Pianta, R. C., Hamre, B., & Stuhlman, M. (2003). Relationships between teachers and children. In W. Reynolds & G. Miller (Eds.), *Handbook of psychology: Vol. 7. Educational psychology* (pp. 199–234). New York: Wiley.

Price, J. M., & Dodge, K. A. (1989). Peers' contributions to children's social maladjustment: Description and intervention. In T. J. Berndt & G. W. Ladd (Eds.), *Peer relationships in child development* (pp. 341–370). New York: Wiley.

Prinstein, M., Rancourt, D., Guerry, J., & Browne, C. (2009). Peer reputations and psychological adjustment. In K. Rubin, W. Bukowski, & B. Laursen (Eds.), *Handbook on peer relationships* (pp. 548–567). New York: Guilford Press.

Raver, C. (2012). Low-income children's self-regulation in the classroom: Scientific inquiry for social change. *American Psychologist, 67*, 681–689.

Reid, M., Landesman, S., Treder, R., & Jaccard, J. (1989). "My family and friends": Six- to twelve-year-old children's perceptions of social support. *Child Development, 60*, 896–910.

Resnick, G. (2010). Project Head Start: Quality and links to child outcomes. In A. Reynolds, A. Rolnick, M. Englund, & J. Temple (Eds.), *Childhood programs and practices in the first decade of life: A human capital integration* (pp. 121–156). New York: Cambridge University Press.

Reynolds, D. R. (1995). Rural education: Decentering the consolidation debate. In E. N. Castle (Ed.), *The changing American countryside: Rural people and places* (pp. 451–480). Lawrence: University Press of Kansas.

Roeser, R., Urdan, T., & Stephens, J. (2009). School as a context of student motivation and achievement. In K. R. Wentzel & A. Wigfield (Eds.), *Handbook of motivation at school* (pp. 381–410). New York: Taylor & Francis.

Rubin, K. H., Bukowski, W., & Parker, J. G. (1998). Peer interactions, relationships, and groups. In W. Damon (Series Ed.) & N. Eisenberg (Vol. Ed.), *Handbook of child psychology: Vol. 3. Social, emotional, and personality development* (5th ed., pp. 619–700). New York: Wiley.

Rumberger, R. W. (1995). Dropping out of middle school: A multilevel analysis of students and schools. *American Educational Research Journal, 32*, 583–625.

Ryan, A., & Shim, S. (2008). An exploration of young adolescents' social achievement goals and social adjustment in middle school. *Journal of Educational Psychology, 100*, 672–687.

Ryan, R. M. (1993). Agency and organization: Intrinsic motivation, autonomy, and the self in psychological development. In J. Jacobs (Ed.), *Nebraska Symposium on Motivation* (Vol. 40, pp. 1–56). Lincoln: University of Nebraska Press.

Sabol, T. J., & Pianta, R. C. (2013). Relationships between teachers and children. In W. Reynolds & G. Miller (Eds.), *Handbook of psychology: Vol. 7. Educational psychology* (2nd ed., pp. 199–211). Hoboken, NJ: Wiley.

Saft, E. W., & Pianta, R. C. (2001). Teachers' perceptions of their relationships with students: Effects of child age, gender, and ethnicity of teachers and children. *School Psychology Quarterly, 16*, 125–141.

Sagi, A., Koren-Karie, N., Gini, M., Ziv, Y., & Joels, T. (2002). Shedding further light on the effects of various types and quality of early child care on infant–mother attachment relationship: The Haifa study of early child care. *Child Development, 73*, 1166–1186.

Salmivalli, C., Garandeau, C., & Veenstra, R. (2012). KiVa Anti-Bullying Program: Implications for school adjustment. In A. M. Ryan & G. W. Ladd (Eds.), *Peer relationships and adjustment at school* (pp. 279–307). Charlotte, NC: Information Age.

Scheerens, J., & Bosker, R. J. (1997). *The foundations of educational effectiveness.* Oxford, UK: Elsevier.

Schunk, D., & Pajares, F. (2009). Self-efficacy theory. In K. R. Wentzel & A. Wigfield (Eds.), *Handbook of motivation at school* (pp. 35–54). New York: Taylor & Francis.

Schunk, D., & Zimmerman, B. (1997). Social origins of self-regulatory competence. *Educational Psychologist, 32*, 195–208.

Schwartz, D., Gorman, A. H., Nakamoto, J., & McKay, T. (2006). Popularity, social acceptance, and aggression in adolescent peer groups: Links with academic performance and school attendance. *Developmental Psychology, 42,* 1116–1127.

Schweinhart, L. J., Barne, H. V., Weikart, D. P., Barnett, W. S., & Epstein, A. S. (1993). *Significant benefits: The High/Scope Perry Preschool Study through age 27.* Ypsilanti, MI: High/Scope Press.

Sederberg, C. H. (1987). Economic role of school districts in rural communities. *Research in Rural Education, 4,* 125–130.

Shonkoff, J. P., & Phillips, D. A. (2000). *From neurons to neighborhoods: The science of early childhood development.* Washington, DC: National Academy Press.

Slavin, R. (2011). Instruction based on cooperative learning. In R. Mayer & P. Alexander (Eds.), *Handbook of research on learning and instruction* (pp.344–360). New York: Routledge.

Smetana, J., & Bitz, B. (1996). Adolescents' conceptions of teachers' authority and their relations to rule violations in school. *Child Development, 67,* 1153–1172.

Toro, P. A., Cowen, E. L., Gesten, E. L., Weissberg, R. P., Rapkin, B. D., & Davidson, E. (1985). Social environmental predictors of children's adjustment in elementary school classrooms. *American Journal of Community Psychology, 13,* 353–363.

Tu, K. M., Erath, S. A., & Flanagan, K. S. (2012). Can socially adept friends protect peer-victimized early adolescents against lower academic competence? *Journal of Applied Developmental Psychology, 33,* 24–30.

Valeski, T. N., & Stipek, D. J. (2001). Young children's feelings about school. *Child Development, 72,* 1198–1213.

Vandell, D. L., Belsky, J., Burchinal, M., Steinberg, L., & Vandergrift, N. (2010). Do effects of early child care extend to age 15 years?: Results from the NICHD study of early child care and youth development. *Child Development, 81,* 737–756.

Vazsonyi, A., Belliston, L., & Flannery, D. (2004). Evaluation of a school-based, universal violence prevention program: Low-, medium-, and high-risk children. *Youth Violence and Juvenile Justice, 2,* 185–206.

Verasalo, M., Tuomivaara, P., & Lindeman, M. (1996). 15-year-old pupils' and their teachers' values, and their belief about the values of an ideal pupil. *Educational Psychology, 16,* 35–47.

Vitaro, F., Boivin, M., & Bukowski, W. M. (2009). The role of friendship in child and adolescent psychosocial development. In K. H. Rubin, W. M. Bukowski, & B. Laursen (Eds.), *Handbook on peer interactions, relationships, and groups* (pp. 568–585). New York: Guilford Press.

Weinstein, R. S. (2002). *Reaching higher: The power of expectations in schooling.* Cambridge, MA: Harvard University Press.

Wentzel, K. R. (1989). Adolescent classroom goals, standards for performance, and academic achievement: An interactionist perspective. *Journal of Educational Psychology, 81,* 131–142.

Wentzel, K. R. (1991). Social competence at school: Relations between social responsibility and academic achievement. *Review of Educational Research, 61,* 1–24.

Wentzel, K. R. (2002). Are effective teachers like good parents?: Interpersonal predictors of school adjustment in early adolescence. *Child Development, 73,* 287–301.

Wentzel, K. R. (2004). Understanding classroom competence: The role of social-motivational and self-processes. In R. Kail (Ed.), *Advances in child development and behavior* (Vol. 32, pp. 214–242). San Diego, CA: Academic Press.

Wentzel, K. R. (2005). Peer relationships, motivation, and academic performance at school. In A. J. Elliot & C. S. Dweck (Eds.), *Handbook of competence and motivation* (pp. 279–296). New York: Guilford Press.

Wentzel, K. R. (2009). Students' relationships with teachers as motivational contexts. In K. Wentzel & A. Wigfield (Eds.), *Handbook of motivation at school* (pp. 301–322). Mahwah, NJ: Erlbaum.

Wentzel, K. R. (2012). Adolescents' relationships with teachers and peers. In T. Wubbels, J. van Tartwijk, P. den Brok, & J. Levy (Eds.), *Interpersonal relationships in education* (pp. 17–36). Rotterdam: Sense Publishers.

Wentzel, K. R. (2013). School adjustment. In W. Reynolds & G. Miller (Eds.), *Handbook of psychology: Vol. 7. Educational psychology* (pp. 213–232). New York: Wiley.

Wentzel, K. R., Baker, S. A., & Russell, S. L. (2012). Young adolescents' perceptions of teachers' and peers' goals as predictors of social and academic goal pursuit. *Applied Psychology: An International Review, 61*(4), 605–633.

Wentzel, K. R., Barry, C., & Caldwell, K. (2004). Friendships in middle school: Influences on motivation and school adjustment. *Journal of Educational Psychology, 96*, 195–203.

Wentzel, K. R., Battle, A., Russell, S., & Looney, L. (2010). Social supports from teachers and peers as predictors of academic and social motivation. *Contemporary Educational Psychology, 35*, 193–202.

Wentzel, K. R., & Caldwell, K. (1997). Friendships, peer acceptance, and group membership: Relations to academic achievement in middle school. *Child Development, 68*, 1198–1209.

Wentzel, K. R., Filisetti, L., & Looney, L. (2007). Adolescent prosocial behavior: The role of self-processes and contextual cues. *Child Development, 78*, 895–910.

Wentzel, K. R., Monzo, J., Williams, A. Y., & Tomback, R. M. (2007, April). *Teacher and peer influence on academic motivation in adolescence: A cross-sectional study.* Paper presented at the biennial meeting of the Society for Research in Child Development, Boston.

Wentzel, K. R., & Wigfield, A. (2009). *Handbook of motivation at school.* New York: Taylor & Francis.

What Works Clearinghouse. (2007). Caring School Community. Retrieved from *www.ies.ed.gov/ncee/wwc.*

Youniss, J. (1994). Children's friendship and peer culture: Implications for theories of networks and support. In F. Nestmann & K. Hurrelmann (Eds.), *Social networks and social support in childhood and adolescence* (pp. 75–88). Berlin: de Gruyter.

CHAPTER 12

Media as Agents of Socialization

Sara Prot
Craig A. Anderson
Douglas A. Gentile
Wayne Warburton
Muniba Saleem
Christopher L. Groves
Stephanie C. Brown

You were never there for me, were you mother? You expected Mike
and Carol Brady to raise me! I'm the bastard son of Claire Huxtable!
I am a Lost Cunningham! I learned the facts of life from watching
The Facts of Life! Oh God!
—Jim Carrey as Ernie "Chip" Douglas
in the movie *The Cable Guy* (1996)

Unlike Chip Douglas from the movie *The Cable Guy*, most children are not raised exclusively by television, without support from parents, teachers, and other caregivers. Nonetheless, media play an increasingly significant role as socializing agents in the lives of children and adolescents. Over the past 10 years, media consumption among youth has grown steadily. There have been significant increases in time spent watching television, listening to music, playing video games, and using the Internet and cell phones (Harris Interactive, 2008; Jones & Fox, 2009; Rideout, Foehr, & Roberts, 2010). Youth in the United States now use media for an average of 7.5 hours a day (Rideout et al., 2010).

The mass media explosion that began in the 1950s has dramatically changed the environment in which children are raised. Electronic media provide children with a variety of new learning opportunities and broaden the range of events children experience. Socialization is no longer restricted to the influences of family, peers, and other people in children's immediate surroundings. Indeed, most everything we experience as humans has an impact on the way the brain becomes wired, just as the things we eat have an impact on our body. As with a food diet, it is important to consider issues such as amount, content, and age-appropriateness when it comes to a media diet (Warburton, 2012a). Although most research has focused on potential negative effects of some types of media, it is equally important to examine positive effects of a "healthy" media diet (Warburton & Highfield, 2012).

In the short term, media use affects behavior through priming cognitions and eliciting affect, increasing arousal and prompting imitation (C. A. Anderson et al., 2003; Paik & Comstock, 1994). In the long term, media influence beliefs, perceptions, behavioral scripts, and affective traits, bringing about lasting changes in personality (Gentile, Groves, & Gentile, 2014; Huesmann & Kirwil, 2007). Significant effects of media use have been demonstrated in a wide range of domains of socialization, including violence, helping, and education (overviewed in Table 12.1). This chapter broadly summarizes research findings concerning entertainment-focused *mass* media as agents of socialization. We do not include media that have been specifically designed to teach educational content or health-related behaviors. Some teaching/learning-based targeted media products have been found to teach their content successfully and represent a positive development in technology use, but they fall outside the scope of this chapter. First, we describe the general learning model (GLM), a useful theoretical framework for understanding socialization mechanisms. Next, we review relevant research on mass media and socialization. Finally, we identify key questions for future research.

The General Learning Model

The GLM (Barlett & Anderson, 2013; Buckley & Anderson, 2006; Gentile et al., 2014)—derived from the general aggression model (C. A. Anderson & Bushman, 2002; DeWall, Anderson, & Bushman, 2012)—is a useful framework for understanding short- and long-term media effects. It describes processes through which personal characteristics and environmental stimuli affect social behaviors in short-term contexts. It also shows how long-term attitudes, beliefs, and behavioral tendencies are formed through repeated exposure to various types of social encounters (including media use). We pay special attention to long-term learning processes because they are the key to media influences on socialization. Nonetheless, we describe short-term processes as well.

In any immediate situation, social behaviors are influenced by both person factors (e.g., personality, mood, genetic predispositions) and situation factors (e.g., media use, the physical environment, other people's actions). Person factors and situation factors influence one's present internal state—active cognitions, affect, and state of arousal. For example, playing a prosocial video game primes prosocial cognitions and increases positive affect (Greitemeyer & Osswald, 2009; Saleem, Anderson, & Gentile, 2012a, 2012b). These internal states jointly influence appraisal and decision-making processes. For instance, increased positive affect may increase benign (rather than hostile) attributions in an ambiguous social encounter. Such immediate appraisals occur automatically and require little mental effort. In contrast, people engage in reappraisal only when sufficient mental resources are available and when the immediate appraisal is perceived as both important and unsatisfactory (Buckley & Anderson, 2006). Thus, normal appraisal and decision-making processes can result in either impulsive or thoughtful actions of many types, prosocial and antisocial. In turn, that action influences the current social situation, essentially starting a new social episode.

TABLE 12.1. A Summary of Main Research Findings on Mass Media as Agents of Socialization

Positive effects	Evidence[a]
Prosocial (nonviolent) media	
Increase prosocial behavior	Fairly strong causal, both short and long term
Increase empathy	Moderate causal, both short and long term
Decrease aggression	Fairly strong causal short term
Civic engagement	Weak causal, only cross-sectional support
Educational media teach specific knowledge and skills	Fairly strong causal, short and long term
Media can promote multicultural awareness and weaken stereotypes	Weak short- and long-term evidence
Social media promote social networking	Weak long-term evidence, conflicting evidence of negative effects on social functioning
Parental involvement in media use protects against negative media effects	Moderate correlational long-term effects, weak experimental long-term evidence

Negative effects	Evidence[a]
Violent media	
Increase aggressive behavior	Very strong causal, both short and long term
Increase violent behavior	Fairly strong long term; moderate causal short term
Increase aggressive cognitions	Very strong causal, both short and long term
Increase aggressive affect	Very strong causal, both short and long term
Desensitize to violence	Very strong causal, both short and long term
Decrease empathy	Very strong causal, both short and long term
Decrease prosocial behavior	Very strong causal, both short and long term
Civic engagement	Weak causal, only cross-sectional support
Risk-glorifying media	
Increase positive attitudes toward risky behaviors	Fairly strong causal, short and long term
Increase likelihood of risky behaviors in real life	Fairly strong causal, short and long term
Stereotypical portrayals of women and ethnic minorities strengthen stereotypes	Fairly strong causal, short and long term

Other domains in need of research	
Identity development	Effects of cell phones, texting, and sexting
Social networking and social functioning	MMORPGs
Media and brain function	

[a]*Strong evidence*: Over 20 methodologically strong studies exist that provide evidence of the effect; *moderate evidence*: A total of 10 to 20 methodologically strong studies exist that provide evidence of the effect; *weak evidence*: Less than 10 methodologically strong studies exist that provide evidence of the effect; *causal evidence*: Multiple methodologically strong studies provide clear evidence of causality.

Through repeated priming and reinforcement of specific knowledge structures, exposure to any type of experience can lead to lasting influences on personality and social development (see Figure 12.1). Long-term effects occur through three interrelated processes: changes in cognitive constructs, cognitive-emotional constructs, and emotional constructs. Cognitive constructs include perceptual schemata, beliefs, and behavioral scripts. For example, long-term exposure to media violence leads to the development of a *hostile attribution bias*, a tendency to perceive other people's harmful actions as hostile rather than accidental (C. A. Anderson, Gentile, & Buckley, 2007). Violent media use also increases beliefs that aggression is an appropriate response (Möller & Krahé, 2009). Cognitive-emotional constructs include attitudes and stereotypes. For example, long-term exposure to media violence is associated with proviolence attitudes (Funk, Baldacci, Pasold, & Baumgardner, 2004). Stereotypical portrayals of racial groups in mass media influences real-world evaluations of minorities (Lett, Dipietro, & Johnson, 2004; Saleem & Anderson, 2013). Emotional constructs include conditioned emotions and affective traits. High exposure to media violence leads to desensitization and reduced empathy toward victims of violence (Carnagey, Anderson, & Bushman, 2007; Krahé & Möller, 2010; Mullin & Linz, 1995). These same psychological processes explain how

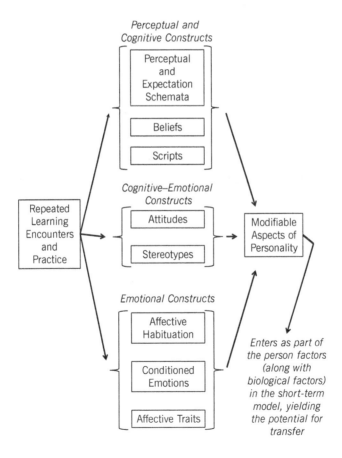

FIGURE 12.1. Long-term processes in the general learning model. From Gentile, Groves, and Gentile (2014). Copyright 2014 by Oxford University Press. Reprinted by permission.

prosocial media use increases empathy (Gentile et al., 2009; Greitemeyer, Osswald, & Brauer, 2010). In summary, people learn attitudes, beliefs, and behaviors from social interactions, real and fictional. What types of beliefs and behaviors are learned from media is largely determined by content.

Empirical Evidence of Socializing Influences of Mass Media

Negative Media Effects

Effects of Violent Media

Effects of media violence on aggression and related outcomes have received a huge amount of attention and are well understood. Experimental, correlational, and longitudinal studies, even experimental intervention studies, confirm that violent media exposure is a causal risk factor for aggression (C. A. Anderson et al., 2010; C. A. Anderson, Berkowitz, et al., 2003; Bushman & Huesmann, 2012). Such effects have been found for movies, television shows (Huesmann, Moise-Titus, Podolski, & Eron, 2003), video games (C. A. Anderson et al., 2010), music (C. A. Anderson, Carnagey, & Eubanks, 2003), and even violent comic books (Kirsh & Olczak, 2002). They have been replicated across age, culture, and research teams.

EXPERIMENTAL EVIDENCE

Experimental research renders a clear picture of the immediate causal influence of media violence exposure on aggression. Many experiments show that even brief violent media exposure can lead to immediate increases in aggressive thoughts, hostile affect, and aggressive behavior. Such effects have been achieved with a variety of different aggression measures, including delivery of aversive noise blasts; administration of painful electric shocks; increases in pushing, hitting, and kicking observed during free play; and forcing hot sauce on a person who is known to dislike spicy foods. Experimental studies have also indicated that exposure to media violence leads to physiological desensitization to violence and decreases in empathy and prosocial behavior (Carnagey et al., 2007; Krahé et al., 2011). For example, one experimental study found that playing a violent video game for 20 minutes made participants slower and less likely to help a victim injured in a fight (Bushman & Anderson, 2009).

One key short-term mechanism involves priming. Simply presenting individuals with images of guns primes aggressive thoughts and increases later aggressive behavior; the types of guns having the biggest impact depends on one's life experience with guns (hunters vs. nonhunters) (Bartholow, Anderson, Carnagey, & Benjamin, 2005). The effects of a single episode of media violence exposure can dissipate quickly (Barlett, Branch, Rodeheffer, & Harris, 2009), but repeated exposure leads to more lasting changes in emotions, cognition, and behavior (i.e., learning).

CORRELATIONAL AND LONGITUDINAL EVIDENCE

Correlational studies demonstrate long-term effects by revealing significant associations between habitual violent media use and real-life aggressive behaviors. For example, preschoolers who typically watch violent television shows tend to exhibit more aggressive play tendencies (hitting, pushing, taking other children's toys; D. G. Singer & Singer, 1976). Children's use of violent media is also associated with perceptions of violence as a legitimate means for solving problems (Dominick & Greenberg, 1972). Of course, drawing causal conclusions from correlational data is risky because of potential confounds, which is why many correlational studies include statistical controls. For example, violent video game use is associated with violent behavior even after researchers control for numerous potential confounds, such as psychopathy (DeLisi, Vaughn, Gentile, Anderson, & Shook, 2013).

Longitudinal studies show that exposure to media violence leads to long-term increases in aggression (C. A. Anderson, Berkowitz, et al., 2007; Christakis & Zimmerman, 2007; Eron, Huesmann, Lefkowitz, & Walder, 1972). Huesmann and colleagues (2003) found that children who viewed more televised violence became more aggressive adults 15 years later, irrespective of how aggressive they had been as children. Long-term violent media use also leads to chronic desensitization to violence, reductions in empathy and prosocial behavior, and increases in aggressive thinking (e.g., C. A. Anderson et al., 2010).

META-ANALYTIC EVIDENCE

Meta-analyses integrate data from multiple studies and provide a comprehensive picture of violent media effects. In the media violence domain, over a dozen meta-analytic reviews have explored the effects of media violence (e.g., C. A. Anderson et al., 2010; Bushman & Huesmann, 2006; Paik & Comstock, 1994). Overall, these meta-analyses provide consistent evidence of small- to moderate-size effects of media violence on aggression, and on other theoretically relevant variables.

Effects of Risk-Glorifying Media

Media often glorify risk-taking behaviors, such as reckless driving, smoking, binge drinking, and unprotected sex. To give a few examples, the television show *Jackass* features young men engaging in a series of dangerous stunts such as pole vaulting over a sewage pit and getting tattooed on a buggy ride. Racing video games such as *Need for Speed*, *Burnout*, and *Road Rash* reward players for reckless driving. Several recent studies indicate that exposure to such risk-glorifying media impacts both risk-taking inclinations and actual risk-taking behaviors (Fischer, Greitemeyer, Kastenmüller, Vogrincic, & Sauer, 2011; Wills, Sargent, Gibbons, Gerrard, & Stoolmiller, 2009). These effects have been apparent in different types of visual media, including advertisements, movies, and video games. In this section, we pay special attention to two types of risk-taking behaviors that are influenced by media use: substance use and risky sexual behaviors.

SUBSTANCE USE

Positive portrayals of substance use that do not show negative consequences are frequent in the media. Some examples include alcohol advertisements (Ellickson, Collins, Hambarsoomians, & McCaffrey, 2005), and portrayals of alcohol use in movies and television shows (Wills et al., 2009).

Experimental studies indicate significant short-term effects of media that glorify substance use. For example, viewing movies that portray drinking in a positive light causes an increase in participants' expectations that drinking alcohol will lead to positive outcomes, such as camaraderie (Kulick & Rosenberg, 2001). After viewing film sequences that include smoking, people report greater likelihood of smoking in the future (Hines, Saris, & Throckmorton-Belzer, 2000).

Correlational studies, including some prospective studies, have found significant associations between exposure to risk-glorifying media and substance use in real life. For example, exposure to alcohol use in movies is related to early-onset and binge drinking among adolescents (Hanewinkel, Tanski, & Sargent, 2007; Sargent, Wills, Stoolmiller, Gibson, & Gibbons, 2006). Longitudinal studies yield similar effects. For example, early exposure to alcohol marketing predicts underage drinking (Collins, Ellickson, McCaffrey, & Hambarsoomians, 2007). Tobacco industry advertising predicts adolescent smoking onset (Pierce, Choi, Gilpin, Farkas, & Berry, 1998; Pierce, Lee, & Gilpin, 1994). Adolescents' exposure to alcohol use in movies predicts increased alcohol consumption and alcohol-related problems measured years later (Wills et al., 2009). Similar longitudinal effects have been shown for smoking (Dalton et al., 2003; Wills et al., 2009).

SEXUAL CONTENT

Learning about sexuality is a normative maturational achievement in adolescence. Unfortunately, a substantial number of adolescents report that they do not get adequate information about sexuality from parents and schools (J. D. Brown, Greenberg & Burkel-Rothfuss, 1993). This is one reason why mass media play a major role in the sexual socialization of most adolescents (Strasburger, 2005). Indeed, research has shown that half of all adolescents actively seek sexual content when choosing media (Bleakley, Hennessy, & Fishbein, 2011).

Sexual content is frequent in the media, especially in movies, sitcoms, and music (Kunkel, Eyal, Finnerty, Biely, & Donnerstein, 2005; Kunkel et al., 2007). However, portrayals of sexuality in the media often are unrealistic. Although over 75% of prime-time television shows have sexual content, they address the risks and responsibilities of sexual activity in only 14% of cases (Kunkel et al., 2005).

Frequent viewing of sexual content on television leads adolescents to overestimate the number of their peers who are sexually active (Buerkel-Rothfuss & Strouse, 1993; Ward & Rivadeneyra, 1999). Exposure to sexual content also changes teens' sexual expectations, attitudes, and intentions (Aubrey, Harrison, Kramer, & Yellin, 2003; L'Engle, Brown & Kenneavy, 2006; Ward, 2002). For example, males who view more sexual content in television shows are more likely to expect a broad range of sexual activities in relationships, whereas females who view a lot of sexual content in television shows are more likely to expect to initiate sex earlier in relationships (Ward & Rivadeneyra, 1999). Some research suggests that the impact of the media on sex-related "knowledge" is greater than the impact of family, peers, and school (Lou et al., 2012).

Studies also indicate significant effects on sexual behavior. Exposure to sexual content in different media (television shows, movies, music, and Internet sites) is linked to more actual sexual activity among adolescents (Bleakley et al., 2011). Exposure to a lot of sexual content on television predicts becoming sexually active at a younger age (Collins et al., 2004). Particularly alarming is the recent longitudinal finding that exposure to violent X-rated material leads to increased sexually aggressive behavior by children and adolescents (Ybarra, Mitchell, Hamburger, Diener-West, & Leaf, 2011).

It is important to note that not all sexual media content has such negative effects. Media that convey accurate information about sexuality and include socially responsible messages effectively educate people about sexuality and promote responsible sexual behaviors (Brodie et al., 2001; Collins, Elliott, Berry, Kanouse, & Hunter, 2003; DuRant, Wolfson, LaFrance, Balkrishnan, & Altman, 2006).

Media and Stereotypes

Stereotypes are sets of socially shared beliefs about traits that are characteristic of members of a social category (Greenwald & Banaji, 1995). From a social cognitive view, stereotypes are a part of people's schemata about social categories (Fiske & Taylor, 1991). Like other elements of an individual's world, schema, race, and gender stereotypes are influenced by what he or she observes across contexts (in the family, in the peer group, in the mass media). Social cognitive models explain how observations of media can influence individuals' understanding of the social world (e.g., Bandura, 1986; Barlett & Anderson, 2013; Berkowitz, 1990; Crick & Dodge, 1994; Gentile et al., 2014). Specifically, media are powerful socializing agents that provide initial or reinforcing information to create cognitive structures and associations between social groups and certain shared characteristics (Entman & Rojecki, 2000). Through repeated media exposure, individuals form associative links between a social group (e.g., black males) and the stereotypical characteristics (e.g., criminality). Eventually these associations become automatized; when the social group category is activated, the associated stereotypes are automatically activated as well (Dixon & Azocar, 2007). Media-based ethnic stereotypes are especially influential for individuals who do not have direct contact with depicted minority members (Fujioka, 1999).

Media and Ethnic-Minority Stereotypes

Even though ethnic minorities make up over 40% of the U.S. population, their representation in American TV and film roles was about 27.5% in 2008 (McNary, 2009). Unfortunately, most of these ethnic-minority representations are negative (Children Now, 2001; Greenberg, Mastro, & Brand, 2002; Mastro & Behm-Morawitz, 2005; Mastro & Greenberg, 2000). The most widely studied group in U.S. media has been African Americans (Harris, 2004). Several researchers have found that the mainstream media juxtapose African American characters with social problems, welfare, crime, poverty, drugs, and violence (e.g., Abraham, 2003). Other ethnic groups are underrepresented in the media. Despite the growing Latino population in the United States (17% of the total population in 2011), Latinos represent only 2–4% of characters on prime-time TV (Mastro & Greenberg, 2000) and a mere 1% of lead characters in top grossing, U.S motion pictures (Eschholz, Bufkin, & Long, 2002). Additionally, Latinos tend to be portrayed in negative or narrow roles when they do occur (Greenberg et al., 2002). Although limited (between 1 and 3% of characters on prime-time U.S. television), the portrayal of Asian Americans seems to be more positive than that of other ethnic groups (Harris, 2004). Since September 11, 2001, depictions of Arabs have increased in U.S. media, but most of these portrayals are negative, associating Arabs with terrorism, violence, and aggression (Shaheen, 2009). Negative Arab stereotypes are present in newspapers, television shows, movies,

Web animations, and even children's literature (Nacos & Torres-Reyna, 2007; Nisbet, Ostman, & Shanahan, 2008; Schmidt, 2006; Van Buren, 2006). In video games, Arabs are almost always depicted as terrorists (Dill, Gentile, Richter, & Dill, 2005; Machin & Suleiman, 2006; Sisler, 2008).

Several studies examined the effects of media-based ethnic stereotypes on attitudes toward those groups. Overall, these studies indicate that even a single exposure to stereotypes in the media can influence real-world evaluations of minorities (Dixon, 2006, 2007), provoke stereotypical responses (Gilliam & Iyengar, 2000), and guide intergroup outcomes (Mastro, 2003). For example, negative portrayals of African Americans significantly influence the evaluations of African Americans in general (Mastro & Tropp, 2004).

Portrayal of ethnic minorities in U.S. television news is more negative than that in fictional programming (Greenberg et al., 2002). When Dixon and Linz (2000) examined 20 weeks of news programming from Southern California, they found that African American perpetrators were overrepresented (37%) compared to actual Southern California crime reports (21%). Such stereotypical depictions have a negative impact on the majority's perceptions of and attitudes toward the stereotyped groups. For instance, overrepresentations of African American criminals on local and network news can lead to strong mental associations between this group and criminality, creating the perception of African Americans as violent and deviant (Dixon, 2008). In an experimental study, Johnson, Olivo, Reed, and Ashburn-Nardo (2009) found that stereotypical media depictions of African Americans after Hurricane Katrina decreased empathy and prosocial responding (i.e., policy support aimed at helping Katrina victims). Similarly, the amount of television news viewing subsequent to the September 11, 2001, attacks was associated with college students' negativity toward Muslim peers (Lett et al., 2004).

Many video games undermine perceptions of minority groups, first, by excluding them from taking on main character roles, and second, portraying them through stereotypical images (Children Now, 2001). A content analysis revealed that over 68% of main characters are European American, with 11% African American and 11% Latino (Dill et al., 2005). Empirical research in this area is limited, but the effects of video game-based stereotypes on attitudes should theoretically be the same as that of other forms of media. Indeed, Saleem and Anderson (2013) recently found that playing a video game portraying Arab as terrorists increased college students' anti-Arab bias and their perceptions of Arabs as aggressive.

MEDIA AND GENDER STEREOTYPES

Media depictions of gender are also problematic. Content analyses of video games reveal that the majority of characters are males (70%), and female characters are often presented as highly sexualized (Beasley & Collins-Standley, 2002; Dill et al., 2005). The Screen Actors Guild noted that male actors receive the majority of TV roles, especially in the supporting category, with about two roles for every female role (McNary, 2009). Content analyses of popular films reveal similar trends (Smith & Cook, 2012). Additionally, in 2011, women held only 34.4% of all jobs in prime-time programs as opposed to 47% of the actual labor force.

In one experimental study, men who were exposed to media-based stereotypical portrayals of women found victims of sexual harassment and rape less credible than men who exposed to nonstereotypical portrayals of women (Murphy, 1998). A meta-analysis of 31 studies revealed a positive correlation between exposure to media-based gender stereotypes and gender-stereotypical attitudes and behaviors (Oppliger, 2007). Furthermore, exposure to physical appearance ideals in the media is associated with poor body image (Dohnt & Tiggemann, 2006) and self-destructive behaviors such as pathogenic dieting practices (Thomsen, Weber, & Brown, 2002). For example, researchers have found that media variables accounted for 15–33% of the variance in measures of adolescent girls' desire for thinness and their body dissatisfaction, bulimic behaviors, and thin-ideal endorsements (Botta, 1999).

Positive Media Effects

Effects of Prosocial Media

The positive impact of media on *prosocial behavior* (defined as voluntary behavior intended to benefit another) has received much less research attention than negative effects of media. But there is a growing research base, much of which is provided by the same research teams that study effects of violent media. Existing studies show consistent effects across research study types and media types; exposure to prosocial media can lead to increases in prosocial behavior in both the short and the long term.

MEDIA WITHOUT PROSOCIAL MESSAGES

Interestingly, media do not need to have a prosocial message to promote prosocial behavior. Media that create a positive mood may facilitate helping behaviors without providing any sort of overt guidance. In particular, music without lyrics can create or enhance desired mood states or counteract undesired ones, and can imbue feelings such as tranquility, peacefulness, and happiness, as well as other positive emotions (see Bruner, 1990; Roberts, Christenson, & Gentile, 2003). Music that induces a positive mood can have a number of positive effects, including increases in helping behavior (Fried & Berkowitz, 1979; North, Tarrant, & Hargreaves, 2004) and decreases in anger, aggressive thoughts, and aggressive behaviors (Krahé & Bieneck, 2012). Similarly, in a recent experiment, Whitaker and Bushman (2012) found that participants who played a relaxing video game that did not have overt prosocial messages behaved less aggressively and more helpfully than those who had just played violent or neutral games.

MEDIA WITH PROSOCIAL MESSAGES

Most research on prosocial effects has looked at media that either provide prosocial messages or model prosocial behavior. Early television studies found that watching prosocial television was positively associated with children's helpful behavior and prosocial attitudes (Mares & Woodard, 2005; Rosenkoetter, 1999; Sprafkin & Rubinstein, 1979). Furthermore, in one longitudinal study, D. Anderson and colleagues (2000) found that children who regularly watched the prosocial television show *Blue's Clues* had greater increases in prosocial behavior over time than children who did not watch it.

VIDEO GAMES

Several recent studies have examined the impact of playing prosocial characters in nonviolent video games (*Super Mario Sunshine, Chibi Robo, Firefighters: Saving Lives*).

For example, playing a prosocial video game can lead to significant decreases in hurtful behavior and increases in helpful behaviors (Gentile et al., 2009; Greitemeyer, Agthe, Turner, & Gschwendtner, 2012; Saleem et al., 2012a). Other prosocial game effects found in experimental studies include increasing the player's likelihood of helping an experimenter with a mundane task (Whitaker & Bushman, 2012); coming to the aid of a female experimenter being harassed by an ex-boyfriend (Greitemeyer & Osswald, 2010); increasing positive emotions (Saleem et al., 2012b), empathy (Greitemeyer et al., 2010), and prosocial thinking (e.g., Greitemeyer & Osswald, 2010; Narvaez, Mattan, Mac-Michael, & Sqillace, 2008); and reducing hostility-related thoughts and emotions (e.g., Greitemeyer & Osswald, 2009; Greitemeyer et al., 2010; Saleem et al., 2012b).

Longitudinal and cross-sectional studies of prosocial video games are fewer in number but yield findings consistent with theory and the experimental studies. Prosocial video game play is positively correlated with cooperation, helping, and sharing, even when other factors that can affect prosocial behavior are taken into account (Gentile et al., 2009; Linder & Gentile, 2009). Importantly, more recent studies have tracked such changes over time. For example, Gentile and colleagues (2009) found that increases in prosocial behavior were linked with prosocial game playing over a 3- to 4-month period. Prot and colleagues (2014) assessed TV and video game habits, empathy, and prosocial behavior over a 2-year period in a large sample of Singaporean children. They found that early exposure to prosocial TV and video games led to increased prosocial behavior, that this effect was partly mediated by increases in empathy, and that violent media had the opposite effects.

MUSIC

Experiments using music with prosocial lyrics have yielded similar results. Compared to music with neutral lyrics, music with lyrics about helping and cooperation leads to increases in prosocial thoughts, greater empathy, and greater helping in the laboratory (Greitemeyer 2009a, 2009b), as well as kinder behavior in the real world (i.e., increases in tipping at a restaurant; see Jacob, Guéguen, & Boulbry, 2010). Prosocial lyrics also have been shown to reduce aggression-related thoughts and feelings and aggressive behavior, primarily through reductions in aggression-related feelings and increased empathy (Greitemeyer, 2009a, 2011).

OVERALL FINDINGS

Regardless of media or study type, recent evidence converges to show that nonviolent media with prosocial content have a positive effect on behaviors that help others. The behavioral effects appear mediate changes in thoughts and feelings.

Effects of Educational Media

Even though spending time with entertainment media can harm children's school performance (C. A. Anderson et al., 2007; Sharif & Sargent, 2006; Weis & Cerankosky, 2010), educational media can improve a variety of academic skills. Longitudinal studies have shown that educational television can have long-term educational benefits (D. Anderson et al., 2000; Ennemoser & Schneider, 2007). Educational program viewing predicts development of reading competencies in early and middle childhood (Ennemoser & Schneider, 2007). Viewing educational programs at a preschool age is associated with better grades and reading more books in adolescence (D. Anderson et al., 2000). Interestingly, interactive shows that prompt children to engage actively, such as *Blue's Clues* and *Dora the Explorer*, may be especially effective teachers (Linebarger & Walker, 2005).

Educational video games may also have significant educational benefits. Video games have several characteristics that make them effective teachers: They require active participation, provide clear goals, give immediate feedback, adapt to the student's level, and encourage distributed learning (Gentile & Gentile, 2008). Educational video games have been used to teach children and adolescents a range of school subjects, such as mathematics, reading, and biology (Corbett, Koedinger, & Hadley, 2001; Murphy et al., 2002). Educational games can also be used to teach youth about specific health conditions and encourage health-promoting behaviors (S. J. Brown et al., 1997; Kato, Cole, Bradlyn, & Pollock, 2008; Lieberman, 2001).

In addition, numerous studies demonstrate that media can be purposefully used as a positive socializing influence (Lemieux, Fisher, & Pratto, 2008; Singhal, Cody, Rogers, & Sabido, 2004). For example, researchers have found that watching the television show *Barney & Friends* can teach children norms of polite social behavior (J. L. Singer & Singer, 1998). Findings from several studies indicate that responsible sexual behavior can be promoted through music (Lemieux et al., 2008), radio drama (Valente, Kim, Lettenmaier, Glass, & Dibba, 1994) and television shows (Collins et al., 2003).

Positive Effects on Ethnic Stereotypes and Gender Socialization

Just as stereotypes in the media increase stereotypical thinking by consumers of those media, exposure to counterstereotypical media exemplars can reduce stereotypical attitudes (Bodenhausen, Schwarz, Bless, & Wänke, 1995; Dasgupta & Greenwald, 2001; Ramasubramanian, 2011). However, note that even a very positive portrayal may contribute to misconceptions. For example, some white viewers of *The Cosby Show* cited the Huxtables as examples of why affirmative action is no longer necessary (Jhally & Lewis, 1992).

Media also can have positive effects on gender role socialization and gender stereotyping. Repeated TV appearances of women in traditionally male occupations can lead to more open attitudes in preteen girls toward considering these occupations (Wroblewski & Huston, 1987). Listening to music with proequality lyrics leads to more positive attitudes and behavior toward women (Greitemeyer, Hollingdale, & Traut-Mattausch, 2012).

Parental Involvement in Media Use

Parental involvement in media use can act as a protective factor to promote positive effects of media and mitigate negative effects (Gentile, Nathanson, Rasmussen, Reimer, & Walsh, 2012; Nathanson, 1999, 2004). However, the type of parental involvement matters. Three types of parental involvement in media use have been identified: active mediation, restrictive monitoring, and coviewing.

Active mediation includes conversations with children, in which parents explain or discuss media content. Active mediation predicts several positive outcomes, such as enhanced learning from television (Valkenburg, Krcmar, & deRoos, 1998) and skepticism toward televised news (Austin, 1992). Active mediation has also been linked with reduced negative effects of advertising (Buijzen & Valkenburg, 2005), news (Buijzen, Walma van der Molen, & Sondij, 2007), and violent media content (Nathanson, 1999, 2004).

Restrictive monitoring involves posing explicit rules about media content and media time. Restrictions on time use yield both lower media consumption (Atkin, Greenberg, & Baldwin, 1991; Rideout et al., 2010) and better school performance (Gentile, Coyne, & Walsh, 2011; Gentile, Lynch, Linder, & Walsh, 2004). Having rules that restrict violent media content may mitigate media violence effects, beyond the direct effect on reducing time spent on violent media, perhaps by conveying family antiviolence attitudes (C. A. Anderson et al., 2007; Grusec, 1973; Nathanson, 1999).

Coviewing involves watching television or playing video games with children. Several studies suggest that coviewing may enhance effects of both positive and negative media content. Coviewing educational television has been shown to enhance children's learning (Salomon, 1977). On the other hand, coviewing of violent television can exacerbate media violence effects (Nathanson & Cantor, 2000).

Given the significant effects of parental involvement in media use, it is worrying that many parents do not monitor their children's media consumption. Only 52% of children in the United States report that their parents have rules concerning computer use, 46% for television use, 30% for video game use, and 26% for music (Rideout et al., 2010).

Emerging Socialization Domains and Effects

In this section, we briefly review several emerging domains in which modern media clearly are involved in socialization, but research is sparse or inconclusive.

Cell Phones, Texting, and Sexting

Cell phone use by young people has increased dramatically. Today, 78% of U.S. adolescents own cell phones, compared to only 45% in 2004 (Lenhart, Hitlin, & Madden, 2005; Madden, Lenhart, Duggan, Cortesi, & Gasser, 2013). About 33% of 8- to 10-year-olds use cell phones (Rideout et al., 2010). Young people average 30 minutes a day talking on a cell phone and send about 60 text messages (Lenhart, 2012; Rideout et al., 2010). Surprisingly, only 14% of parents set rules about texting, and only 27% limit the time spent on voice calls (Rideout et al., 2010).

Texting is a popular mode of communication by children and adolescents (Lenhart, Ling, Campbell, & Purcell, 2010). The majority of text messages are used to enhance and maintain intimate relationships, especially in friendships and in romantic relationships (Thurlow & Brown, 2002). Adolescents also use texting as a means of civic engagement (Lenhart et al., 2008). Voice calls are more commonly used to communicate with parents (Lenhart et al., 2010). Cell phones provide a way for parents to monitor and provide support to their children. There is limited mixed correlational evidence concerning impact on socialization, with some positive and some negative effects (Weisskirch, 2009). In summary, using cell phones does not necessarily lead to better (or poorer) parenting, parent–child relationships, or socialization experiences. High cell phone and texting use by youth has led to concerns about potential adverse effects (Zhao, Qiu, & Xie, 2012), but research has lagged.

One concern that is receiving attention is sexting—sending sexually explicit or suggestive images via cell phones (Mitchell, Finkelhor, Jones, & Wolak, 2012). About 15% of U.S. adolescents report having received messages with sexual content, whereas 4% report sending them (Lenhart, 2009). Older adolescents are more likely to send sexual photographs (8% among 17-year-olds compared to 4% among 12-year-olds). Thus, sexting is not a normative behavior, but a sizable minority does engage in it. Such behavior merits research attention given that it can result in considerable distress both for youth receiving images and for youth appearing in images (Mitchell et al., 2012). Recently, researchers have begun exploring the contexts in which sexting occurs, motivations for sexting, and associations between sexting and risky sexual behaviors. Sexting most commonly happens in existing romantic relationships, but it is sometimes also done as a prank or as a means to start a new relationship (Mitchell et al., 2012). One-third of such incidents have been found to be related to aggravating factors, such as alcohol or drug use (Mitchell et al., 2012). There is some evidence that sexting may lead to other risky sexual behaviors, but this research is currently limited to cross-sectional correlational studies (Benotsch, Snipes, Martin, & Bull, 2013). Of course, there are numerous reports of how sexting is used to embarrass and harass other youth, occasionally leading to suicide. Longitudinal studies are needed both to examine predictors and consequences of sexting and to explore prevention and intervention methods.

Media and Identity Development

A key part of human development is the creation of both a unique identity—a distinctive set of attributes, beliefs, desires, and principles that individuals think distinguishes them from others—and a group identity (Fearon, 1999). Identity formation is a particularly salient task for teens (Erikson, 1968), a group also characterized by considerable media use. The media with which children and youth identify can become incorporated into their personal and social identities (Warburton, 2012b), for good or ill.

Although a preference for any type of media can become incorporated into a person's identity, research most often examines the role of music preference. Music that a child likes may provide messages for how to behave (both in lyrics and video clips), and admired musicians may behave in ways that can be imitated. Thus, preferred music and musicians can influence a child's beliefs, feelings, and behavioral tendencies, and these in turn can become part of who children "think they are" (Warburton, 2012b). As Roe noted in 1996, "Music plays a central role in the process of identity construction of young people. This process includes not only elements of personal identity but also important aspects of national, regional, cultural, ethnic, and gender identity" (p. 85).

Given the extensive research showing causal long-term effects of antisocial and prosocial media on behavior, it is reasonable to expect corresponding positive and negative effects on identity development. However, more research is needed on this topic.

Media and Social Networking

Social Networking Media and Microblogs

More than half of U.S. teenagers log into their favorite social networking site at least once a day; almost one-fourth of them log in 10 times a day or more (O'Keeffe &

Clarke-Pearson, 2011). Clearly, social networking through websites, such as Facebook and LinkedIn, and microblogs, such as Twitter, play an important role in developing and maintaining social relationships for many people (Rideout et al., 2010). Whether the effects of these new socialization techniques are generally positive or negative for youth is unclear, and this probably is too broad a question. Social media have some well-publicized problems, including privacy issues, predatory behavior, and cyberbullying (Barlett et al., 2014). But, they also play a positive role in many people's everyday lives. For example, O'Keeffe and Clarke-Pearson (2011) suggest that social networking media provide youth with opportunities for (1) engaging with the wider community (through volunteering), (2) developing creativity through the sharing of artistic endeavors, (3) sharing and developing ideas, (4) developing increased tolerance through the expansion of social networks to include greater diversity, and (5) fostering one's individual identity and unique social skills. It is important to add that social networking has also been linked with enhanced learning opportunities (Borja, 2005; Boyd, 2008), better access to health information, and better health outcomes (increased adherence to medical treatments; see Krishna, Boren, & Balas, 2009). But, research on long-term positive and negative effects is relatively sparse.

Multimedia Devices and Massive Multiplayer Online Role-Playing Games

Multimedia technology such as broadband-capable mobile devices also make it possible to reach out to another person at any time of the night or day using speech, e-mail, text messaging, picture images, or person-to-person video conferencing. Such devices markedly increase the options for direct and delayed interpersonal communication, and therefore the potential for connectedness between a person and his or her social networks (Warburton & Highfield, 2012). But whether this increased accessibility results in better, poorer, or mixed outcomes for youth development is unclear.

Massive multiplayer online role-playing games (MMORPGs) such as *World of Warcraft* and *Star Wars: The Old Republic* are online video games that can have millions of subscribers and hundreds of thousands of players at any given moment. MMORPGs have become increasingly popular; one of the attractive features is the opportunity for social networking. For example, in *World of Warcraft*, players typically gather into guilds that work together within the game, and multiple players from the same guild can connect to each other in real time via audio headphones. Of course, such online communication can also lead to negative consequences. That is, online communication does not always lead to benefits equal to face-to-face communication and can result in lowered well-being (Pea et al., 2012).

Conclusion

The rapid expansion of research on media effects has increased our understanding of the roles media play in the socialization process. Media have significant socializing influences across a wide range of domains, such as aggression, stereotyping, helping, sexual behaviors, education, social networking, and identity development. The findings can be understood within the framework of the GLM, which delineates the processes through which media can affect social behavior in short-term and long-term contexts. The GLM emphasizes the fact that media effects are complex and depend on content, structure, time, and context. Media effects can be harmful, such as the effects of violent media on aggression and the effects of stereotypical media portrayals of groups on stereotypes and behaviors toward outgroups. Media effects can also be beneficial, such as the effects of prosocial media use on helping. Parental involvement can be a protective factor that helps to foster positive media effects and ameliorate negative media effects.

Media psychology research has broadened over the past 20 years. Early studies focused on media violence effects, but several other lines of research have grown, such as media effects on risky behaviors and positive media effects on social networking and identity development. The rapid expansion of research in the field of media psychology has been accompanied by an overall trend toward better methodological quality in the field (Prot & Anderson, 2013). An especially important development is the increasing number of high-quality longitudinal studies, which demonstrate long-term, cumulative effects of media use on socialization (Gentile et al., 2009; Krahé & Möller, 2010). Methodological diversity also is increasing. For example, researchers have begun exploring how media affect brain function (Bailey, West, & Anderson, 2011; Hummer et al., 2010). Finally, recent studies demonstrate that the science of media effects can yield effective interventions that promote healthier media habits and ameliorate negative media effects on socialization (Möller, Krahé, Busching, & Krause, 2012).

In our view, several research areas within this field represent fruitful avenues for future research. One research question that merits further attention is that of age as a moderator of media effects. A large proportion of studies on socializing influences of mass media have been conducted on college-age adolescent and young adult populations, both for practical reasons and because of ethical concerns. More studies on children are needed to elucidate developmental differences in specific media effects. Further research also is needed on the neural bases of media effects. Finally, additional studies examining the impact of new technologies on socialization (e.g., cell phones and the Internet) are needed.

In summary, a broad research literature demonstrates that media are powerful socializing agents that can lead to numerous positive and negative outcomes. Given the extraordinary amount of time of children and adolescents spend interacting with media, increasing our understanding of both positive and negative media effects is an important research goal for practical reasons. Findings concerning the socializing influences of mass media have implications for theory development, for public policy decisions, and for developing interventions that can promote healthier media habits among youth.

REFERENCES

Abraham, L. (2003). Media stereotypes of African Americans. In P. M. Lester & S. D. Ross (Eds.), *Images that injure: Pictorial stereotypes in the media* (2nd ed., pp. 87–92). Westport, CT: Praeger.

Anderson, C. A., Berkowitz, L., Donnerstein, E., Huesmann, R. L., Johnson, J., Linz, D., et al. (2003). The influence of media violence on youth. *Psychological Science in the Public Interest, 4*, 81–110.

Anderson, C. A., & Bushman, B. J. (2002). Human aggression. *Annual Review of Psychology, 53*, 27–51.

Anderson, C. A., Carnagey, N. L., & Eubanks, J. (2003). Exposure to violent media: The effects of songs with violent lyrics on aggressive thoughts and feelings. *Journal of Personality and Social Psychology, 84,* 960–971.

Anderson, C. A., Gentile, D. A., & Buckley, K. E. (2007). *Violent video game effects on children and adolescents: Theory, research, and public policy.* New York: Oxford University Press.

Anderson, C. A., Shibuya, A., Ihori, N., Swing, E. L., Bushman, B. J., Sakamoto, A., et al. (2010). Violent video game effects on aggression, empathy, and prosocial behavior in Eastern and Western countries. *Psychological Bulletin, 136,* 151–173.

Anderson, D., Bryant, J., Wilder, A., Santomero, A., Williams, M., & Crawley, A. M. (2000). Researching *Blue's Clues:* Viewing behavior and impact. *Media Psychology, 2,* 179–194.

Atkin, C., Greenberg, B., & Baldwin, T. (1991). The home ecology of children's television viewing: Parental mediation and the new video environment. *Journal of Communication, 41,* 40–52.

Aubrey, J. S., Harrison, K., Kramer, L., & Yellin, J. (2003). Variety versus timing: Gender differences in college students' expectations as predicted by exposure to sexually oriented television. *Communication Research, 30,* 432–460.

Austin, E. W. (1992). Parent–child TV interactions: The importance of perspective. *Journal of Broadcasting and Electronic Media, 36,* 359–361.

Bailey, K., West, R., & Anderson, C. A. (2011). The influence of video games on social, cognitive, and affective information processing. In J. Decety & J. Cacioppo (Eds.), *Handbook of social neuroscience* (pp. 1001–1011). New York: Oxford University Press.

Bandura, A. (1986). *Social foundations of thought and action: A social cognitive theory.* Englewood Cliffs, NJ: Prentice-Hall.

Barlett, C. P., & Anderson, C. A. (2013). Examining media effects: The general aggression and general learning models. In E. Scharrer (Ed.), *Media effects/media psychology* (pp. 1–20). New York: Blackwell-Wiley.

Barlett, C. P., Branch, O. L., Rodeheffer, C. D., & Harris, R. H. (2009). How long do the short-term violent video game effects last? *Aggressive Behavior, 35,* 225–236.

Barlett, C. P., Gentile, D. A., Anderson, C. A., Suzuki, K., Sakamoto, A., Kumazaki, A., et al. (2014). Cross-cultural differences in cyberbullying behavior: A short-term longitudinal study. *Journal of Cross-Cultural Psychology, 45*(2), 300–313.

Bartholow, B. D., Anderson, C. A., Carnagey, N. L., & Benjamin, A. J., Jr. (2005). Interactive effects of life experience and situational cues on aggression: The weapons priming effect in hunters and nonhunters. *Journal of Experimental Social Psychology, 41,* 48–60.

Beasley, B., & Collins-Standley, T. C. (2002). Shirts vs. skins: Clothing as an indicator of gender stereotyping in video games. *Mass Communication and Society, 5,* 279–293.

Benotsch, E. G., Snipes, D. J., Martin, A. M., & Bull, S. S. (2013). Sexting, substance use, and sexual risk behavior in young adults. *Journal of Adolescent Health, 52,* 307–313.

Berkowitz, L. (1990). On the formation and regulation of anger and aggression: A cognitive-neoassociationistic analysis. *American Psychologist, 45,* 494–503.

Bleakley, A., Hennessy, M., & Fishbein, M. (2011). A model of adolescents' seeking of sexual content in their media choices. *Journal of Sex Research, 48*(4), 37–48.

Bodenhausen, G. V., Schwarz, N., Bless, H., & Wänke, M. (1995). Effects of atypical exemplars on racial beliefs: Enlightened racism or generalized appraisals? *Journal of Experimental Social Psychology, 31,* 48–63.

Borja, R. R. (2005, December 14). "Blogs" catching on as tool for instruction: Teachers use interactive Web pages to hone writing skills. Retrieved March 7, 2013, from *www.edweek.org/ew/articles/2005/12/14/15blogs.h25.html?qs=borja.*

Botta, R. A. (1999). Television images and adolescent girls' body image disturbance. *Journal of Communication, 49,* 22–41.

Boyd, D. (2008). *Taken out of context: American teen sociality in networked publics.* Berkeley: University of California.

Brodie, M., Foehr, U., Rideout, V., Baer, N., Miller, C., Flournoy, R., et al. (2001). Communicating health information through the entertainment media. *Health Affairs, 20,* 1–8.

Brown, J. D., Greenberg, B. S., & Burkel-Rothfuss, N. L. (1993). Mass media, sex, and sexuality. *Adolescent Medicine, 4*, 511–525.

Brown, S. J., Lieberman, D. A., Gemeny, B. A., Fan, Y. C., Wilson, D. M., & Pasta, D. J. (1997). Educational video game for juvenile diabetes: Results of a controlled trial. *Medical Informatics, 22*(1), 77–89.

Bruner, G. C. (1990). Music, mood and marketing. *Journal of Marketing, 54*, 94–104.

Buckley, K. E., & Anderson, C. A. (2006). A theoretical model of the effects and consequences of playing video games. In P. Vorderer & J. Bryant (Eds.), *Playing video games—motives, responses, and consequences* (pp. 363–378). Mahwah, NJ: Erlbaum.

Buerkel-Rothfuss, N. L., & Strouse, J. S. (1993). Media exposure and perceptions of sexual behaviors: The cultivation hypothesis moves to the bedroom. In B. S. Greenberg, J. D. Brown, & N. L. Buerkel-Rothfuss (Eds.), *Media, sex, and the adolescent* (pp. 225–247). Cresskill, NJ: Hampton Press.

Buijzen, M., & Valkenburg, P. M. (2005). Parental mediation of undesired advertising effects. *Journal of Broadcasting and Electronic Media, 49*, 153–165.

Buijzen, M., Walma van der Molen, J. H., & Sondij, P. (2007). Parental mediation of children's emotional responses to a violent news event. *Communication Research, 34*, 212–230.

Bushman, B. J., & Anderson, C. A. (2009). Comfortably numb: Desensitizing effects of violent media on helping others. *Psychological Science, 20*, 273–277.

Bushman, B. J., & Huesmann, L. R. (2006). Short-term and long-term effects of violent media on aggression in children and adults. *Archives of Pediatrics and Adolescent Medicine, 160*, 348–352.

Bushman, B. J., & Huesmann, L. R. (2012). Effects of violent media on aggression. In D. G. Singer & J. L. Singer (Eds.), *Handbook of children and the media* (2nd ed., pp. 249–272). Thousand Oaks, CA: Sage.

Carnagey, N. L., Anderson, C. A., & Bushman, B. J. (2007). The effect of video game violence on physiological desensitization to real-life violence. *Journal of Experimental Social Psychology, 43*, 489–496.

Children Now. (2001). *Fair play?: Violence, gender and race in video games*. Los Angeles: Author.

Christakis, D. A., & Zimmerman, F. J. (2007). Violent television viewing during preschool is associated with antisocial behavior during school age. *Pediatrics, 120*, 993–999.

Collins, R. L., Ellickson, P., McCaffrey, D., & Hambarsoomians, K. (2007). Early adolescent exposure to alcohol advertising and its relationship to underage drinking, *Journal of Adolescent Health, 40*, 527–534.

Collins, R. L., Elliott, M. N., Berry, S. H., Kanouse, E., & Hunter, S. B. (2003). Entertainment television as a healthy sex educator: The impact of condom-efficacy information in an episode of Friends. *Pediatrics, 112*, 1115–1121.

Collins, R. L., Elliott, M. N., Berry, S. H., Kanouse, D. E., Kunkel, D., Hunter, S. B., et al. (2004). Watching sex on television predicts adolescent initiation of sexual behavior. *Pediatrics, 114*, e280–e289.

Corbett, A. T., Koedinger, K. R., & Hadley, W. (2001). Cognitive tutors: From the research classroom to all classrooms. In P. S. Goodman (Ed.), *Technology enhanced learning* (pp. 235–263). Mahwah, NJ: Erlbaum.

Crick, N. R., & Dodge, K. A. (1994). A review and reformulation of social information-processing mechanisms in children's social adjustment. *Psychological Bulletin, 115*, 113–126.

Dalton, M. A., Sargent, J. D., Beach, M. L., Titus-Ernstoff, L., Gibson, J. J., Ahrens, M. B., et al. (2003). Effects of viewing smoking in movies on adolescent smoking initiation: A cohort study. *Lancet, 362*, 281–285.

Dasgupta, N., & Greenwald, A. G. (2001). On the malleability of automatic attitudes: Combating automatic prejudice with images of admired and disliked individuals. *Journal of Personality and Social Psychology, 81*, 800–814.

DeLisi, M., Vaughn, M. G., Gentile, D. A., Anderson, C. A., & Shook, J. (2013). Violent video games, delinquency, and youth violence: New evidence. *Youth Violence and Juvenile Justice, 11*, 132–142.

DeWall, C. N., Anderson, C. A., & Bushman, B. J. (2012). Aggression. In I. Weiner (Ed.), *Handbook of psychology* (Vol. 5, 2nd ed., pp. 449–466). New York: Wiley.

Dill, K. E., Gentile, D. A., Richter, W. A., & Dill, J. C. (2005). Violence, sex, race and age in popular video games: A content analysis. In E. Cole & J. Henderson Daniel (Eds.), *Featuring females: Feminist analyses of the media* (pp. 115–130). Washington, DC: American Psychological Association.

Dixon, T. L. (2006). Schemas as average conceptions: Skin tone, television news exposure, and culpability judgments. *Journalism and Mass Communication Quarterly, 83*, 131–149.

Dixon, T. L. (2007). Black criminals and White officers: The effects of racially misrepresenting law breakers and law defenders on television news. *Media Psychology, 10*, 270–291.

Dixon, T. L. (2008). Crime news and racialized beliefs: Understanding the relationship between local news viewing and perceptions of African Americans and crime. *Journal of Communication, 58*, 106–125.

Dixon, T. L., & Azocar, C. L. (2007). Priming crime and activating blackness: Understanding the psychological impact of the overrepresentation of Blacks as lawbreakers on television news. *Journal of Communication, 57*, 229–253.

Dixon, T. L., & Linz, D. (2000). Overrepresentation and underrepresentation of African American and Latinos as law breakers on television news. *Journal of Communication, 50*, 131–154.

Dohnt, H., & Tiggemann, M. (2006). The contribution of peer and media influences to the development of body satisfaction and self-esteem in young girls: A prospective study. *Developmental Psychology, 42*, 929–936.

Dominick, J. R., & Greenberg, B. S. (1972). Attitudes towards violence: The interaction of television exposure, family attitudes, and social class. In G. A. Comstock & E. A. Rubinstein (Eds.), *Television and social behavior: Vol. III. Television and adolescent aggressiveness* (pp. 314–335). Washington, DC: U.S. Government Printing Office.

DuRant, R. H., Wolfson, M., LaFrance, B., Balkrishnan, R., & Altman, D. (2006). An evaluation of a mass media campaign to encourage parents of adolescents to talk to their children about sex. *Journal of Adolescent Health, 38*, 2981–2989.

Ellickson, P. L., Collins, R. L., Hambarsoomians, K., & McCaffrey, D. F. (2005). Does alcohol advertising promote adolescent drinking?: Results from a longitudinal assessment. *Addiction, 100*, 235–246.

Ennemoser, M., & Schneider, W. (2007). Relations of television viewing and reading: Findings from a 4-year longitudinal study. *Journal of Educational Psychology, 99*, 349–368.

Entman, R., & Rojecki, A. (2000). *The black image in the white mind.* Chicago: University of Chicago Press.

Erikson, E. H. (1968). *Identity: Youth and crisis.* New York: Norton.

Eron, L. D., Huesmann, L. R., Lefkowitz, M. M., & Walder, L. O. (1972). Does television violence cause aggression? *American Psychologist, 27*, 253–263.

Eschholz, S., Bufkin, J., & Long, J. (2002). Symbolic reality bites: Women and racial/ethnic minorities in modern film. *Sociological Spectrum, 22*, 299–334.

Fearon, J. D. (1999). *What is identity (as we now use the word)?* Unpublished manuscript, Stanford University, Stanford, CA. Retrieved March 14, 2013, from *www.stanford.edu/~jfearon/papers/iden1v2.pdf.*

Fischer, P., Greitemeyer, T., Kastenmüller, A., Vogrincic, C., & Sauer, A. (2011). The effects of risk-glorifying media exposure on risk-positive cognitions, emotions, and behaviors: A meta-analytic review. *Psychological Bulletin, 137*(3), 367–390.

Fiske, S. T., & Taylor, S. E. (1991). *Social cognition* (2nd ed.). New York: McGraw-Hill.

Fried, R., & Berkowitz, L. (1979). Music hath charms . . . and can influence helpfulness. *Journal of Applied Social Psychology, 9*, 199–208.

Fujioka, Y. (1999). Television portrayals and African-American stereotypes: Examination of television effects when direct contact is lacking. *Journalism and Mass Communication Quarterly, 76,* 52–75.

Funk, J. B., Baldacci, H. B., Pasold, T., & Baumgardner, J. (2004). Violence exposure in real-life, video games, television, movies, and the Internet: Is there desensitization? *Journal of Adolescence, 27*(1), 23–39.

Gentile, D. A., Anderson, C. A., Yukawa, N., Saleem, M., Lim, K. M., Shibuya, A., et al. (2009). The effects of prosocial video games on prosocial behaviors: International evidence from correlational, longitudinal, and experimental studies. *Personality and Social Psychology Bulletin, 35,* 752–763.

Gentile, D. A., Coyne, S. M., & Walsh, D. A. (2011). Media violence, physical aggression and relational aggression in school age children: A short-term longitudinal study. *Aggressive Behavior, 37,* 193–206.

Gentile, D. A., & Gentile, J. R. (2008). Violent video games as exemplary teachers: A conceptual analysis. *Journal of Youth and Adolescence, 37,* 127–141.

Gentile, D. A., Groves, C. L., & Gentile, J. R. (2014). The general learning model: Unveiling the learning potential of video games. In F. C. Blumberg (Ed.), *Learning by playing: Frontiers of video gaming in education* (pp. 121–142). New York: Oxford University Press.

Gentile, D. A., Lynch, P. J., Linder, J. R., & Walsh, D. A. (2004). The effects of violent video game habits on adolescent hostility, aggressive behaviors, and school performance. *Journal of Adolescence, 27,* 5–22.

Gentile, D. A., Nathanson, A. I., Rasmussen, E. E., Reimer, R. A., & Walsh, D. A. (2012). Do you see what I see?: Parent and child reports of parental monitoring. *Family Relations, 61,* 470–487.

Gilliam, F. D., Jr., & Iyengar, S. (2000). Prime suspects: The influence of local television news on the viewing public. *American Journal of Political Science, 44,* 560–574.

Greenberg, B. S., Mastro, D., & Brand, J. E. (2002). Minorities and the mass media: Television into the 21st century. In J. Bryant & D. Zillmann (Eds.), *Media effects: Advances in theory and research* (2nd ed., pp. 333–352). Hillsdale, NJ: Erlbaum.

Greenwald, A. G., & Banaji, M. R. (1995). Implicit social cognition: Attitudes, self-esteem, and stereotypes. *Psychological Review, 102,* 4–27.

Greitemeyer, T. (2009a). Effects of songs with prosocial lyrics on prosocial behaviour: Further evidence and a mediating mechanism. *Personality and Social Psychology Bulletin, 35,* 1500–1511.

Greitemeyer, T. (2009b). Effects of songs with prosocial lyrics on prosocial thoughts, affect, and behavior. *Journal of Experimental Social Psychology, 45,* 186–190.

Greitemeyer, T. (2011). Exposure to music with prosocial lyrics reduces aggression: First evidence and test of the underlying mechanism. *Journal of Experimental Social Psychology, 47,* 28–36.

Greitemeyer, T., Agthe, M., Turner, R., & Gschwendtner, C. (2012). Acting prosocially reduces retaliation: Effects of prosocial video games on aggressive behaviour. *European Journal of Social Psychology, 42,* 235–242.

Greitemeyer, T., Hollingdale, J., & Traut-Mattausch, E. (2012). Changing the track in music and misogyny: Listening to music with pro-equality lyrics improves attitudes and behavior toward women. *Psychology of Popular Media Culture.*

Greitemeyer, T., & Osswald, S. (2009). Prosocial video games reduce aggressive cognitions. *Journal of Experimental Social Psychology, 45,* 896–900.

Greitemeyer, T., & Osswald, S. (2010). Effects of prosocial video games on prosocial behavior. *Journal of Personality and Social Psychology, 98,* 211–221.

Greitemeyer, T., Osswald, S., & Brauer, M. (2010). Playing prosocial video games increases empathy and decreases *schadenfreude. Emotion, 6,* 796–802.

Grusec, J. E. (1973). Effects of co-observer evaluations on imitation: A developmental study. *Developmental Psychology, 8,* 141.

Hanewinkel, R., Tanski, S. E., & Sargent, J. D. (2007). Exposure to alcohol use in motion pictures and teen drinking in Germany. *International Journal of Epidemiology, 36,* 1068–1077.

Harris Interactive. (2008). Teenagers: A generation unplugged. Retrieved January 15, 2013, from *http://files.ctia.org/pdf/hi_teenmobilestudy_researchreport.pdf.*

Harris, R. J. (2004). *A cognitive psychology of mass communication.* Mahwah, NJ: Erlbaum.

Hines, D., Saris, R. N., & Throckmorton-Belzer, L. (2000). Cigarette smoking in popular films: Does it increase viewers' likelihood to smoke? *Journal of Applied Social Psychology, 30,* 2246–2269.

Huesmann, L. R., & Kirwil, L. (2007). Why observing violence increases the risk of violent behavior in the observer. In D. Flannery (Ed.), *The Cambridge handbook of violent behavior and aggression* (pp. 545–570). Cambridge, UK: Cambridge University Press.

Huesmann, L. R., Moise-Titus, J., Podolski, C. P., & Eron, L. D. (2003). Longitudinal relations between childhood exposure to media violence and adult aggression and violence: 1977–1992. *Developmental Psychology, 39*(2), 201–221.

Hummer, T. A., Wang, Y., Kronenberger, W. G., Mosier, K. M., Kalnin, A. J., Dunn, D. W., et al. (2010). Short-term violent video game play by adolescents alters prefrontal activity during cognitive inhibition, *Media Psychology, 13,* 136–154.

Jacob, C., Guéguen, N., & Boulbry, G. (2010). Effects of songs with prosocial lyrics on tipping behavior in a restaurant. *International Journal of Hospitality Management, 29,* 761–763.

Jhally, S., & Lewis, J. (1992). *Enlightened racism:* The Cosby Show, *audiences and the myth of the American dream.* Boulder, CO: Westview.

Johnson, J. D., Olivo, N. G., Reed, N., & Ashburn-Nardo, L. (2009). Priming media stereotypes reduces support for social welfare policies: The mediating role of empathy. *Personality and Social Psychology Bulletin, 35,* 463–476.

Jones, S., & Fox, S. (2009). Generations online in 2009. Retrieved January 15, 2013, from *www. pewinternet.org/reports/2009/generations-online-in-2009.aspx.*

Kato, P. M., Cole, S. W., Bradlyn, A. S., & Pollock, B. H. (2008). A video game improves behavioral outcomes in adolescents and young adults with cancer: A randomized trial. *Pediatrics, 122,* 305–317.

Kirsh, S. J., & Olczak, P. V. (2002). The effects of extremely-violent comic books on social information processing. *Journal of Interpersonal Violence, 17*(11), 1160–1178.

Krahé, B., & Bieneck, S. (2012). The effect of music-induced mood on aggressive affect, cognition and behavior. *Journal of Applied Social Psychology, 42,* 271–290.

Krahé, B., & Möller, I. (2010). Longitudinal effects of media violence on aggression and empathy among German adolescents. *Journal of Applied Developmental Psychology, 31,* 401–409.

Krahé, B., Möller, I., Huesmann, L. R., Kirwil, L., Felber, J., & Berger, A. (2011). Desensitization to media violence: Links with habitual media violence exposure, aggressive cognitions and aggressive behavior. *Journal of Personality and Social Psychology, 100,* 630–646.

Krishna, S., Boren, S. A., & Balas, E. A. (2009). Healthcare via cell phones: A systematic review. *Telemedicine and eHealth, 15,* 231–240.

Kulick, A. D., & Rosenberg, H. (2001). Influence of positive and negative film portrayals of drinking on older adolescents' alcohol outcome expectancies. *Journal of Applied Social Psychology, 31,* 1492–1499.

Kunkel, D., Eyal, K., Finnerty, K., Biely, E., & Donnerstein, E. (2005). *Sex on TV 4.* Menlo Park, CA: Henry J. Kaiser Family Foundation.

Kunkel, D., Farrar, K. M., Eyal, K., Biely, E., Donnerstein, E., & Rideout V. (2007). Sexual socialization messages in entertainment television: Comparing content trends 1997–2002. *Media Psychology, 9,* 595–622.

Lemieux, A. F., Fisher, J. D., & Pratto, F. (2008). A music-based HIV prevention intervention for urban adolescents. *Health Psychology, 27,* 349–357.

L'Engle, K. L., Brown, J. D., & Kenneavy, K. (2006). Mass media are an important context for adolescents' sexual behavior. *Journal of Adolescent Health, 36*(3), 186–192.

Lenhart, A. (2009). Teens and sexting. Pew Internet & American Life Project Report. Retrieved from *http://pewinternet.org/~/media//files/reports/2009/pip_teens_and_sexting.pdf.*

Lenhart, A. (2012). Teens, smartphones & texting. Pew Internet & American Life Project Report.

Retrieved from *http://pewinternet.org/~/media//files/reports/2012/pip_teens_smartphones_and_texting.pdf.*

Lenhart, A., Hitlin, P., & Madden, M. (2005). Teens and technology. Pew Internet & American Life Project Report. Retrieved from *www.pewinternet.org/~/media//files/reports/2005/pip_teens_tech_july2005web.pdf.pdf.*

Lenhart, A., Kahne, J., Middaugh, E., Macgill, A. R., Evans, C., & Vitak, J. (2008). Teens' video games, and civics. Pew Internet & American Life Project. Retrieved July 5, 2010, from *www.pewinternet.org/reports/2008/teens-video-games-and-civics.aspx.*

Lenhart, A., Ling, R., Campbell, S., & Purcell, K. (2010). Teens and mobile phones. Pew Internet & American Life Project Report. Retrieved from *http://pewinternet.org/~/media//files/reports/2010/pip-teens-and-mobile-2010-with-topline.pdf.*

Lett, M. D., Dipietro, A. L., & Johnson, D. I. (2004). Examining effects of television news violence on college students through cultivation theory. *Communication Research Reports, 21,* 39–46.

Lieberman, D. A. (2001). Management of chronic pediatric diseases with interactive health games: Theory and research findings. *Journal of Ambulatory Care Management, 24,* 26–38.

Linder, J. R., & Gentile, D. A. (2009). Is the television rating system valid?: Indirect, verbal, and physical aggression in programs viewed by fifth grade girls and associations with behavior. *Journal of Applied Developmental Psychology, 30,* 286–297.

Linebarger, D. L., & Walker, D. (2005). Infants' and toddlers' television viewing and language outcomes. *American Behavioral Scientist, 48,* 624–625.

Lou, C., Cheng, Y., Gao, E., Zuo, X., Emerson, M. R., & Zabin, L. S. (2012). Media's contribution to sexual knowledge, attitudes, and behaviors for adolescents and young adults in three Asian cities. *Journal of Adolescent Health, 50*(3), 26–36.

Machin, D., & Suleiman, U. (2006). Arab and American computer war games: The influence of a global technology on discourse. *Critical Discourses Studies, 3,* 1–22.

Madden, M., Lenhart, A., Duggan, M., Cortesi, S., & Gasser, U. (2013). Teens and Technology 2013. Pew Internet & American Life Project Report. Retrieved from *http://pewinternet.org/~/media//files/reports/2013/pip_teensandtechnology2013.pdf.*

Mares, M. L., & Woodard, E. (2005). Positive effects of television on children's social interactions: A meta-analysis. *Media Psychology, 7,* 301–322.

Mastro, D. (2003). A social identity approach to understanding the impact of television messages. *Communication Monographs, 70,* 98–113.

Mastro, D., & Behm-Morawitz, E. (2005). Latino representation on primetime television. *Journalism and Mass Communication Quarterly, 82,* 110–130.

Mastro, D., & Greenberg, B. S. (2000). The portrayal of racial minorities on prime time television. *Journal of Broadcasting and Electronic Media, 44,* 690–703.

Mastro, D. E., & Tropp, L. R. (2004). The effects of interracial contact, attitudes, and stereotypical portrayals on evaluations of Black television sitcom characters. *Communication Research Reports, 21,* 119–129.

McNary, D. (2009). SAG stats: Diversity lags. Retrieved March 1, 2013, from *www.variety.com/article/vr1118010361/?categoryid=1055&cs=1.*

Mitchell, K. J., Finkelhor, D., Jones, L. M., & Wolak, J. (2012). Prevalence and characteristics of youth sexting: A national study. *Pediatrics, 129,* 13–20.

Möller, I., & Krahé, B. (2009). Exposure to violent video games and aggression in German adolescents: A longitudinal analysis. *Aggressive Behavior, 35,* 75–89.

Möller, I., Krahé, B., Busching, R., & Krause, C. (2012). Efficacy of an intervention to reduce the use of media violence and aggression: An experimental evaluation with adolescents in Germany. *Journal of Youth and Adolescence, 41,* 105–120.

Mullin, C. R., & Linz, D. (1995). Desensitization and resensitization to violence against women: Effects of exposure to sexually violent films on judgments of domestic violence victims. *Journal of Personality and Social Psychology, 69,* 449–459.

Murphy, R. F., Penuel, W. R., Means, B., Korbak, C., Whaley, A., & Allen, J. E. (2002). *E-DESK:*

A review of recent evidence on the effectiveness of discrete educational software (Prepared for Planning and Evaluation Service, U.S. Department of Education.) Princeton, NJ: SRI International.

Murphy, S. T. (1998). The impact of factual versus fictional media portrayals on cultural stereotypes. In E. Katz & J. J. Strange (Eds.), *Annals of the American Academy of Political and Social Science* (Vol. 560, pp. 165–178). Thousand Oaks, CA: Sage.

Nacos, B. L., & Torres-Reyna, O. (2007). *Fueling our fears: Stereotyping, media coverage and public opinion of Muslim Americans.* Lanham, MD: Rowman & Littlefield.

Narvaez, D., Mattan, B., MacMichael, C., & Sqillace, M. (2008). Kill bandits, collect gold or save the dying: The effects of playing a prosocial video game. *Media Psychology Review, 1*(1). Retrieved March 8, 2013, from *http://mprcenter.org/mpr/index.php?option=com_content &view=article&id=35&Itemid=121.*

Nathanson, A. I. (1999). Identifying and explaining the relationship between parental mediation and children's aggression. *Communication Research, 26*, 124–143.

Nathanson, A. I. (2004). Factual and evaluative approaches to modifying children's responses to violent television. *Journal of Communication, 54*, 321–336.

Nathanson, A. I., & Cantor, J. (2000). Reducing the aggression-promoting effect of violent cartoons by increasing children's fictional involvement with the victim: A study of active mediation. *Journal of Broadcasting and Electronic Media, 44*, 125–142.

Nisbet, E. C., Ostman, R., & Shanahan, J. (2008). Public opinion toward Muslim Americans: Civil liberties and the role of religiosity, ideology, and media use. In A. Sinno (Ed.), *Muslims in Western politics* (pp. 161–199). Bloomington: Indiana University Press.

North, A. C., Tarrant, M., & Hargreaves, D. J. (2004). The effects of music on helping behavior: A field study. *Environment and Behavior, 36*(2), 266–275.

O'Keeffe, G. S., & Clarke-Pearson, K. (2011). The impact of social media on children, adolescents, and families. *Pediatrics, 127*, 800–804.

Oppliger, P. A. (2007). Effects of gender stereotyping on socialization. In R. W. Preiss, B. M. Gayle, N. Burrell, M. Allen, & J. Bryant (Eds.), *Mass media effects research: Advances through meta-analysis* (pp. 199–214). Mahwah, NJ: Erlbaum.

Paik, H., & Comstock, G. (1994). The effects of television violence on antisocial behavior: A meta-analysis. *Communication Research, 21*(4), 516–546.

Pea, R., Nass, C., Meheula, L., Rance, M., Kumar, A., Bamford, H., et al. (2012). Media use, face-to-face communication, media multitasking, and social well-being among 8- to 12-year-old girls. *Developmental Psychology, 48*(2), 327–336.

Pierce, J. P., Choi, W., Gilpin, E., Farkas, A., & Berry, C. (1998). Tobacco industry promotion of cigarettes and adolescent smoking. *Journal of the American Medical Association, 279*, 511–515.

Pierce, J. P., Lee, L., & Gilpin, E. A. (1994). Smoking initiation by adolescent girls, 1944 through 1988: An association with targeted advertising. *Journal of the American Medical Association, 271*, 608–611.

Prot, S., & Anderson, C. A. (2013). Research methods, design, and statistics in media psychology. In K. Dill (Ed.), *The Oxford handbook of media psychology* (pp. 109–136). New York: Oxford University Press.

Prot, S., Gentile, D. G., Anderson, C. A., Suzuki, K., Swing, E., Lim, K. M., et al. (2014). Long-term relations between prosocial media use, empathy and prosocial behavior. *Psychological Science, 25*(2), 358–368.

Ramasubramanian, S. (2011). The impact of stereotypical versus counterstereotypical media exemplars on racial attitudes, causal attributions, and support for affirmative action. *Communication Research, 38*, 497–516.

Rideout, V. J., Foehr, U. G., & Roberts, D. F. (2010). *Generation M2: Media in the lives of 8–18 year olds.* Merlo Park, CA: Henry J Kaiser Foundation.

Roberts, D. F., Christenson, P. G., & Gentile, D. A. (2003). The effects of violent music on children and adolescents. In D. A. Gentile (Ed.), *Media violence and children: A complete guide for parents and professionals* (pp. 153–170). Westport, CT: Praeger.

Roe, K. (1996). Music and identity among European youth: Music as communication. In P. Rutten (Ed.), *Music in Europe* (pp. 85–97). Brussels: European Music Office.

Rosenkoetter, L. I. (1999), The television situation comedy and children's prosocial behavior. *Journal of Applied Social Psychology, 29,* 979–993.

Saleem, M., & Anderson, C. A. (2013). Arabs as terrorists: Effects of stereotypes within violent contexts on attitudes, perceptions and affect. *Psychology of Violence, 3,* 84–99.

Saleem, M., Anderson, C. A., & Gentile, D. A. (2012a). Effects of prosocial, neutral, and violent video games on children's helpful and hurtful behaviors. *Aggressive Behavior, 38,* 281–287.

Saleem, M., Anderson, C. A., & Gentile, D. A. (2012b). Effects of prosocial, neutral, and violent video games on college students' affect. *Aggressive Behavior, 38,* 263–271.

Salomon, G. (1977). Effects of encouraging Israeli mothers to co-observe *Sesame Street* with their five-year-olds. *Child Development, 48,* 1146–1151.

Sargent, J. D., Wills, T. A., Stoolmiller, M., Gibson, J., & Gibbons, F. X. (2006). Alcohol use in motion pictures and its relation with teen drinking. *Journal of Studies on Alcohol, 67,* 54–65.

Schmidt, C. S. (2006). Not just Disney: Destructive stereotypes of Arabs in children's literature. In D. A. Zabel (Ed.), *Arabs in the Americas: Interdisciplinary essays on the Arab Diaspora* (pp. 169–182). New York: Peter Lang.

Shaheen, J. G. (2009). *Reel bad Arabs: How Hollywood vilifies a people.* Brooklyn, NY: Olive Branch Press.

Sharif, I., & Sargent, J. D. (2006). Association between television, movie, and video game exposure and school performance. *Pediatrics, 118*(4), e1061–e1070.

Singer, D. G., & Singer, J. L. (1976). Family television viewing habits and the spontaneous play of pre-school children. *American Journal of Orthopsychiatry, 46,* 496–502.

Singer, J. L., & Singer, D. G. (1998). *Barney & Friends* as entertainment and education. In J. K. Asamen & G. Berry (Eds.), *Research paradigms, television, and social behavior* (pp. 305–367). Thousand Oaks, CA: Sage.

Singhal, A., Cody, M. J., Rogers, E. M., & Sabido, M. (2004). *Entertainment–education and social change: History, research, and practice.* Mahwah, NJ: Erlbaum.

Sisler, V. (2008). Digital Arabs: Representation in video games. *European Journal of Cultural Studies, 11,* 203–220.

Smith, S. L., & Cook, C. A. (2012). Gender stereotypes: An analysis of popular films and TV. Geena Davis Institute for Gender and Media. Retrieved October 1, 2013, from *www.seejane.org/downloads/gdigm_gender_stereotypes.pdf.*

Sprafkin, J. N., & Rubinstein, E. A. (1979). Children's television viewing habits and prosocial behavior: A field correlational study. *Journal of Broadcasting, 23,* 265–276.

Strasburger, V. C. (2005). Adolescents, sex and the media: Ooooo, Baby, Baby—a Q & A. *Adolescent Medicine, 16,* 269–288.

Thomsen, S. R., Weber, M. M., & Brown, L. (2002). The relationship between reading beauty and fashion magazines and the use of pathogenic dieting methods among adolescent females. *Adolescence, 37*(145), 1–18.

Thurlow, C., & Brown, A. (2002). Generation txt?: The sociolinguistics of young people's text-messaging. *Discourse Analysis Online, 1*(1). Retrieved from *www.crispinthurlow.net/papers/Thurlow%282003%29-DAOL.pdf.*

Valente, T. W., Kim, Y. M., Lettenmaier, C., Glass, W., & Dibba, Y. (1994). Radio promotion of family planning in the Gambia. *International Family Planning Perspectives, 20,* 96–100.

Valkenburg, P. M., Krcmar, M., & deRoos, S. (1998). The impact of a cultural children's program and adult mediation on children's knowledge of and attitudes toward opera. *Journal of Broadcasting and Electronic Media, 42,* 315–326.

Van Buren, C. (2006). Critical analysis of racist post 9/11 Web animations. *Journal of Broadcasting and Electronic Media, 50,* 537–554.

Warburton, W. A. (2012a). Growing up fast and furious in a media saturated world. In W. A. Warburton & D. Braunstein (Eds.), *Growing up fast and furious: Reviewing the impacts of violent and sexualised media on children* (pp. 1–33). Sydney: Federation Press.

Warburton, W. A. (2012b). How does listening to Eminem do me any harm?: What the research says about music and anti-social behaviour. In W. A. Warburton & D. Braunstein (Eds.), *Growing up fast and furious: Reviewing the impacts of violent and sexualised media on children* (pp. 85–115). Sydney: Federation Press.

Warburton, W. A., & Highfield, K. (2012). Children, media and technology. In J. Bowes, K. Hodge, & R. Grace (Eds.), *Children, families and communities* (pp. 142–161). London: Oxford University Press.

Ward, L. M. (2002). Does television exposure affect emerging adults' attitudes and assumptions about sexual relationships?: Correlational and experimental confirmation. *Journal of Youth and Adolescence, 31*, 1–15.

Ward, L. M., & Rivadeneyra, R. (1999). Contributions of entertainment television to adolescents' sexual attitudes and expectations: The role of viewing amount versus viewer conceptual issues. *European Journal of Social Psychology, 23*, 39–52.

Weis, R., & Cerankosky, B. C. (2010). Effects of video-game ownership on young boys' academic and behavioral functioning: A randomized, controlled study. *Psychological Science, 21*(4), 463–470.

Weisskirch, R. S. (2009). Parenting by cell phone: Parental monitoring of adolescents and family relations. *Journal of Youth and Adolescence, 38*, 1123–1139.

Whitaker, J. L., & Bushman, B. J. (2012). "Remain calm. Be kind.": Effects of relaxing video games on aggressive and prosocial behavior. *Social Psychological and Personality Science, 3*, 88–92.

Wills, T. A., Sargent, J. D., Gibbons, F. X., Gerrard, M., & Stoolmiller, M. (2009). Movie exposure to alcohol cues and adolescent alcohol problems: A longitudinal analysis in a national sample. *Psychology of Addictive Behaviors, 23*(1), 23–35.

Wroblewski, R., & Huston, A. C. (1987). Televised occupational stereotypes and their effects on early adolescents: Are they changing? *Journal of Early Adolescence, 7*, 283–298.

Ybarra, M. L., Mitchell, K. J., Hamburger, M., Diener-West, M., & Leaf, P. J. (2011). X-rated material and perpetration of sexually aggressive behavior among children and adolescents: Is there a link? *Aggressive Behavior, 37*, 1–18.

Zhao, Y., Qiu, N., & Xie, N. (2012). Social networking, social gaming, texting. In D. G. Singer & J. L. Singer (Eds.), *Handbook of children and the media* (2nd ed., pp. 97–112). Thousand Oaks, CA: Sage.

CHAPTER 13

New-Employee Organizational Socialization
Adjusting to New Roles, Colleagues, and Organizations

Allison M. Ellis
Talya N. Bauer
Berrin Erdogan

The process of socialization is one that occurs throughout the life span as we enter into new phases of our lives, new relationships, and new locations. And, without a doubt, entry into a new job is no exception because it constitutes a major transition each time a person changes organizations to start a new job. In fact, census data indicate that, on average, at least in the United States, this type of new job transition occurs 11.3 times in a person's lifetime (U.S. Bureau of Labor Statistics, 2012). It is not surprising, then, that considerable research on organizational behavior and industrial/organizational psychology has been concerned with the specific socialization process that occurs when one enters into a new job or new organization. *Organizational socialization* refers to the "process by which newcomers [to an organization] make the transition from being organizational outsiders to being insiders" (Bauer, Bodner, Erdogan, Truxillo, & Tucker, 2007, p. 707). In other words, it is the process of learning the ropes within a new organization (Van Maanen & Schein, 1979). In practice, this refers to the extent to which newcomers acquire the knowledge, skills, and functional understanding of their new jobs, make connections with others in the organization, and garner insight into the culture, processes, and people in their new organization. Importantly, organizational socialization has been recognized as a joint process wherein organizations encourage newcomers to accept and adapt to aspects of the organizational culture and established way of doing things, while newcomers actively seek information in an effort to understand and facilitate their own adjustment (Bauer, Morrison, & Callister, 1998). In other words, it relates to the individual, job, group, and organizational levels of analysis. In this chapter, we review the research on organizational socialization, pointing out important trends and findings, and highlighting the many levels of socialization within organizations.

Why Does Organizational Socialization Matter?

In 1998, Bauer and colleagues pointed to four reasons why organizational socialization is important to organizations: First, they noted that the costs to organizations that fail to socialize employees effectively are great. In particular, they noted that organizations that are unsuccessful at socializing employees can expect to pay the price in the form of high turnover. Turnover occurs for a number of reasons, but for new employees, turnover is often the result of unmet expectations (Wanous, 1980) or poor perceived fit with the job or the organization (Kammeyer-Mueller, Wanberg, Glomb, & Ahlburg, 2005). Second, effective socialization can lay the groundwork for a committed and productive workforce. Indeed, effective socialization has been related to increased job satisfaction, organizational commitment, and job performance (Saks & Ashforth, 1997). Third, socialization is a key factor in transmitting an organization's cultural norms and values to new employees (Cable & Parsons, 2001) and vice versa (Cable, Gino, & Staats, 2013). In many ways this is one of the most important aspects of socialization, in that it ensures a common understanding and set of goals among organizational members, and provides employees with important information about expected attitudes and behaviors. Finally, it is also an important vehicle for providing new employees with information regarding relevant organizational politics and power dynamics that enable them to be successful in their new work role.

In today's workplace, these points are perhaps more relevant than ever (Wanberg, 2012). The work context of the 21st century is characterized by turbulent economic times, rapid technological change, and the advent of flexible work schedules that pose many new challenges for organizations in terms of effectively integrating new employees into the organization. For instance, as communications technology continues to evolve, it is ever more commonplace for employees to work from their homes, coffee shops, or remote offices, with little or no direct contact with their colleagues and supervisor (Kossek & Michel, 2011), making the effective integration of employees more challenging. Furthermore, continued economic hardships have changed the context of work such that employees may worry about the security of their position or may enter jobs for which they are overqualified. These factors, coupled with the uncertainty associated with changing jobs or careers, have important implications for not only employee and organizational effectiveness but also employee health and well-being (Probst, 2005). Thus, understanding how organizational socialization practices can effectively build and contribute to cultural norms and values within the organization, facilitate positive adjustment for employees, and transmit expectations for behavior and performance is essential to coping with many of the challenges that face organizations and their employees today.

Socialization and Organizational Fit throughout the Life Course

Work in adult life contributes to one's security and identity and may dramatically affect the individual's physical and psychological well-being. Over the life course, workforce participation may span a period of five or more decades. During this time, individuals develop and mature, learn new job skills, build domains of task knowledge and specific work competencies, and form, modify, and dissolve powerful relational attachments.
—KANFER, CHEN, AND PRICHARD (2008, p. 2)

In the preceding quotation, Kanfer and colleagues point out the importance of work as a source of security and self-concept for individuals throughout their life span. In other words, it is a major source of individual identity. Although, historically, the organizational literature has placed little emphasis on the effects of aging on work behavior, recent years have seen a surge in interest on the topic (e.g., Avery, McKay, & Wilson, 2007). In large part, this is due to the dramatic demographic changes in the workforce, wherein the population of workers over age 40 is burgeoning and economic factors have contributed to older individuals' postponing retirement and staying employed full-time for longer (Alley & Crimmins, 2007). Simultaneously, young adults are continuing to enter the workforce with their own set of values, skills, and needs. Thus, unlike ever before, the work context is increasingly multigenerational and diverse.

This juxtaposition has made salient the role of age and development as it relates to the work context. Accordingly, organizational research has begun to focus increasingly on the factors that impact work motivation, job attitudes, and employee well-being at various stages of the life course (cf. Chen & Kanfer, 2006; Ng & Feldman, 2010). A corresponding increase in scholarly examination of the meaning of work for individuals (Wrzesniewski, Dutton, & Debebe, 2003), prosocial impact (Grant, 2008), and the role that work plays in individuals' lives (Wrzesniewski, McCauley, Rozin, & Schwartz, 1997) has brought important questions to the forefront about how work contributes to one's sense of self and appeals to one's changing skills, identities, and needs throughout the life span.

The application of developmental theories to organizational behavior has provided important insights into the role of work in employees' lives (Baltes & Finkelstein, 2011). For instance, socioemotional selectivity theory (Carstensen, Isaacowitz, & Charles, 1999) posits that with changes in development throughout the life span of a worker, different values are likely to be more or less salient. As a case in point, younger adults are more likely to strive toward career goals that are in accordance with their need for building social and psychological resources. Conversely, older adults tend to value emotion regulation goals (i.e., goals aimed at maintaining positive emotional experiences), which causes them to focus their efforts on work tasks that bring opportunities for maintaining the valued social networks that are meaningful to them. Similarly, in late career, employees are likely to be less interested in financial attainment and more interested in work that is in alignment with their values and talents, and provides increased autonomy and flexibility (Baltes & Finkelstein, 2011). Other researchers (e.g., Mainiero & Sullivan, 2005) have proposed that while challenge is important in one's early career, balance becomes increasingly important midcareer, when employees take on additional familial or other responsibilities outside the work domain. Finally, Mainiero and Sullivan argue that, in one's late career, authenticity (i.e., being true to oneself) becomes increasingly salient for employees. Together these frameworks provide a more nuanced understanding of the importance of the work role in terms of identity, meaning, and providing a sense of integration and competence for employees—needs that Deci and Ryan (1985) suggest are fundamental to individual well-being.

It follows, then, that to the extent that employees derive meaning and information about their own self-identity from their work role, they will look to employment options that reinforce and support those notions of the self (Schneider, 1987). Drawing on this idea, scholarly work examining the role of perceived person–environment fit has provided important information about understanding employee motivation, job attitudes, and performance (Kristof-Brown, Zimmerman, & Johnson, 2005). This line of inquiry has informed our understanding of what attracts employees to a given organization

(Chapman, Uggerslev, Carroll, Piasentin, & Jones, 2005), as well as how socialization practices can impact these perceptions and subsequent outcomes. For instance, the attraction–selection–attrition (ASA; Schneider, 1987) model suggests that people will be attracted to other individuals, groups, or organizations that are similar to themselves and reinforce their self-image. Similarly, those individuals who exhibit characteristics congruent with those of the group are more likely to be selected into and accepted by the group. In turn, meta-analytic results support the notion that to the extent that there is perceived fit between a person and his or her environment (e.g., organization, job, team), job attitudes, including commitment to the environment and a willingness to stay, are enhanced (Kristof-Brown et al., 2005).

Although the bulk of organizational socialization research has focused on employees transitioning to new organizations (Bauer & Erdogan, 2011), a life span perspective makes salient the need to expand scholarly attention to include transitions within organizations as employees move throughout occupational roles (e.g., from supervisee to supervisor). Together these insights have relevance for the way organizations approach socialization and other formal practices, especially with regard to facilitating the congruence between employees' needs, values, and identities with organizationally relevant belief and value systems. Moreover, the study of organizational socialization provides a unique context in which to understand better how people make decisions and interpret their environment in relation to their own values, needs, and ideals. Specifically, major transitions in employment (i.e., job changes) represent a highly uncertain period that can bring these aspects of identity to the forefront for employees. Effective integration and adjustment with an organization (i.e., effective socialization) that provides reinforcement of those values can signal to employees their fit with the organization, thereby providing a source of motivation, commitment, and well-being for them.

The Socialization Process

Rather than being a single "thing," organizational socialization is a process. Figure 13.1 illustrates that the socialization process includes both the influence of insiders and the organization on a new employee, as well as the influence exerted by the new employee on insiders and the organization. This reciprocal process, termed the *interactionist perspective* (Reichers, 1987), is an important point of view that describes both directions of influence. In the following sections we review prevalent theoretical frameworks used to describe and understand the socialization process, as well as relevant empirical literature investigating these assumed relationships.

Organizational Learning and the Reduction of Uncertainty

Klein and Heuser (2008) emphasized learning across organizational levels (i.e., organization, work group, job) as a key component of effective organizational socialization. Accordingly, research aimed at understanding organizational socialization has primarily taken two perspectives with regard to learning: (1) focusing on the factors that facilitate learning (e.g., organizational tactics) during socialization, and (2) assessing what is actually learned by newcomers. As an example of the latter, a scale developed by Chao, O'Leary-Kelly, Wolf, Klein, and Gardner (1994) assesses the extent to which newcomers

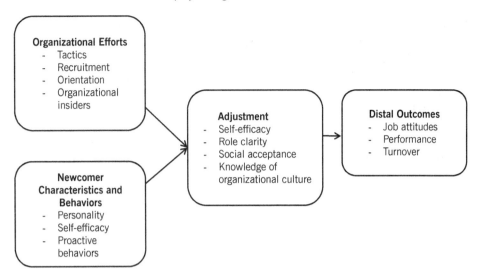

FIGURE 13.1. Antecedents and outcomes of organizational socialization.

have achieved a working knowledge of the organizational history, language, people, and so forth, at different points within the first year of employment. In contrast to cultural knowledge, other scholars have emphasized the role of learning as it pertains to effective reduction of ambiguities related to work tasks, as well as social and behavioral expectations associated with one's new role in an organization.

In the latter case, uncertainty reduction theory (Berger & Calabrese, 1975) has provided a useful framework for understanding what constitutes effective organizational socialization. Originally developed to explain the psychological processes relevant to strangers meeting for the first time, uncertainty reduction theory has been applied to the introduction of new employees to their employing organization. The theory posits that individuals progress through three phases in the process of figuring out where they stand in a new relationship. Phase 1 is the *entry phase*, in which individuals seek readily available or observable information about the other. This phase is followed by Phase 2, the *personal phase*, in which individuals seek information not readily available (e.g., values, beliefs, or attitudes of the other). Finally, in Phase 3, the *exit phase*, individuals negotiate plans for future interactions (i.e., whether or not the relationship will continue).

In the context of a new employment contract, newcomers may garner readily available information during the recruitment and selection processes (Phase 1); however it is during the socialization process (i.e., Phase 2), once newcomers have come on board, that they are able to realize important aspects of the organizational culture that are not readily available (e.g., social norms, justice climate). In addition, this secondary phase is essential to reduce the inherent stress associated with entering a new job for employees. Particularly, by increasing clarity and perceived competence around work tasks and social relationships, effective socialization can drastically alter the extent to which employees feel able and willing to stay in their new role. Based on the information gathered in this phase, newcomers transfer to the exit phase (i.e., Phase 3) in which they come to a conclusion regarding their willingness to remain with an organization.

Building on this framework, successful adjustment of newcomers can be understood as the extent to which employees perceive clarity in their role (i.e., the extent to which newcomers understand job tasks and task priorities), self-efficacy (i.e., newcomers' beliefs that they are capable and can be effective in their role), and acceptance by insiders (i.e., feeling accepted, liked, and trusted by peers), all of which assess the extent to which the organizational socialization process has enabled newcomers to successfully "learn the ropes" of the new organization. In turn, effective adjustment is related to a host of more distal outcomes relevant for organizations and employees. The following section reviews the literature with regard to important organizational and individual predictors of effective socialization, along with key outcomes both proximal and distal to the socialization process.

Antecedents of Adjustment

Organizational Efforts

Organizational efforts as they relate to the process of organizational socialization refer to those formal or informal efforts by the organization and its members to influence the experience of new employees. These efforts can range from a one-time new-employee orientation to complex and integrated socialization systems that include traditional human resources procedures (i.e., recruitment and selection processes) with formalized training and mentoring programs. The following sections review some of the ways in which organizations exert influence on the experience and adjustment of newcomers.

TACTICS

One of the most frequently discussed and studied aspects of new-employee socialization is that of organizational socialization tactics. Van Maanen and Schein (1979) introduced the concept of *organizational socialization tactics*, which they defined as occurring on six dimensions: (1) collective versus individual socialization (i.e., the extent to which newcomers go through the socialization process as a group with common experiences, or as individuals with unique experiences); (2) formal or informal socialization (i.e., the extent to which newcomers are segregated from current employees while they undergo the socialization process, or are working directly with current employees acquiring information on the job); (3) sequential or random training steps (i.e., the extent to which the process, or sequence, in which new material and tasks are presented to new employees is previously determined and known to new employees); (4) fixed or variable sequencing of training (i.e., the extent to which knowledge of timetables is known to new employees); (5) serial or disjunctive tactics (i.e., the extent to which experienced employees serve as role models to newcomers); and (6) investiture or divestiture (i.e., the extent to which newcomers receive positive or negative support from current organizational members). Subsequent research by Jones (1986) and others has organized these tactics along a continuum of institutionalized (i.e., the combination of collective, formal, sequential, fixed, serial, and investiture tactics) and individualized tactics (i.e., individual, informal, random, variable, disjunctive, divestiture). Interestingly, newcomers tend to prefer institutionalized tactics—perhaps due to the structure they provide, which helps to decrease uncertainty in the short run (Ashforth & Saks, 1996).

RECRUITMENT

The recruitment process is important in and of itself because it is a primary determinant of whether or not an applicant takes a job (Ployhart, 2006). For example, Walker and colleagues (2013) found that job seekers were influenced by the interactions they had with organizations that served to maintain their interest throughout recruitment. However, the recruitment process is especially important in that it is truly the start of the newcomers' relationship with the organization. What happens during recruitment sets up newcomers' expectations in terms of what organizational life will be like upon entry (Fisher, 1986; Wanous, 1980). To the degree that these expectations are met, socialization should be more effective. For example, Bauer and Green (1994) found that accurate preview information was related to lower role conflict and higher feelings of acceptance by new research scientists working toward their PhDs in the hard sciences. Kammeyer-Mueller and Wanberg (2003) found similar results in a study of newcomers from seven different organizations, in which newcomers' preentry knowledge about the organization was related to task mastery, role clarity, integration with the work group, political knowledge, and lower work withdrawal at a follow-up time point. These findings are consistent with the work on realistic job previews (e.g., Breaugh, 1983), which refers to providing applicants with accurate information about what the job will actually be like (expected work tasks, the social environment, company culture, etc.) during the recruitment phase. Thus, it is clear that what happens during recruitment and the information received by newcomers, along with the accuracy of their expectations, constitute important aspects of the relationship they form with their new organization. This is especially true once the newcomers start work with the organization, and as the comparison between old expectations or beliefs and new experiences becomes more and more salient.

ORIENTATIONS

When a new employee starts a job, one of the first formal activities is the new-employee orientation (NEO). In the past, the NEO was considered the main vehicle for helping newcomers adjust. Only in the recent past have organizations come to think of socialization and *onboarding* (i.e., bringing new employees on board and up to speed in their new work roles) as a long-term process comprising many interrelated and coordinated parts. Nevertheless, NEO remains an important aspect of the socialization process because research indicates that those who attend them tend to be more successfully socialized than those who do not (Klein & Weaver, 2000). Orientations that focus more attention on helping the new employee feel comfortable and welcome, and that provide the basics, such as where to get additional information, are rated as more effective than those that focus on filling out forms and doing basic paperwork (Shepherd, 2013). In addition, according to recent research, orientations that focus on the new employee and what he or she brings to the organization are more effective than more traditional orientations that focus primarily on positive features of the organization itself (Cable et al., 2013). Part of the effectiveness of NEO is that it helps individuals connect to one another. Work on the difference between remote and in-person NEO attendance shows that those attending remotely were reported to be less well socialized (Wesson & Gogus, 2005). Overall, the NEO is an important part of socialization because it occurs so early in the relationship

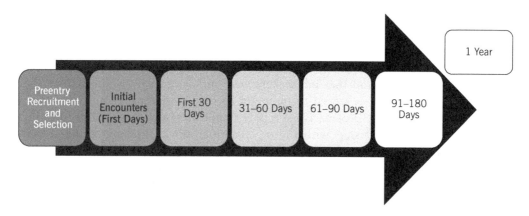

FIGURE 13.2. The socialization process unfolds over a newcomer's first year. Darker gray boxes indicate the more intense socialization time periods, such that pre-entry and the first 30 days tend to be more intense transitions than the period between 180 days and 1-year postentry.

with the organization. However, socialization factors continue to make a difference over the first 90 days and beyond (see Figure 13.2).

ORGANIZATIONAL INSIDERS

A key aspect of newcomer organizational socialization success or failure revolves around organizational insiders (i.e., current organizational members) because socialization does not take place in a vacuum (Van Maanen & Schein, 1979). Research on relationships with coworkers (Nelson & Quick, 1991; Settoon & Adkins, 1997), leaders (Bauer & Green, 1998; Filstad, 2004; Major, Kozlowski, Chao, & Gardner, 1995; Payne, Culbertson, Boswell, & Barger, 2008; Sluss & Thompson, 2012), and mentors (Green & Bauer, 1995) has shown that they are important aspects of adjustment and socialization outcomes. For example, Nelson and Quick (1991) found that interactions with supervisors and colleagues were the most helpful aspect of socialization, as well as the most readily available socialization support received, relative to eight other potential sources of support, including formal orientations and training sessions, assigned mentors and other newcomers, and support staff. Korte (2010) conducted a qualitative study highlighting the importance of building relationships with coworkers for successful socialization; results showed that learning about coworkers, earning their respect, and socializing with them helped facilitate better adjustment for new employees. Relatedly, Bauer and Green (1996) found that for new college graduates entering a variety of industries, forming high-quality relationships with their direct leaders was critical to their success. They also found that for newcomers, actively engaging with those tasks delegated to them by their leaders was an important way to build their relationship with them (Bauer & Green, 1996). Similarly, Chen (2005) and Chen and Klimoski (2003) showed the importance of newcomers' communication, understanding, and integration into their team early in their tenure, for facilitating newcomer performance. While there are many positive ways insiders may help newcomers adjust to their new role, job, workgroup, and organization, there are also ways that insiders may derail the success of newcomers. For example, Kammeyer-Mueller, Wanberg, Rubstein, and Song (2013) found that newcomers who were undermined by supervisors as part of their new-employee experience had higher turnover risks. They also found that insider support for newcomers declined after 90 days, which gives further credence to the idea that the first 90 days are critical in a newcomer's adjustment process (Bauer et al., 1998).

SUMMARY

Together the preceding research indicates that organizational efforts are an important category of antecedents to effective organizational socialization. These efforts refer to a variety of methods, including organizational tactics that range from highly institutionalized tactics, characterized by formal and systematic socialization processes, to individualized tactics that rely primarily on one-on-one, on-the-job training and informal means of adjustment. Other efforts include recruitment processes that occur early in the socialization process, before an employee has formally entered the organization, and NEO programs that directly provide newcomers with information about the job and organization, and initial opportunities for networking with other newcomers. Finally, organizational efforts include formal (e.g., mentors) or informal (e.g., work-group members) interactions with current organizational members that can facilitate effective adjustment of new employees by providing information about the job, role, or larger organizational culture.

Newcomer Characteristics and Behaviors

Although organizational efforts are important for effective socialization, newcomers themselves are active participants in the socialization process and play an essential role in their own adjustment to new organizations. According to the interactionist perspective (Reichers, 1987), characteristics and actions taken by newcomers interact with and reciprocally influence the organization and its members. Research examining the role of the newcomer has tended to focus on either key personality factors that relate to increased adjustment behaviors or on uncovering the behaviors themselves in which newcomers engage. The following sections describe specific characteristics of newcomers that have been identified in the research literature as important to adjustment. In addition, newcomer proactive behaviors are discussed in terms of their contribution to successful organizational socialization.

NEWCOMER PERSONALITY

Bauer and Erdogan (2011) noted that, across studies, a proactive personality consistently plays an important role in the experience of newcomers. *Proactive personality*, as discussed by Crant (2000), refers to a stable tendency to take action on one's environment for the purpose of bringing about change and is associated with a high desire for control. Those with proactive personalities are more likely to seek out and identify opportunities for constructive change that make them more successful in their careers in general (Seibert, Kraimer, & Crant, 2001). With regard to the socialization process, newcomers with higher proactive personality are more motivated to learn (Major, Turner, & Fletcher, 2006), and more likely to take initiative and seek out information and opportunities to learn relevant skills, develop relationships with their peers, and engage in other self-initiated behaviors that facilitate their own integration into the new organizational system. For example, in a sample of 589 employees in the manufacturing, food distribution, health care, and education industries, Kammeyer-Mueller and Wanberg (2003) found that newcomer proactive personality was positively related to increased task mastery, group integration, and political knowledge regarding the organization, which in turn was related to decreased work withdrawal and increased organizational commitment.

Aspects of the five-factor model of personality have also been investigated with respect to newcomer adjustment. Findings indicate that those higher in Extraversion (i.e., social, gregarious, assertive) and Openness to Experience (i.e., curious, intelligent, adventurous) exhibit higher levels of adjustment, in part due to their willingness to engage in important proactive socialization behaviors such as information seeking and building relationships with others (Wanberg & Kammeyer-Mueller, 2000). Investigating this relationship further, Gruman and Saks (2011) found that in a sample of 243 undergraduates, personality factors were related to preference for different socialization tactics, as well as intentions to engage in proactive behavior. More specifically, results showed that those who scored high on Agreeableness preferred more institutionalized socialization tactics and reported increased intentions to engage in relationship building. Those high on Extraversion and proactive personality reported a greater intention to be proactive on the job, specifically, in the form of general socializing and networking behavior with respect to the former, and seeking feedback, building a relationship with their boss, networking, and negotiating job changes with respect to the latter.

Recently, Harrison, Sluss, and Ashforth (2011) found that trait curiosity was related to newcomer socialization and adjustment. They studied both specific (i.e., narrow and direct forms of exploration) and diversive curiosity (i.e., broad and indirect forms of exploration). Specific curiosity was related to information-seeking behaviors, whereas diversive curiosity was related to positive framing (i.e., cognitively reframing events as opportunities and challenges). These results indicate that individual curiosity matters, and that the relationships between curiosity and adjustment indicators are not universal. In other words, how adjustment is affected depends on which facet of curiosity is studied.

NEWCOMER SELF-EFFICACY

Other research has identified additional newcomer characteristics important for effective socialization and adjustment. For example, Gruman, Saks, and Zweig (2006) conducted a longitudinal study examining the role of newcomer *self-efficacy* (defined in the referenced study as the extent to which newcomers felt confident in the tasks, role, work group, and organizational domains of the job), proactive behaviors, and socialization outcomes in a sample of 140 students enrolled in a cooperative management program, in which students alternated between school terms and work terms. Findings revealed that together with socialization tactics, newcomer self-efficacy positively predicted newcomer proactive behaviors, including feedback seeking, information seeking, and general socializing, among others. In turn, these behaviors were positively related to more distal socialization outcomes such as perceptions of fit with the job and organization, job satisfaction, and organizational commitment.

OTHER NEWCOMER CHARACTERISTICS

Finally, a recent study has suggested a link between employees' attachment style and their propensity to engage in proactive behaviors at work (Wu & Parker, 2012). Among a sample of Taiwanese students, Wu and Parker showed that relationship anxiety in adult-hood moderated the intraindividual relation between *core self-evaluations* (CSEs; i.e., a global judgment about an individual's own worth, ability, and effectiveness across situations) and *future orientation* (i.e., consideration of future events and a propensity to take action relative to those events), and the outcome, proactive behavior, which was assessed monthly. Results showed that for those with low relationship anxiety, the magnitude of the positive relation between CSEs and proactive behavior was enhanced, whereas for those high in relationship anxiety, this relation was weaker. Conversely, students with low relationship anxiety showed a weaker positive relation between future orientation and proactive behavior than those with high relationship anxiety. These authors concluded that for those with high relationship anxiety "behaving proactively might be a good way to approach future goals, but the fragility of their self-concepts does not help them sustain proactive actions" (p. 528). Furthermore, they argued that positive social environments that protect against threats of loss may be functional in promoting proactive behaviors among these employees. These findings are interesting because, whereas the study does not assess proactivity among new employees, one might expect that fears associated with relationships and social interactions might be even more salient for new employees who have yet to establish high-quality relationships in the workplace. Although these findings occur only in a single study, they point to the importance of understanding employee behavior within the larger social context of work, as well as appreciation for human development and experience across the life span.

Newcomer Proactive Behaviors

As indicated earlier, new employee characteristics facilitate adjustment largely through their impact on employee proactive behaviors during organizational socialization (Wanberg & Kammeyer-Mueller, 2000). Building on this notion, Ashford and Black (1996) developed a taxonomy of newcomer proactive behaviors identifying the following as relevant to newcomer adjustment: information seeking, feedback seeking, general socializing, networking, building relationships with one's boss, negotiating job changes, and positive framing. In a test of their model, the authors found that building a relationship with one's boss and positive framing predicted positive job performance. Information seeking, general socializing, and negotiating job changes were related to job satisfaction. In addition, some newcomer proactive behaviors were associated with increased desire for control, indicating that newcomers may use these tactics as a way to exert control over their new environment. The majority of empirical literature investigating proactive behaviors among newcomers has focused on information seeking and feedback seeking (Bauer et al., 2007) because these behaviors are viewed as crucial to the learning and adjustment process necessary for effective socialization.

INFORMATION SEEKING

Unlike those who may passively wait to be engaged in the socialization process, newcomers who actively seek out information about their work role and environment are more likely to garner a better understanding about expected behaviors and interdependencies among work roles; they are more likely to have more interaction with their coworkers and/or supervisor, thereby providing opportunities for additional resources in the form of both information and support from colleagues. Accordingly, Bauer and colleagues

(2007) conducted a meta-analysis in which they tested a model of newcomer adjustment during organizational socialization. They found that newcomers who proactively sought out information about their work role and organization exhibited more positive organizational adjustment in the form of increased role clarity, self-efficacy, and social acceptance. In addition, information seeking was found to positively relate to more distal outcomes of the socialization process, including job performance, job satisfaction, organizational commitment, and intentions to remain with the organization.

FEEDBACK SEEKING

Feedback seeking is another way in which newcomers garner information about their new environment. While information seeking can include both active and passive modes of gathering information, feedback seeking represents a truly active attempt to understand how others in the work environment view a newcomer's behavior. In turn, feedback provided by one's supervisor and coworkers is thought to reduce uncertainty associated with the new role, thereby decreasing stress. Accordingly, in a three-wave longitudinal study, Wanberg and Kammeyer-Mueller (2000) found that newcomers who solicited feedback from their supervisors and coworkers were more likely to report higher job satisfaction and less likely to leave their job several months later. They also reported positive relations between making an effort to build relationships at work and feelings of social integration, role clarity, and job satisfaction, and negative relations with intentions to leave their job.

JOB CRAFTING AND IDIOSYNCRATIC DEALS

Other proactive behaviors identified in the organizational literature that are likely to be relevant to the process of organizational socialization include job crafting (Wrzesniewski & Dutton, 2001) and the development of idiosyncratic deals (Rousseau, 2001). *Job crafting* refers to the process of modifying one's work tasks, cognitions, or relationships for the purpose of developing increased meaning and significance in work. Original conceptualizations of job crafting (Wrzesniewski & Dutton, 2001) were developed to understand better how individuals cope with marginalized work tasks (e.g., a nurse bathing an older adult patient). However, subsequent research has indicated that employees in a range of occupational positions and industries engage in job-crafting behaviors (e.g., Petrou, Demerouti, Peeters, Schaufeli, & Hetland, 2012; Tims, Bakker, & Derks, 2012). Researchers theorized that how individuals think about and apply meaning to their work impacts their commitment and willingness to engage in the work. Together these concepts recognize the role of newcomers and their own beliefs and cognitions with regard to facilitating not only adjustment to their new role but also the ongoing desire to stay with the organization or within a given role.

Similarly, the development of idiosyncratic deals (i-deals) refers to the process of employees negotiating terms of employment and benefits on behalf of themselves (Rousseau, 2001). Investigations surrounding the development of i-deals have ranged from examining how exceptional employees negotiate flexibility in scheduling to opportunities for professional development, to changes in job tasks and design (Hornung, Rousseau, Glaser, Angerer, & Weigl, 2010). From an organizational socialization standpoint, employees who successfully negotiate changes to their employment contracts are more likely to experience increased perceptions of fit with the job, satisfaction, and ultimately are more likely to stay with the organization, although there remains a significant need for additional empirical work to substantiate these statements.

SUMMARY

A second category of antecedents that are important to effective organizational socialization includes the personality and unique individual differences that newcomers bring to their new work environment, and the self-initiated behaviors in which they engage to facilitate their own adjustment. Research suggests that characteristics such as extraversion and proactive personality are important individual differences that predict which employees are more likely to take initiative and engage in proactive behaviors that assist in the process of adjustment. The primary focus of socialization researchers has been on acts such as information seeking and feedback seeking, in terms of their relations with socialization outcomes; however, new research indicates that other behaviors, such as job crafting and negotiation of i-deals, are important avenues for future investigation.

Outcomes of Adjustment

Proximal/Adjustment Indicators

Adjustment indicators refer to proximal outcomes of the socialization process that signify effective organizational socialization and adjustment to the new work role. These factors are often measured early on in the socialization process (Bauer et al., 1998) and represent the extent to which newcomers feel sure of what is expected of them, confident in their own ability to meet those expectations, and that they have the needed support and social resources to flourish in their new role. For example, Bauer and colleagues (2007) reviewed the socialization literature and found support for their model identifying role clarity, self-efficacy, and acceptance by organizational insiders as important indicators of adjustment for newcomers. Other research includes knowledge of organizational culture as a fourth indicator of adjustment (Bauer & Erdogan, 2011). The following reviews each of these adjustment indicators in more detail.

ROLE CLARITY

Role clarity refers to the extent to which one understands his or her role (Katz & Kahn, 1978). Research on work stress has pointed to the detrimental impact that *role stress* (i.e., role ambiguity and role conflict) has on employee performance and well-being (Gilboa, Shirom, Fried, & Cooper, 2008). This finding carries through to less traditional modes of performance as well; role stressors are negatively related to organizational citizenship behaviors (e.g., helping coworkers; Eatough, Chang, Miloslavic, & Johnson, 2011). Furthermore, the stress related to confusion regarding one's role can spill over into the nonwork domain and contribute to increased levels of work–family conflict (Allen, Herst, Bruck, & Sutton, 2000). While these findings refer to employees in general, role ambiguity may be particularly problematic for newcomers. For example, empirical findings show that role clarity early on in an employee's tenure is related to higher job satisfaction and organizational commitment (Adkins, 1995; Bauer & Green, 1994). Moreover, role clarity has been shown to be a significant predictor of newcomer behaviors, including higher levels of newcomer performance and reduced turnover (Bauer et al., 2007).

SELF-EFFICACY

As indicated earlier in the chapter, research has identified self-efficacy as an important newcomer characteristic for predicting socialization at work. Other scholars (e.g., Bauer et al., 2007) have conceptualized self-efficacy as an indicator, in and of itself, of effective adjustment. From this latter perspective, self-efficacy can be understood as a proximal outcome of effective socialization practices, and a predictor of more distal attitudes and behaviors. For example, research has indicated the importance of self-efficacy in predicting the extent to which newcomers actively engage in the socialization process, as well as subsequent attitudes and behavior on the job, such as perceptions of fit with the job and organization, job satisfaction, and organizational commitment (Gruman et al., 2006). In addition to providing newcomers the confidence to engage in proactive socialization behaviors, self-efficacy has implications for motivation to learn during training (Colquitt, LePine, & Noe, 2000) and has been found to partially mediate the relations between new employee training and job satisfaction, organization commitment, and intentions to quit. Moreover, from a stress perspective, belief in one's capability can be conceptualized as a psychological resource that moderates the negative impact of stress and may facilitate increased engagement in the work role (Demerouti, Bakker, Nachreiner, & Schaufeli, 2001).

SOCIAL ACCEPTANCE

Social acceptance by organizational insiders is a third factor that has been found to be a relevant indicator of effective adjustment during the socialization process (Bauer et al., 2007). *Social acceptance* refers to the extent to which one feels a part of, and integrated into, the social fabric of the environment. Scholarly work by Deci and Ryan (1985) has noted that a sense of relatedness and belonging to the social environment is a fundamental human need that, when satisfied, contributes to increased intrinsic motivation and self-determination. Other research indicates the roles of social support and a sense of belonging in the workplace as important resources that can be leveraged in times of stress (Viswesvaran, Sanchez, & Fisher, 1999). For newcomers, a feeling of being accepted by other organizational insiders may serve as a source of instrumental support to the extent that newcomers are able to access important information that facilitates their own performance and functioning within the group. Moreover, feeling like an accepted member of a group is likely to lead to increased attraction to the group, enhancing perceptions of fit and intentions to stay (Schneider, 1987). Empirical work supporting this assertion indicates that social acceptance is positively related to job satisfaction, organizational commitment, and intentions to remain with the organization, as well as increased performance (Bauer et al., 2007).

KNOWLEDGE OF ORGANIZATIONAL CULTURE

Finally, knowledge of organizational culture, including an understanding of how an organization functions, is an important part of transitioning from an organizational outsider to an insider. The research in this area considers newcomers who better understand the social and functional systems relevant to an organization to be better adjusted and better prepared to be successful in their work role. A popular socialization scale by Chao and colleagues (1994) measures six dimensions relevant to the socialization process: performance proficiency, politics, language, people, organizational goals and values, and history. *Performance proficiency* refers to an understanding of the work role and performance-relevant expectations. *Politics* refers to an understanding of the social culture of the work environment, including power structures within the organization. Comprehension of appropriate jargon, slang and other language specific to the organization are key to the *language* dimension. Similar to social acceptance discussed earlier, the *people* dimension refers to the extent to which the newcomer has been able to form meaningful relationships within the work environment. *Organizational goals and values* measures the extent to which the newcomer has been able to garner an understanding of the organization's overarching aims and missions. Finally, *history* refers to understanding of the organization's past traditions, customs, and other culturally relevant experiences and history. Together these dimensions are indicative of effective socialization practices, in that they assess the extent to which newcomers are able to understand, internalize, and participate in the organizational culture.

SUMMARY

Adjustment indicators represent proximal outcomes of the socialization process and include role clarity, self-efficacy, social acceptance, and knowledge of organizational culture. Thus, successful organizational socialization occurs when organizational efforts and individual behaviors effectively address and aid in the development of these indicators.

Distal Outcomes

Distal outcomes are long-term attitudinal and behavioral changes that result from the joint efforts of organizations and newcomers throughout the socialization process. Ultimately, the goal of organizational socialization is to integrate newcomers effectively into the organization, such that they feel competent in their skills, supported by the organization and its members, and committed to high performance and longevity with the organization. Thus, examining distal outcomes of the socialization process provides insight into the effectiveness of various modes of socialization across contexts and time. The primary focus of research in the organizational socialization literature on distal outcomes has been on examining attitudinal outcomes, followed by newcomer behaviors relevant to organizational and individual effectiveness. The following briefly reviews both.

JOB ATTITUDES

Employee job attitudes are important to organizations in terms of their relations with individual performance-related behaviors, as well as important outcomes in and of themselves. Within organizational behavior and industrial/organizational psychology, the most commonly studied job attitudes are job satisfaction, organizational commitment, and intentions to leave the organization (i.e., turnover intentions; Schleicher, Hansen, & Fox, 2011), and this trend is reflected in the organizational socialization literature as well (Bauer & Erdogan, 2012). With regard to newcomers, job attitudes are important in that they provide insight into future employee performance and how likely it is that an employee will stay with the organization. For example, job satisfaction has been positively related to both in-role performance (i.e., performance of assigned job tasks) and extrarole performance (i.e., behaviors that are not formally recognized by the reward systems but support the social and psychological work context; Riketta, 2008). Similarly, organizational commitment is an important predictor of turnover intentions, actual turnover, and job performance (Meyer, Stanley, Herscovitch, & Topolnytsky, 2002).

Research has supported the impact of aspects of the organizational socialization process on job attitudes. For example, Saks, Uggerslev, and Fassina (2007) conducted a meta-analysis of the literature examining organizational socialization tactics and newcomer adjustment; their results indicated that formalized organizational tactics, especially those related to facilitating social and interpersonal adjustment for employees, were significant positive predictors of job attitudes, including job satisfaction and organizational commitment, and negative predictors of intentions to quit. Moreover, their results support partial mediation in which organizational tactics relate to these distal socialization outcomes through more proximal adjustment indictors (i.e., lower role conflict and role ambiguity) and perceptions of fit with the job and/or organization. Wanberg and Kammeyer-Mueller (2000) examined the role of newcomer proactivity with regard to adjustment outcomes. Their results indicated that new employees who engaged in greater feedback seeking were more satisfied with their jobs. Similarly, those who actively attempted to build relationships with others in their workplace reported higher job satisfaction and lower intentions to turnover. Results of Bauer and colleagues' (2007) meta-analysis provide further support for the relations between both organizational and newcomer socialization tactics and job attitudes. Results showed that both organizational socialization tactics and information seeking are positively related to job satisfaction, organizational commitment, and intentions to remain with the organization.

EMPLOYEE BEHAVIORS

Also relevant to the socialization process are actual employee behaviors, including job performance and turnover. Results from numerous studies point to the importance of organizational socialization in facilitating increased employee effectiveness on the job and decreased turnover (Bauer et al., 1998). For example, Bauer and colleagues (2007) found support for the relation between newcomer information seeking and job performance. Saks and colleagues (2007) demonstrated significant relations between organizational tactics, namely, those that are categorized as investiture, institutionalized, content, and social (i.e., formalized institutionalized tactics), and newcomer performance. Additionally, feedback seeking, one type of proactive behavior in which newcomers may engage, has been significantly and negatively related to actual turnover behavior (Wanberg & Kammeyer-Mueller, 2000). Significant and positive relations with job performance, and significant negative relations with actual turnover and previously discussed adjustment indicators have been reported in a meta-analysis by Bauer and colleagues. More recent research suggests that organizational socialization processes that appeal to newcomers' sense of identity and unique value may be an important factor in explaining how and under what conditions formal processes facilitate effective adjustment and impact distal outcomes (Cable et al., 2013).

Bauer and Erdogan (2012) discuss other potential outcomes of the socialization process that have been examined less often, or not at all, in the organizational literature but may have important relations to the organizational socialization process. These possible outcomes include perceptions of job or organizational fit, employee stress and well-being, ethical work behavior, organizational change, work–life conflict, life satisfaction, perceived overqualification, changes in organizational relationships, and leader stress and well-being. Thus, there is substantial room to expand our current understanding of the role of the organizational socialization process and additional organizational- and employee-relevant outcomes.

SUMMARY

Distal outcomes of the socialization process include both employee job attitudes and performance on the job. Job attitudes include organizational commitment and job satisfaction, as well as intentions to stay with or leave the organization, all of which have implications for employee behavior. Behaviors including task performance and helping behaviors at work are commonly assessed and conceptualized as outcomes of effective organizational socialization practices. Other behaviors, such as whether or not employees actually leaves the organization, are considered important outcomes of effective socialization practices.

Future Research Directions

Many opportunities for future research in the area of organizational socialization exist. Research within the field of organizational socialization is rapidly evolving, and researchers continue to face important questions, such as how organizational values and cultural norms are transmitted through electronic means in our changing technological environment. While there has been some preliminary work regarding the role of technology and socialization (e.g., Wesson & Gogus, 2005), we know little about this topic. The degree to which technology helps or hinders the adjustment process for newcomers is a key question that remains to be answered.

Another key question is how an organization ensures high commitment and productivity when employees work from home or remote locations. As telecommuting becomes more and more prevalent, it is important to understand how socialization takes place in remote contexts. It may be that the process simply takes longer, but it may also be the case that the organizational socialization process fundamentally differs depending on the work setting. Similarly, it will be important for future research to understand better the other side of the coin, which is how telecommuting may impact the development of identity and sense of belonging experienced by newcomers. Without further research into this evolving work context, we cannot know which is more likely the case for the millions of remote workers.

Furthermore, how can organizations ensure that they are inclusive, so that older and minority workers feel integrated into the social context of work to the same extent as other employees? It seems that in an aging workforce, factors influencing newcomer adjustment for older and younger workers may vary. Identifying which organizational efforts or newcomer initiatives may result in more successful socialization of newcomers at different stages of their careers and lives is a key research direction. In addition, it is important to examine whether the theories of socialization currently in use continue to explain the socialization process of these particular newcomers. Similarly, as the composition of the workforce changes to include more cultural and demographic diversity, exploring the predictive validity of current models of socialization will be important.

So little work has been done on stress as an important aspect of socialization as both a process and as an outcome that a key remaining question is how socialization practices can reduce the stress and uncertainty associated with entering a new job. These challenges are increasingly relevant for organizations in today's workplace and in many ways can be addressed by effective organizational socialization. In addition to stress, *well-being* (e.g., overall sense of competence, fit, and certainty that may impact functioning in both work and nonwork domains) of the newcomer is likely to be affected by newcomer socialization process. During the early days of the socialization process, newcomers experience a significant amount of uncertainty and lack of confidence, which likely results in stress and reduces newcomer well-being. Stress may also have crossover effects impacting the newcomer's family members and close others. In other words, the effects of newcomer socialization may go beyond influencing work behavior of the newcomer to affect newcomer and family member well-being. Such effects, if identified, would increase the critical importance of effective management of newcomer socialization from the perspective of newcomers, organizations, and society at large.

Finally, we note the relative lack of attention to the way that organizational socialization is embedded into the larger constellation of socialization throughout the life span. We encourage research that identifies ways in which types of adjustment relate to, and the degree to which they help or hinder, one another. For example, is it possible for newcomers to adjust fully within an organization if they are not fully adjusted in other aspects of their lives? Taking a longer term perspective would also be useful because little research has addressed how organizational socialization in one organization affects adjustment in another organization. Given that this transition occurs so frequently, on average, for individuals, the more we learn about the effect of past transitions on future ones, the more we will be able to help both individuals and organizations identify best practices and contingency and boundary conditions to help aid in organizational socialization success.

Conclusion

In this chapter, we have reviewed the organizational literature on newcomer socialization. The process of socialization is a function of organizational efforts such as adopting different approaches toward socializing newcomers, orientation programs, and recruitment techniques employed by the organization, as well as newcomers' effects on this process through their personality traits and proactive behaviors. Indicators of newcomer adjustment and proximal outcomes of the socialization process include role clarity, self-efficacy, social acceptance, and knowledge of the organizational culture. In turn, this adjustment to the new job has implications for job attitudes, performance, and turnover of the newcomer. Taken together, the organizational socialization literature suggests that the early days a newcomer spends at work in the process of learning about their new job and organization matter and constitute an important socialization experience.

REFERENCES

Adkins, C. L. (1995). Previous work experience and organizational socialization: A longitudinal examination. *Academy of Management Journal, 38*, 839–862.

Allen, T. D., Herst, D. E., Bruck, C. S., & Sutton, M. (2000). Consequences associated with work-to-family conflict: A review and agenda for future research. *Journal of Occupational Health Psychology, 5*, 278–308.

Alley, D., & Crimmins, E. (2007). The demography of aging and work. In K. S. Schultz & G. A. Adams (Eds.), *Aging and work in the 21st century* (pp. 7–24). Mahwah, NJ: Erlbaum.

Ashford, S. J., & Black, J. S. (1996). Proactivity during organizational entry: The role of desire for control. *Journal of Applied Psychology, 81*, 199–214.

Ashforth, B. K., & Saks, A. M. (1996). Socialization tactics: Longitudinal effects on newcomer adjustment. *Academy of Management Journal, 39*, 149–178.

Avery, D. R., McKay, P. F., & Wilson, D. C. (2007). Engaging the aging workforce: The relationship between perceived age similarity, satisfaction with co-workers, and employee engagement. *Journal of Applied Psychology, 92*, 1542–1556.

Baltes, B. B., & Finkelstein, L. M. (2011). Contemporary empirical advancements in the study of aging in the workplace. *Journal of Organizational Behavior, 32*, 151–154.

Bauer, T. N., Bodner, T., Erdogan, B., Truxillo, D., & Tucker, J. S. (2007). Newcomer adjustment during organizational socialization: A meta-analytic review of antecedents, outcomes, and methods. *Journal of Applied Psychology, 92*, 707–721.

Bauer, T. N., & Erdogan, B. (2011). Organizational socialization: The effective onboarding of new employees. In S. Zedeck, H. Aguinis, W. Cascio, M. Gelfand, K. Leung, S. Parker, et al. (Eds.), *APA handbook of I/O psychology* (Vol. 3, pp. 51–64). Washington, DC: American Psychological Association Press.

Bauer, T. N., & Erdogan, B. (2012). Organizational socialization outcomes: Now and into the future. In C. Wanberg (Ed.), *Organizational socialization* (pp. 97–112). Oxford, UK: Oxford University Press.

Bauer, T. N., & Green, S. G. (1994). The effect of newcomer involvement in work-related activities: A longitudinal study of socialization. *Journal of Applied Psychology, 79*, 211–223.

Bauer, T. N., & Green, S. G. (1996). Development of leader–member exchange: A longitudinal test. *Academy of Management Journal, 39*, 1538–1567.

Bauer, T. N., Morrison, E. W., & Callister, R. R. (1998). Organizational socialization: A review and directions for future research. In G. R. Ferris (Ed.), *Research in personnel and human resource management* (Vol. 16, pp. 149–214). Greenwich, CT: JAI Press.

Berger, C. R., & Calabrese, R. J. (1975). Some explorations in initial interaction and beyond: Toward a developmental theory of interpersonal communication. *Human Communication Research, 1*, 99–112.

Breaugh, J. A. (1983). Realistic job previews: A critical appraisal and future research directions. *Academy of Management Review, 8*, 612–619.

Cable, D. M., Gino, F., & Staats, B. R. (2013). Breaking them in or eliciting their best?: Reframing socialization around newcomers' authentic self-expression. *Administrative Science Quarterly, 58*, 1–36.

Cable, D. M., & Parsons, C. K. (2001). Socialization tactics and person-organization fit. *Personnel Psychology, 54*, 1–23.

Carstensen, L. L., Isaacowitz, D. M., & Charles, S. T. (1999). Taking time seriously: A theory of socioemotional selectivity. *American Psychologist, 54*, 165–181.

Chao, G. T., O'Leary-Kelly, A. M., Wolf, S., Klein, H. J., & Gardner, P. D. (1994). Organizational socialization: Its content and consequences. *Journal of Applied Psychology, 79*, 730–743.

Chapman, D. S., Uggerslev, K. L., Carroll, S. A., Piasentin, K. A., & Jones, D. A. (2005). Applicant attraction to organizations and job choice: A meta-analytic review of the correlates of recruiting outcomes. *Journal of Applied Psychology, 90*, 928–944.

Chen, G. (2005). Newcomer adaptation in teams: Multilevel antecedents and outcomes. *Academy of Management Journal, 48,* 101–116.

Chen, G., & Kanfer, R. (2006). Toward a systems theory of motivated behavior in work teams. *Research in Organizational Behavior, 27,* 223–267.

Chen, G., & Klimoski, R. J. (2003). The impact of expectations on newcomer performance in teams as mediated by work characteristics, social exchanges, and empowerment. *Academy of Management Journal, 46,* 591–607.

Colquitt, J. A., LePine, J. A., & Noe, R. A. (2000). Toward an integrative theory of training motivation: A meta-analytic path analysis of 20 years of research. *Journal of Applied Psychology, 85,* 678–707.

Crant, J. M. (2000). Proactive behavior in organizations. *Journal of Management, 26,* 274–276.

Deci, E. L., & Ryan, R. M. (1985). *Intrinsic motivation and self-determination in human behavior.* New York: Plenum.

Demerouti, E., Bakker, A. B., Nachreiner, F., & Schaufeli, W. B. (2001). The job demands–resources model of burnout. *Journal of Applied Psychology, 86,* 499–512.

Eatough, E. M., Chang, C., Miloslavic, S. A., & Johnson, R. E. (2011). Relationships of role stressors with organizational citizenship behavior: A meta-analysis. *Journal of Applied Psychology, 96,* 619–632.

Filstad, C. (2004). How newcomers use role models in organizational socialization. *Journal of Workplace Learning, 16,* 396–409.

Fisher, C. D. (1986). Organizational socialization: An integrative review. In K. M. Rowland & G. R. Ferris (Eds.), *Research in personnel and human resources management* (Vol. 4, pp. 101–145). Greenwich, CT: JAI Press.

Gilboa, S., Shirom, A., Fried, Y., & Cooper, C. (2008). A meta-analysis of work demand stressors and job performance: Examining main and moderating effects. *Personnel Psychology, 61,* 227–271.

Grant, A. (2008). Does intrinsic motivation fuel the prosocial fire?: Motivational synergy in predicting persistence, performance, and productivity. *Journal of Applied Psychology, 93,* 48–58.

Green, S. G., & Bauer, T. N. (1995). Supervisory mentoring by advisers: Relationships with Ph.D. student potential, productivity, and commitment. *Personnel Psychology, 48,* 537–561.

Gruman, J. A., & Saks, A. M. (2011). Socialization preferences and intentions: Does one size fit all? *Journal of Vocational Behavior, 79,* 419–427.

Gruman, J. A., Saks, A. M., & Zweig, D. L. (2006). Organizational socialization tactics and newcomer proactive behaviors: An integrative study. *Journal of Vocational Behavior, 69,* 90–104.

Harrison, S. H., Sluss, D. M., & Ashforth, B. E. (2011). Curiosity adapted the cat: The role of trait curiosity in newcomer adaptation. *Journal of Applied Psychology, 96,* 211–220.

Hornung, S., Rousseau, D. M., Glaser, J., Angerer, P., & Weigl, M. (2010). Beyond top-down and bottom-up work redesign: Customizing job ontent through idiosyncratic deals. *Journal of Organizational Behavior, 31,* 187–215.

Jones, G. R. (1986). Socialization tactics, self-efficacy, and newcomers' adjustments to organizations. *Academy of Management Journal, 29,* 262–279.

Kammeyer-Mueller, J., Wanberg, C., Rubstein, A., & Song, Z. (2013). Support, undermining, and newcomer socialization: Fitting in during the first 90 days. *Academy of Management Journal, 56*(4), 1104–1124.

Kammeyer-Mueller, J. D., & Wanberg, C. R. (2003). Unwrapping the organizational entry process: Disentangling multiple antecedents and their pathways to adjustment. *Journal of Applied Psychology, 88,* 779–794.

Kammeyer-Mueller, J. D., Wanberg, C. R., Glomb, T. M., & Ahlburg, D. (2005). The role of temporal shifts in turnover processes: It's about time. *Journal of Applied Psychology, 90,* 664–658.

Kanfer, R., Chen, G., & Prichard, R. (2008). Work motivation: Forgoing new perspectives and directions in the post-millennium. In R. Kanfer, G. Chen, & R. D. Prichard (Eds.), *Work motivation: Past, present, and future* (pp. 601–632). New York: Routledge.

Katz, D., & Kahn, R. L. (1978). *The social psychology of organizations*. New York: Wiley.

Klein, H. J., & Heuser, A. E. (2008). The learning of socialization content: A framework for researching orientating practices. *Research in personnel and human resources management* (Vol. 27, pp. 279–336). Greenwich, CT: JAI Press.

Klein, H. J., & Weaver, N. A. (2000). The effectiveness of an organization-level orientation training program in the socialization of new hires. *Personnel Psychology, 53*, 47–66.

Korte, R. (2010). "First, get to know them": A relational view of organizational socialization. *Human Resource Development International, 13*, 27–43.

Kossek, E., & Michel, J. (2011). Flexible work schedules. In S. Zedeck, H. Aguinis, W. Cascio, M. Gelfand, K. Leung, S. Parker, et al. (Eds.), *APA handbook of I/O psychology* (Vol. 1, pp. 535–572). Washington, DC: American Psychological Association Press.

Kristof-Brown, A. K., Zimmerman, R. D., & Johnson, E. C. (2005). Consequences of individuals' fit at work: A meta-analysis of person–job, person–organization, and person–group, and person–supervisor fit. *Personnel Psychology, 58*, 281–342.

Mainiero, L. A., & Sullivan, S. E. (2005). Kaleidoscope careers: An alternate explanation for the "opt-out" revolution. *Academy of Management Perspectives, 19*, 106–123.

Major, D., Kozlowski, S. W. J., Chao, G. T., & Gardner, P. D. (1995). A longitudinal investigation of newcomer expectations, early socialization outcomes, and the moderating effects of role development factors. *Journal of Applied Psychology, 80*, 418–431.

Major, D. A., Turner, J. E., & Fletcher, T. D. (2006). Linking proactive personality and the Big Five to motivation to learn and developmental activity. *Journal of Applied Psychology, 91*, 927–935.

Meyer J. P., Stanley, D. J., Herscovitch, L., & Topolnytsky, L. (2002). Affective, continuance, and normative commitment to the organization: A meta-analysis of antecedents, correlates, and consequences. *Journal of Vocational Behavior, 61*, 20–52.

Nelson, D. L., & Quick, J. C. (1991). Social support and newcomer adjustment in organizations: Attachment theory at work? *Journal of Organizational Behavior, 12*, 543–554.

Ng, T., & Feldman, D. C. (2010). The relationships of age with job attitudes: A meta-analysis. *Personnel Psychology, 63*, 677–718.

Payne, S. C., Culbertson, S. S., Boswell, W. R., & Barger, E. J. (2008). Newcomer psychological contracts and employee socialization activities: Does perceived balance in obligations matter? *Journal of Vocational Behavior, 73*, 465–472.

Petrou, P., Demerouti, E., Peeters, M. C., Schaufeli, W. B., & Hetland, J. (2012). Crafting a job on a daily basis: Contextual correlates and the link to work engagement. *Journal of Organizational Behavior, 33*, 1120–1141.

Ployhart, R. E. (2006). Staffing in the 21st century. *Journal of Management, 32*, 868–897.

Probst, T. M. (2005). Economic stressors. In J. Barling, K. Kelloway, & M. Frone (Eds.), *Handbook of work stress* (pp. 267–297). Thousand Oaks, CA: Sage.

Reichers, A. E. (1987). An interactionist perspective on newcomer socialization rates. *Academy of Management Review, 12*, 278–287.

Riketta, M. (2008). The causal relation between job attitudes and performance: A meta-analysis of panel studies. *Journal of Applied Psychology, 93*, 472–481.

Rousseau, D. M. (2001). Schema, promise and mutuality: The building blocks of the psychological contract. *Journal of Occupational and Organizational Psychology, 74*, 511–541.

Saks, A. M., & Ashforth, B. E. (1997). Organizational socialization: Making sense of past and present as a prologue for the future. *Journal of Vocational Behavior, 51*, 234–279.

Saks, A. M., Uggerslev, K. L., & Fassina, N. E. (2007). Socialization tactics and newcomer adjustment: A meta-analytic review and test of a model. *Journal of Vocational Behavior, 70*, 413–446.

Schleicher, D. J., Hansen, S. D., & Fox, K. E. (2011). Job attitudes and work values. In S. Zedeck, H. Aguinis, W. Cascio, M. Gelfand, K. Leung, S. Parker, et al. (Eds.), *APA handbook of*

I/O psychology (Vol. 3, pp. 137–189). Washington, DC: American Psychological Association Press.

Schneider, B. (1987). The people make the place. *Personnel Psychology, 40,* 437–453.

Seibert, S. E., Kraimer, M. L., & Crant, J. M. (2001). What do proactive people do?: A longitudinal model linking proactive personality and career success. *Personnel Psychology, 54,* 845–874.

Settoon, R. P., & Adkins, C. L. (1997). Newcomer socialization: The role of supervisors, coworkers, friends and family members. *Journal of Business and Psychology, 11,* 507–516.

Shepherd, W. (2013). Onboarding at Huntington National Bank [Webcast]. Retrieved April 24, 2013, from *www.conference-board.org/webcasts/ondemand/webcastdetail.cfm?webcastid=2980.*

Sluss, D. M., & Thompson, B. S. (2012). Socializing the newcomer: The mediating role of leader–member exchange. *Organizational Behavior and Human Decision Processes, 119,* 114–125.

Tims, M., Bakker, A. B., & Derks, D. (2012). Development and validation of the job crafting scale. *Journal of Vocational Behavior, 80,* 173–186.

U.S. Bureau of Labor Statistics. (2012). Number of jobs held, labor market activity, and earnings growth among the youngest baby boomers: Results from a longitudinal survey. Retrieved May 29, 2013, from *www.bls.gov/news.release/pdf/nlsoy.pdf?.*

Van Maanen, J., & Schein, E. H. (1979). Toward a theory of organizational socialization. *Research in Organizational Behavior, 1,* 209–264.

Viswesvaran, C., Sanchez, J. I., & Fisher, J. (1999). The role of social support in the process of work stress: A meta-analysis. *Journal of Vocational Behavior, 54,* 314–334.

Walker, H. J., Bauer, T. N., Cole, M. S., Bernerth, J. B., Feild, H. S., & Short, J. C. (2013). Is this how I will be treated?: Reducing uncertainty through recruitment interactions. *Academy of Management Journal, 56*(5), 1325–1347.

Wanberg, C. R. (2012). Facilitating organizational socialization: An introduction. In C. Wanberg (Ed.), *The Oxford handbook of organizational socialization* (pp. 17–21). New York: Oxford University Press.

Wanberg, C. R., & Kammeyer-Mueller, J. D. (2000). Predictors and outcomes of proactivity in the socialization process. *Journal of Applied Psychology, 85,* 373–385.

Wanous, J. (1980). *Organizational entry: Recruitment, selection, and socialization of newcomers.* Reading, MA: Addison-Wesley.

Wesson, M. J., & Gogus, C. I. (2005). Shaking hands with a computer: An examination of two methods of organizational newcomer orientation. *Journal of Applied Psychology, 90,* 1018–1026.

Wrzesniewski, A., & Dutton, J. E. (2001). Crafting a job: Revisioning employees as active crafters of their work. *Academy of Management Review, 26,* 179–201.

Wrzesniewski, A., Dutton, J. E., & Debebe, G. (2003). Interpersonal sensemaking and the meaning of work. *Research in Organizational Behavior, 25,* 93–135.

Wrzesniewski, A., McCauley, C. R., Rozin, P., & Schwartz, B. (1997). Jobs, careers, and callings: People's relations to their work. *Journal of Research in Personality, 31,* 21–33.

Wu, C., & Parker, S. K. (2012). The role of attachment styles in shaping proactive behaviour: An intra-individual analysis. *Journal of Occupational and Organizational Psychology, 85,* 523–530.

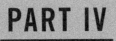

PART IV

BIOLOGICAL ASPECTS
OF SOCIALIZATION

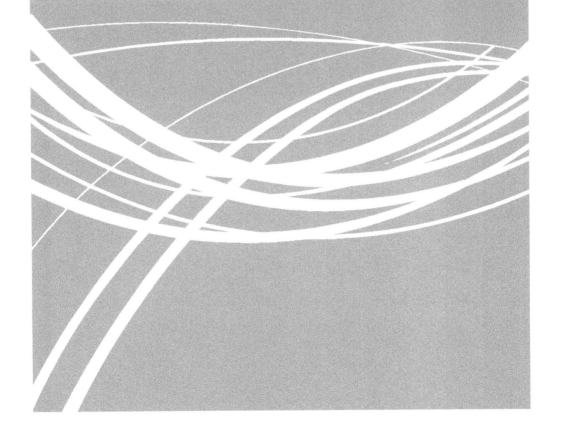

CHAPTER 14

An Evolutionary Approach to Socialization

Daphne Blunt Bugental
Randy Corpuz
David A. Beaulieu

In this chapter, we extend our understanding of socialization by making use of theoretical approaches drawn from evolutionary theory (parental investment theory and life history theory), approaches that have not regularly been integrated with socialization theory. By doing so, we believe that we add breadth to our understanding of the many ways in which parents influence the developing child. As noted by the editors of this volume, socialization is concerned with the various processes by which the young are assisted in becoming effective members of their society. Socialization focuses on parenting tactics and parent–child transactions as the key intermediary process in the child's acquisition of relevant skills and knowledge. Evolutionary psychology emphasizes the role of evolved adaptations that influence parent–child transactions. In doing so, it emphasizes parental allocation of resources and protective efforts that predict the child's subsequent health and resilience. We view the two approaches as complementary in their shared focus on the platforms and pathways that predict the young becoming effective adults within their local environment.

Approaches to Socialization

One of the earliest approaches to socialization was social learning theory (Bandura, 1977). From this perspective, children's behaviors are influenced by their observation of the outcome of the behaviors and interactions of others, and by the vicarious reinforcement patterns that follow from these observations. Later on, social information-processing theory was employed as a framework for socialization. Children acquire cognitive representations (or schemas) of social relationships (Baldwin, 1992), in particular, their relationships with their parents.

As attention increasingly turned to the effects of children on their socializing experiences, increased attention was given to biological influences. This included genetic influences on child temperament, patterns that influenced differences in their receptivity to socialization (Belsky, 2005). Subsequently, attention was given to the hormonal (as well as behavioral) responses of both parents and offspring to each other, for example, hormonal responses of parents prior to and immediately following the birth of an infant (e.g., Fleming, Ruble, Krieger, & Wong, 1997; Storey, Walsh, Quinton, & Wynne-Edwards, 2000) as well as infants' hormonal response to their parents' actions (e.g., Bugental, Schwartz, & Lynch, 2010). Regardless of the theoretical approach taken, concern with the role of parents in their children's development has increasingly taken a transactional approach (Sameroff, 2009). From this perspective, there is a continuing two-way influence between parents and their children.

Evolutionary theory first became relevant to parental influences as a result of *parental investment theory*, which posits the presence of computational mechanisms that include (1) assessment of the available resources that parents may use to enhance the welfare of their young, and (2) the reproductive value of a particular child (e.g., the likelihood that the child will survive to produce healthy progeny) versus the reproductive value of their other (current or future) children. Parental investment theory adds to socialization theory in that parental investment of time and resources in the young includes efforts to promote child health and to influence the probability of growing up to produce healthy progeny.

Life history theory—an approach that has origins in biology, demography, anthropology, and, more recently, within psychology—adds to socialization theory. It posits that the young calibrate their physiological and behavioral development as adaptive responses to features of their environment, including the environment provided by their parents. This theoretical approach has been employed extensively in evolutionary developmental psychology (a field highlighted in a special issue of *Developmental Psychology*, 2012, edited by Ellis & Bjorklund).

Socialization theory has focused on parental efforts to prepare children to manage the tasks of social life. Evolutionary theory focuses on the ways in which parents implicitly prepare their offspring for the kind of environment they are likely to experience at older ages and to respond in ways that optimize reproductive success.

Formulations of Evolutionary Psychology

Before turning to parental investment theory and life history theory as examples of an evolutionary approach to parental influences, it may be useful to consider some of the basic concepts of evolutionary psychology, along with the terminology employed therein.

Proximate versus Ultimate Causation

An important distinction between standard socialization theory and evolutionary approaches to socialization involves the different levels of causal analysis they emphasize. Standard socialization theory focuses primarily on proximate causation (*how* processes operate in socializing transactions to yield offspring who are likely to be socially competent adults). In contrast, evolutionary theory gives greater attention to ultimate causation (*why* particular parenting transactions had an adaptive advantage in our ancestral past, as defined by the number of healthy, surviving progeny they produced).

While ultimate explanations describe the "function" of a given trait (e.g., hunger functions to signal that the body is low on calories), proximate explanations describe the process by which this function is carried out (e.g., brain regions associated with hunger release hormones that communicate and alter other parts of the body to facilitate a search for food). Specific to childrearing, proximate explanations focus on ontogeny. Such explanations focus on the ways in which observed responses can be accounted for by socialization, development, or genetic factors. In contrast, ultimate explanations focus on how observed behavior can be explained by forces operating in our evolutionary past. In utilizing evolutionary explanations, social scientists are concerned with (1) the phylogenetic history of a response pattern (exploring patterns shown both across and within species) and (2) the adaptive advantage of that response pattern within the organism's evolutionary past. The two levels of analysis are complementary, and joint consideration of both explanations affords the possibility of a more complete explanation of human processes (Scott-Phillips, Dickins, & West, 2011).

In addition, any change that appears within one generation will only be passed on to future generations if the carriers of that change mate successfully and have progeny who themselves mate and bear healthy offspring. While most alterations to genes (i.e., mutations) lead to either detrimental or neutral changes in one's phenotype, genes that lead to traits that increase (on average) the probability of survival and reproduction will increase in frequency within the population. In some cases, a change will emerge as an *adaptation*, which is a naturally selected trait that demonstrates better ways of *solving* a problem associated with survival and/or reproduction. When the carriers of an adaptation go on to leave descendants (more successfully, on average and across multiple generations, than others), the adaptation is passed along; thus, we speak of enhanced *reproductive success*. The adaptations that are currently part of our human endowment are the results from generations of natural selection.

Although adaptations must always be understood as applicable to our evolutionary past, evolutionarily minded research remains important because those adaptations continue to strongly influence the cognitions, emotions, and actions of both parents and offspring in the present time. However, under some circumstances, adaptations may no longer provide benefits in contemporary times. As an example, most Western parents discover (to their dismay) that their very young children strongly resist nighttime separation from parents, in particular in a room by themselves. They are in actual fact perfectly safe under these circumstances in present times. However, in our evolutionary past, even brief separations were life threatening by virtue of the constant threat from predators. It was essential that infants and young children vigorously signal their parents in ways that strongly motivated the maintenance of continuous contact. As such, natural selection selected an *evolutionary design* (a term used to describe mechanisms that are effective in solving specific adaptive problems) that ensures a child's safety throughout the night.

Evolutionary Trade-Offs

Adaptations and the implementation of adaptations involve trade-offs (e.g., Dawkins, 1982). In our evolutionary past, individuals, in order to be reproductively successful, would have needed to divide their energy, time, and resources between many competing problems. Although all such efforts served the same basic ultimate function (i.e., survival and reproduction), the immediate function would have varied (e.g., selecting food, avoiding predators). Reproductively successful individuals would have constantly balanced their allocation of time, effort, and resources in solving the competing problems they continuously faced across their life histories. For example, the allocation of exceptionally high effort to self-maintenance and self-protection would have limited the ability to allocate effort to reproductive activity. Likewise, the allocation of high effort in mating activity would have limited the availability of efforts for either self-maintenance or care of the young.

Parental Investment Theory

Next we consider one way in which evolutionary theory adds to socialization theory. In this review, we use the term *parental investment* to refer to the construct first introduced by Trivers (1972, 1974), and more fully developed by Daly and Wilson (1984, 1988). Parental investment theory emerged within an evolutionary framework and is concerned with factors that predict the extent to which parents provide for the well-being of the young, thus increasing their chances of successful survival to reproductive age.

Parental investment processes seen among humans overlap parental care patterns generally observed in mammals as a whole. This includes parents' provision for the basic needs of their young. As the most basic feature, it involves the provision of shelter and sustenance. Beyond this, there are many other ways in which parents may manifest their investment in the young. For example, Keller (2000) proposed that parental investment in infancy might include body contact and carrying, stimulus provision, and face-to-face contact.

Early Formulations

Sex Differences

An initial concern of evolutionary psychologists was the different ways that males and females (in our evolutionary past) would have best served their own reproductive success in their investment decisions (Buss, 1994; Trivers, 1972). They pointed out that there are differential trade-offs for males and females in making investment decisions. In order to reproduce, males are obligated to invest only their sperm and the time needed to engage in copulation, whereas females must invest a very large amount of time and energy (e.g., 9 months of gestation). From an evolutionary perspective, it is not surprising that, in many species, fathers provide less parental care than mothers (e.g., Buss, 1994).

Biological Relatedness

Empirical evidence has shown that parents are more likely to invest in children to whom they are biologically related. In support of this, it has been shown that parents are more likely to abuse their stepchildren than their biological children (e.g., Daly & Wilson, 1984, 1988; Lightcap, Kurland, & Burgess, 1982). This relation between abuse and biological relatedness remains even when one controls for potential confounds such as socioeconomic status (SES), maternal age, and family size (Daly & Wilson, 1988). In addition, parents show lower levels of investment (e.g., amount of financial resources, contact time) in their stepchildren than in their biological children (Anderson, Kaplan, Lam, & Lancaster, 1999; Zwoch, 1999).

Parental efforts to ensure the biological relatedness of the young before investing in parental care are of particular concern for theories of *paternal* investment (Geary, 2000). For women, doubts concerning relatedness of offspring are nonexistent. Males can never be 100% certain that a child is theirs. Indeed, empirical evidence that has emerged indicates that males are more influenced than females by cues of biological relatedness. For instance, men, more than women, are influenced by facial resemblance in their response to infant faces (e.g., feelings of parental care) in a hypothetical child adoption task (Volk & Quinsey, 2002). In another test of the hypothesis, Platek, Burch, Panyavin, Wasserman, and Gallup (2002) asked adults to judge the faces of children for attractiveness, for their adoptive preferences, for the child with whom they would most like to spend time, for the child on whom they would be willing to spend money, and for the child for whom they would least resent paying child support. Judgments (unbeknown to the judges) were based on photographs of children that were either morphed with the judge's own face or with the face of a stranger. Males expressed more willingness to invest in a child whose face had been morphed with their own face. Women were less influenced by facial resemblance. This observed difference between the sexes is an example of a process that is more easily explained by evolutionary theory than by learning theory.

Discriminative Investment in Offspring

Daly and Wilson (1988) extended notions of parental investment by addressing the selective investment patterns shown by parents as a result of (1) the resources available to parents, and (2) the characteristics of the child, for example, cues to the child's health and probable survival. From this standpoint, parental investment is concerned with the amount of time, effort, and resources expended in the care of one child, in comparison with the amount of time, effort, and resources invested in other children (or possible future children), or the individual's own personal interests (a zero-sum conceptualization). This approach to parental investment theory considers parental mechanisms that ultimately facilitate the reproductive success of the sum total of all surviving offspring.

More Recent Formulations

Bugental, Beaulieu, and Corpuz (2011), operationalized parental investment on the basis of differential allocation of resources that included time, attention, emotion, and cognition. Other researchers (e.g., De Baca, Figueredo, & Ellis, 2012; Schlomer, Del Giudice, & Ellis, 2011), using the same evolutionary principles, operationalized parental investment in terms of parental effort, as measured by the Parental Effort Scales, an instrument that has its foundation in life history theory. Although different research groups have measured this construct in different ways, the theoretical origins are the same for all measures, and the findings obtained are similar.

How are parental resources defined? Because the notion of parental investment developed within evolutionary psychology and evolutionary biology, systematic attention was given to variables that influence the extent to which parents invest in the care of the young. As one parameter, interest turned to the differential investment of parents under different circumstances. Parental investment changes as a function of the resources available to provide for the young.

Parental resources take many forms. At the most basic level, they include the ability of parents to provide for the basic needs of their young (e.g., provision of sustenance). In contemporary times, economic resources serve as a basic marker of access to many kinds of resources that are important for the caregiving process. In addition, the availability of supportive others represents an important resource for parents. This may involve an extended network of supportive others who provide assistance at a socioemotional level, as well as at the level of assistance, in direct care of the young. Indeed, it has been suggested that the family itself evolved as a means of facilitating the shared reproductive success of kin (MacDonald, 1988). Resources also come in other forms, for example, parenting skills that can be passed on intergenerationally (Chen & Kaplan, 2001).

Extensive observations have been made of the differential patterns of investment made by parents whose resources differ. For example, parental lack of resources was identified in Belsky's (1993) review of the literature as an important contributor to physical abuse and neglect. It is well known that maltreatment of children is more likely to occur at lower socioeconomic levels (e.g., Gelles, 1992). In addition, parents living in poverty may respond with reduced investment patterns as a function of the high level of instability (i.e., lack of access to stable resources) and powerlessness (i.e., overall inability to acquire resources).

Reproductive Value of the Young

As another area of interest that has received attention in parental investment theory is the characteristics of the young. Across evolutionary history, children have provided early cues to their health, and therefore the likelihood that they would survive to become parents themselves. Reference is made to child "value" in the sense that children vary in the probability that they would have enhanced the reproductive success of their parents in humans' ancestral past. Whereas some children demonstrate cues indicating good health and the higher probability of future reproductive benefits, other children provide cues that they would pose a cost (or relatively small benefit) to parents' reproductive success (e.g., Daly & Wilson, 1984). Thus, from an evolutionary perspective, parents would be expected to show differential investment in children based on early indicators of their potential costs and benefits.

Particular attention has been given to the reduced parental investment that is typically shown for children who manifest some kind of physical or medical anomaly or health problem early in life. In addition, children who show crying anomalies (e.g., anomalous pitch properties) provide cues to their health (Boukydis & Lester, 1998); that is, the quality of crying provides reliable cues to the infant's fitness. Children who have visible (or audible) indications of abnormalities early in life provide cues to high reproductive costs for their parents. Costs may occur at many different levels. That is, the child could be expected to be less likely to survive and, even if he or she did survive, would require greater care than other children (posing a threat to the parents' ability to care for other existing or possible progeny). As summarized by Hagen (1999), even mild birth disorders (e.g., prematurity) in actual fact are predictors of later morbidity and mortality.

Historical accounts provide evidence that infanticide of children with physical abnormalities has been common across the history of Western civilization (Moseley, 1986). Daly and Wilson (1984) gave attention to the kinds of children in today's world that are more likely to be abandoned or killed at birth. They pointed out that children who demonstrate some type of physical abnormality or health problem at birth are at high risk for abandonment or infanticide in many traditional cultures. They also went on to document the prevalence of such outcomes (including infanticide) even in modern countries with strict laws against infanticide and child maltreatment. Furthermore, there is a substantial literature providing evidence of the higher levels of abuse and neglect experienced by children in industrialized countries who manifest medical, learning, or physical disorders (e.g., Bugental, 2003; Sullivan & Knutson, 2000).

An example that captures the nature of parental responses to such children is provided by Weiss (1994, 1998), who compared children given up at birth for adoption based on their potential medical problems. Some of the children had problems with visible components (e.g., spina bifida), whereas others had problems that were just as medically severe but without visible components (e.g., heart problems). Parents were found to base their decisions (keeping the child or relinquishing the child for adoption) on the visibility of the child's disorder rather than its actual severity (which therefore reflected perceptually based cues to risk rather than medically indicated risk). Whereas only 7% of children with medical problems that had no visible components were relinquished for adoption, roughly 67% of children with visible medical conditions were relinquished. Such children were sometimes viewed as "monsters" (Weiss, 1994, p. 476). In addition, they were seen as a source of stigma and shame for the family.

Why should the visibility of a medical condition be so important in such parenting decisions? Parenting decisions evolved to take into consideration offspring cues that would have been reliably associated with reproductive success. However, the evolutionary design for sensitivity to child cues originates in our ancestral past—a time when medical knowledge was unavailable as a basis for predicting a child's later outcomes. From this perspective, visible cues to health are expected to carry more weight than medical predictions.

Finally, the same child may have a different value based on that parent's options. A mother may easily invest in even a very high-risk child if she is unlikely to bear other children (e.g., impending menopause). Supporting this position, older mothers are less likely to neglect, abuse, or kill their infants than younger mothers (Daly & Wilson, 1988; Lee & George, 1999).

Interactive Effects of Parental Resources and Child Value

Relatively recently, attention has turned not only to the independent factors that serve to influence the probability of parental investment in a high-risk (or costly) child but also to the combination of factors that increase the probability of parental investment in such a child (Bugental & Beaulieu, 2003). This represents a "contingent model" of parental investment. When parents have low resources, preferential levels of parental investment are given to high-value offspring. In this case, parents maximize their outcomes by investing in the child most likely to survive. However, among parents with high resources, higher levels of parental investment are given to low-value offspring. In this case, less healthy (low-value) children are provided with the extra investment that is needed for their survival—without any loss to healthy (high value) children, who are also guaranteed sufficient parental resources. The net effect is that all children are more likely to survive.

Evidence for a Contingent Model of Parental Investment from Nonhumans

As an important step in providing evidence for an interactional model, Davis and Todd (1999) conducted a computer simulation study in which they assessed the total size (i.e., weight) of a surviving brood of birds based on the differential feeding strategies shown with high-value (large) versus low-value (small) chicks under different conditions of food accessibility (a key resource). As anticipated, the success of feeding strategies was contingent upon the availability of food. When food was scarce, the best strategy (i.e., the strategy that led to the greatest number of surviving chicks) was to feed the largest chick first. In contrast, the best strategy when food was plentiful was to feed the smallest chick first. Naturalistic observations of the feeding pattern of birds have produced supportive evidence for this interactive pattern (e.g., Gottlander, 1987). These studies with birds, then, indicate that differential investment processes can appear in the absence of the capability for reflective appraisal processes.

Evidence for a Contingent Model of Parental Investment among Humans

What do we know about the interactive influences of offspring value and parental resources amongst humans? Belsky (1993) suggested that when resources are scarce, parents should show preferential investment based on the child's reproductive potential; thus, those children who show lower potential are more likely to be subjected to maltreatment when living in a low-resource environment. Similarly, Mann (1992) suggested that parents lacking resources must be selective in their allocation of scarce resources, and are therefore particularly likely to invest selectively in offspring with high reproductive potential. In support of this, parents in poverty areas are more likely than parents in more affluent areas to withhold nutrients from sickly children (Schepher-Hughes, 1985).

Bugental and colleagues expanded on previous research by systematically testing the interactive effects of parental resources and child value. Their proposed model focused on parental responses to medically at-risk children (e.g., infants born prematurely). Such children provided cues in our evolutionary past to a reduced chance of survival to adulthood, and even in the present time, they are more likely than other children to have later medical problems (e.g., Gross, Spiker, & Haymes, 1997; Picard, Del Dotto, & Breslau, 2000; Schmitz & Reif, 1994). As noted earlier, parents with low resources cannot easily "afford" to invest in high-risk children. On the other hand, parents with high resources can "afford" to invest in a high-risk child without any threat to their ability to provide simultaneous high-quality care to other offspring or potential offspring. For such parents, reproductive success in our evolutionary past might have been highest when they invested disproportionately in a high-risk child.

Beaulieu and Bugental (2008) tested the contingent model by comparing the parental investment patterns of depressed mothers (conceptualized as low in emotional or attention resources) versus nondepressed mothers (conceptualized as higher in emotional or attention resources) with infants born at high or low medical risk. Mothers were shown pictures of items that would be valuable to them (e.g., perfume) and items that would be valuable to the child (e.g., an educational toy). They then were asked to list their top three

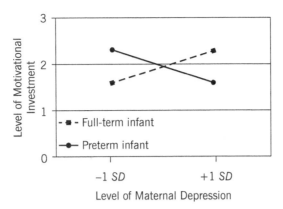

FIGURE 14.1. Parental motivational investment as a function of maternal depression and child risk. Regression lines are plotted for families in which maternal depression was 1 *SD* above and 1 *SD* below the mean. Investment scores reflect the proportion of benefits allocated to child versus self.

preferences for a gift to be received later. The more likely mothers were to pick a gift relevant for a child (as opposed to a gift for herself), the higher the parental investment score. The effects are shown in Figure 14.1. As predicted, depressed mothers provided lower levels of investment with high-risk infants, and high levels of investment were provided by nondepressed mothers with high-risk infants. The reverse effect is shown with low-risk infants.

Experimental Test of Evolutionary Approach to Parental Investment

Intervention programs offer an opportunity for assessing predicted effects when experiences are introduced experimentally. As an example of this, Bugental and her colleagues (2002) conducted a community-based program directed toward reducing child abuse and enhancing child health. Mothers were randomly assigned to a "cognitive reframing" condition or one of two control conditions. In the reframing condition, mothers were assisted in resolving caregiving challenges and finding ways to gain access to needed resources within the community.

Analyses were conducted (Bugental, Beaulieu, & Silbert-Geiger, 2010) to determine the effects of this early intervention on parental investment and child health outcomes. Children's health outcomes were assessed at age 3. Parents in the cognitive reframing condition showed higher levels of investment (amount of time providing care) to their at-risk child than did parents in the comparison conditions. Time spent in care provision mediated this relation among medically high-risk children. In the evolutionary past, elevations in the quality of a given child's health would also have predicted an increased probability that this child survives to reproductive age.

It is important to assess the extent to which parents make investment decisions without their own awareness, which suggests some level of automatic processing. To this end, Corpuz and Bugental (2013) employed an experimental manipulation that primed parents for thoughts of high or low resources, thus allowing a test of shifts in their projected investment patterns. When primed for decreasing financial resources in the general economy, parents subsequently showed preferential investment of time and money in low-risk children. However, when primed for increasing financial resources, parents showed preferential investment in high-risk children.

Summary

We have presented evidence across species and methods suggesting that parental investment in their offspring is best explained by a contingent model that gives joint consideration to resources available to the parent and the reproductive risk level of the young. Although early parental investment research made use of an additive model (parental resources, combined with risk level of the young), more recent findings suggest an interactive model.

Life History Theory:
Biological Sensitivity and Calibration of Children to Their Environment

Life history theory is concerned with the ways that individuals adjust their strategies across the life course so as to be responsive to environmental cues regarding threats versus positive opportunities within the environment. Threats may include high indications of morbidity or mortality within their local environment (e.g., high level of medical problems and high violence). Opportunities may include the accessibility of resources (e.g., social and economic resources).

The theory's influence can be seen across a variety of research fields, such as biology, anthropology, demography, nutrition, medicine, and (most recently) psychology. Life history theory relies on the principles of natural selection and the adaptations that contribute to the reproductive success of any organism, including humans. Environments characterized by threat (harsh and/or unpredictable) and by opportunity (safe and/or predictable) have been present across our ancestral history, and the young respond adaptively to either type of environment. Boyce and Ellis (2005) suggested that the context sensitivity shown by young children evolved as a means of calibrating their developmental trajectories to fit the characteristics of their early environment; that is, their responses serve to optimize their reproductive success. More recently, Del Giudice, Hinnant, Ellis, and El-Sheikh (2012) focused on the adaptive calibration of children's physiological responses to a novel task as a function of their early history of stress in the family.

Slow to Fast Continuum

Strategies are thought to exist along a *slow* to *fast* continuum—terms that indicate the relative tempo of one's development and reproduction (Ellis & Bjorklund, 2012). Slow continuum strategists are characterized by long-term planning, later reproduction, and fewer (but more stable) sexual relationships. When the environment is stable and resources are readily available, and the rates of mortality are low, a slow strategy is most adaptive. Slow continuum strategists have fewer children, which allows for greater and more prolonged investment (e.g., effort and time for socialization) in each child in order to ensure that he or she is well prepared to compete for resources (e.g., high-quality food, jobs, mates). Fast continuum life histories are marked by the opposite pattern. Faced with the risk of dying prior to reproduction, fast continuum strategists are rewarded (in terms of reproductive success) for reproducing early. These individuals, on average, mature faster, reproduce soon after sexual maturation, and seek uncommitted and less stable sexual relationships.

The Central Role of Children's Sensitivity to Early Environment

Early in life, children make use of cues that derive primarily from their experience in families, such as the amount of investment they receive from their parents (ranging from high provisioning by parents to high levels of neglect or harsh discipline). Life history theory supposes that very young children monitor specific environmental inputs—cues that would have allowed a developing child to predict the (social and physical) condition of their adult environment. Any developmental adaptations that allowed children some predictive power over what to expect in their adult environment would be favored by increasing their ability to align their phenotype with the challenges expected to persist in the local ecology.

Children should possess mechanisms that are receptive to a specific set of cues that offers reliable information (based on the underlying, long-standing correlation between an appreciable cue and the state of the environment for which this cue appears more often than not) about the harshness or unpredictability of the environment. For example, harsh parenting occurs in response to harsh environments (Quinlan & Quinlan, 2007). Children can use such parental harshness as a cue that the broader environment is harsh. Subsequently, they calibrate their development to adapt better to this harsh environment.

Cues That Indicate the Level of Environmental Harshness or Unpredictability

Critical differences exist between environments that are harsh and/or uncertain and environments that are relatively stable and safe. Modern indices of where a person's environment fits on this continuum can be summed by one's SES, a proxy for the relative condition of one's local ecology (Belsky, Schlomer, & Ellis, 2012; Simpson, Griskevicius, Kuo, Sung, & Collins, 2012). In low-SES environments, people routinely endure stressors such as multiple job changes, frequent residence changes, variable resource availability, parental stress accompanying the lack of resources, unstable domestic relationships, and increased criminality. These stressors are largely absent or occur with much less frequency in high-SES environments.

The quality of parental investment that children receive is a key mechanism through which they receive information about the levels of stress and support in their broader environment. The informational value of parental investment has been demonstrated across a range of cultures. In a study by Quinlan and Quinlan (2007), low levels of parental investment were correlated with ecological stress (i.e., warfare, famine, pathogens), whereas high levels of parental time, attention, and sensitive care were correlated with more stable environments. Low parental investment or harsh parenting has also been found to be reliably associated with fast continuum life history traits such as early puberty and sexual debut, adolescent pregnancy, and shorter life expectancy (see Ellis, Figueredo, Brumbach, & Schlomer, 2009, for review). Low parental investment (or harsh parenting) signals high levels of morbidity and mortality to offspring and provides a reliable cue for a child to use as the basis for accelerated life history strategies.

Another reliable indicator of an unpredictable environment is the number of parent changes a child endures. Multiple studies have found that a relatively high number of total parental transitions is correlated with an earlier age of sexual debut (among girls) as well as higher rates of premarital sex and pregnancy (e.g., Albrecht & Teachman, 2003; Wu, 1996).

Life history theory has increasingly provided the basis for predicting the processes involved in the child's adaptive calibration of environmental cues that have implications for morbidity/mortality and ease of access to resources. Although these processes may reflect events in the broader environment, they typically follow more directly from events in the family. Parents from low-resource, risky environments are more likely to show responses that predict child aggression (e.g., parental modeling of aggressive behavior, maternal aggressive values; Dodge, Pettit, & Bates, 1994). At the same time, these practices may set children on an "optimal" course for early mating and childbearing. Belsky and Pluess (2012) found that the link between early environmental unpredictability and the number of sexual partners reported later in life was mediated by maternal depressive symptoms (a condition that often results is exceedingly low levels of parental investment) and maternal sensitivity (or the lack thereof). Children raised in unpredictable environments had mothers who were more depressed and provided less sensitive care—both indicators that children can reliably use as cues to the nature of the environment in which they are likely to develop. It is this systematic relation between a set of cues received early in life (e.g., exposure to harsh parenting as a child) and one's physiological and psychological development (e.g., early sexual maturity and decreased levels of investment in one's own children as an adult) that life history theory can help to explain.

A Critical Period for Life History Calibration

Theoretical and empirical work suggests that life history strategies (across species) are most beneficial to an organism the earlier in life that they are calibrated (e.g., Belsky, Steinberg, & Draper, 1991; Simpson & Belsky, 2008). A growing body of research supports the existence of an apparent "critical period" early in a person's life that is used to assay the condition of the environment and use the information gathered at this early stage to adjust one's life history trajectory toward a strategy that aligns well with the anticipated adult environment (e.g., Del Giudice & Belsky, 2011; Ellis et al., 2003; Simpson & Belsky, 2008).

Simpson and colleagues (2012), utilizing data collected from 1,364 mothers and their children, found that the strongest predictor of "fast" life history strategies at age 23 was whether one's childhood environment (between the ages of 0 and 5 years) was unpredictable—determined by the frequency of residential changes, parent employment changes, and parental transitions (i.e., divorce and remarriage). The more unstable the early childhood environment, the higher children's scores on measures of aggression and delinquency, the earlier they reached sexual maturity, and the greater number of total lifetime sexual partners reported—indicating a fast life history trajectory that appears to have been calibrated in response to a very early sampling of the environment. The level of environmental harshness and unpredictability reported between ages 6 and 16, despite moderate correlations with earlier childhood environments, did not predict any of these behaviors associated with a fast life history orientation.

Recent experimental work further supports the idea of a sensitive period for life history calibration that exists early in life. Griskveicius and colleagues (2013) found that how one responds to indicators of current resource scarcity depends critically on childhood SES, *not* current SES. Individuals who grew up in relatively wealthier environments responded to cues of current resource scarcity (news reports on the economy) with less risky and less impulsive decisions on temporal discounting tasks and were also slower to approach temptations (reaching for desirable products). The opposite was true for all three dependent variables in individuals who grew up in poor SES environments. In addition, these researchers found that level of oxidative stress (the imbalance between the adaptive production of oxygen and the damage that may occur in the overproduction of free radicals) serves as a potential biological marker of suboptimal rearing environments; that is, it serves as an indicator of early stress and the diversion of resources away from body maintenance. Oxidative stress has also been found to be related to life history. For example, research participants with high levels of oxidative stress took more risks when confronted with negative information about the economy.

In related research, Griskevicius, Delton, Robertson, and Tybur (2011) found that, in response to a threatening stimuli (a mortality cue), individuals who reported having low SES as children wanted to have their own children sooner, while participants who grew up in high-SES environments elected to delay reproduction when faced with threatening stimuli. Once again, this divergence in life history strategies was *not* related to current SES.

Taken together, this recent (albeit early) work on human life history strategies suggests that a critical period for adaptive calibration of strategies does exist, and it appears to occur fairly early in one's development (early childhood). These results are consistent with other work in the biomedical field that demonstrates adult stress has different effects on one's health as a function of an individual's childhood SES and *not* a function of current SES (e.g., Cohen, Janicki-Deverts, Chen, & Matthews, 2010). Much more work is needed to tease apart the relative influence of early, middle, and late childhood, as well as adolescence, on adult life history strategies. Placing a premium on early specialization does impose costs, however (e.g., increased risk of miscalibration due to less time to "assay" the environment before committing to a trajectory, and the high cost of "shifting" strategies if required). These costs should also be considered in future research that assesses the relative utility of an early sensitive period.

Empirical Support for Life History Predictions

In addition to the empirical findings we discussed earlier, a growing body of work has consistently shown that higher levels of familial and ecological stress early in life predict developmental outcomes such as early sexual maturation, increased promiscuity, early age of first intercourse, greater risk taking, and a generally decreased prosocial orientation (see Belsky et al., 2012, for a detailed review). Evidence for the tenets of life history theory from humans first emerged in empirical work focused on young children's unique sensitivity to their early environment, particularly their home environment. Early work by Belsky and colleagues (1991) provided preliminary evidence that children make use of cues from their environment (without awareness) in ways that influence their later development; that is, children's early life history may be seen as diagnostic with respect to the nature of the world that they may anticipate as adults. If, for example, children are reared without a father, the absence of protection might suggest the possibility that the world is dangerous and poses many hazards. In this case, their reproductive success (in our evolutionary past) would have best been achieved by demonstrating a pattern that is consistent with a faster trajectory—high involvement in early mating activity and early parenting. This life history orientation may serve to promote an individual's early reproductive success while diminishing their proclivity for long-term mating and/or prolonged, high-quality care of their young.

Low SES has been found to predict a wide range of fast life history strategies, such as early sexual debut (Ellis et al., 2003), adolescent pregnancy and childbearing (Miller, Benson, & Galbraith, 2001), high offspring number (Vining, 1986), and low levels of parental investment per child (Belsky et al., 1991). Another piece of evidence for the existence of mechanisms that differentially orient individuals toward reproduction earlier and/or more often comes from Hogan and Kitagawa (1985), who found that the number of children born to married women was 2.9 in high-quality neighborhoods, 3.7 in medium-quality neighborhoods, and 5.9 in low-quality neighborhoods—correlational support that fast life histories are indeed played out in response to modern environments that may be harsh or unpredictable. In another study, the variation in life expectancy at the time of a mother's birth accounted for 74% of the variance in a mother's age at first birth (Low, Hazel, Parker, & Welch, 2008) which corresponds with earlier work that found a similar relationship in mothers in harsh Chicago neighborhoods (Daly & Wilson, 1988). Although correlational studies cannot be interpreted in terms of direction of effects, these findings do indicate that higher mortality rates are associated with faster life history strategies in modern environments. More work using innovative longitudinal and experimental designs is needed.

Research on Nonhumans

Current understanding of the causal relations within these processes has come, in part, from controlled experiments using nonhuman animals. While rats allow researchers to answer many questions using methods that would not be permitted with human subjects, researchers should always heed caution when using a species with a completely different phylogenic history to try to pinpoint the operation of adaptive mechanisms in our own species. Nonetheless, the findings from the work on maternal behavior as it relates to outcomes of rat pups offer some insight into the possible mechanisms that selection can produce.

Meaney and colleagues (e.g., Liu, Diorio, Day, Francis, & Meaney, 2000) found strong support for the idea that rats vary their response to the current environment as a result of cues provided by the level of maternal investment they received as pups. In one study, the researchers exposed a group of female rats to stressors and compared them to a group of females that were not exposed to these stressors. Once these females became mothers, the stressed mothers displayed low levels of licking, grooming, and arched back nursing—investment behaviors that are known to regulate a rat pup's stress response system, brain development, and cognitive performance. The pups of stressed mothers appeared to utilize this lack of parental investment as a critical ecological cue. These pups showed lower levels of glucocorticoid receptor expression, among other physiological indicators of an up-regulated stress response. As a result, their behaviors and development were affected; these pups were more defensive, vigilant, and experienced earlier puberty and increased sexual behavior—all components of a coordinated physiological and psychological life history adjustment.

Importantly, those rats (second generation) raised by stressed mothers showed reduced parental investment in their own pups (third generation)—an apparent cross-generational transmission of the stress response (Francis, Diorio, Liu, & Meaney, 1999). This result could not have been due to any direct genetic effects because the rat pups were cross-fostered and randomly assigned to maternal rearing conditions in the original experiment. In rats, parents communicate environmental conditions to their pups (i.e., stressful environment leads to reduced parental investment). Pups, in turn, respond by adjusting their cognitive and physiological development in an adaptive manner (increased stress response and accelerated pubertal development). When these pups become parents themselves, through diminished parental investment, they continue to guide offspring development toward adaptive strategies best fitted for stressful environments (Cameron et al., 2005). This cross-generational transmission of adaptive responses to stressful environments may be influenced by modification to epigenetic markers (selective activation–deactivation) of regulatory switches that are maintained in subsequent generations.

It has also been found that rats raised by stressed mothers display cognitive impairments under normal, stress-free conditions. These rats are outperformed by rat pups of nonstressed mothers on tasks that demonstrate learning and memory. However, this pattern reverses when the environment is experimentally altered. Those rats raised by stressed mothers outperform the nonstressed group when the cognitive tasks also includes stressors intended to interfere with cognitive performance (see Oitzl, Champagne, van der Veen, & De Kloet, 2010, for a review of this research). In high-stress environments, at least in terms of cognition, these studies point to the benefits of "matching" an individual's phenotype to the anticipated levels of stress in the environment.

The previously discussed cognitive performance results demonstrate that it may be the mismatch itself of a rat's rearing environment to the testing environment that imposes the costs to cognitive performance. That is, it cannot be assumed that pups of stressed mothers were cognitively inferior due to disturbances in development or perturbation in their rearing. These findings also contradict, at least in rats, the idea that nurturing environments are (by default) always able to enrich the cognitive development of dependent offspring. The notion that early stressors better prepare an individual for later environments that contain stress is not unique to life history theory. Garmezy's (1991) stress inoculation model (and supporting evidence) emphasizes the idea that during development, mild stressors may positively influence developmental outcomes, in part because these stressors allow the individual to develop the ability to cope better with stressful situations later in life.

Developmental Mismatch

As mentioned throughout this chapter, one's life history orientation is determined by specific cues present in one's early environment. This design runs the risk of the organism's strategy not being appropriately aligned with the actual condition of the adult environment if, for example, one's early and later environments are vastly different.

When it comes to the rats used in the previously mentioned studies, mothers appear to be adaptively tuned early and remain resistant to any malleability in their environment because such fluctuations would have been rare. This design feature is not pathological in any sense; rather, it is adaptive in the context of natural selection. The environment for which these rat mothers were originally primed is most likely the environment in which they will raise their many offspring. Any changes in environment that will lead to modifications in maternal behavior, and therefore changes in the developmental programming of future generations (outside of the laboratory), will be gradual and necessarily under-whelming because this modification to match "new" environments takes place over mul-tiple generations—a phenomenon known as *phenotypic inertia* (Kuzawa, 2005).

For long-lived species such as humans, however, environments can and do change within a single generation, leading to the increased likelihood of developmental mis-matches. Developmental mismatches can also be expected to be more prevalent in societ-ies that have recently experienced or are currently experiencing a demographic transition. Thus, developmentally plastic mechanisms that rely on cues from the early environment may be costly when the early environment is an unreliable predictor of events at older ages. For example, heightened levels of vigilance and stress reactivity may persist even after children from initially harsh environments are adopted into supportive and resource abundant households (e.g., Gunnar, Morison, Chisholm & Schuder, 2001; Marshall & Kenney, 2009).

Research on general health, immune functioning and nutrition has found similar instances of developmental mismatch. Early environments consisting of stressors that chronically activate a child's stress response system continue to challenge a child's immune system even well after the child has moved to a new, improved environment (Shirtcliff, Coe, & Pollak, 2009). In societies that have experienced a rapid transition toward rela-tively greater environmental safety (e.g., through clean drinking water, increased access to health care, and access to readily available sources of food), researchers have found that the transitions have unintentionally also led to increases in the susceptibility to certain diseases (e.g., cardiovascular), increased risk of obesity and diabetes, allergies, and compromised immune function (Barker, 1994; Kuzawa, 2005) due to the mismatch between what individuals in these societies were prepared for in their environment (food scarcity) and the environment they ended up inhabiting (where food is readily available).

In a world of perfectly accurate information, environmental cues would correlate in lockstep with behavioral strategies that respond to such cues (aggression would *only* appear in environments that were unpredictable or dangerous). Short of this perfectly accurate information, a person must rely on the extent to which a given cue is more likely to appear in one type of environment than in another. The fit between one's life history trajectory (based on early cues) and the adult environment in which these strategies may play out is a matter of probability. When it comes to adaptive calibration, the costlier error is to deviate too far away from the trajectory that would have, on average, been the adaptive path of development during humans' evolutionary history.

Remediation in Current Times

Despite the reproductive advantage of some of children's responses (e.g., aggression) to risky environments, there are personal costs to the children themselves as well as those around them (which is especially true in more modern environments). Thus, intervention efforts may be employed to prevent such outcomes by reducing the sources of stress in children's very early environment. Bugental, Schwartz, and colleagues (2010) provided experimental evidence supporting adaptive calibration theory. That is, preterm infants (who are particularly sensitive to their environment) showed both the best health out-comes (when parents received an intervention that increased their cognitive resources) and the worst health outcomes, if the parents participated in a control condition. Ellis and colleagues (2012) made use of life history theory in designing an intervention for reducing aggression and risk taking in teenagers who live in high risk environments. They argued for and demonstrated the utility of using an intervention that works with, rather than against, teenagers' motivations. Therefore, evolutionary theories can be used to good advantage in designing interventions that help parents and youth to facilitate behavioral outcomes that are consistent with values in Western cultures.

Summary

Life history theory facilitates a paradigm shift in thinking about how environments influence child development. Whereas more traditional approaches view high-risk environments as negatively influencing children's well-being, a life history approach suggests that children's risky behaviors reflect adaptations to risky environments. A child's seemingly maladaptive behavior (by today's standards) should be construed as behavior that is well adapted (in the evolutionary sense) to stressful environmental conditions; that is, a child following a fast life history strategy in a risky environment has a better chance of reproductive success.

Researchers interested in finding better answers to the bases of a child's developmental trajectory may benefit by viewing early environmental influences as important cues that the child uses to calibrate an (evolutionarily) adaptive and coordinated life history strategy. The child, rather than being a passive participant in a given ecology, is an active perceiver of environmental cues. The human child is designed to hone in on and utilize relevant cues to adjust physiological and psychological development along a slow-to-fast life history continuum. Ancestral humans undoubtedly encountered stressful environments, and life history theory supposes that contemporary children, given cues to harsh environments, show behaviors that would have been an adaptive response to this environment in our ancestral past. Thus, there is an important frame shift—where behaviors shown by the young in response to the environment provided by their parents are thought of as adaptive calibration to the world in which they may expect to live.

This area of interest is still in its infancy, and there are many questions still to be answered. For example, although there has been rather consistent evidence that children reared under high-threat conditions do reach sexual maturity at a younger age than children who receive greater protective care, the hormonal route through which this process occurs in unclear. In addition, it has been suggested that there is better evidence for the role of supportive parental care as a predictor of delayed puberty than for the role of a harsh environment as a predictor of early puberty (Ellis, McFadyen-Ketchum, Dodge, Petttit, & Bates, 1999). These theoretical notions need further investigation before these processes can be fully understood.

Conclusions

In this chapter, we have argued that the predictions made by evolutionary theory share considerable ground with socialization theory in terms of goals seen as valuable in a child's early experience. However, we argue that evolutionary theory provides a new model that affords a better accounting of the contingent nature of the relationship between children and parents based on parental access to resources and children's cues to health and likelihood of surviving.

The evolutionary model accounts for similarities observed across cultures and across species. Evolutionary psychology has focused on ultimate causation in terms of adaptations that have evolved to solve recurrent problems within our evolutionary history. As such, it is concerned with the "design" of the experience-expectant brain (as the means by which evolutionary design is implemented). In contrast, standard socialization theory has been concerned with proximate causation across the life course.

Together, parental investment and children's calibration to their environment can be thought of as transactional in nature. That is, parents differentially invest in the young in a way that (in our evolutionary past) would have fostered parents' reproductive success. In conjunction with this, children respond differentially to the environment created by their early history (a process that serves to foster their reproductive success). Observable transactional effects emerge as a function of (1) parent–child engagement in negotiating both shared and conflicting interests, and (2) epigenetics, in which consideration is given to differential gene expression as a result of the response shown by both parents and children to their social and physical environment, as well as the specific environment that children and parents create for each other. From this perspective, children's outcomes as a result of their parenting history should be understood as involving bidirectional relations between biological and experiential factors (e.g., Bjorklund, Yunger, & Pellegrini, 2002).

Evolutionary thought was described as offering a unique advantage by providing a framework for understanding the biological design or blueprints for socialization—both in terms of children's receptivity and the facilitative efforts typically offered by caregivers (or other agents of socialization).

It should be noted that an evolutionary approach is in no way seen as providing a contemporary moral justification for parental responses that, although adaptive in human evolutionary past, impose costs in contemporary society. Thus, traditional socialization theories consider some frequently observed patterns of parenting (e.g., neglect) as pathological, immoral, or illegal, as opposed to optimizing the reproductive success of the parent under certain types of harsh conditions. Resolving the moral dilemma brought about by selective parental investment involves possible resolutions such as the introduction of early interventions. Interventions that foster the resource acquisition ability of parents (even those from a highly disadvantaged background) promote the later outcomes of their children.

Both evolutionary and standard socialization theories have been concerned with the differences that occur in different "domains" or "contexts" (e.g., Bugental, 2000; Grusec & Davidov, Chapter 7, this volume). We have suggested here that evolutionary thought offers the greatest advantage in accounting for the processes that occur within provisioning (i.e., providing for both the physical and health needs of the young). In addition, it informs our understanding of the emotional level of investment made by parents, and the resultant effects on children's early stress levels and later cognitive abilities (Bugental et al., 2011).

We have suggested here that parents' selective investment influences the life outcomes of their children in ways that are dependent on their local environment. Up to this point, parental investment theory has been more concerned with the reasons for and effects of parental failure to invest in their children. We hope to have shown that it also represents a new way of thinking about the ways parents act to enhance the life outcomes of their children. Consistent with life history theory, evolutionary theory also accounts for the adaptive calibration of children in ways that ultimately optimize their reproductive success.

The integration of different fields (evolutionary psychology, standard socialization theory, developmental neuroscience, and epigenetics) is increasingly understood as providing the most complete picture of the developing child (Boyce & Ellis, 2005; Burgess & Drais, 1999). As has been argued in the past, we believe that it is time to bring evolutionary thought into the mainstream of socialization theory.

REFERENCES

Albrecht, C., & Teachman, J. D. (2003). Childhood living arrangements and the risk of premarital intercourse. *Journal of Family Issues, 24,* 867–894.

Anderson, K. G., Kaplan, H., Lam, D., & Lancaster, J. (1999). Paternal care by genetic fathers and stepfathers II: Reports by Xhosa high school students. *Evolution and Human Behavior, 20,* 433–451.

Baldwin, M. W. (1992). Relational schemas and the processing of social information. *Psychological Bulletin, 112,* 461–484.

Bandura, A. (1977). *Social learning theory.* Englewood Cliffs, NJ: Prentice-Hall.

Barker, D. J. P. (1994). *Mothers, babies, and disease in later life.* London: BMJ Publishing Group.

Beaulieu, D. A., & Bugental, D. B. (2008). Contingent parental investment: An evolutionary framework for understanding early interaction between mothers and children. *Evolution and Human Behavior, 29,* 249–255.

Belsky, J. (1993). Etiology of child maltreatment: A developmental–ecological analysis. *Psychological Bulletin, 114,* 413–434.

Belsky, J. (2005). Differential susceptibility to rearing influences: An evolutionary hypothesis and some evidence. In B. J. Ellis & D. F. Bjorklund (Eds.), *Origins of the social mind: Evolutionary psychology and child development* (pp. 139–163). New York: Guilford Press.

Belsky, J., & Pluess, M. (2012). Differential susceptibility to long-term effects of quality of child care on externalizing behavior in adolescence. *International Journal of Behavioral Development, 36*(1), 2–10.

Belsky, J., Schlomer, G. L., & Ellis, B. J. (2012). Beyond cumulative risk: Distinguishing harshness and unpredictability as determinants of parenting and early life history strategy. *Developmental Psychology, 48*(3), 662–673.

Belsky, J., Steinberg, L., & Draper, P. (1991). Childhood experience, interpersonal development, and reproductive strategy: An evolutionary theory of socialization. *Child Development, 62,* 647–670.

Bjorklund, D. R., Yunger, J. L., & Pellegrini, A. D. (2002). The evolution of parenting and evolutionary approaches to childrearing. In M. H. Bornstein (Ed.), *Handbook of parenting: Vol. 2. Biology and ecology of parenting* (pp. 3–30). Mahwah, NJ: Erlbaum.

Boukydis, C. F. Z., & Lester, B. M. (1998). Infant crying, risk status and social support in families of preterm and term infants. *Early Development and Parenting, 7,* 31–40.

Boyce, W. T., & Ellis, B. J. (2005). Biological sensitivity to context: I. An evolutionary-developmental theory of the origins and functions of stress reactivity. *Development and Psychopathology, 17*(2), 271–301.

Bugental, D. B. (2000). Acquisition of the algorithms of social life: A domain-based approach. *Psychological Bulletin, 126*(2), 187.

Bugental, D. B. (2003). *Thriving in the face of childhood adversity.* New York: Psychology Press.

Bugental, D. B., & Beaulieu, D. A. (2003). A bio-social-cognitive approach to understanding and promoting the outcomes of children with medical and physical disorders. In R. Kail (Ed.), *Advances in child development and behavior* (Vol. 31, pp. 329–361). New York: Academic Press.

Bugental, D. B., Beaulieu, D. A., & Corpuz, R. (2011). Parental investment in caregiving. In S. L. Brown, R. M. Brown, & L. S. Penner (Eds.), *Moving beyond self-interest* (pp. 153–165). New York: Oxford University Press.

Bugental, D. B., Beaulieu, D. A., & Silbert-Geiger, A. A. (2010). Increases in parental investment and child health as a result of an early intervention. *Journal of Experimental Child Psychology, 106,* 30–40.

Bugental, D. B., Ellerson, P. C., Lin, E. K., Rainey, B., Kokotovic, A., & O'Hara, N. (2002). A cognitive approach to child abuse prevention. *Journal of Family Psychology, 16,* 243–258.

Bugental, D. B., Schwartz, A., & Lynch, C. (2010). Effects of an early family intervention on children's memory: The mediating effects of cortisol levels. *Mind, Brain, and Education, 4,* 159–170.

Burgess, R. L., & Drais, A. A. (1999). Beyond the "Cinderella effect": Life history theory and child maltreatment. *Human Nature, 10,* 373–398

Buss, D. M. (1994). *The evolution of desire.* New York: Basic Books.

Cameron, N. M., Champagne, F. A., Parent, C., Fish, E. W., Ozaki-Kuroda, K., & Meaney, M. J. (2005). The programming of individual differences in defensive responses and reproductive strategies in the rat through variations in maternal care. *Neuroscience and Biobehavioral Reviews, 29,* 843–865.

Chen, Z., & Kaplan, H. H. (2001). Intergenerational transmission of constructive parenting. *Journal of Marriage and the Family, 63,* 17–31.

Cohen, S., Janicki-Deverts, D., Chen, E., & Matthews, K. A. (2010). Childhood socioeconomic status and adult health. *Annals of the New York Academy of Sciences, 1186*(1), 37–55.

Corpuz, R., & Bugental, D. B. (2013). *Parental investment in child welfare within a shifting economy.* Manuscript submitted for publication.

Daly, M., & Wilson, M. (1984). A sociobiological analysis of human infanticide. In G. Hausfater & S. B. Hrdy (Eds.), *Infanticide: Comparative and evolutionary perspectives* (pp. 4887–5020). New York: de Gruyter.

Daly, M., & Wilson, M. (1988). *Homicide.* New York: de Gruyter.

Davis, J. N., & Todd, P. M. (1999). Parental investment by simple decision rules. In G. Gigerenzer & P. M. Todd (Eds.), *Simple heuristics that make us smart* (pp. 309–326). New York: Oxford University Press.

Dawkins, R. (1982). *The extended phenotype.* San Francisco: Freeman.

De Baca, T. T., Figueredo, A. J., & Ellis, B. J. (2012). An evolutionary analysis of variation in parental effort: Determinants and assessment. *Parenting: Science and Practice, 12,* 94–104.

Del Giudice, M., & Belsky, J. (2011). The development of life history strategies: Toward a multistage theory. *Development, 2*(1), 154–176.

Del Giudice, M., Hinnant, J. B., Ellis, B. J., & El-Sheikh, M. (2012). Adaptive patterns of stress responsivity: A preliminary investigation. *Developmental Psychology, 48*(3), 775.

Dodge, K. A., Pettit, G. S., & Bates, J. E. (1994). Socialization mediators of the relation between socioeconomic status and child conduct problems. *Child Development, 65,* 649–665.

Ellis, B. J., Bates, J. D., Dodge, K. A., Fergusson, D. M., Horwood, L. J., Pettit, G. S., et al. (2003). Does father absence place daughters at special risk for early sexual activity and teenage pregnancy? *Child Development, 74,* 801–821.

Ellis, B. J., & Bjorklund, D. F. (2012). Beyond mental health: An evolutionary analysis of development under risky and supportive environmental conditions: An introduction to the special section. *Developmental Psychology, 48,* 591–597.

Ellis, B. J., Del Giudice, M., Dishion, T. J., Figueredo, A. J., Gray, P., Griskevicius, V., et al. (2012). The evolutionary basis of risky adolescent behavior: Implications for science, policy, and practice. *Developmental Psychology, 48,* 598–623.

Ellis, B. J., Figueredo, A. J., Brumbach, B. H., & Schlomer, G. L. (2009). Fundamental dimensions of environmental risk. *Human Nature, 20*(2), 204–268.

Ellis, B. J., McFadyen-Ketchum, S., Dodge, K. A., Pettit, G. S., & Bates, J. E. (1999). Quality of early family relationships and individual differences in the timing of pubertal maturation in girls: A longitudinal test of an evolutionary model. *Journal of Personality and Social Psychology, 77,* 387–401.

Fleming, A. S., Ruble, D., Krieger, H., & Wong, P. Y. (1997). Hormonal and experiential correlates of maternal responsiveness during pregnancy and the puerperium in human mothers. *Hormones and Behavior, 31,* 134–158.

Francis, D., Diorio, J., Liu, D., & Meaney, M. J. (1999). Nongenomic transmission across generations of maternal behavior and stress responses in the rat. *Science, 286*(5442), 1155–1158.

Garmezy, N. (1991). Resilience in children's adaptation to negative life events and stressed environments. *Pediatric Annals, 20*(9), 459–460, 463–466.

Geary, D. C. (2000). Evolution and proximate expression of human parental investment. *Psychological Bulletin, 126,* 55–77.

Gelles, R. J. (1992). Poverty and violence toward children. *American Behavioral Scientist, 35,* 258–274.

Gottlander, K. (1987). Parental feeding behavior and sibling competition in the pied flycatcher Ficedula hypoleuca. *Ornis Scandanavica, 18,* 269–276.

Griskevicius, V., Ackerman, J. M., Cantú, S. M., Delton, A. W., Robertson, T. E., Simpson, J. A., et al. (2013). When the economy falters, do people spend or save?: Responses to resource scarcity depend on childhood environments. *Psychological Science, 24*(2), 197–205.

Griskevicius, V., Delton, A. W., Robertson, T. E., & Tybur, J. M. (2011). Environmental contingency in life history strategies: The influence of mortality and socioeconomic status on reproductive timing. *Journal of Personality and Social Psychology, 100*(2), 241–254.

Gross, R. T., Spiker, D., & Haymes, C. W. (1997). *Helping low birth weight, premature babies: The Infant Health and Development Program.* Palo Alto, CA: Stanford University Press.

Gunnar, M. R., Morison, S. J., Chisholm, K. I. M., & Schuder, M. (2001). Salivary cortisol levels in children adopted from Romanian orphanages. *Development and Psychopathology, 13*(3), 611–628.

Hagen, E. H. (1999). The functions of postpartum depression. *Evolution and Human Behavior, 20*(5), 325–359.

Hogan, D. P., & Kitagawa, E. M. (1985). The impact of social status, family structure, and neighborhood on the fertility of black adolescents. *American Journal of Sociology, 90,* 825–855.

Keller, H. (2000). Human parent–child relationships from an evolutionary standpoint. *American Behavioral Scientist, 43,* 957–969.

Kuzawa, C. W. (2005). Fetal origins of developmental plasticity: Are fetal cues reliable predictors of future nutritional environments? *American Journal of Human Biology, 17*(1), 5–21.

Lee, B. J., & George, R. M. (1999). Poverty, early childbearing and child maltreatment: A multinomial study. *Child and Youth Services Review, 21,* 755–780.

Lightcap, J. L., Kurland, J. A., & Burgess, R. L. (1982). Child abuse: A test of some predictions from evolutionary theory. *Ethology and Sociobiology, 3,* 61–67.

Liu, D., Diorio, J., Day, J. C., Francis, D. D., & Meaney, M. J. (2000). Maternal care, hippocampal neurogenesis, and cognitive development in rats. *Nature Neuroscience, 3,* 799–806.

Low, B. S., Hazel, A., Parker, N., & Welch, K. B. (2008). Influences on reproductive lives. Unexpected ecological underpinnings. *Cross-Cultural Research, 42,* 201–219.

MacDonald, K. B. (1988). *Social and personality development: An evolutionary synthesis.* New York: Plenum Press.

Mann, J. (1992). Nurturance or negligence: Maternal psychology and behavioral preference among preterm twins. In J. H. Barkow, L. Cosmides, & J. Tooby (Eds.), *The adapted mind: Evolutionary psychology and the generation of culture* (pp. 367–390). Oxford, UK: Oxford University Press.

Marshall, P. J., & Kenney, J. W. (2009). Biological perspectives on the effects of early psychosocial experience. *Developmental Review, 29*(2), 96–119.

Miller, B. C., Benson, B., & Galbraith, K. A. (2001). Family relationships and adolescent pregnancy risk: A research synthesis. *Developmental Review, 21,* 1–38.

Moseley, K. L. (1986). The history of infanticide in Western society. *Issues in Law and Medicine, 1,* 345–361.

Oitzl, M. S., Champagne, D. L., van der Veen, R., & De Kloet, E. R. (2010). Brain development under stress: Hypotheses of glucocorticoid actions revisited. *Neuroscience and Biobehavioral Reviews, 34*(6), 853–866.

Picard, K. M., Del Dotto, J. E., & Breslau, N. (2000). Prematurity and low birthweight. In K.

O. Yestes & M. D. Ris (Eds.), *Pediatric neuropsychology: Research, theory, and practice* (pp. 237–251). New York: Guilford Press.

Platek, S. M., Burch, R. L., Panyavin, I. B., Wasserman, B. H., & Gallup, G. G., Jr. (2002). Reactions to children's faces: Resemblance affects males more than females. *Evolution and Human Behavior, 23,* 159–166.

Quinlan, R. J., & Quinlan, M. B. (2007). Evolutionary ecology of human pair-bonds. *Cross-Cultural Research, 41,* 149–169.

Sameroff, A. (2009) *Transactional processes in development.* Washington, DC: American Psychological Association.

Schepher-Hughes, N. (1985). Culture, scarcity, and maternal thinking: Maternal detachment and infant survival in a Brazilian shantytown. *Ethos, 13,* 291–317.

Schlomer, G. L., Del Giudice, M., & Ellis, B. J. (2011). Parent–offspring conflict theory: An evolutionary framework for understanding conflict within human families. *Psychological Review, 118,* 496–521.

Schmitz, K., & Reif, L. (1994). Reducing prenatal risk and improving birth outcomes: The public health nursing role. *Public Health Nursing, 11,* 174–180.

Scott-Phillips, T. C., Dickins, T. E., & West, S. A. (2011). Evolutionary theory and the ultimate-proximate distinction in the human behavioral sciences. *Perspectives on Psychological Science, 6*(1), 38–47.

Shirtcliff, E. A., Coe, C. L., & Pollak, S. D. (2009). Early childhood stress is associated with elevated antibody levels to herpes simplex virus type 1. *Proceedings of the National Academy of Sciences, 106*(8), 2963–2967.

Simpson, J. A., & Belsky, J. (2008). Attachment theory within a modern evolutionary framework. In P. R. Shaver & J. Cassidy (Ed.), *Handbook of attachment: Theory, research, and clinical applications* (2nd ed., pp. 131–157). New York: Guilford Press.

Simpson, J. A., Griskevicius, V., Kuo, S. I., Sung, S., & Collins, W. A. (2012). Evolution, stress, and sensitive periods: The influence of unpredictability in early versus late childhood on sex and risky behavior. *Developmental Psychology, 48*(3), 674–686.

Storey, A. E., Walsh, C. J., Quinton, R. L., & Wynne-Edwards, K. E. (2000). Hormonal correlates of paternal responsiveness in new and expectant fathers. *Evolution and Hunan Behavior, 21,* 79–95.

Sullivan, P. M., & Knutson, J. F. (2000). Maltreatment and disabilities: A population-based epidemiological study. *Child Abuse and Neglect, 24,* 1257–1273.

Trivers, R. (1972). Parental investment and sexual selection. In B. Campbell (Ed.), *Sexual selection and the descent of man, 1871–1971* (pp. 136–179). Chicago: Aldine.

Trivers, R. L. (1974). Parent–offspring conflict. *Integrative and Comparative Biology, 14,* 249–264.

Vining, D. R., Jr. (1986). Social versus reproductive success: The central problem of human sociobiology. *Behavior and Brain Science, 9,* 167–216.

Volk, A., & Quinsey, V. L. (2002). The influence of infant facial cues on adoption preferences. *Nature, 13,* 437–455.

Weiss, M. (1994). Nonperson and nonhome: Territorial seclusion of appearance-impaired children. *Journal of Contemporary Ethnography, 22,* 463–487.

Weiss, M. (1998). Parents' rejection of their appearance-impaired newborns: Some critical observations regarding the social myth of bonding. *Marriage and Family Review, 27,* 191–209.

Wu, L. L. (1996). Effects of family instability, income, and income instability on the risk of a premarital birth. *American Sociological Review, 61,* 386–406.

Zwoch, K. (1999). Family type and investment in education: A comparison of genetic and stepparent families. *Evolution and Human Behavior, 20,* 453–464.

CHAPTER 15

Socialization, Genetics, and Their Interplay in Development

Reut Avinun
Ariel Knafo-Noam

The study of socialization substantially contributes to identification of the underpinnings of personality and psychopathology, and to the promotion of children's healthy development and well-being. However, the lion's share of psychological research to date has investigated the environment as the force shaping development, and has therefore focused on the "nurture" while neglecting the "nature" part of the equation. Indeed, even though the age-old debate of nature versus nurture has turned into the realization that nature and nurture contribute to development synergistically (Plomin & Asbury, 2005), the integration of knowledge from quantitative genetic and, later, molecular studies into psychological research is only beginning to happen in a new wave of studies. In this chapter we review some of these studies and attempt to provide a glimpse of the intricate web of influences that mold child development.

Throughout their development, children are exposed to many socialization agents, including siblings, peers, school, and the media. However, children's first caregiving figures are usually the parents, who are considered to have long-standing effects on child development (Belsky & de Haan, 2011). Most of psychology's grand theories allocated an important role to parents in children's personality and psychopathology development (for historical reviews, see Grusec & Kuczynski, 1997; Maccoby, 1992). Therefore, many researchers have chosen to study the influence of parental behavior on child outcomes. As a consequence, most of the research reviewed in this chapter concerns parents.

We start by discussing parenting, and the meaning of parenting effects on children's development in light of gene–environment correlations (rGE; when the environment to which the individual is exposed is associated with his or her genotype through passive, evocative, or active processes) and gene–environment interactions (G × E; when an outcome is affected by the nonadditive contributions of the developing person's genetics and his or her environment). We present research from both quantitative genetic and molecular research designs. Quantitative genetic designs rely on genetic similarities between family members in order to estimate genetic and environmental effects on a variable (e.g., temperament). Molecular genetic designs look for associations between a variable of interest (e.g., parenting) and DNA variation across individuals (work reviewed in this chapter typically deals with genes that relate to the modulation of brain processes that involve the activity of dopamine, serotonin, oxytocin, and vasopressin, which have all been associated with social behavior in different species). We then describe epigenetic and other processes in which environmental effects can leave their mark on the developing person through their effect on biological factors. Finally, we discuss both G × E and rGE with regard to socialization processes outside the home, most notably school and peers. Table 15.1 provides a description of key genetic concepts relevant to socialization.

Parenting

As noted, much of the research on socialization has focused on parents, and different parenting styles have been associated with different child outcomes (Baumrind, 1971). However, because children and their parents share 50% of their genetic material, determining the direction of effects between parenting styles and child outcomes is challenging. In brief, the mere sharing of genes between biological parents and their children can lead to associations between parental behavior and child behavior (Knafo & Jaffee, 2013). Furthermore, as in other relationships, the parent–child relationship is bidirectional. Therefore, genetically influenced characteristics of children can affect and shape the parental behavior they experience. These phenomena have been termed rGE and are described in further detail below.

Gene–Environment Correlations

In order to partition the variance of individual differences in a certain trait to environmental and genetic effects, many behavioral genetic studies take advantage of the genetic difference between monozygotic (MZ) twins, who share 100% of their genes, and dizygotic (DZ) twins, who share on average 50% of their genetic material. The twin design assumes that if MZ twins are more similar than DZ twins, then the individual differences in the characteristic examined are influenced by heritability (Table 15.1). Similarity beyond this genetic effect is attributed to the environment the twins share (shared or common environment effect), and any differences between the twins are ascribed to nonshared environment, which also includes measurement error (Plomin, DeFries, McClearn, & McGuffin, 2008).

However, environmental and genetic effects are usually intertwined to such an extent that it is quite difficult to disentangle them. This is portrayed in findings that indicate measures of the environment can be affected by genetic influences (Kendler & Baker, 2007). This notion may seem paradoxical when first encountered because environmental and genetic influences are usually presented as independent from one another

TABLE 15.1. Definitions of Main Terms and Means of Testing

Term	Definition	Possible means of testing
Heritability	The proportion of phenotypic variance in a certain population and context that can be attributed to genetic differences within the population.	Designs including relatives relying on group differences in degree of communality in genetic or environmental factors. The most common is the classic twin design, comparing monozygotic and dizygotic twins to partition the variance of a phenotype into genetic effects, shared environmental effects, and nonshared environmental effects (which also include measurement error).
Gene–environment correlation (rGE)	The case of an association between an individual's genotype and an environment.	
Passive rGE	Occurs when there is a sporadic association between an environment and an individual's genotype that is due to a shared genotype between the individual (e.g., child) and the person providing the environment (e.g., parent).	Compare associations between an environmental variable (e.g., parenting) and a behavioral phenotype (e.g., externalizing) in genetically related and unrelated dyads of parents and children.
Evocative rGE	Refers to responses that are evoked from the environment by genetically influenced characteristics.	1. A twin design estimating genetic effects on an environmental variable (e.g., parenting). 2. Test for an association between an individual's candidate gene and an environmental variable, while controlling for the same gene in the person that provides the environment (i.e., eliminate passive rGE).
Active rGE	Refers to instances in which individuals select their environment (e.g., friends, university) based on their genetic tendencies.	1. A twin design estimating genetic effects on an environmental variable that is chosen by the individual. 2. Test for an association between an individual's candidate gene and an environment that is chosen by them, while controlling for the same gene in the person that provides the environment (i.e., eliminate passive rGE).
Gene–environment interaction ($G \times E$)	Refers to instances in which the influence of genetics changes according to the environment (or vice versa).	1. If the heritability estimate in a quantitative genetic design changes depending on environmental conditions. 2. The presence of a statistical interaction between a measured environment (e.g., risk exposure) and a genotype (e.g., presence of a certain allele) in predicting an outcome.
Diathesis stress	The notion that some individuals are more vulnerable to adverse environments than others, due to an endogenous "risk" characteristic. If the risk factor is genetic, constitutes a case of $G \times E$.	If the effect of a certain allele on an outcome changes for the worse when it is combined with the negative end of an environmental spectrum, and does not change for the better when it is combined with the positive end. Noncarriers of the allele show weaker or no association between the environmental variable and the outcome.

(continued)

TABLE 15.1. *(continued)*

Term	Definition	Possible means of testing
Vantage sensitivity	The notion that some individuals are more sensitive than others to beneficial environments. If the sensitivity factor is genetic, constitutes a case of G × E.	If the effect of a certain allele on an outcome changes for the better when it is combined with the positive end of an environmental spectrum, and does not change for the worse when it is combined with the negative end. Noncarriers of the allele show weaker or no association between the environmental variable and the outcome.
Differential susceptibility	The notion that some individuals are more sensitive than others to the effects of both adverse and beneficial environments. The presence of putative "plasticity alleles" indicates G × E.	If the effect of a certain allele on an outcome changes for the worse when it is combined with the negative end of an environmental spectrum, and changes for the better when it is combined with the positive end, while noncarriers of the allele show weaker or no association between the environmental variable and the outcome.
Epigenetics	Biological changes that can affect gene expression without changes to the DNA sequence.	Test whether DNA methylation at a certain site changes the expression of a gene and whether it is associated with behavior or with an environmental variable.
Telomere research	Telomeres are the repetitive DNA sequences at each end of the chromosomes that protect against genomic instability. They shorten in somatic tissues with each cell division and are considered to be the molecular clock of the life span of cells, since the cell cycle halts once they become senescent.	Test whether there is an association between telomere length and life events.

(Saudino, 1997), but consider the following examples. Even experiences that seem most random, such as getting struck by lightning or breaking a wrist, may be influenced by risk taking and impulsive behaviors that have genetic origins (Bezdjian, Baker, & Tuvblad, 2011).

As mentioned, genetic associations with the environment have been titled gene–environment correlations (rGE). The idea that genes and the environment are interrelated was first discussed decades ago (Plomin, DeFries, & Loehlin, 1977; Scarr & McCartney, 1983). Although increasing numbers of studies have utilized sequential analyses or longitudinal designs to make inferences about the directions of associations between measures taken from parents and children, it is still uncommon for researchers to recognize that the shared genes of parents and children might contribute to the development of correspondence of their behaviors or other characteristics over time. Thus, evidence for rGE may affect our interpretation of previous research that supported unidirectional parent → child conclusions. Three types of rGE have been proposed (Plomin et al., 1977; Scarr & McCartney, 1983): passive, evocative, and active.

Passive rGE

Passive rGE is the phenomenon in which an association between an environment and an individual is at least partly explained by a shared genotype between the individual (e.g., a child) and the person providing the environment (e.g., a socialization agent). For example, both children's prosocial behavior (Knafo, Israel, & Ebstein, 2011) and parents' warmth (Neiderhiser et al., 2004) have been shown to be heritable. If the genes responsible for prosocial behavior and personal warmth overlap, then a positive correlation between parents' warmth and children's prosocial behavior may be partly explained in terms of their genetic relatedness (Knafo & Jaffee, 2013). This type of rGE is called *passive* because no direct influence of parents and children on each other is required to create a correlation between the environment (e.g., parenting) and the child's behavior. Passive rGE is relevant to any socialization agent who shares a genotype with the target individual (e.g., biological siblings, grandparents).

Findings concerning passive rGE may have important implications for psychological research because they sometimes provide an alternative explanation for correlation between parenting or the home environment and child behavior, an explanation that relies on shared genetics instead of causality. The home environment is affected by the parents' characteristics, which, like parenting, are influenced by the parents' genetic makeup. When the same genetic makeup is inherited by the children and affects their behavior, it may lead to spurious correlations between parenting/home environment and child behavior (Price & Jaffee, 2008).

QUANTITATIVE FINDINGS THAT SUPPORT PASSIVE rGE

One approach to the investigation of passive rGE is to compare associations between dyads of parents and children who are either genetically related or unrelated. If an association is seen only in the related dyads, this suggests that shared genetic factors account for the association. When both genetic and environmental factors contribute, the association is present in both dyads but will be greater in the genetically related parent–child dyads. This approach was employed in a reexamination of the relatively established link between smoking during pregnancy and children's attention-deficit/hyperactivity disorder (ADHD) (Thapar et al., 2009). The researchers found that the association between smoking during pregnancy and children's ADHD is only significant in related mother–child dyads, which supports passive rGE, and implies that the tendency to smoke is genetically related to ADHD symptomatology. Although the sample of smoking mothers used in Thapar and colleagues' (2009) study was small, the findings are in line with research on siblings discordant for maternal smoking during pregnancy, which demonstrates that both siblings are at risk for ADHD (D'Onofrio et al., 2008).

Another study, employing similar methodology, focused on the link between parent and offspring depressive symptoms in early to middle childhood (Rice, Lewis, Harold, & Thapar, 2013). The findings supported a passive rGE, so that reduced parental positivity partially mediated the parent–child continuity in depression, but only in genetically related parent–child pairs. Thus, the association between child depressive symptoms and reduced parental positivity is partly due to shared genotype with the parent (Rice et al., 2013).

It is also possible to examine passive rGE in a children-of-twins (CoT) design, which takes advantage of the fact that the child of an MZ twin shares 50% of his or her DNA with both the parent and the parent's cotwin but is provided a direct rearing environment only by the biological parents. The situation for DZ twins is similar, although in this case the child shares 25% of his or her DNA with the parent's cotwin. The comparison of MZ child–aunt/uncle and DZ child–aunt/uncle correlations in the phenotypes of choice (e.g., parental and child depression) estimates the genetic and environmental components of intergenerational transmission. A higher MZ avuncular correlation compared with the DZ avuncular correlation suggests the importance of genetic factors, and equal correlations suggest that environmental factors are responsible for the intergenerational association. For example, by applying the CoT design, Silberg, Maes, and Eaves (2010) demonstrated that the association between parental depression and children's conduct disorder is partly accounted for by passive rGE.

MOLECULAR GENETIC FINDINGS SUPPORTING PASSIVE rGE

As mentioned earlier, passive rGE research is very limited, and we are not aware of molecular genetic studies that have investigated it. Nonetheless, studies that examine the genetic underpinnings of parental behavior are suggestive because they target genes that have been associated with various social behaviors, some of them in children, and therefore open the door to the possibility of rGE. For example, variation in the oxytocin receptor (*OXTR*) gene has been associated with maternal sensitivity (Bakermans-Kranenburg & van IJzendoorn, 2008; Feldman et al., 2012) and with attachment in infants (Chen, Barth, Johnson, Gotlib, & Johnson, 2011); variation in the vasopressin receptor 1A (*AVPR1A*) has been associated with maternal focused support (Avinun, Ebstein, & Knafo, 2012) and with preschoolers' altruistic behavior (Avinun et al., 2011); and variation in the serotonin transporter gene has been associated with maternal sensitivity (Bakermans-Kranenburg & van IJzendoorn, 2008) and with depression in children (Nobile et al., 2004).

The few studies of passive rGE that have been carried out demonstrate the importance of this line of research by providing part of the explanation for known environment–child–outcome associations. Research on other forms of rGE (nonpassive) is also in its infancy but can likewise shed important light on developmental and socialization processes.

Evocative rGE

Evocative rGE refers to instances in which an individual's genetically influenced behavior affects the environment. For example, a child characterized by high levels of antisocial behavior, a trait showing substantial heritability, may elicit more harsh discipline from parents than a child who is low in antisocial behavior. Evocative rGE can also be tackled with both twin and molecular genetic studies.

QUANTITATIVE FINDINGS SUPPORTING EVOCATIVE rGE

A children-as-twins design can be used to assess the similarity in socialization (e.g., parenting) received by MZ and DZ twins. The heritability estimate obtained for the studied socialization variable in this method reflects nonpassive (i.e., active and evocative) rGE effects (Neiderhiser et al., 2004). This estimate, which is based on differences between MZ and DZ twins, cannot reflect passive rGE because passive rGE does not lead to differences between children's socialization experiences. Genetic effects on parenting can be demonstrated by a higher correlation of the parenting received by MZ compared with DZ twins.

Various children-as-twins studies have investigated the portion of variance in parental behavior that is explained by the child's genotype. Findings show that evocative rGE can account for up to 60% of the variance in parental behavior (Mackinnon, Henderson, & Andrews, 1991). The proportion of variance explained varies greatly from study to study, depending, for example, on children's ages and the assessment method used. As children grow older, it appears that their evocative effect on parents grows stronger (Elkins, McGue, & Iacono, 1997). This increase might be expected given that children gain independence and freedom as they grow up, which most likely corresponds with being more influential in the familial environment. The effect of assessment method was demonstrated in one study that used both parental self-reports and observations (Deater-Deckard, 2000). Heritability estimates were 55% for individual differences in negative affect, as measured by self-reports, and 6% for the same parental behavior when evaluated by observations, a pattern that has also been found in other studies (reviewed in Avinun & Knafo, 2014; Kendler & Baker, 2007). A possible explanation for this pattern is that extreme behaviors that are rated in questionnaires affect parenting more substantially than the relatively limited set of behaviors that can be detected during observations of parent–child interactions.

Since the heritability estimate in the twin design is based on the difference between MZ and DZ twins' covariances, it may be inflated if parents base their ratings on the perception of their twins' zygosity, and not on true zygosity. That is, parents may be influenced by thinking that their twins are MZ or DZ, and not by actual genetic similarities or differences. However, research shows that MZ and DZ twins' correlations that are based on the reports of parents who are misinformed regarding their children's zygosity do not significantly differ from correlations that are based on reports of correctly informed parents (Cohen, Dibble, & Grawe, 1977; Lytton, 1980; Scarr, 1968). Hence, a greater similarity in the treatment of MZ twins is most likely the result of their identical genetics that evokes similar responses from the environment.

Studies have also examined specific child behaviors that may affect parenting, by employing the children-as-twins design and introducing a child behavior into the model that possibly mediates the evocative effect (i.e., heritability). For instance, among 5-month-old infant twins, maternal hostile–reactive behaviors were moderately accounted for by genetic factors in the infant, an association mediated by infant difficult behavior (Boivin et al., 2005). Another study focused on mother-reported corporal punishment and maltreatment in 5-year-old twins living in England and Wales (Jaffee et al., 2004). Results showed that children's experience of corporal punishment was mediated by the same genetic factors that predisposed them to antisocial behavior. Thus, aggressive and oppositional behavior of children evoked more frequent physical punishment.

Another way to examine evocative rGE is to study adoptive families. Adoptions enable researchers to differentiate between heritable (biological parents) and environmental (adoptive parents) effects on the adoptee's behavior. For example, Ge and colleagues (1996) demonstrated that parental behavior of adoptive parents was associated with the psychiatric status of the adoptee's biological parents, and that this association was mediated by the adoptee's behavior. More specifically, adoptees born to parents with psychopathologies were more hostile and antisocial, and their adoptive parents used more harsh discipline and were less nurturing and involved (also see O'Connor, Deater-Deckard, Fulker, Rutter, & Plomin, 1998). The interpretation of these findings is that having genes of parents with psychopathologies affects adoptees' behavior, and therefore the parental behavior of adoptive parents as well.

Longitudinal cross-lagged studies (i.e., studies that measure and assess the relation between two phenotypes in at least two time points) have also been conducted in an attempt to understand causality in the bidirectional parent–child relationship. This approach allows researchers to predict a child variable based on parenting, while controlling for prior levels of the child variable, and vice versa. Yet it is crucial to keep in mind that time precedence is not necessarily indicative of causality (Reiss, 1995). Not all genetic tendencies manifest at birth (e.g., Knafo & Plomin, 2006), and it is also possible for children to be involved in relationships with peers that lead to an increase in their innate tendencies and therefore to an increase in parents' responses to them.

There are also cross-lagged studies that incorporate behavioral genetic methods and are therefore more suited to the determination of causality. For instance, in an innovative biometric cross-lagged design, Burt, McGue, Krueger, and Iacono (2005) examined the links between externalizing behavior and parent–child conflict as assessed by twins and their parents at ages 11 and 14 years. The design enabled the investigation of the genetic and environmental contributions to both phenotypes at both ages, and also the genetic and environmental contributions to their continuity and change, and to their cross-lagged bidirectional effects (by treating them as phenotypes). The results revealed three primary findings. First, the stability of conflict and externalizing behavior over time is largely a result of child genetic factors. Second, there appears to be a bidirectional relation between conflict and externalizing behavior over time, such that both conflict and child externalizing behavior at age 11 independently predict the other 3 years later. Finally, the results are consistent with the notion that parent–child conflict partially results from parents' responses to their child's heritable externalizing behavior, while simultaneously contributing to child externalizing behavior via environmental mechanisms.

One caveat regarding this study is that conflict, which was assessed by items such as "My parent often irritates me" and "I treat others with more respect than I treat my parent," is not a measurement of parenting per se. Since it involves characteristics of the child, it is difficult to determine whether the influences found for externalizing behavior on conflict indeed represent an influence of the child on the parent. Notably, however, another study, which implemented the same biometrical cross-lagged design but examined the relation between child antisocial behavior at ages 4 and 7 years and parental negativity, also found evidence of bidirectional effects (Larsson, Viding, Rijsdijk, & Plomin, 2008).

MOLECULAR GENETIC FINDINGS SUPPORTING EVOCATIVE rGE

To our knowledge, only two molecular genetic studies have examined the link between children's genotype and the parenting they experience, while also taking into account the parents' genotype in order to rule out passive rGE (Mills-Koonce et al., 2007; Pener-Tessler et al., 2013). Mills-Koonce and colleagues (2007) demonstrated that children who were carriers of A1 allele of the *Taq1A* polymorphism of the dopamine receptor D2 (*DRD2*), which has been associated with decreased reward sensitivity and addiction (Munafò, Clark, Johnstone, Murphy, & Walton, 2004; Munafò, Matheson, & Flint, 2007), exhibited greater negative mood during parent–child interactions and had mothers who were less sensitive. Importantly, the authors also demonstrated that the mothers' *DRD2* genotype was not associated with maternal sensitivity or with the child's mood, thus ruling out the possibility of passive rGE that is based on mothers and children sharing their *DRD2* genotype.

Pener-Tessler and colleagues (2013) demonstrated that the association between boys' serotonin transporter gene polymorphism (*5-HTTLPR*) genotype and maternal positivity was mediated by the child's self-control: Boys who carried the short allele of *5-HTTLPR* exhibited higher levels of self-control and received higher levels of positive parenting. Although mothers' genotype did affect their behavior toward boys, the finding of an evocative rGE remained significant after including the mothers' genotype in the model.

Evocative rGE stresses the role children play in the family environment (and other environments). It shows that children's genetically based characteristics influence their surrounding environments, a phenomenon that should always be considered in interventions aimed at improving child outcomes. Furthermore, similar to passive rGE, acknowledging evocative rGE helps to further the understanding of cause and effect in the parent–child relationship, and sheds new light on previous psychological theories to the extent that it demonstrates the importance of recognizing the interplay between environment and genes.

Active rGE

Active rGE refers to instances where individuals choose their environment (e.g., friends, hobbies) based on their genetic tendencies. Because active rGE is less relevant to parent–child relationships, we elaborate on this issue in a later section that is devoted to other socialization agents.

Gene–Environment Interactions

Various Approaches to G × E and Supporting Molecular Genetic Studies

Developmental theorists have proposed the idea of goodness of fit, in which the environment (e.g., parenting) should be matched with the characteristics of the developing child in order to obtain optimal development (Chess & Thomas, 1999). Recently, much research effort has been devoted to children's genotype as one variable that can affect the outcome of environmental influences. Additionally, new theories that have emerged postulate that some individuals may be more affected by the environment than others.

The process termed G × E refers to instances in which the environment influences the outcome of genetics (and vice versa). The presence of G × E may provide answers to questions such as why does parental abuse have a substantial negative effect on some children but not others? Why do interventions work better for some individuals? And why does psychological therapy help certain patients more? Three compatible approaches exist for conceptualizing the nature of the genetic susceptibility to the environment (somewhat resembling earlier approaches such as *organismic specificity*, which stresses the

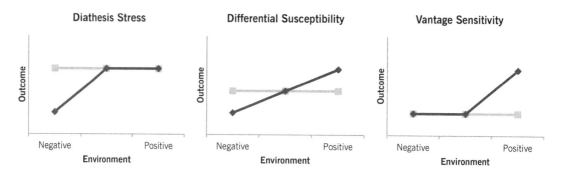

FIGURE 15.1. A schematic illustration of three different forms of gene–environment interactions. In each of these, the moderation can reflect a genetic or a nongenetic variable, such as a temperament dimension.

importance of individual differences in predicting the effect of an environmental stimulus; Wachs & Gandour, 1983): diathesis stress, differential susceptibility, and vantage sensitivity (Figure 15.1).

DIATHESIS STRESS

The *diathesis stress* approach (also referred to as *dual risk*) postulates that there are risk factors, and in the context of G × E "risk alleles," that render individuals carrying them more vulnerable to the environment (i.e., more sensitive to adversities and therefore more likely to develop psychopathologies and/or physical problems). The focus of this approach on risk stems from the fact that, historically, most researchers have been interested in the prevention of disorders and diseases. For example, in an influential study, Caspi and colleagues (2003) tried to provide an answer to one of the most interesting questions in mental health—why stressful experiences lead to depression in some but not all people. Since depression is one of the leading causes of disability, finding its underlying causes has the potential to improve the lives of many individuals. Their results indicated that a combination of carrying the short *5-HTTLPR* allele and experiencing stressful events in adulthood (e.g., employment, financial, health, and relationship problems) or childhood maltreatment increases the risk of depression. The finding has been supported by a recent meta-analysis (Karg, Burmeister, Shedden, & Sen, 2011; but see Risch et al., 2009).

DIFFERENTIAL SUSCEPTIBILITY

The *differential susceptibility* theory states that positive and nurturing environments are also likely to affect genetic outcomes, and that it is probable that some individuals are just more sensitive to environmental influences in a "for better and for worse" manner (Belsky, Bakermans-Kranenburg, & van IJzendoorn, 2007). The rationale behind this theory from an evolutionary stand point is that since the future cannot be predicted, the best way to maximize fitness is by producing two types of children, so-called *orchids* and *dandelions* (Ellis, Boyce, Belsky, Bakermans-Kranenburg, & van IJzendoorn, 2011). The orchid metaphor refers to highly reactive individuals who tend to change according to the environment, while the dandelion metaphor refers to resilient individuals who are less susceptible to environmental influences and can function similarly under various conditions. Orchids decline/wither under unfavorable conditions and thrive/flourish under favorable conditions, whereas dandelions are resilient and less affected by their environment. Notably, because multiple genes are involved in susceptibility, and because individuals are exposed to diverse environmental factors, the same individual may be both resilient and susceptible depending on genotype and context.

For instance, Luijk and colleagues (2011) examined the link between the mineralocorticoid receptor (MR; associated with the stress response), maternal sensitivity, and secure attachment in infants. The findings revealed that infants carrying the minor *MR* allele (G) were more securely attached if their mothers showed more sensitive responsiveness and less securely attached if their mothers showed extremely insensitive behaviors. These associations were not significant for carriers of the AA genotype of *MR* (dandelions).

In another study, Hankin and colleagues (2011) examined whether an interaction between the *5-HTTLPR* polymorphism and positive parenting can predict positive affect. Their results indicated that youth who carried two copies of the short *5-HTTLPR* allele exhibited significantly lower levels of positive affect when they experienced unsupportive parenting, and significantly higher levels of positive affect when they experienced supportive parenting. In contrast, youth carrying the long *5-HTTLPR* allele showed relatively consistent levels of positive affect across both the supportive and unsupportive parenting environments.

VANTAGE SENSITIVITY

A more recent approach to G × E is the *vantage sensitivity* theory (Pluess & Belsky, 2013), which postulates that there are instances in which certain alleles may only be affected by positive environments (making it a complementary approach to diathesis stress and the concept of "risk alleles"). As mentioned in the article that introduced the theory (Pluess & Belsky, 2013), there have been no studies yet that tested it directly and examined reactions of individuals carrying certain alleles to both positive and negative environmental influences. Nonetheless, if the lack of a positive environment can be considered as negative (as in some diathesis stress studies in which the lack of a negative environment was considered to be positive), then there are studies of interventions that can provide examples of vantage sensitivity. For example, Bakermans-Kranenburg, van IJzendoorn, Pijlman, Mesman, and Juffer (2008) investigated whether a variation in the third exon of the dopamine receptor D4 (*DRD4*) gene interacts with a video-feedback parenting intervention to reduce externalizing behavior in a sample of 1- to 3-year-old children randomly assigned to treatment condition. Providing support for vantage sensitivity, the intervention proved effective in decreasing externalizing behavior, but only for children carrying the 7-repeat allele of the *DRD4* gene. Children without the 7-repeat allele did not benefit from the intervention. Thus, it is possible that some children are more susceptible to environmental interventions aimed at improving social functioning.

G × E Supported by Quantitative Genetic Designs

G × E can also be detected in quantitative genetic studies. The environment can reduce the heritability estimate found in twin studies by preventing the realization of one's genetic potential. For instance, in a study of genetic and environmental influences on verbal IQ, it has been shown that the educational level of parents moderates the heritability estimate of verbal IQ (Rowe, Jacobson, & Van den Oord, 1999). The heritability of verbal IQ was much higher in high-education households (i.e., the average educational level attained by both residential parents exceeded high school) than in low-education households (.74 and .26, respectively). This finding demonstrates how the environment can constrain one's genetic potential by not providing the appropriate context for development.

Another example comes from a study of the effects of perceived relationship with parents on the heritability of positive and negative emotionality (Krueger, South, Johnson, & Iacono, 2008). The results indicated that perceived parental regard significantly affected the heritability estimate. Specifically, the heritability of positive emotionality increased with higher levels of perceived parental regard. Similarly, the heritability of negative emotionality increased with higher levels of perceived parental regard, and decreased with higher levels of perceived parental conflict. These findings demonstrate the important influence of the environment in moderating genetic tendencies, and how, when it comes to complex traits, genetic influence does not equal determinism. Thus, parents may help their children by providing a nurturing environment that can moderate genetic tendencies.

$G \times E$ further entangle the links between genes and environment to the point that they may reduce the accuracy of quantitative genetic models' estimations of genetic and environmental influences. Twin study estimates of environmental and genetic effects may include a $G \times E$ component. Particularly, interaction between genes and the shared-environment leads to an increased heritability estimate, and interaction between genes and the nonshared environment lead to an increased nonshared environment estimate (Purcell, 2002). Thus, $G \times E$ may, in part, account for the low estimations of the shared environment component found in most quantitative genetic studies.

Furthermore, $G \times E$ may also explain the mystery of the *missing heritability* (Zuk, Hechter, Sunyaev, & Lander, 2012), which refers to the heritability of common traits and diseases that remains unexplained despite the efforts made by genomewide association studies (GWAS). At the moment GWAS have only managed to explain a small proportion of heritability in different traits and disorders. It has been suggested that $G \times E$ may lead to inflated heritability estimates (Zuk et al., 2012), leading researchers to invest their time in wild goose chases. For example, if MZ twins evoke more similar responses from their environment than DZ twins, as was shown in evocative rGE studies, then it is possible that they will only become more similar as they grow older because the interaction between their identical genes and similar environments will yield a stronger similarity between them with time. On the other hand, DZ twins will become less similar due to their different genes and differentiating environments (again, the product of both rGE and $G \times E$). The difference between the MZ and DZ twins' correlations, which in fact is attributable to both genes and environment, will lead to inflated heritability estimates. Indeed, this fits perfectly with the increase in heritability with age, which is consistently shown in studies of human traits (Elkins et al., 1997; Knafo & Plomin, 2006; Knafo, Zahn-Waxler, Van Hulle, Robinson, & Rhee, 2008). Consequently, one should consider all heritability estimates to include, in addition to genetic effects, the contributions of the environment's interplay with genetics.

Another important contribution is that $G \times E$ theories may provide part of the explanation for the difficulty in replicating findings that show main effects of genes.

Considering the complexity of human behavior, it is most likely that many genes affect any given behavior interdependently, and that their influence is dependent on environmental conditions. Therefore, findings of main effects may be the result of a certain alignment of genes and circumstances, and only represent the involvement of any particular gene in an intricate web of influence.

Biological Embedding of the Environment

Epigenetics

Epigenetic (*epi* translates to "above" in Greek) modifications constitute an additional regulatory layer on top of the DNA sequence. The DNA is organized into units referred to as *nucleosomes*, each of which contains about 150 base pairs wrapped around a core region of histone proteins. This restrictive configuration is maintained, in part, by electrostatic bonds between the positively charged histones and the negatively charged DNA. Modifications of these bonds through mechanisms such as DNA methylation modulate gene transcription and expression. DNA methylation in mammals involves the addition of a methyl group to a cytosine in a relatively stable chemical bond that leads to the silencing of gene transcription (Meaney, 2010). Thus, the epigenome plays an important part in the modulation of gene expression. There is still considerable debate around how many of these changes are heritable across generations of organisms (Grossniklaus, Kelly, Ferguson-Smith, Pembrey, & Lindquist, 2013). In any case, epigenetic changes may be one way in which the environment leaves its mark on an organism. Recent studies indeed show that experiences, including those relevant to socialization, such as parental behavior, can lead to epigenetic changes in mature cells. We provide some examples below.

Studies in rats have indicated that variation in maternal care during the first postnatal week affects the development of cognitive, behavioral, and endocrine responses of offspring (Fish et al., 2006). The individual differences in dams' maternal care are mainly shown in licking and grooming (LG) of pups and arched-back nursing (ABN; a particular form of nursing behavior). Compared to pups of low LG-ABN dams, pups of high LG-ABN dams show a decreased stress response, enhanced spatial memory, increased glucocorticoid receptor expression in the hippocampus (leading to an increased regulation of the stress response), and increased synaptogenesis in the hippocampus (Fish et al., 2006). These effects are also evident when pups are cross-fostered (Weaver et al., 2004), thus demonstrating that they are not due to genetic inheritance. In pups of low LG-ABN dams, methylation levels are higher in the promoter region of the glucocorticoid receptor (Weaver et al., 2004), which is consistent with the lower glucocorticoid receptor expression level and heightened stress response that characterize them. Importantly, these behavioral and endocrine effects are still present in adulthood.

It has been suggested that epigenetic mechanisms can provide the basis for parental effects that increase the chances of offspring survival (Meaney, 2010). It is possible that parental signals program offspring by leading to certain epigenetic modifications. These modifications in turn increase fitness by making offspring better fit their current and future surrounding environment. In order for parental programming to be adaptive, there should be a high degree of fidelity between the quality of the environment and parental care; otherwise, there will be a mismatch between the individual's attributes and environmental conditions. This is in line with research showing, for example, that parental behavior tends to be negative under adverse conditions. Under conditions of poverty, what is considered as neglectful and negative parenting (Evans, 2004) may prepare the offspring for adverse surroundings by causing elevated levels of glucocorticoids, fearfulness, and vigilance. These responses promote detection of potential threat and avoidance learning, which are potentially helpful in an environment where one has to struggle for survival. Moreover, energy reserves are mobilized in a way that is better suited to cope with nutrient deprivation, and glucocorticoid levels provide protection against septic shock, which is a threat in impoverished environments that may be associated with multiple sources of infection (Meaney, 2010).

Meaney (2010, p. 67) suggests that "there is no single form of ideal parenting"; rather, there are various "ideals" that depend on environmental conditions. In evolutionary terms, the ultimate measure of success for any phenotypic trait is the degree to which it enhances the probability for reproductive success. Indeed, phenotypic variation is crucial for enhancing fitness within the diversity of species-typical environments encountered, and a behavior that is nonadaptive under a certain environmental condition may be adaptive under another (Boyce, Sokolowski, & Robinson, 2012; Bugental, Corpuz, & Beaulieu, Chapter 14, this volume).

Evidence in humans for epigenetic variation that correlates with environmental differences (unlike, e.g., variation that is responsible for cell differentiation or X chromosome inactivation) is beginning to surface. McGowan and colleagues (2009) compared three groups of males: victims of suicide who had a history of childhood abuse, victims of suicide who had no such history, and individuals who died suddenly of other causes. In all cases, there was no medical or paramedical intervention that could have altered methylation levels. McGowan and colleagues found higher methylation levels in the promoter region of the glucocorticoid receptor in hippocampal samples from the suicide victims compared with controls, but only if suicide was accompanied by a developmental history of child maltreatment. The higher methylation levels were associated with lower levels of glucocorticoid receptor messenger ribonucleic acid (mRNA). Lower glucocorticoid receptor expression corresponds with a decreased modulation of the stress response. Thus, these findings, albeit not causal, indicate a link between extremely harsh parental behavior and alterations in the offspring's stress response caused by epigenetic processes.

The association between a history of abuse and the stress response was further examined in a study that focused on childhood trauma and its interaction with the FK506 binding protein 5 (FKBP5) gene in predicting posttraumatic stress disorder (PTSD; Klengel et al., 2012). FKBP5 is associated with glucocorticoid receptor activity. The results of the study demonstrated that carriers of a certain variant of an FKBP5 polymorphism were more likely to have lower methylation levels at a different FKBP5 site if they had a history of childhood abuse. Lower methylation levels at this site lead to higher FKBP5 expression levels, which may lead to a dysregulated stress response that puts individuals at risk for developing conditions such as PTSD. Interestingly, this was not shown for exposure to adult trauma, which suggests an early critical period for the described epigenetic effects.

Epigenetic patterns may provide one explanation for the relatively low replicability rate in molecular genetic studies. A study of adults who were adopted in the first few months after birth examined the combined effect of *5-HTTLPR* allelic variation and levels of methylation of the 5-HTT promoter on levels of unresolved loss or trauma (van IJzendoorn, Caspers, Bakermans-Kranenburg, Beach, & Philibert, 2010). Results indicated that methylation levels moderated the influence of the *5-HTTLPR* genotype.

As mentioned, another important aspect of epigenetic changes is that they may be heritable. Reprogramming of the epigenome occurs in each generation, so that epigenetic marks (e.g., methylation) are cleared in order to enable the fertilized egg to develop into any type of cell (epigenetic modifications are involved in cellular differentiation; unlike the genome, they differ between tissues and make the creation of numerous cellular identities, e.g., liver cells and heart cells, possible). However, it is possible that this clearance is not always complete, and that, in some cases, transgenerational epigenetic inheritance occurs. In other words, the DNA can be inherited with a few marks left by the environment. There is evidence for this process from other mammals and flies (Daxinger & Whitelaw, 2012), and the evolutionary explanation behind it may be that it prepares the next generation for its future environment, thus providing a mechanism for a rapid form of adaptive evolution (Chong & Whitelaw, 2004). There is suggestive evidence for the inheritance of environmentally induced epigenetic changes in humans. For example, research on the Dutch famine of 1944–1945 revealed an increase in neonatal adiposity and poorer health in the grandchildren of women who were pregnant during the famine (Painter et al., 2008). Nonetheless, further research is needed to understand the underlying causes of these phenomena, especially in humans.

In summary, epigenetics is one more important contributor to the molding of social behavior. Epigenetic processes further the understanding of variation in genetic influences, since they function as an extra layer of gene expression modulation. Interestingly, it appears that some genetic variants are more susceptible to epigenetic changes than others (Klengel et al., 2012), which means that they may also be more susceptible to the environment and therefore possibly provide a part of the explanation for the mechanism behind G × E (van IJzendoorn, Bakermans-Kranenburg, & Ebstein, 2011). Finally, although epigenetic research on the effects of human parenting is still in its infancy, the implications of this research are far-reaching. Epigenetic modifications may be one way through which environmental forces, such as socialization, leave their mark on the DNA. Through the changes in genetic expression, brain activity changes and subsequently affects psychopathology and personality. Although epigenetic research does have its challenges (e.g., because epigenetic modifications differ between cell types, measuring them in one type of cells does not necessarily indicate their magnitude or position in another), it appears to hold promise for the understanding of how the environment can modify our genetic programming.

Telomere Research

Telomere science is an emerging field that can shed further light on the developmental influences of parental behavior. *Telomeres* are the repetitive DNA sequences at each end of the chromosomes that protect against genomic instability. They shorten in somatic tissues with each cell division and are considered to be the molecular clock of the life span of cells because the cell cycle halts once they become senescent (a form of cellular aging; Bekaert, 2005; Harley, Futcher, & Greider, 1990). Shortened telomeres have been linked to several age-related diseases and early mortality (Shalev, Entringer, et al., 2013). Recently, research on erosion of telomeres has opened a new pathway to understanding how life events, including negative or stressful socialization experiences, affect development biologically. For example, Shalev, Moffitt, and colleagues (2013) examined the effect of domestic violence, frequent bullying victimization, and physical maltreatment, as reported by mothers, on the erosion rate of telomere length in children aged 5–10 years. Results demonstrated a cumulative effect of violence exposure, so that children who experienced higher levels of violence showed accelerated telomere length erosion. Furthermore, some research suggests that telomeres may be susceptible to maternal stress during pregnancy. Entringer and colleagues (2011) published the first human study of the association between maternal exposure to severe psychosocial stress during pregnancy and offspring telomere length in young adulthood. The effect equated approximately to an additional 3.5 years of cellular aging in prenatally stressed offspring. In a second, smaller prospective study, Entringer and colleagues (2013) found that maternal pregnancy-specific stress (worries about the health of the unborn child) assessed in early pregnancy significantly predicted newborn leukocyte telomere length. Such findings of biological embedding of early social adversity will become increasingly important and sophisticated in the next few years (Boyce et al., 2012).

Beyond Parents:
The Interplay of Genetic Influences with Other Socialization Agents

Up to this point, we have mostly reviewed research on rGE, G × E, and epigenetics that involves parental behavior. However, other socialization agents, such as siblings, teachers, and peers, should be considered as well. The environment outside the home can constitute a major part of the individual's life from an early stage in development given that the child's life includes day care, school, and afterschool activities. The behavior of the individual is shaped not only by social interactions with parents but also social interactions with peers. Genetic research on interactions with peers is relatively scarce, since researchers tend to put more emphasis on the role of parents in child development. Nonetheless, we provide a few examples that demonstrate how the interplay of children's genetics and the peer environment can affect the course of development as well.

rGE Beyond Parents

Peers differ from parents as socializing agents in many respects. One important aspect is highly relevant to rGE: To some extent, peers are chosen by the individual. Twin research on children's social problems suggests that the way children are treated by their peers is in part evoked by their own genetically influenced behavior. For example, in a children-as-twins design, Benish-Weisman, Steinberg, and Knafo (2010) found that at the age of 3, variation in children's mother-reported peer problems was substantially influenced by heritability (44%), which suggests that genetically influenced child behaviors evoke negative reactions from peers. Benish-Weisman and colleagues further found that these genetic influences on peer problems were partly the same as those influencing negative emotionality (in boys only), and low sociability and activity. Similarly, children's disruptive behavior has been shown to evoke negative peer relations, in an evocative rGE process (Boivin et al., 2013). Together, these studies show how genetically influenced behaviors affect peer relationships. (Notably, some of these evocative influences may also represent active influences, i.e., may be related to the selection of peers by the individual.)

Another twin study examined possible evocative influences on teachers (Houts, Caspi, Pianta, Arseneault, & Moffitt, 2010). It was shown that individual differences in teachers' ratings of the amount of effort each 12-year-old child required (i.e., the frequency with which they needed to intervene with the child in the classroom) were substantially influenced by the child's genetics (56%). Furthermore, by using mother, teacher, and observer reports, it was demonstrated that children who were rated as more inattentive and hyperactive at age 5 required more teacher effort at age 12, and that these behaviors partly mediated the genetic effect of the child on the teacher's behavior, providing yet another example of how our genetically influenced behaviors affect the way our environment treats us.

An innovative molecular genetic rGE study (Burt, 2009) investigated whether likability is associated with a variation in the $5\text{-}HT_{2A}$ serotonin receptor gene, and whether this association is mediated by rule-breaking behavior. The sample comprised male college students, placed into groups of five and asked collectively to plan two parties and complete a brief series of brain teasers (anagrams, puzzles, etc.). After the group interaction, participants were asked to rate how much they liked each of the other participants. Furthermore, observer reports, based on the group interaction, and self-reports were used to determine the level of rule-breaking behavior. Results showed that the polymorphism in the $5\text{-}HT_{2A}$ serotonin receptor gene significantly affected likability, and that part of this association was mediated through rule-breaking behavior, so that increased levels of rule breaking corresponded with higher levels of likability. Thus, as may be expected, genetically affected behavior of individuals affects how much others in their environment will like them.

As mentioned earlier, active rGE is more relevant to interactions with nonkin because it involves the active selection of one's environment. Various studies have shown that people tend to surround themselves with others who resemble them, in other words, that "birds of a feather flock together" (McPherson, Smith-Lovin, & Cook, 2001). This phenomenon, termed *homophily*, refers to the principle that contact between similar people occurs at a higher rate than contact among dissimilar people. Homophily and the gain in independence as people grow older provide part of the explanation for the increase in heritability of temperament and cognitive abilities that is seen with age. In other words, if individuals select their environment based on their genetically influenced characteristics, then these choices (e.g., selecting similar friends or deciding to surround oneself with books and devote a lot of time to reading) are likely to make these characteristics more salient.

Recently, Fowler, Settle, and Christakis (2011) investigated the effects of measured genes on homophily and heterophily ("opposites attract") among friends. While controlling for sex, age and race, the *DRD2 Taq1A* polymorphism, which has been associated with reward sensitivity and addiction (Munafò et al., 2004, 2007), was found to be associated with homophily. In addition, a variation in the *CYP2A6* (cytochrome P450 2A6) gene, which was associated with openness (Waga & Iwahashi, 2007), was found to be associated with heterophily. These findings suggest that whereas there are certain genotypes that increase our tendency to seek individuals who resemble us, there are also genotypes that increase our tendency to seek the company of our opposites. Such genetically influenced relationships may later modulate individuals' heritable characteristics and either enhance or reduce them.

Results of genetically informative designs have indicated that affiliation with delinquent peers is genetically influenced (Cleveland, Wiebe, & Rowe, 2005; Neiderhiser, Marceau, & Reiss, 2013). In an attempt to identify one of the specific genes responsible for the tendency to associate with delinquent peers, Beaver, Wright, and DeLisi (2008) focused on variation in the dopamine transporter gene (*DAT1*). Peer delinquency was assessed by relying on three questionnaire items that pertain to peers' smoking and alcohol use. In addition, familial risk was assessed according to adolescents' reports of their mothers' involvement, attachment (both reverse coded), and disengagement. Results indicated that male adolescents with high familial risk who were carriers of a certain *DAT1* variant were more likely to associate with delinquent peers. Thus, there is some preliminary evidence for active rGE, but further research is needed in order to distinguish between active and evocative rGE, and to uncover the specific genes involved in these processes.

G × E Beyond Parents

G × E is not restricted to interactions between children's genotypes and parental behavior. Other environments are also important contributors to the molding of behavior.

G × E in Molecular Genetic Studies

Several studies have shown how the influence of peer relationships can interact with the influence of certain alleles and direct the course of development toward one path instead of another (Brendgen, 2012). For instance, Lee (2011) found that affiliation with deviant peers was more strongly associated with overt antisocial behavior for boys who were carriers of the high-activity allele of the monoamine oxidase A (*MAOA*) gene, than for boys who were carriers of the low-activity allele. Importantly, *MAOA* was not associated with deviant peer affiliation, suggesting absence of rGE with respect to this particular gene. Thus, results indicated that carriers of the high-activity allele who had deviant friends were more likely to show overt antisocial behavior. Similar results were shown with the *BDNF* gene, such that carriers of a certain genotype who affiliated with aggressive peers in childhood showed increased risk for being aggressive in adolescence (Kretschmer, Vitaro, & Barker, 2014). Therefore, at least in some cases, the susceptibility of the individual to peer influences depends on the genotype.

G × E in Quantitative Genetic Studies

There is also evidence for G × E from quantitative genetic studies that examined environments other than parents. For example, in a twin study that estimated genetic liability to aggression based on the cotwins' aggression status and the pair's zygosity, it has been shown that not only do genetic liability and having aggressive friends predict aggression, but their interaction is also a significant predictor (Van Lier et al., 2007). Specifically, high levels of aggression in kindergarten children were most likely when genetically vulnerable children interacted with aggressive friends.

Davis, Haworth, Lewis, and Plomin (2012) explored how geographical location can affect the influence of nature and nurture on a phenotype. The study sample comprised families of twins from England and Wales. When the twins were 12 years old, data on their cognitive abilities and behavioral traits were collected from parents and teachers. The United Kingdom postcodes gave accurate location to a subneighborhood scale. Results showed that the extent of the genetic and environmental influences on the attributes measured changed according to location. For instance, classroom behavior problems were found to be more influenced by the nonshared environment in London compared with other areas in the United Kingdom. The explanation suggested by the authors for this finding was that London is characterized by the highest variability in socioeconomic status (SES).

It is easy to imagine how deprived environments can suppress genetic tendencies, but other, more subtle variations in the environment can also affect development. For example, it has been shown that physical activity moderates the effect of genetics on body mass index, so that higher levels of physical activity correspond with lower heritability estimates (Mustelin, Silventoinen, Pietiläinen, Rissanen, & Kaprio, 2008). Hence, people living in an area in which it is culturally common to exercise might not express their individual inherited vulnerabilities for obesity. Indeed, positive environments can suppress genetic tendencies. Social norms and laws can limit genetic susceptibility to substance abuse or aggression. It has been shown that in U.S. states with a high tax on cigarettes, the heritability of daily smoking among adolescents is lower (Boardman, 2009). Such findings have important repercussions because they imply that when genetic studies are conducted to identify variants that influence complex traits, the area from which the sample is recruited will influence the power of the analysis to detect the variants: Recruiting in areas where the trait of interest is more heritable is likely to improve power to detect the effects of individual genetic variants. More importantly, perhaps, it should be taken into account that one complexity of G × E phenomena is that genetic and environmental estimates are often specific to the context in which they are measured.

Concluding Remarks

The concept of genetics and heritability still tends to raise warning signs that read "Beware, determinism" in people's minds. But, similar to the environment, heritability is only one ingredient in the blend that makes us who we are. When it comes to personality, cognitive abilities, and other complex traits, the heritability component in quantitative genetic studies never amounts to 100%. The environment, which includes all of our surroundings, from bacteria, nutrition, weather, and *in utero* conditions to psychosocial factors, also plays a crucial role in development. As a consequence, the joint contribution of genes and environment is the real story behind development, a story into which we have tried to provide a glimpse in this chapter.

The outcome of socialization is affected by the interaction of socialization experiences with the inherited characteristics of the individual, who may be relatively resistant or susceptible to these experiences. Furthermore, socialization experiences are affected by the individual who, in many instances, selects and evokes them, whether intentionally or unintentionally. Therefore, socialization should be seen as an interactive process and not as independent from the individual. One of the consequences of this realization is that we should expect different individuals to respond differently to the same experience. Thus, it should be acknowledged that when it comes to interventions (or any socialization experience), no single intervention can produce the same result for everyone. Integrating knowledge from different fields and conducting interdisciplinary research holds great promise for our understanding of child development and for developing interventions and socialization contexts that are sensitive to the specific characteristics of each child.

ACKNOWLEDGMENTS

Preparation of this chapter was supported by Starting Grant No. 240994 from the European Research Council to Ariel Knafo. We thank Lior Abramson, Maayan Davidov, Shany Edelman, Liat Hasenfratz, Ellen Moss, Josh Moss, Yael Paz, Roni Pener-Tessler, and Idan Shalev for their comments on an earlier version of this chapter.

REFERENCES

Avinun, R., Ebstein, R. P., & Knafo, A. (2012). Human maternal behaviour is associated with arginine vasopressin receptor 1A gene. *Biology Letters, 8*(5), 894–896.

Avinun, R., Israel, S., Shalev, I., Gritsenko, I., Bornstein, G., Ebstein, R. P., et al. (2011). AVPR1A variant associated with preschoolers' lower altruistic behavior. *PLoS ONE, 6*(9), e25274.

Avinun, R., & Knafo, A. (2014). Parenting as a reaction evoked by children's genotype: A meta-analysis of children-as-twins studies. *Personality and Social Psychology Review, 18*(1), 87–102.

Bakermans-Kranenburg, M. J., & van IJzendoorn, M. (2008). Oxytocin receptor (OXTR) and serotonin transporter (5-HTT) genes associated with observed parenting. *Social Cognitive and Affective Neuroscience, 3*(2), 128–134.

Bakermans-Kranenburg, M. J., van IJzendoorn, M. H., Pijlman, F. T. A., Mesman, J., & Juffer, F. (2008). Experimental evidence for differential susceptibility: Dopamine D4 receptor polymorphism (DRD4 VNTR) moderates intervention effects on toddlers' externalizing behavior in a randomized controlled trial. *Developmental Psychology, 44*(1), 293–300.

Baumrind, D. (1971). Current patterns of parental authority. *Developmental Psychology, 4*(1, Pt. 2), 1–103.

Beaver, K. M., Wright, J. P., & DeLisi, M. (2008). Delinquent peer group formation: Evidence of a gene × environment correlation. *Journal of Genetic Psychology, 169*(3), 227–244.

Bekaert, S. (2005). Telomere length: The biological clock reviewed. *BioTech International, 17*(5), 8–10.

Belsky, J., Bakermans-Kranenburg, M. J., & van IJzendoorn, M. H. (2007). For better and for worse differential susceptibility to environmental influences. *Current Directions in Psychological Science, 16*(6), 300–304.

Belsky, J., & de Haan, M. (2011). Annual research review: Parenting and children's brain development: The end of the beginning. *Journal of Child Psychology and Psychiatry, 52*(4), 409–428.

Benish-Weisman, M., Steinberg, T., & Knafo, A. (2010). Genetic and environmental links between children's temperament and their problems with peers. *Israel Journal of Psychiatry and Related Sciences, 47*(2), 144–151.

Bezdjian, S., Baker, L. A., & Tuvblad, C. (2011). Genetic and environmental influences on impulsivity: A meta-analysis of twin, family and adoption studies. *Clinical Psychology Review, 31*(7), 1209–1223.

Boardman, J. D. (2009). State-level moderation of genetic tendencies to smoke. *American Journal of Public Health, 99*(3), 480–486.

Boivin, M., Brendgen, M., Vitaro, F., Forget-Dubois, N., Feng, B., Tremblay, R. E., et al. (2013). Evidence of gene–environment correlation for peer difficulties: Disruptive behaviors predict early peer relation difficulties in school through genetic effects. *Development and Psychopathology, 25*, 79–92.

Boivin, M., Pérusse, D., Dionne, G., Saysset, V., Zoccolillo, M., Tarabulsy, G. M., et al. (2005). The genetic–environmental etiology of parents' perceptions and self-assessed behaviours toward their 5-month-old infants in a large twin and singleton sample. *Journal of Child Psychology and Psychiatry, 46*(6), 612–630.

Boyce, W. T., Sokolowski, M. B., & Robinson, G. E. (2012). Toward a new biology of social adversity. *Proceedings of the National Academy of Sciences, 109*(Suppl. 2), 17143–17148.

Brendgen, M. (2012). Genetics and peer relations: A review. *Journal of Research on Adolescence, 22*(3), 419–437.

Burt, A. (2009). A mechanistic explanation of popularity: Genes, rule breaking, and evocative gene–environment correlations. *Journal of Personality and Social Psychology, 96*(4), 783–794.

Burt, S. A., McGue, M., Krueger, R. F., & Iacono, W. G. (2005). How are parent–child conflict and childhood externalizing symptoms related over time?: Results from a genetically informative cross-lagged study. *Development and Psychopathology, 17*(1), 145–165.

Caspi, A., Sugden, K., Moffitt, T. E., Taylor, A., Craig, I. W., Harrington, H. L., et al. (2003). Influence of life stress on depression: Moderation by a polymorphism in the 5-HTT gene. *Science, 301*, 386–389.

Chen, F. S., Barth, M. E., Johnson, S. L., Gotlib, I. H., & Johnson, S. C. (2011). Oxytocin receptor (OXTR) polymorphisms and attachment in human infants. *Frontiers in Psychology, 2*, 200.

Chess, S., & Thomas, A. (1999). *Goodness of fit: Clinical applications from infancy through adult life.* Philadelphia: Brunner/Mazel.

Chong, S., & Whitelaw, E. (2004). Epigenetic germline inheritance. *Current Opinion in Genetics and Development, 14*(6), 692–696.

Cleveland, H. H., Wiebe, R. P., & Rowe, D. C. (2005). Sources of exposure to smoking and drinking friends among adolescents: A behavioral-genetic evaluation. *Journal of Genetic Psychology, 166*(2), 153–169.

Cohen, D. J., Dibble, E., & Grawe, J. M. (1977). Parental style: Mothers' and fathers' perceptions of their relations with twin children. *Archives of General Psychiatry, 34*(4), 445–451.

D'Onofrio, B. M., Hulle, C. A., Waldman, I. D., Rodgers, J. L., Harden, K. P., Rathouz, P. J., et al. (2008). Smoking during pregnancy and offspring externalizing problems: An exploration of genetic and environmental confounds. *Development and Psychopathology, 20*(1), 139–164.

Davis, O., Haworth, C., Lewis, C., & Plomin, R. (2012). Visual analysis of geocoded twin data puts nature and nurture on the map. *Molecular Psychiatry, 17*(9), 867–874.

Daxinger, L., & Whitelaw, E. (2012). Understanding transgenerational epigenetic inheritance via the gametes in mammals. *Nature Reviews Genetics, 13*(3), 153–162.

Deater-Deckard, K. (2000). Parenting and child behavioral adjustment in early childhood: A quantitative genetic approach to studying family processes. *Child Development, 71*(2), 468–484.

Elkins, I. J., McGue, M., & Iacono, W. G. (1997). Genetic and environmental influences on parent–son relationships: Evidence for increasing genetic influence during adolescence. *Developmental Psychology, 33*(2), 351–363.

Ellis, B. J., Boyce, W. T., Belsky, J., Bakermans-Kranenburg, M. J., & van IJzendoorn, M. H. (2011). Differential susceptibility to the environment: An evolutionary–neurodevelopmental theory. *Development and Psychopathology, 23*(1), 7–28.

Entringer, S., Epel, E. S., Kumsta, R., Lin, J., Hellhammer, D. H., Blackburn, E. H., et al. (2011). Stress exposure in intrauterine life is associated with shorter telomere length in young adulthood. *Proceedings of the National Academy of Sciences, 108*(33), E513–E518.

Entringer, S., Epel, E. S., Lin, J., Buss, C., Shahbaba, B., Blackburn, E. H., et al. (2013). Maternal psychosocial stress during pregnancy is associated with newborn leukocyte telomere length. *American Journal of Obstetrics and Gynecology, 208*(2), 134e1–134e7.

Evans, G. W. (2004). The environment of childhood poverty. *American Psychologist, 59*(2), 77–92.

Feldman, R., Zagoory-Sharon, O., Weisman, O., Schneiderman, I., Gordon, I., Maoz, R., et al. (2012). Sensitive parenting is associated with plasma oxytocin and polymorphisms in the OXTR and CD38 genes. *Biological Psychiatry, 72*(3), 175–181.

Fish, E. W., Shahrokh, D., Bagot, R., Caldji, C., Bredy, T., Szyf, M., et al. (2006). Epigenetic programming of stress responses through variations in maternal care. *Annals of the New York Academy of Sciences, 1036*(1), 167–180.

Fowler, J. H., Settle, J. E., & Christakis, N. A. (2011). Correlated genotypes in friendship networks. *Proceedings of the National Academy of Sciences, 108*(5), 1993–1997.

Ge, X., Conger, R. D., Cadoret, R. J., Neiderhiser, J. M., Yates, W., Troughton, E., et al. (1996). The developmental interface between nature and nurture: A mutual influence model of child antisocial behavior and parent behaviors. *Developmental Psychology, 32*(4), 574–589.

Grossniklaus, U., Kelly, B., Ferguson-Smith, A. C., Pembrey, M., & Lindquist, S. (2013). Transgenerational epigenetic inheritance: How important is it? *Nature Reviews Genetics, 14*(3), 228–235.

Grusec, J. E., & Kuczynski, L. E. (1997). *Parenting and children's internalization of values: A handbook of contemporary theory.* New York: Wiley.

Hankin, B., Nederhof, E., Oppenheimer, C., Jenness, J., Young, J., Abela, J., et al. (2011). Differential susceptibility in youth: Evidence that *5-HTTLPR* × positive parenting is associated with positive affect "for better and worse." *Translational Psychiatry, 1*(10), e44.

Harley, C. B., Futcher, A. B., & Greider, C. W. (1990). Telomeres shorten during ageing of human fibroblasts. *Nature, 345*, 458–460.

Houts, R. M., Caspi, A., Pianta, R. C., Arseneault, L., & Moffitt, T. E. (2010). The challenging pupil in the classroom: The effect of the child on the teacher. *Psychological Science, 21*(12), 1802–1810.

Jaffee, S. R., Caspi, A., Moffitt, T. E., Polo-Tomas, M., Price, T. S., & Taylor, A. (2004). The limits of child effects: Evidence for genetically mediated child effects on corporal punishment but not on physical maltreatment. *Developmental Psychology, 40*(6), 1047–1057.

Karg, K., Burmeister, M., Shedden, K., & Sen, S. (2011). The serotonin transporter promoter variant (5-HTTLPR), stress, and depression meta-analysis revisited: Evidence of genetic moderation. *Archives of General Psychiatry, 68*(5), 444–454.

Kendler, K. S., & Baker, J. H. (2007). Genetic influences on measures of the environment: A systematic review. *Psychological Medicine, 37*(5), 615–626.

Klengel, T., Mehta, D., Anacker, C., Rex-Haffner, M., Pruessner, J. C., Pariante, C. M., et al. (2012). Allele-specific FKBP5 DNA demethylation mediates gene-childhood trauma interactions. *Nature Neuroscience, 16*(1), 33–41.

Knafo, A., Israel, S., & Ebstein, R. P. (2011). Heritability of children's prosocial behavior and differential susceptibility to parenting by variation in the dopamine receptor D4 gene. *Developmental Psychopathology, 23*(1), 53–67.

Knafo, A., & Jaffee, S. R. (2013). Gene–environment correlation in developmental psychopathology. *Development and Psychopathology, 25*(1), 1–6.

Knafo, A., & Plomin, R. (2006). Prosocial behavior from early to middle childhood: Genetic and environmental influences on stability and change. *Developmental Psychology, 42*(5), 771–786.

Knafo, A., Zahn-Waxler, C., Van Hulle, C., Robinson, J. L., & Rhee, S. H. (2008). The developmental origins of a disposition toward empathy: Genetic and environmental contributions. *Emotion, 8*(6), 737–752.

Kretschmer, T., Vitaro, F., & Barker, E. D. (2014). The association between peer and own aggression is moderated by the BDNF val-met polymorphism. *Journal of Research on Adolescence, 24*(1), 177–185.

Krueger, R. F., South, S., Johnson, W., & Iacono, W. (2008). The heritability of personality is not always 50%: Gene–environment interactions and correlations between personality and parenting. *Journal of Personality, 76*(6), 1485–1522.

Larsson, H., Viding, E., Rijsdijk, F. V., & Plomin, R. (2008). Relationships between parental negativity and childhood antisocial behavior over time: A bidirectional effects model in a longitudinal genetically informative design. *Journal of Abnormal Child Psychology, 36*(5), 633–645.

Lee, S. S. (2011). Deviant peer affiliation and antisocial behavior: Interaction with monoamine oxidase a (MAOA) genotype. *Journal of Abnormal Child Psychology, 39*(3), 321–332.

Luijk, M. P., Tharner, A., Bakermans-Kranenburg, M. J., van IJzendoorn, M. H., Jaddoe, V. W., Hofman, A., et al. (2011). The association between parenting and attachment security is moderated by a polymorphism in the mineralocorticoid receptor gene: Evidence for differential susceptibility. *Biological Psychology, 88*(1), 37–40.

Lytton, H. (1980). *Parent–child interaction: The socialization process observed in twin singleton families.* New York: Plenum Press.

Maccoby, E. E. (1992). The role of parents in the socialization of children: An historical overview. *Developmental Psychology, 28*(6), 1006–1017.

Mackinnon, A., Henderson, A., & Andrews, G. (1991). The Parental Bonding Instrument: A measure of perceived or actual parental behavior? *Acta Psychiatrica Scandinavica, 83*(2), 153–159.

McGowan, P. O., Sasaki, A., D'Alessio, A. C., Dymov, S., Labonté, B., Szyf, M., et al. (2009). Epigenetic regulation of the glucocorticoid receptor in human brain associates with childhood abuse. *Nature Neuroscience, 12*(3), 342–348.

McPherson, M., Smith-Lovin, L., & Cook, J. M. (2001). Birds of a feather: Homophily in social networks. *Annual Review of Sociology, 27*, 415–444.

Meaney, M. J. (2010). Epigenetics and the biological definition of gene × environment interactions. *Child Development, 81*(1), 41–79.

Mills-Koonce, W. R., Propper, C. B., Gariepy, J. L., Blair, C., Garrett-Peters, P., & Cox, M. J. (2007). Bidirectional genetic and environmental influences on mother and child behavior: The family system as the unit of analyses. *Development and Psychopathology, 19*(4), 1073–1087.

Munafò, M. R., Clark, T. G., Johnstone, E. C., Murphy, M. F. G., & Walton, R. T. (2004). The genetic basis for smoking behavior: A systematic review and meta-analysis. *Nicotine and Tobacco Research, 6*(4), 583–597.

Munafò, M. R., Matheson, I., & Flint, J. (2007). Association of the DRD2 gene Taq1A polymorphism and alcoholism: A meta-analysis of case–control studies and evidence of publication bias. *Molecular Psychiatry, 12*(5), 454–461.

Mustelin, L., Silventoinen, K., Pietiläinen, K., Rissanen, A., & Kaprio, J. (2008). Physical activity reduces the influence of genetic effects on BMI and waist circumference: A study in young adult twins. *International Journal of Obesity, 33*(1), 29–36.

Neiderhiser, J. M., Marceau, K., & Reiss, D. (2013). Four factors for the initiation of substance use by young adulthood: A ten-year follow-up twin and sibling study of marital conflict, monitoring, siblings and peers. *Development and Psychopathology, 25*(1), 133–149.

Neiderhiser, J. M., Reiss, D., Pedersen, N. L., Lichtenstein, P., Spotts, E. L., Hansson, K., et al. (2004). Genetic and environmental influences on mothering of adolescents: A comparison of two samples. *Developmental Psychology, 40*(3), 335–351.

Nobile, M., Cataldo, M. G., Giorda, R., Battaglia, M., Baschirotto, C., Bellina, M., et al. (2004). A case-control and family-based association study of the 5-HTTLPR in pediatric-onset depressive disorders. *Biological Psychiatry, 56*(4), 292–295.

O'Connor, T. G., Deater-Deckard, K., Fulker, D., Rutter, M., & Plomin, R. (1998). Genotype-environment correlations in late childhood and early adolescence: Antisocial behavioral problems and coercive parenting. *Developmental Psychology, 34*(5), 970–981.

Painter, R., Osmond, C., Gluckman, P., Hanson, M., Phillips, D., & Roseboom, T. (2008). Transgenerational effects of prenatal exposure to the Dutch famine on neonatal adiposity and health in later life. *BJOG: An International Journal of Obstetrics and Gynaecology, 115*(10), 1243–1249.

Pener-Tessler, R., Avinun, R., Uzefovsky, F., Edelman, S., Ebstein, R. P., & Knafo, A. (2013). Boys' serotonin transporter genotype affects maternal behavior through self-control: A case of evocative gene–environment correlation. *Development and Psychopathology, 25*, 151–162.

Plomin, R., & Asbury, K. (2005). Nature and nurture: Genetic and environmental influences on behavior. *Annals of the American Academy of Political and Social Science, 600*(1), 86–98.

Plomin, R., DeFries, J. C., & Loehlin, J. C. (1977). Genotype–environment interaction and correlation in the analysis of human behavior. *Psychological Bulletin, 84*(2), 309–322.

Plomin, R., DeFries, J., McClearn, G., & McGuffin, P. (2008). *Behavioral genetics* (Vol. 5). New York: Worth.

Pluess, M., & Belsky, J. (2013). Vantage sensitivity: Individual differences in response to positive experiences. *Psychological Bulletin, 139*(4), 901–916.

Price, T. S., & Jaffee, S. R. (2008). Effects of the family environment: gene-environment interaction and passive gene-environment correlation. *Developmental Psychology, 44*(2), 305–315.

Purcell, S. (2002). Variance components models for gene–environment interaction in twin analysis. *Twin Research, 5*(6), 554–571.

Reiss, D. (1995). Genetic influence on family systems: Implications for development. *Journal of Marriage and the Family, 57*, 543–560.

Rice, F., Lewis, G., Harold, G. T., & Thapar, A. (2013). Examining the role of passive gene–environment correlation in childhood depression using a novel genetically sensitive design. *Development and Psychopathology, 25*(1), 37–50.

Risch, N., Herrell, R., Lehner, T., Liang, K. Y., Eaves, L., Hoh, J., et al. (2009). Interaction between the serotonin transporter gene (5-HTTLPR), stressful life events, and risk of depression. *Journal of the American Medical Association, 301*, 2462–2471.

Rowe, D. C., Jacobson, K. C., & Van den Oord, E. J. C. G. (1999). Genetic and environmental influences on vocabulary IQ: Parental education level as moderator. *Child Development, 70*(5), 1151–1162.

Saudino, K. J. (1997). Moving beyond the heritability question: New directions in behavioral genetic studies of personality. *Current Directions in Psychological Science, 6*(4), 86–90.

Scarr, S. (1968). Environmental bias in twin studies. *Biodemography and Social Biology, 15*(1), 34–40.

Scarr, S., & McCartney, K. (1983). How people make their own environments: A theory of genotype environment effects. *Child Development, 54*(2), 424–435.

Shalev, I., Entringer, S., Wadhwa, P. D., Wolkowitz, O. M., Puterman, E., Lin, J., et al. (2013). Stress and telomere biology: A lifespan perspective. *Psychoneuroendocrinology, 38*(9), 1835–1842.

Shalev, I., Moffitt, T., Sugden, K., Williams, B., Houts, R., Danese, A., et al. (2013). Exposure to violence during childhood is associated with telomere erosion from 5 to 10 years of age: A longitudinal study. *Molecular Psychiatry, 18*(5), 576–581.

Silberg, J. L., Maes, H., & Eaves, L. J. (2010). Genetic and environmental influences on the transmission of parental depression to children's depression and conduct disturbance: An extended Children of Twins study. *Journal of Child Psychology and Psychiatry, 51*(6), 734–744.

Thapar, A., Rice, F., Hay, D., Boivin, J., Langley, K., Van Den Bree, M., et al. (2009). Prenatal smoking might not cause attention-deficit/hyperactivity disorder: Evidence from a novel design. *Biological Psychiatry, 66*(8), 722–727.

van IJzendoorn, M. H., Bakermans-Kranenburg, M. J., & Ebstein, R. P. (2011). Methylation matters in child development: Toward developmental behavioral epigenetics. *Child Development Perspectives, 5*(4), 305–310.

van IJzendoorn, M. H., Caspers, K., Bakermans-Kranenburg, M. J., Beach, S. R. H., & Philibert, R. (2010). Methylation matters: Interaction between methylation density and serotonin transporter genotype predicts unresolved loss or trauma. *Biological Psychiatry, 68*(5), 405–407.

Van Lier, P., Boivin, M., Dionne, G., Vitaro, F., Brendgen, M., Koot, H., et al. (2007). Kindergarten children's genetic vulnerabilities interact with friends' aggression to promote children's own aggression. *Journal of the American Academy of Child and Adolescent Psychiatry, 46*(8), 1080–1087.

Wachs, T. D., & Gandour, M. J. (1983). Temperament, environment, and six-month cognitive-intellectual development: A test of the organismic specificity hypothesis. *International Journal of Behavioral Development, 6*(2), 135–152.

Waga, C., & Iwahashi, K. (2007). CYP2A6 gene polymorphism and personality traits for NEO-FFI on the smoking behavior of youths. *Drug and Chemical Toxicology, 30*(4), 343–349.

Weaver, I. C. G., Cervoni, N., Champagne, F. A., D'Alessio, A. C., Sharma, S., Seckl, J. R., et al. (2004). Epigenetic programming by maternal behavior. *Nature Neuroscience, 7*(8), 847–854.

Zuk, O., Hechter, E., Sunyaev, S. R., & Lander, E. S. (2012). The mystery of missing heritability: Genetic interactions create phantom heritability. *Proceedings of the National Academy of Sciences, 109*(4), 1193–1198.

CHAPTER 16

Temperament, Parenting, and Social Development

John E. Bates
Gregory S. Pettit

Temperament and parenting are important for understanding individual differences in children's social development. Researchers using the constructs of temperament, parenting, and social development aim to build models with accurate predictions about future social adaptations. Such models ultimately advance prevention and early treatment of problems in social development. In this chapter we describe findings and models of how temperament and parenting are involved in children's social development. Findings on how temperament and parenting are empirically related allow enrichment of both kinds of concept, and findings on the joint and independent contributions of temperament and parenting to children's social development allow us to refine and enrich our concepts of individual differences in social development.

Temperament Concepts

Temperament is an umbrella term for biologically based individual differences in behavior that become children's basic personality (Rothbart, 2011; Zuckerman, 1991). In the relatively short history of the study of temperament in developmental science, dating from the early 1960s (e.g., Thomas, Chess, Birch, Herzig, & Korn, 1963), there have been many conceptual and operational definitions of temperament (Rothbart & Bates, 1998). We accept that the concept of temperament is not sharply defined (Wachs & Bates, 2010). However, over the past few decades, the various definitions have been coalescing into several broad dimensions or factors (Rothbart & Bates, 2006). At the broadest level, we can describe *temperament* as individuals' deeply rooted predispositions toward emotional reactivity and self-regulation. *Reactivity* refers to differences in the speed and intensity with which one reacts to relevant situations with positive emotions (e.g., interest, approach, or dominance) and negative emotions, sometimes with and other times without distinctions between distress arising from fear or anger; *self-regulation* refers to differences in the extent or efficiency with which one regulates attention, emotion, and behavior (Rothbart & Bates, 2006). Thus, the domain of temperament can be summarized in three dimensions: positive emotionality, negative emotionality, and self-regulation. At the same time that concepts of temperament have been coalescing into a limited set of dimensions, however, operational measures of temperament have been expanding. For example, although questionnaires and structured observations of behavior are still the most frequently employed measures, increasing numbers of studies have used basic biological markers that can stand for temperament, including electrophysiological measures, such as vagal tone and electroencephalography (EEG), and specific genes. The dimensionality of caregiver reports of temperament, and to some extent ratings of behavior in batteries of laboratory tasks, has been explored in studies that factor-analyze many temperament concepts—showing how variables are related and not related to one another. However, we have not seen comparable studies with arrays of biological markers, so we are less certain as to the dimensional meanings of these measures. There are some conventions in measurement of temperament (e.g., Bates, Schermerhorn, & Petersen, 2012; Rothbart & Bates, 2006), but there is no single standard measure or set of measures. Nor is the complex network of temperament completely mapped.

Temperament Concepts in Developmental Context

An important part of the difficulty in mapping temperament is that as social behavior becomes more complex with development, the phenotypes used to define temperament become increasingly complex, too, at least for development from infancy to middle childhood. It appears that along with considerable stability of temperament measures across ages, individuals' rank-order positions on temperament traits also change detectably. Negative emotionality may change across development partly as the result of good self-regulation traits coming online with maturation of brain, motor skills, and cognition, which allows children with higher levels of self-regulation to modulate the expression of previously high levels of negative emotion. Negative emotionality may also change as the result of environmental adaptations (e.g., parents learning to prevent the triggers of a child's negative emotion). Variance in temperamental positive emotionality is relatively strongly associated with variance in the environment from early in infancy (Goldsmith, Buss, & Lemery, 1997), so we would expect changes in temperament due to both maturation of self-regulation and environmental influences. Self-regulation traits themselves would also likely change, due to both biological development (Rothbart, 2011) and environmental pressures, for example, due to neurohormonal and brain structure changes at puberty, as well as environmental influences, such as transition to middle school (Bates et al., 2012; Neyer & Lehnart, 2007). In this chapter, we ask how child temperament might play a role in the development of parenting, how parenting might play a role in the development of temperament, and how both temperament and parenting are involved in child social development. These questions have fairly broad theoretical interest (Collins, Maccoby, Steinberg, Hetherington, & Bornstein, 2000; Lengua & Wachs, 2012; Molfese, Rudasill, & Molfese, 2013). Temperament concepts may be considered in relation to other important aspects of the environment, too, such as nutrition, toxins, chronic stressors, and social factors beyond parenting (Lengua & Wachs, 2012; Schermerhorn et al., 2013), but here we focus on what are probably the most proximal correlates of children's temperament: parenting variables.

Parenting Concepts

We regard differences in parenting as the most important factors in the child's social environment, especially at early ages (Maccoby, 1992). We do not think of parenting concepts as marking only qualities independent of the child. Just as with temperament, individual differences in parenting are now seen as part of the biopsychosocial network of factors; parenting differences may be related to genetic differences that influence parental personality (Collins et al., 2000; Dodge & Pettit, 2003; Moffitt & Caspi, 2007). Nevertheless, there is evidence from genetic studies that effects of the social environment on child development are not merely attributable to genetic overlap between parents and their children (Ganiban, Saudino, Ulbricht, Neiderhiser, & Reiss, 2008; Goldsmith, Lemery, Buss, & Campos, 1999), and researchers have suggested processes through which parenting could influence temperament (e.g., Bates et al., 2012). Parenting differences have been described in terms of both stylistic qualities, such as responsiveness, restrictiveness, and affection, and deliberate, goal-directed practices, such as proactive control or context-relevant teaching of social skills (Goodnight, Bates, Pettit, & Dodge, 2008; Ladd & Pettit, 2002; Mize & Pettit, 1997). One key dimension of parenting is warmth, which typically includes affection, nurturance, and responsiveness. A second key dimension, control, has sometimes been divided into autonomy-suppressing and autonomy-supporting dimensions, with the latter sometimes included with warmth and emotionally positive involvement (Bugental & Grusec, 2006; Maccoby & Martin, 1983).

A measurement challenge in elucidating the impact of parenting on development is that as children's social development proceeds, behavioral markers of a given aspect of parenting change, just as behavioral markers of temperament change. This does not preclude inferences about continuity and development—there are, in fact, many longitudinal, cross-time correlations between conceptually related qualities of both temperament and parenting—but it does suggest caution in generalizing the meaning of measures of parenting at one stage of development to meanings at another stage. This chapter describes the ways in which temperament and parenting join in helping to explain children's individual differences in social development. The literature focuses primarily on development of social adjustment, often in terms of internalizing and externalizing behavior problems, but it sometimes considers other adjustment outcomes, such as mature self-regulation and empathy, especially in recent research. The chapter builds especially on two previous chapters that considered the same issues, one in the previous edition of this handbook on socialization (Bates & Pettit, 2007) and the other in a handbook on temperament (Bates et al., 2012). We summarize in this chapter some key points of the previous chapters and consider them further in light of the more recent literature.

In this chapter we consider four questions:

1. Does temperament influence the development of parenting?
2. Does parenting influence the development of temperament?

3. Do temperament and parenting additively complement one another in predicting child social development?

4. Do temperament and parenting interact with one another in predicting child social development?

Our interest in development leads us to prefer longitudinal rather than cross-sectional evidence on these questions. We also prefer data from real lives rather than experimental manipulations because experiments have difficulty capturing the time scale and experiential depth of social development in their simulations of postulated mechanisms. The first two questions address the fundamental meanings of both temperament and parenting in the context of development. The third and fourth questions address the ways in which temperament and parenting are involved in social development. The first three questions involve the building of additive, linear models. The fourth, the subject of a burgeoning literature, involves nonlinear, multiplicative processes.

Does Temperament Influence the Development of Parenting?

Why should temperament influence parenting? Parenting may involve stable traits, but theoretically those traits can be modified by experience, and child behavior is a major part of that experience. Dominant theoretical models all admit some likelihood of child–parent transactional influences (Bell, 1968; Sameroff, 2009). Multiple research projects have tested for such processes (Bates, 1987; Kiff, Lengua, & Zalewski, 2011). We have addressed this literature in reviews recently (Bates & Pettit, 2007; Bates et al., 2012), and this chapter builds on conclusions from those reviews, as well as others, including Lengua and Wachs (2012). The best evidence that temperament might influence parenting would be the temperament–parenting linkage across development that controls for the initial level of a parenting variable. This is often shown by a partial correlation between time 1 temperament and time 2 parenting, with researchers controlling for time 1 parenting. It is also sometimes shown in a cross-lagged correlation, in which temperament predicts the part of the variance in parenting at time 2 that remains after researchers control for the time 1 parenting and its concurrent link to time 1 temperament. A few studies also control for initial levels of temperament (or parenting) in analyses of individual growth trajectories, and a few also consider cross-lagged processes across more than two waves of data collection. However, evidence like this is not always available. There is considerable change across development in a child's needs and capabilities; hence, parenting repertoires change. The meaning of a parenting style or strategy varies from one developmental era to another. Nevertheless, there is likely some developmental coherence in parenting just as in child adaptations (Sroufe & Rutter, 1984) and, indeed, there are correlations of parenting variables across time. For example, Haltigan, Roisman, and Fraley (2013) found a correlation of .45 between age-appropriate composite measures of maternal sensitivity (warmth, nonhostility, and autonomy support) assessed at early childhood and at age 10 years. This is a substantial but far from perfect continuity. We think it is prudent, therefore, for purposes of evaluating cross-time influences, to be cautious about equating parenting variables in infancy to parenting variables in later childhood. This leads us not to expect that we will find many instances of infant temperament influencing changes in parenting in toddlerhood or beyond. Therefore, studies of infancy-era temperament and later parenting could have an especially hard time establishing that infant temperament influences changes in parenting in toddlerhood or beyond. In this chapter, we emphasize studies that include autoregressive controls for initial levels of parenting (and/or temperament). However, because of the possible lack of equivalence of the measures across developmental eras, we do recognize that causal inferences must be tempered.

Negative Reactivity → Parenting

First, we consider the possible influence of child negative emotionality on parental warmth. There have been multiple relevant findings but no clear answer to the question of whether early child negative emotionality predicts later parental warmth (Bates et al., 2012). The valence of the relation—whether negative reactivity predicts more or less warmth—seems to depend on the ages of the children, the measures, and the samples, and the research is not definitive. According to a meta-analysis by Paulussen-Hoogeboom, Stams, Hermanns, and Peetsma (2007), child negative emotionality tends to be associated with lower parental warmth, but we are also aware of studies that suggest that in infancy, especially for samples with higher socioeconomic status (SES), negative emotionality is associated with higher levels of parental warmth (Bates, Olson, Pettit, & Bayles, 1982; Crockenberg, 1986). Also making the answer nondefinitive, the relevant studies have largely lacked autoregressive controls. In a recent study with such controls, Scaramella, Sohr-Preston, Mirabile, Robison, and Callahan (2008) found that high levels of distress at age 12 months predicted reductions in maternal supportive parenting from ages 12–24 months. At this point, although it appears that child negative emotionality might lead to the development of lower levels of parent warmth, the literature has not established this definitively and hints at the possibility that instances of negative emotionality may produce more warmth, at least in children's early months of life.

Second, we consider the possible influence of child negative reactivity on parental control. Child negative reactivity has been found to predict parental control, mostly in studies without autoregressive controls, with earlier negative emotionality associated with high parental control in toddlers and preschoolers (Bates et al., 2012; Frankel & Bates, 1990; Gauvain & Fagot, 1995; C. L. Lee & Bates, 1985). Child negative reactivity also predicted, with autoregressive controls, increases in parents' inconsistency in control for elementary school-age children (Lengua, 2006; Lengua & Kovacs, 2005). The Scaramella and colleagues (2008) study also considered parental control variables, and found that early distress did *not* predict change in maternal harsh discipline. We note this null finding as an occasion for mentioning our assumption that considerable numbers of relevant effects are tested and not found. Some null findings are mentioned in the context of the articles reporting some significant effects, but we doubt that all have been reported. In the interests of space considerations in this chapter, at this early stage of research, it seems productive to give more attention to emerging patterns of findings across studies— replication is key—and to give less attention to nonfindings that may or may not be in the literature. We mention in this chapter some nonfindings that have caught our interest, and if a replicated pattern of nonfindings does emerge, we hope to notice it more properly in the future.

Fear/Inhibition → Parenting

As previously mentioned, some studies measuring specific aspects of negative emotionality have distinguished between fearful tendencies and general negative emotionality. The dimension of fearful temperament involves distress, withdrawal, and inhibition of activity in contexts with new people and strange objects. Enough studies have considered concurrent associations between child fearful temperament and parenting that a meta-analysis has been done by Paulussen-Hoogeboom and colleagues (2007), but the pattern in the studies does not suggest much of a correlation. Longitudinal studies are less numerous, but there have been some studies in which child fearfulness or inhibited tendencies predict more maternal warmth, even when researchers controlled for early parenting (Lengua, 2006; Lengua & Kovacs, 2005). Lengua (2006) also found evidence that in the transition into adolescence, fearfulness predicts reduced parental inconsistency in control. On the other hand, earlier in development, Rubin, Nelson, Hastings, and Asendorpf (1999) found that parents' perceptions of child shyness at age 2 predicted lower levels of parents' self-reported encouragement of child independence at age 4, even when they controlled for initial levels of encouragement of independence and continuity in child shyness. More recently, Natsuaki and colleagues (2013) found that high child social wariness at 18 months predicted lower levels of structured parenting at 27 months (directiveness in a cleanup task), even when they controlled for parenting at 18 months and changes in child social wariness. Aside from the use of a cross-lagged design, another factor that makes the Natsuaki and colleagues study especially interesting is that it involved adoptive children and their parents, thereby ruling out a shared-genes explanation for the apparent child temperament effect. Any correlation, even one in a cross-lagged model, can reflect more than child or parent effects. Shared genes may be an alternative explanation, so it is good to see this tested and ruled out.

Angry Temperament → Parenting

Another aspect of negative emotionality that has been distinguished from general negative emotionality and from fearfulness is anger, which often occurs in situations where the child's approach or mastery efforts have been frustrated. Child frustration/anger may affect parenting, as suggested by previous studies showing concurrent correlations (e.g., Kochanska, Friesenborg, Lange, & Martel, 2004), in which higher levels of child anger/frustration are associated with lower levels of supportive parenting and higher levels of negative parenting. We had not previously found many relevant longitudinal studies, however (Bates et al., 2012). This absence could stem from several possible factors. We think an ideal measurement of temperament would separate angry emotionality from more general distress and from fearful emotionality, but such distinctions in measurement are relatively infrequent. In infants' early months, it is hard to separate anger and other forms of distress, and this is when temperament has often been assessed. However, in addition to the possible measurement issues and our own incomplete search of the literature, the explanation could also involve a file-drawer problem. One can imagine different kinds of parents responding differently to early anger and its absence, and children differing on the other temperament traits that frame their level of anger. Some parents might respond to angry tendencies by becoming more warm, strategic, and proactive than they had been. Others might grow in irritability, inconsistency, and harsh reactivity.

Research might specify the ways in which demographic and personality factors shape parents' responses to child temperament. For example, in the study by Hastings and Rubin (1999), punitively controlling responses to hypothetical child aggressive behavior were found to depend on the interaction of the child's angry temperament and the parents' own authoritarian attitudes. Perhaps across families the associations between angry temperament and the development of parenting are very small, and clear moderators have not yet been discovered (see our later section on moderator effects), so simple angry temperament → parenting findings that do not reach significance may not as often be submitted for publication. We did, however, find one recent study that found a general effect, consistent with a temperament effect: In a study of children in middle childhood, E. H. Lee, Zhou, Eisenberg, and Wang (2013) found that higher levels of child anger/frustration predicted increased levels of later authoritarian parenting, even when the researchers controlled for earlier parenting.

Positive Emotional Reactivity → Parenting

Bates and colleagues (2012) were unable to conclude whether a child's early positive emotionality (i.e., level of joy, interest, and approach) affects the development of parenting. A number of cross-sectional studies have shown concurrent correlations between positive reactivity and parental interest and warmth (Bates et al., 2012), but we found only two relevant prospective studies, one of which found no influence of infants' joy on parenting (Kochanska et al., 2004) and the other of which, controlling for earlier maternal acceptance, did find that child positive emotionality in middle childhood predicted more maternal acceptance of the child. Parents have multiple ways to respond to children's joyfulness, interest, and social warmth (and their absence). Parents' personality and their child's other traits may moderate the implications of the child's positive emotionality. So perhaps there is in fact not a simple effect of child positive emotionality on parenting. However, in a recent study, Bridgett, Laake, Gartstein, and Dorn (2013) suggested that infants who score high on a smiling and laughing temperament scale from ages 4 to 12 months have mothers who use less negative parenting (less mother-reported lax, overreactive, and overtalkative discipline) at 18 months, given the researchers' controls for earlier mother personality, even without controls for earlier parenting. At this time, as with the effects of angry temperament, we are not able to draw a conclusion about the effects of positive reactivity upon parenting.

Self-Regulation → Parenting

There have been many studies on cross-sectional associations between early child effortful control traits and parenting (Bates et al., 2012; Karreman, van Tuijl, van Aken, & Deković, 2006). There is an association between better child regulation and more positive and less negative parenting. Too few longitudinal studies have addressed early childhood temperamental self-regulation to ascertain a clear effect on parenting, but an interesting one by Kennedy, Rubin, Hastings, and Maisel (2004) considered effects of child self-regulation ability, as indexed by vagal tone. Vagal tone indexes heart rate changes linked with respiration, and is regarded as a good estimate of parasympathetic nervous system influence on the heart and a marker of emotion regulation at the physiological level. Kennedy and colleagues found that higher child vagal tone (more parasympathetic regulation) predicted more supportive mothering, as well as less restrictive mothering, even when they controlled for earlier mothering. These findings converge with a set of similar longitudinal results related to child self-regulation from middle and late childhood into early adolescence and later parenting (e.g., Lengua, 2006), with researchers controlling for earlier parenting (see Bates et al., 2012). Several newer studies by Eisenberg and her colleagues support the general trend, especially with regard to qualities of parental control: First, Eisenberg and colleagues (2010) showed that child effortful control at age 18 months predicted mothers' use of more cognitive tactics than directive tactics to assist the child in a teaching task at 30 months, controlling for initial values; and similarly, effortful control at age 30 months predicted parenting at 42 months in the same way. A notable nonreplication, however, came from Taylor, Eisenberg, Spinrad, and Widaman (2013), who, using the same sample, failed to find that child effortful control predicted later intrusive parenting across several laboratory tasks. Finally, E. H. Lee and colleagues (2013) found that children's effortful control inversely predicted parents' authoritarian parenting, controlling for earlier authoritarian parenting. However, interestingly, child temperament did not significantly predict an alternative dimension of parenting, authoritative parenting—a variable that presumably combines warmth with effective control, as opposed to the more negatively focused authoritarian parenting.

Summary

In summary, there is evidence that child temperament may shape the development of parenting. Fearful and general negative emotionality and self-regulation appear to influence changes in parenting. Angry emotionality and positive emotionality do not do so as definitively, and it is not yet clear why these variables should have less impact on the development of parenting than fearfulness and general negative emotionality.

Does Parenting Influence the Development of Child Temperament?

The notion that parenting may shape child temperament may challenge the most basic view of temperament as a stable trait. However, although temperament traits, as commonly measured, are indeed relatively stable, individuals also do show some changes in rank-order position on temperament variables (Rothbart & Bates, 2006), so it is reasonable to ask whether experience, including parent–child relations, might alter temperament. Perhaps ordinary experiences with parenting would have little effect on the deeper genetic underpinnings of temperament, but in multiple ways they could affect the behavioral phenotypes that are measured by temperament scales (Bates, 1989).

Parenting → Negative Reactivity

Evidence has suggested that higher levels of parental sensitive, warm parenting predict later decreases in child negative reactivity, even when researchers control for initial levels (Bates et al., 2012). A few studies have provided evidence that higher levels of harsh control lead to increased child negative reactivity, even when researchers control for initial temperament. Examples include Belsky, Fish, and Isabella (1991) and Braungart-Rieker, Hill-Soderlund, and Karrass (2010). An additional study partly confirms and partly disconfirms this pattern: Scaramella and colleagues (2008) found that in a small sample of toddlers, maternal harsh control in response to child noncompliance at age 12 months predicted increased child negative reactivity across several laboratory tasks at 24 months, given researchers' controls for initial level of child negative reactivity, but mother supportive parenting did not produce change in child negative reactivity.

Parenting → Fear/Inhibition

Two patterns observed in the literature (Bates et al., 2012) are that low parental sensitive responsiveness predicted increased fear, when researchers controlled for initial levels (e.g., Pauli-Pott, Mertesacker, & Beckmann, 2004), and the inverse, first shown by Arcus (2001) and Park, Belsky, Putnam, and Crnic (1997), that challenging parenting leads to reduced levels of fearfulness over time. By characterizing parenting in the second pattern as challenging we summarize a somewhat diverse set of variables across studies, ranging from directive to somewhat (but not harshly) negative. In one recent study supporting the second pattern, Natsuaki and colleagues (2013) reported that fathers' highly structured parenting (directiveness during a cleanup task) at 18 months predicted lower levels of social wariness at 27 months, with researchers' controlling for initial levels of social wariness and changes in structured parenting. In another study, which supports both patterns, Booth-LaForce and Oxford (2008) found in the large, National Institute of Child Health and Human Development Study of Early Child Care and Youth Development (NICHD SECCYD) sample of school-age children that insensitive parenting led to both to increasing and decreasing trajectories of social withdrawal and not to a continuously low social withdrawal, even with controls for earlier child temperamental shyness or inhibitory control. This is perhaps the first demonstration of both of the prior patterns in a single study, a set of effects made possible by a creative use of growth mixture modeling. We do not know why some children showed one pattern and others showed the opposite. However, it is possible that unmeasured moderating qualities of either parenting or child temperament could have altered the implications of the insensitive parenting measure. Finally, Rapee, Kennedy, Ingram, Edwards, and Sweeney (2010) provide a relevant experimental result indicating that a parenting intervention focused on decreasing overprotectiveness and increasing mastery of feared situations changed parent-reported child anxiety symptoms, but not child temperamental inhibition in a structured laboratory situation. This finding converges with a few similar, prior findings (e.g., Sheeber, 1995) that indicate parent-focused treatments can produce changes in child problem behavior without affecting temperamental dispositions that are associated with the problem behavior. It also provides evidence that parenting does not necessarily influence change in child temperament, despite studies we have reviewed that do show parenting effects on temperament.

Parenting → Angry Temperament

Bates and colleagues (2012) found no studies showing the effect of parenting on angry temperament. However, in a more recent study, E. H. Lee and colleagues (2013) found that not only did child temperament predict changes in parenting, as mentioned previously, but also parenting predicted changes in child temperament: Authoritarian parenting (self-reported harsh and noninductive discipline) led to increased anger/frustration and reduced effortful control, with researchers controlling for initial levels.

Parenting → Positive Emotionality

One might expect more parental positivity and responsiveness to lead to growth in positive emotionality in children who are initially low in positive emotionality, which is consistent with the Goldsmith and colleagues (1997) finding in twin research of a strong shared environment component in children's positive emotionality. Such an effect was indeed found in a study by Belsky and colleagues (1991), in which parents' high positive involvement—high overall levels of engagement in observed interactions at age 3 months—did predict increased infant positive emotionality at 9 months of age even after the researchers controlled for positive emotionality at age 3 months. However, Bates and colleagues (2012) found little additional evidence of such effects, and we did not find further studies for the present review.

Parenting → Self-Regulation

Earlier findings suggested that parental warmth leads to increased effortful control, even when researchers control for initial levels of effortful control (Kochanska, Murray, & Harlan, 2000), and harsh parenting leads to reduced levels of effortful control (Eisenberg et al., 1999). Among several more recent studies, one is a nonfinding: Eisenberg and colleagues (2010) reported that parenting measured in a teaching task did not predict later child effortful control changes, although, as mentioned, child effortful control did influence parental teaching tactics over time. The other studies did show parent effects. Taylor and colleagues (2013) found that parental intrusive control predicted lower levels of child effortful control, and E. H. Lee and colleagues (2013) reported a similar effect; researchers in both studies controlled for initial levels of child temperament. Booth-LaForce and Oxford (2008) demonstrated an effect that converges with these two studies, in which insensitive parenting at age 6 months predicted a less securely attached mother–child relationship at 24 months, which in turn predicted lower levels of child inhibitory control at age 54 months, when researchers controlled for child dysregulated temperament at 6 months. Similarly, Bridgett and colleagues (2011) found that a marker of warm involvement—the amount of time mothers spent with their babies at 6 months (playing, holding, bathing, reading, etc.)—predicted child effortful control at 18 months, even when they controlled for the intercept and slope of precursors of effortful control reported by mothers on the Rothbart Infant Behavior Questionnaire across ages 4, 6, 8, 10, and 12 months.

Summary

In summary, there is some evidence that parenting variables predict changes in child temperament over development. Warm parenting has predicted decreases in child negative emotionality, and harsh parenting has predicted increases in negative emotionality. Low warmth has led to higher fear, but challenging parenting has also has led to reduced fear. Finally, evidence supports positive parenting, including high warmth and low harsh control, as a factor in the development of child effortful control.

Transactional and Mediational Models
of Temperament, Parenting, and Adjustment

We have summarized evidence of how temperament and parenting may shape one another. There is enough evidence of linkage between the two constructs that it appears that both are plausible influences on one another. This could support a transactional model (Sameroff, 2009) in which temperament shapes the development of parenting, and parenting shapes the development of temperamental traits. For example, to use the Scaramella and colleagues (2008) findings mentioned previously, we could interpret the results as relevant to the following model: Harsh parenting, which theoretically influences the child's development through the modeling of dysfunctional social skills, reward of coercive behavior, and conflict-induced distress, leads to increases in the child's negative emotional reactivity and, in turn, the negative reactivity makes it more likely that the child would behave in difficult ways, eliciting more negative parenting or making it more likely that the child, ultimately, would not learn skills needed for successful social development. However, Scaramella and colleagues had a two-wave model, so their findings only carry the model to the point of showing, in separate analyses, both temperament → parenting and parenting → temperament effects. Support for a transactional or mediational model would, ideally, come from studies that have three or more measurement occasions, and test mediational processes more explicitly. A few studies do show cascades of temperament influencing parenting development or parenting influencing temperament, which then augments the prediction of an adjustment outcome. Taylor and colleagues (2013), for example, with a three-wave (18, 30, and 42 months) cross-lagged structural model, showed that intrusive parenting influences child effortful control more than child effortful control influences intrusive parenting, and that effortful control mediates some of the negative association between intrusive parenting and ego resiliency. More such tests are needed.

Do Temperament and Parenting
Additively Complement One Another in Predicting Child Adjustment?

Temperament and parenting are often listed in theory as independent factors in social development, but evidence from studies testing both as predictors of child outcomes was thin in our previous reviews (Bates & Pettit, 2007; Bates et al., 2012). We can rectify that in the current review, with many more citations, but our basic conclusion is similar: Some studies show that the two kinds of variables do supplement one another in predictions of child social development outcomes, but others find one or the other, but not both, to predict. This may well be related to the findings just discussed, that temperament and parenting indices often are related. Altogether, for the present review, we read 20 studies testing supplemental prediction. Eleven of these studies showed both a temperament and a parenting variable linearly and independently adding to prediction of a child adjustment outcome (Barker, Oliver, Viding, Salekin, & Maughan, 2011; Booth-LaForce & Oxford, 2008; Bridgett et al., 2011; Kimonis et al., 2006; Kochanska & Kim, 2013; Kochanska, Kim, Barry, & Philibert, 2011; Leve, Kim, & Pears, 2005; Lindhout, Markus, Hoogendijk, & Boer, 2009; Poehlman et al., 2011; Raver, Blair, Willoughby, & the Family Life Project Key Investigators, 2013; Taylor et al., 2013). Nine of the studies reported instances in which a temperament or parenting variable might predict, but not both (Cipriano & Stifter, 2010; Hane, Cheah, Rubin, & Fox, 2008; Hilt, Armstrong, & Essex, 2012; Kim & Kochanska, 2012; Kochanska et al., 2011; Kolak & Volling, 2013; Lewis-Morrarty et al., 2012; Smith et al., 2012; Ursache, Blair, Stifter, & Voegtline, 2013). We do not see any obvious patterns of constructs considered or types of measures differentiating between the two groups of studies. For the time being, we conclude that temperament and parenting variables can sometimes supplement one another in prediction of child outcomes, but often they do not. Aside from possible measurement issues, the inconsistent findings may also have to do with the small-to-moderate correlations between temperament and parenting variables, such as those described in our section on cross-time associations. These could reduce independent effects on the child outcome of either the temperament or parenting variable. It is also worth noting that, typically, neither temperament nor parenting variables in longitudinal studies account for large portions of the variance in the child social development outcome variable. This has led to questions about the possible interactions between temperament and parenting. In fact, our finding of a relatively large number of recent articles with information about additive effects is partly a by-product of the still-accelerating numbers of papers on temperament × parenting interaction effects because studies that consider interaction effects typically use statistical models that also test the additive main effects.

Do Child Temperament and Parenting Interact with One Another in Predicting Child Social Adjustment?

The literature on temperament × parenting interactions in prediction of social development is fast growing but unruly, with many different temperament, parenting, and social development constructs measured, along with many different research designs, each of which has its own limited window into nature. For the sake of comparisons, we group findings primarily by the conceptual category of temperament, as in other sections of the chapter. As with our reviews in the preceding sections, this risks some small distortions because the actual temperament measures of the studies are far from uniform in their operational definitions. However, we are reasonably confident in our interpretations of the measures. When possible, we secondarily group findings by the interacting dimensions of parenting. Also, where possible we further group findings according to the particular outcome dimension. Furthermore, to summarize our reading of the older (still relatively recent) literature (Bates et al., 2012) for ourselves with a sort of cartoon, we formed a somewhat composite description of the interaction that best describes the set of most relevant studies in the literature, with most effects considered in terms of how parenting predicts child adjustment, and how child temperament moderates this prediction. Two forms of interaction dominated these summaries: More often, studies describe a form of the interaction in which at one level of temperament, the effects of parenting on adjustment are enhanced and, at the other level of temperament, the effects of parenting on adjustment are diminished. Often, the social development outcomes were roughly equivalent for children with easier and more challenging temperaments when the parenting was warm and effectively controlling, and outcomes were discrepant for the temperament groups when the parenting was less ideal. This is often called a "fan-shaped," ordinal, or dual-risk interaction. It is also sometimes spoken of as an illustration of a diathesis stress effect, in which a given stress (the presence of negative parenting or the absence of positive parenting) produces psychopathology only in the presence of a temperamental diathesis (adverse temperament or the absence of positive temperament). Once in a while, but not very often, the form of the interaction is a crossover, in which parenting affects child adjustment at both levels of a temperament moderator variable, but the two effects run in opposite directions. Another, less stringent, but increasingly common version of a crossover effect is one in which the social development of one of the temperament groups is good when the parenting is good, and poor when the parenting is poor, whereas in the other group, social development is at a middle level and parenting correlates less strongly with it. For example, for children who are high in negative emotionality, harsh parental control leads to the worst child outcomes and gentle control leads to the best outcomes. For children who are low in negative emotionality, harsh control predicts perhaps a little worse outcome than gentle control, but not as poor as the outcome for highly emotional children, and gentle control predicts an outcome that is not as good as that for highly emotional children. This kind of interaction effect is sometimes spoken of as differential susceptibility to parenting or sensitivity to context (Belsky, Bakermans-Kranenburg, & van IJzendoorn, 2007; Roisman et al., 2012). In a few articles (e.g., Kochanska et al., 2011; Smith et al., 2012), the interaction shape is statistically defined using the graphically helpful "regions of significance" approach.

Child General Negative Emotionality × Parenting

Several studies (e.g., Belsky, Hsieh, & Crnic, 1998; Bradley & Corwyn, 2008; Pluess & Belsky, 2009) indicated a pattern in which children high in negative emotionality did the worst of all children in terms of externalizing behavior when there was high negative or low positive parenting, and children with low general negative emotionality were in the middle, with their externalizing behavior relatively unaffected by the parenting qualities (Bates et al., 2012). Several newer studies can to one degree or another be interpreted as supportive of this general pattern. First, Roisman and colleagues (2012) used the same large data set used by Bradley and Corwyn (2008) and Pluess and Belsky (2010), but they evaluated the interaction effects in a more sophisticated way, considering regions of significance. They also considered the effects on adjustment outcomes across multiple ages. Roisman and colleagues found that for children with difficult temperaments, there were stronger links between early maternal sensitivity (warmth + autonomy support) and later adjustment than for children with easy temperaments, considering six outcome variables rated by both mothers and teachers. Moreover, they found that for teacher-rated outcomes, there were interactions in which difficult children did better than easy children when they had a highly sensitive mother and worse when they had a mother observed to be relatively insensitive. For the mother-rated outcomes, as well as children's performance on an academic skills test, temperament moderated in a simpler way, with higher maternal sensitivity predicting better functioning for all children, but to a stronger degree for the difficult ones. In another study, Poehlmann and colleagues (2011) systematically tested interactions between multiple measures of both temperament and parenting predicting effortful control and behavior problem outcomes of preterm infants followed up as toddlers. Note that toddler effortful control in this study is one of the adjustment outcomes and is not used here as a temperament predictor. Of 36 tests for interaction, 10 were significant. Their findings support a pattern in previous studies described in

Bates and colleagues (2012): Children high in general negative emotionality did better on multiple adjustment outcomes, including more delay of gratification and effortful attention and fewer internalizing and externalizing problems, when their mothers were high in positive affect or low in anger or instrusiveness toward them at age 9 months, and they did significantly worse when their mothers were low in positive affect and high in negative parenting. Low-difficult children (low in negative emotionality, primarily) did not show as clear a relation between parenting and self-regulation and behavior problem outcomes. Poehlmann and colleagues interpreted several interactions as reflecting a crossover. In these, less positive or more negative parenting predicted the least mature delay of gratification or effortful attention in laboratory tasks, or the highest level of externalizing problems, but only for infants seen as difficult by parents or as highly distress-prone by observers. The low-difficult or low-distress infants were not as affected by parenting but appeared to have done a little better, if at all, when their mothers were warmly involved, nonintrusive, or low in anger in terms of parenting. In another study, Kolak and Volling (2013) found that young children's temperamental negative reactivity predicted changes in their internalizing problems following the birth of a sibling, but only when their parents undermined one another's parenting. Kolak and Volling also found that the children's negative emotionality predicted postsibling increases in externalizing problems, but only for those whose two parents were both undermining and unsupportive of one another. Finally, we mention the findings of Hilt and colleagues (2012), in which adolescents' self-reported tendency to ruminate (theoretically a factor in the development of depression) was predicted by the interaction of mother-reported family qualities and child negative emotionality measured in early childhood. The first pattern was that the high-negative children with an overcontrolling parent were the most likely to develop rumination and that low-negative children whose mothers were not overcontrolling had the least rumination of all. This pattern is quite consistent with the pattern in other studies reviewed in this section. The second, rather different pattern was that low-negative children became ruminative only if their family was high on general negativity, while high-negative children became ruminative regardless of the family's level of general negativity. A child with low-negative emotionality in this instance had an advantage in a family with low negativity but a disadvantage in a family with high negativity.

Child Fearfulness × Negative Parenting

There is evidence from several studies that child temperamental fearfulness moderates the links between negative parenting and child externalizing behavior. Higher levels of fearfulness have been found to strengthen the links between harsh versus gentle parenting and the development of conduct problems versus prosocial skills (Kochanska, 1995; Kochanska, Aksan, & Joy, 2007; Lengua, 2008). Harsh parenting predicted high levels of child externalizing behavior and low levels of positive behavior for high-fear children. Harsh versus gentle parenting did not matter much for the low-fear children or, conversely, the level of fear did not matter much when children had gentle or non-negative parenting. One recent study (Hastings et al., 2011) was cross-sectional but found an interesting effect in the interaction of mothers' reported use of punishment and preschoolers' cortisol response to an adult stranger in predicting externalizing problems. Boys with high-punishment mothers and high cortisol measured 20 minutes after meeting the stranger scored highest on externalizing behavior problems, and boys with low punishment mothers and high cortisol responses scored lowest on externalizing behavior. One feasible interpretation of a high-cortisol response at the beginning of an interaction with a stranger is that it reflects stranger anxiety. The child's disposition to anxiety in conjunction with an anxiety-arousing parent–child relationship could interfere with his or her cognitive ability to learn social rules, and hence to develop externalizing problems.[1] The Hastings and colleagues (2011) study also included parent-rated inhibition, which correlated with child internalizing problems and not externalizing problems, as would be expected. However, parent-rated inhibition did not correlate with the cortisol measures, and it did not interact with parenting in its association with the adjustment measures.

Two other recent studies tested somewhat similar models involving the interaction of child fearfulness and parenting. Lewis-Morrarty and colleagues (2012), using a sample with more behaviorally inhibited and more uninhibited children than those in a normal sample, found that behavioral inhibition across ages 1–7 predicted high levels of child social anxiety in adolescence, but only when at age 7 they had mothers who scored high in overcontrol, and not otherwise. We interpret this interaction effect to be similar to the previous pattern, in that fearful children were more poorly adjusted only if they received relatively high levels of parenting that could be broadly construed as negative. In this particular study, overcontrol was intrusive and unresponsive to the child, but not necessarily harsh or punitive. Leve and colleagues (2005) found a rather different pattern, in which temperamentally low-fear girls who received high levels of harsh discipline showed higher externalizing growth than other children, increasing across ages 5–17 years, and the low-fear girls who received low levels of harsh discipline showed the steepest decline in externalizing problems. High-fear girls who received high levels of harsh discipline showed slightly more decline in externalizing behavior than the high-fear girls who experienced low harshness. Put another way, with temperamentally low-fear girls, parents' harsh discipline predicted acting out, which is not an outcome most parents would want. However, for high-fear girls, harsh discipline was associated with no higher trajectories of externalizing, and perhaps even lower, than if they had received mild discipline, with slopes of externalizing behavior ranging from average at very low levels of harsh parenting to about one-fourth of a standard deviation below the mean (a more negative slope) at very high levels of harsh parenting. Although replications of the Leve and colleagues study are needed, a somewhat similar effect has been seen, with the developmental consequences of child fearfulness being moderated by what we call not-too-nice parenting, as we describe later.

Child Fearfulness × Positive Parenting

In prior reviews (Bates et al., 2012; Degnan, Almas, & Fox, 2010), an effect parallel to the interaction between fearfulness and negative parenting in prediction of externalizing problems has been noted for positive parenting (e.g., Lahey et al., 2008). However, the low-fear children appear more sensitive to the beneficial effects of positive parenting than the high-fear children. An excellent example of such research is that of Kochanska and colleagues (2007). We did not find a study like this in our current search, but it remains a practically appealing pattern. We often recommend to parents of low-fear children that they emphasize positive parenting (Bates, 2012), as challenging as this can be. Further confirmation of this pattern will be important.

Child Fearfulness × Not-Too-Nice Parenting

As mentioned, there is a well-replicated main effect of early fearful temperament predicting later anxiety problems. However, far from every infant or young child with a fearful temperament ends up with internalizing problems. We have been especially intrigued by a pattern in which early fearful temperament is less predictive of later internalizing behavior problems when the parents are challenging, such as being somewhat intrusive and frustrating rather than highly supportive (Bates et al., 2012; Fox, Henderson, Marshall, Nichols, & Ghera, 2005), which we have begun to refer to as "not-too-nice" parenting (Bates, 2012). Key examples include Arcus (2001), Park and colleagues (1997), and Willams and colleagues (2009). This does not mean rejecting or denigrating parenting, which would lead to more behavior problems (Rubin, Burgess, Dwyer, & Hastings, 2003), but rather, it appears from the few relevant studies, parenting that includes some negativity. It can be adaptive for young children to be somewhat inhibited in novel situations, but with experience, they ideally should grow in their skills and confidence in situations with novelty. Parents often help this process along, encouraging the child to encounter and master initially fearful situations (Chess & Thomas, 1984; Rubin & Mills, 1991). But in some instances, rather than encourage mastery, parents reinforce the child's negative affect displays by removing or otherwise protecting the child. Through the coercive power of negative reinforcement (e.g., the crying stops when the parent removes the child), protectiveness can become a habit for parents, and across many instances the child therefore fails to learn how to master novelty. As the child accumulates such experiences, his or her lags in self-regulation and social skills relative to other children become further reasons for fear. Temperamentally inhibited children with not-too-nice parents may have more opportunities to extinguish fears and therefore end up with fewer anxiety problems than temperamentally inhibited children with parents who cater to their fears. One new study, by Hastings, Kahle, and Nuselovici (2014), indicated that socially wary children with overprotective mothers later had the highest levels of internalizing problems, especially when they were also low in parasympathetic regulation. We also found the reviews by Degnan and colleagues (2010), Fox and colleagues (2005), and Rapee, Schniering, and Hudson (2009) to be helpful in enriching the theoretical mechanism. They emphasized the pattern as one involving solicitousness—a combination of warmth and high control that may reinforce children's anxious tendencies, along with a failure to encourage development of mastery skills. Thus, although we find the pattern very appealing from a theoretical and clinical perspective, we have to remain tentative about the solidity of the developmental phenomenon and encourage further research.

Child Frustration × Parenting

Children's frustrated emotionality is qualitatively different from fearful emotionality, and one might expect that frequently frustrated children who show it would need different kinds of parenting than do seldom-frustrated children. Previously, we had not seen enough evidence to suggest a clear pattern (Bates et al., 2012), but we were much intrigued by the pattern found by Degnan, Calkins, Keane, and Hill-Soderlund (2008), in which toddlers' high levels of frustration predicted high levels of aggression as far as age 5, but only for toddlers who experienced maternal overcontrol in their visit to the laboratory. More recently, two, relevant articles have appeared. In one study, Kochanska and Kim (2013) found that hard-to-manage 30-month-old children (angry, low effortful control) showed more noncompliance and other behavior problems at 40 months, but only when their mothers were low in responsiveness. Easy-to-manage toddlers tended to end up with low levels of problem behavior or high levels of prosocial behavior no matter how responsive their mothers had been observed to be. In the other study, Kim and Kochanska (2012) found that highly frustrated 7-month-olds actually showed high levels of compliance and self-regulation at 25 months if they had been observed at 15 months to have high levels of responsiveness with their mothers, but with low levels of responsive interactions they turned out to be very low in compliance and self-regulation. Mother–infant responsiveness had little to do with the outcomes for the children who had showed low levels of angry reactivity to frustration and other negative emotionality at 7 months, and these children ended up with moderate levels of compliance and self-regulation. All in all, the patterns reported by Kochanska and Kim are quite similar to those reported by Degnan and colleagues. The two sets of measures are not identical, but they are conceptually related. Also of interest, one of the articles (Kim & Kochanska, 2012) provides evidence that frustration reactivity can be either a good sign for later social development or a bad sign, depending on parenting.

Child Positive Emotionality × Negative and Less-Warm Parenting

Lahey and colleagues (2008) found that hostile parenting predicted child depression or conduct problems, but mainly when the child had low positive emotionality, and not when the child had high positive emotionality. Similarly, Cipriano and Stifter (2010) found that warmly controlling maternal behavior at age 2 predicted parent-rated effortful control of children at age 4 for exuberant (approaching and positively emotional) toddlers. However, effortful control outcomes of nonexuberant (either behaviorally inhibited or low-reactive) toddlers were not as well predicted by warmly controlling maternal behavior. Cipriano and Stifter also found that child effortful control outcomes measured by observation were predicted by low usage of neutral redirection/reasoning behaviors. Mothers who used more neutral-toned redirection/reason with their exuberant toddlers saw less child self-regulation in a laboratory visit 2 years later, whereas mothers who used neutral-redirection/reasoning with behaviorally inhibited or low-reactive children saw neutral or possibly even positive effects on child regulation. In short, this study suggests that self-regulation grows best, for exuberant children, in a warmly controlling or at least not-neutral-reasoning family. This is consistent with Kochanska's (1997) observation of the importance of warmly responsive parenting for the early development of conscience in young children with a highly approach-oriented, fearless temperament.

Child Self-Regulation × Parenting

In the previously noted patterns of child temperamental self-regulation in interaction with parenting to predict later adjustment (Bates et al., 2012), high levels of negative parenting or low levels of positive parenting predicted later behavior problems, but mainly for children who started with poor self-regulation; conversely, poor self-regulation mattered for later behavior problems mainly for those who experienced high levels of negative parenting or low levels of positive parenting (e.g., Bates, Pettit, Dodge, & Ridge,

1998; Degnan et al., 2008; Rubin et al., 2003). Some recent studies support and others do not support the previous pattern. Poehlmann and colleagues (2011) found that a measure theoretically related to effortful control—sustained attention in play with a colored block at 9 months—moderated the prediction from high-positive or nonangry parenting to more mature social development later. Infants who showed high sustained attention in the block task and experienced positive or low-anger mothering later showed better turn taking during a game with the mother than high-attention infants who experienced low positive or angry mothering, and also better turn taking than the low-attention infants. In addition, attentive infants in the block task who experienced maternal positive affect also showed slightly fewer internalizing behavior problems than those with low mother positivity or who were low in attention. If one considers high sustained attention in the block task at age 9 months to reflect a predecessor to effortful control, these three Poehlmann and colleagues findings suggest a pattern that is the opposite of the previously reviewed pattern: It was the highly attentive infant for whom parenting mattered, and the low attentive infant was not affected by parenting. On the other hand, Poehlmann and colleagues also found that low-attention infants with high-intrusive mothers ended up with more internalizing problems than if they had low-intrusive mothers. Those with low attention and highly intrusive mothering had the most internalizing problems of all children. The intrusiveness of the mother did not matter for the high-attentive children, who showed low levels of internalizing problems. This fourth pattern, in which parenting mattered more for predicting later internalizing problems for the inattentive infants, does support the previously reviewed pattern. All four of these patterns have a more a fan shaped than crossover or differential susceptibility shape.

The pattern in the first three attentiveness × parenting effects in Poehlmann and colleagues (2011) is supported by the Hilt and colleagues (2012) study. Young children with high effortful control and overcontrolling mothers had high levels of rumination in adolescence, whereas those with high effortful control and mothers who were not overcontrolling had the lowest level of rumination of all children. This pattern is the opposite of the pattern in which the effect of parenting is strongest for the low self-regulated children, and it is convergent with the pattern in which parenting matters more for children with high effortful control.

In contrast, support for the pattern in which parenting matters more for children with low self-regulation comes from Smith and colleagues (2012). Essentially, they found that the dopamine D4 receptor gene (*DRD4*) 7-repeat allele, believed to be related to impulsivity, magnified the association between high levels of negative parenting and low levels of 3-year-olds' self-regulation—defined as not waiting for turns in a cooperative, tower-building task and not being able to delay eating a candy. However, the genotype did not affect the relation between positive parenting and self-regulation outcome. Also supporting the pattern in which parenting matters more for dysregulated children, Leve and colleagues (2005) found that for temperamentally impulsive girls, parents' harsh discipline predicted acting-out problems, but for low-impulsive girls, harsh discipline predicted no worse, and perhaps better, outcomes than mild discipline. It will be interesting to see how future research finds that child temperamental self-regulation and parenting qualities interact in predicting child adjustment. We especially hope that it clarifies the conditions in which parenting matters more for both attentive and well-regulated and inattentive and dysregulated children.

Summary

In summary, studies showing interactions between child temperament and parenting in predicting child adjustment and other social development outcomes have continued to appear in recent years.

1. Children high in general negativity were at risk from high-negative or low-positive parenting in older studies. Newer studies generally confirmed this pattern.

2. Fearful children were at risk for externalizing problems from negative parenting in older studies. One newer study using cortisol reactivity, which may reflect stress from novelty, and therefore may reflect fearful temperament (Hastings et al., 2011), supports the outline of the older finding. However, another study found that not the children with high fear but those with low fear were most at risk from negative parenting (Leve et al., 2005). We can conclude, provisionally, that fearful children's risk for later problem behavior depends on the level of harsh or intrusively controlling parenting received, and that fearless children's risk depends on level of positive parenting received, and possibly, in some studies, also on level of negative parenting.

3. The pattern of interaction we saw in older studies between positive parenting and child fearfulness was interesting: Low-fear children were at risk for high externalizing and low positive adjustment because of the relative absence of positive parenting. We did not find a recent study on this.

4. We did find a recent study (Hastings et al., 2014) that is at least indirectly supportive of a very interesting pattern of interaction between challenging, "not-too-nice" parenting and fearfulness, in which high fear children were most at risk for internalizing problems when parenting was not challenging, perhaps too compliant and supportive, or overcontrolling in ways that would inhibit mastery learning, and perhaps deficient in opportunities for extinction of maladaptive fears.

5. Children with high frustrated reactivity were at risk because of overcontrolling parenting in an older study, and two newer studies roughly replicate that finding, if one agrees that there is conceptual overlap between parental overcontrol and lack of responsiveness.

6. Children with low positive emotionality were more at risk from negative parenting in a few older findings. In the one newer study we found on positive emotionality as a moderator (Cipriano & Stifter, 2010), children with high positive emotionality were more at risk from lack of positive parenting or heavy use of neutral-toned redirection.

7. In our final pattern, we had observed children with low self-regulation to be at risk for adjustment problems if they experienced high-negative or low-positive parenting. We found three newer studies that essentially confirmed this pattern. We also found three effects (in two studies) with an opposite pattern, in which children with high regulation were the ones who were at risk from high-negative or low-positive parenting. We do not see simple methodological variables, such as the nature of the adjustment construct, that could account for the difference in findings. At this point, we conclude that the evidence for the effects of parenting on children with low self-regulation is a little better than that on children with high self-regulation, but the picture is not yet resolved.

Conclusions

Early in the history of developmental psychology, it was common to think of temperament as nature and parenting as nurture. However, theory and the emerging empirical literature on temperament and parenting give reasons to see these two concepts as developmentally intertwined rather than as discrete influences in children's social development. We now prefer to think of temperament as a multilayered construct involving basic biological elements with experiential overlays, perhaps even to the level of experience-induced changes in biological roots of behavior differences (Bates, 1989). Child temperament measures have been found to predict parenting qualities, even in a handful of studies that control for initial levels of parenting. Nevertheless, the effects are generally modest and there are null findings; cross-study similarities in patterns are relatively few in number; and, with many different ways of operationally defining the research questions, full replications remain rare. The same can be said about parenting as a predictor of changes in child temperament. The findings do strongly hint that temperament and parenting might be seen as describing not just static traits but rather dynamic traits actively involved in the development of both children and parents. For example, a parent of a negatively emotional child might adapt by becoming less supportive over time, and a parent who is harsh may see increases in child negative emotionality across development. Although related, temperament and parenting are separate enough that it is still plausible to ask whether they have independent effects in forecasting child social development. Quite a few studies have now suggested that they do, but a number of studies have not found independent predictions from both variables. The imperfect association between temperament and parenting also allows for interactions between temperament and parenting in predicting social development. We see a number of plausible patterns of moderation by temperament of parenting effects or moderation by parenting of temperament effects. Given the methodological challenges of finding interaction effects, we are impressed to see as much evidence for patterns as we do see. However, just as with the research on temperament effects on parenting, parenting effects on temperament, and independent effects of both temperament and parenting on social development, the research on temperament–parenting moderation effects has many gaps. Studies are needed to clarify the mechanisms through which the observed interactions are found. For example, although the currently dominant theoretical interpretation of the pattern in which parenting produces both the best and the worst outcomes for children with high negative emotionality is that it is due to negative emotionality marking high child sensitivity to context (Bates, Schermerhorn, & Petersen, 2014), it is also possible that other processes could be at work. The actual process might involve parents' ability to respond (or not respond) to child irritability in effective ways. Irritable children with parents who are able to do this might turn out especially well because of their parents' "sensitivity," as much as or more than because of their own sensitivity. Alternatively, the mechanism might actually have more to do with a child's combination of temperament traits, (e.g., positive emotionality × effortful control), and the parenting variable may mainly reflect the child's pattern of behavior. We are now beginning to see studies that evaluate temperament × temperament × environment interactions (Hastings et al., 2014; Schermerhorn et al., 2013). As research improves understanding of social development, it becomes the basis for improved prevention and treatment. Indeed, practitioners are already considering possible applications of temperament, parenting, and temperament

× parenting concepts. As the research advances, and the meanings of temperament and parenting for one another and for social development become more clearly described, we expect that clinical and educational applications of temperament and parenting will become increasingly helpful.

NOTE

1. Another, possibly complementary interpretation is that the high initial cortisol level could reflect distress for the more approach-oriented child, under the assumption that the inhibited child might experience less stress by shrinking back from close interaction (Gunnar, 1994); a young child could be a little afraid of, but also impulsively approach, new people. For such children, punitive parenting could reflect a child effect, and the outcome of behavior problems could be as much due to the child's multidimensional temperament profile as to the child's adverse development in response to negative parenting. Many of the other interactions we review could reflect similar mechanisms. Nevertheless, in the absence of sufficient research to distinguish between these models, we emphasize the interpretation that harsh parenting creates anxiety, which interferes with social learning.

REFERENCES

Arcus, D. (2001). Inhibited and uninhibited children: Biology in the social context. In T. D. Wachs & G. A. Kohnstamm (Eds.), *Temperament in context* (pp. 43–60). Mahwah, NJ: Erlbaum.

Barker, E. D., Oliver, B. R., Viding, E., Salekin, R. T., & Maughan, B. (2011). The impact of prenatal maternal risk, fearless temperament and early parenting on adolescent callous–unemotional traits: A 14-year longitudinal investigation. *Journal of Child Psychology and Psychiatry, 52*(8), 878–888.

Bates, J. E. (1989). Concepts and measures of temperament. In G. A. Kohnstamm, J. E. Bates, & M. K. Rothbart (Eds.), *Temperament in childhood* (pp. 3–26). Chichester, UK: Wiley.

Bates, J. E. (2012). Temperament as a tool in promoting early childhood development. In S. L. Odom, E. P. Pungello, & N. Gardner-Neblett (Eds.), *Infants, toddlers, and families in poverty: Research implications for early child care* (pp. 153–177). New York: Guilford Press.

Bates, J. E. (1987). Temperament in infancy. In J. D. Osofsky (Ed.), *Handbook of infant development* (2nd ed., pp. 1101–1149). New York: Wiley.

Bates, J. E., Olson, S. L., Pettit, G. S., & Bayles, K. (1982). Dimensions of individuality in the mother–infant relationship at six months of age. *Child Development, 53*, 446–461.

Bates, J. E., & Pettit, G. S. (2007). Temperament, parenting, and socialization. In J. E. Grusec & P. D. Hastings (Eds.), *Handbook of socialization: Theory and research* (pp. 153–177). New York: Guilford Press.

Bates, J. E., Pettit, G. S., Dodge, K. A., & Ridge, B. (1998). Interaction of temperamental resistance to control and restrictive parenting in the development of externalizing behavior. *Developmental Psychology, 34*, 982–995.

Bates, J. E., Schermerhorn, A. C., & Petersen, I. T. (2012). Temperament and parenting in developmental perspective. In M. Zentner & R. L. Shiner (Eds.), *Handbook of temperament* (pp. 425–441). New York: Guilford Press.

Bates, J. E., Schermerhorn, A. C., & Petersen, I. T. (2014). Temperament concepts in developmental psychopathology. In M. Lewis & K. Rudolph (Eds.), *Handbook of developmental psychopathology* (3rd ed., pp. 311–329). New York: Guilford Press.

Bell, R. Q. (1968). A reinterpretation of the direction of effects in socialization research. *Psychological Review, 75*(2), 81–95.

Belsky, J., Bakermans-Kranenburg, M. J., & van IJzendoorn, M. H. (2007). For better and for worse: Differential susceptibility to environmental influences. *Current Directions in Psychological Science, 16*, 300–304.

Belsky, J., Fish, M., & Isabella, R. A. (1991). Continuity and discontinuity in infant negative and positive emotionality: Family antecedents and attachment consequences. *Developmental Psychology, 27*(3), 421–431.

Belsky, J., Hsieh, K.-H., & Crnic, K. (1998). Mothering, fathering, and infant negativity as antecedents of boys' externalizing problems and inhibition at age 3 years: Differential susceptibility to rearing experience? *Development and Psychopathology, 10*, 301–319.

Booth-LaForce, C., & Oxford, M. L. (2008). Trajectories of social withdrawal from grades 1 to 6: Prediction from early parenting, attachment, and temperament. *Developmental Psychology, 44*(5), 1298–1313.

Bradley, R. H., & Corwyn, R. F. (2008). Infant temperament, parenting, and externalizing behavior in the first grade: A test of the differential susceptibility hypothesis. *Journal of Child Psychology and Psychiatry, 49*, 124–131.

Braungart-Rieker, J. M., Hill-Soderlund, A. L., & Karrass, J. (2010). Fear and anger reactivity trajectories from 4 to 16 months: The roles of temperament, regulation, and maternal sensitivity. *Developmental Psychology, 46*(4), 791–804.

Bridgett, D. J., Gartstein, M. A., Putnam, S. P., Lance, K. O., Iddins, E., Waits, R., et al. (2011). Emerging effortful control in toddlerhood: The role of infant orienting/regulation, maternal effortful control, and maternal time spent in caregiving activities. *Infant Behavior and Development, 34*, 189–199.

Bridgett, D. J., Laake, L. M., Gartstein, M. A., & Dorn, D. (2013). Development of infant positive emotionality: The contribution of maternal characteristics and effects on subsequent parenting. *Infant and Child Development, 22*(4), 362–382.

Bugental, D. B., & Grusec, J. E. (2006). Socialization processes. In W. Damon & R. M. Lerner (Editors-in-Chief) & N. Eisenberg (Vol. Ed.), *Handbook of child psychology* (pp. 366–428). New York: Wiley.

Chess, S., & Thomas, A. (1984). *Origins and evolution of behavior disorders.* New York: Brunner/Mazel.

Cipriano, E. A., & Stifter, C. A. (2010). Predicting preschool effortful control from toddler temperament and parenting behavior. *Journal of Applied Developmental Psychology, 31*, 221–230.

Collins, W. A., Maccoby, E. E., Steinberg, L., Hetherington, E. M., & Bornstein, M. H. (2000). Contemporary research on parenting: The case for nature and nurture. *American Psychologist, 55*, 218–232.

Crockenberg, S. (1986). Are temperamental differences in babies associated with predictable differences in care giving? *New Directions for Child Development, 31*, 53–73.

Degnan, K. A., Almas, A. N., & Fox, N. A. (2010). Temperament and the environment in the etiology of childhood anxiety. *Journal of Child Psychology and Psychiatry, 51*(4), 497–517.

Degnan, K. A., Calkins, S. D., Keane, S. P., & Hill-Soderlund, A. L. (2008). Profiles of disruptive behavior across early childhood: Contributions of frustration reactivity, physiological regulation, and maternal behavior. *Child Development, 79*(5), 1357–1376.

Dodge, K. A., & Pettit, G. S. (2003). A biopsychosocial model of the development of chronic conduct problems in adolescence. *Developmental Psychology, 39*(2), 349–371.

Eisenberg, N., Fabes, R. A., Shepard, S. A., Guthrie, I. K., Murphy, B. C., & Reiser, M. (1999). Parental reactions to children's negative emotions: Longitudinal relations to quality of children's social functioning. *Child Development, 70*(2), 513–534.

Eisenberg, N., Vidmar, M. A., Spinrad, T. L., Eggum, N. D., Edwards, A., Gaertner, B., et al. (2010). Mothers' teaching strategies and children's effortful control: A longitudinal study. *Developmental Psychology, 46*, 1294–1308.

Fox, N. A., Henderson, H. A., Marshall, P. J., Nichols, K. E., & Ghera, M. M. (2005). Behavioral inhibition: Linking biology and behavior within a developmental framework. *Annual Review of Psychology, 56*, 235–262.

Frankel, K. A., & Bates, J. E. (1990). Mother–toddler problem-solving: Antecedents in attachment, home behavior, and temperament. *Child Development, 61*, 810–819.

Ganiban, J. M., Saudino, K. J., Ulbricht, J., Neiderhiser, J. M., & Reiss, D. (2008). Stability and change in temperament during adolescence. *Journal of Personality and Social Psychology, 95*, 222–236.

Gauvain, M., & Fagot, B. (1995). Child temperament as a mediator of mother–toddler problem solving. *Social Development, 4*(3), 257–276.

Goldsmith, H. H., Buss, K. A., & Lemery, K. S. (1997). Toddler and childhood temperament: Expanded content, stronger genetic evidence, new evidence for the importance of environment. *Developmental Psychology, 33*(6), 891–905.

Goldsmith, H. H., Lemery, K. S., Buss, K. A., & Campos, J. J. (1999). Genetic analyses of focal aspects of infant temperament. *Developmental Psychology, 35*, 972–985.

Goodnight, J. A., Bates, J. E., Pettit, G. S., & Dodge, K. A. (2008). Parents' campaigns to reduce their children's conduct problems: Interactions with temperamental resistance to control. *European Journal of Developmental Science, 2*, 100–119.

Gunnar, M. R. (1994). Psychoendocrine studies of temperament and stress in early childhood: Expanding current models. In J. E. Bates & T. D. Wachs (Eds.), *Temperament: Individual differences at the interface of biology and behavior* (pp. 175–198). Washington, DC: American Psychological Association.

Haltigan, J. D., Roisman, G. I., & Fraley, R. C. (2013). The predictive significance of early caregiving experiences for symptoms of psychopathology through midadolescence: Enduring or transient effects? *Development and Psychopathology, 25*, 209–221.

Hane, A. A., Cheah, C., Rubin, K. H., & Fox, N. A. (2008). The role of maternal behavior in the relation between shyness and social reticence in early childhood and social withdrawal in middle childhood. *Social Development, 17*, 795–811.

Hastings, P. D., Kahle, S., & Nuselovici, J. M. (2014). How well socially wary preschoolers fare over time depends on their parasympathetic regulation and socialization. *Child Development, 85*(4), 1586–1600.

Hastings, P. D., & Rubin, K. H. (1999). Predicting mothers' beliefs about preschool-aged children's social behavior: Evidence for maternal attitudes moderating child effects. *Child Development, 70*(3), 722–741.

Hastings, P. D., Ruttle, P. L., Serbin, L. A., Mills, R. S. L., Stack, D. M., & Schwartzman, A. E. (2011). Adrenocortical responses to strangers in preschoolers: Relations with parenting, temperament, and psychopathology. *Developmental Psychobiology, 53*, 694–710.

Hilt, L. M., Armstrong, J. M., & Essex, M. J. (2012). Early family context and development of adolescent ruminative style: Moderation by temperament. *Cognition and Emotion, 26*, 916–926.

Karreman, A., van Tuijl, C., van Aken, M. A. G., & Deković, M. (2006). Parenting and self-regulation in preschoolers: A meta-analysis. *Infant and Child Development, 15*, 561–579.

Karreman, A., van Tuijl, C., van Aken, M. A. G., & Deković, M. (2008). The relation between parental personality and observed parenting: The moderating role of preschoolers' effortful control. *Personality and Individual Differences, 44*(3), 723–734.

Kennedy, A. E., Rubin, K. H., Hastings, P. D., & Maisel, B. (2004). Longitudinal relations between child vagal tone and parenting behavior: 2 to 4 years. *Developmental Psychobiology, 45*, 10–21.

Kiff, C. J., Lengua, L. J., & Zalewski, M. (2011). Nature and nurturing: Parenting in the context of child temperament. *Clinical Child and Family Psychology Review, 14*, 251–301.

Kim, S., & Kochanska, G. (2012). Child temperament moderates effects of parent–child mutuality on self-regulation: A relationship-based path for emotionally negative infants. *Child Development, 83*, 1275–1289.

Kimonis, E. R., Frick, P. J., Boris, N. W., Smyke, A. T., Cornell, A. H., Farrell, J. M., et al. (2006). Callous–unemotional features, behavioral inhibition, and parenting: Independent predictors of aggression in a high-risk preschool sample. *Journal of Child and Family Studies, 15*(6), 741–752.

Kochanska, G. (1995). Children's temperament, mothers' discipline, and security of attachment: Multiple pathways to emerging internalization. *Child Development, 66,* 597–615.

Kochanska, G. (1997). Multiple pathways to conscience for children with different temperaments: From toddlerhood to age 5. *Developmental Psychology, 33,* 228–240.

Kochanska, G., Aksan, N., & Joy, M. E. (2007). Children's fearfulness as a moderator of parenting in early socialization: Two longitudinal studies. *Developmental Psychology, 43,* 222–237.

Kochanska, G., Friesenborg, A. E., Lange, L. A., & Martel, M. M. (2004). Parents' personality and infants' temperament as contributors to their emerging relationship. *Journal of Personality and Social Psychology, 86*(5), 744–759.

Kochanska, G., & Kim, S. (2013). Difficult temperament moderates links between maternal responsiveness and children's compliance and behavior problems in low-income families. *Journal of Child Psychology and Psychiatry, 54*(3), 323–332.

Kochanska, G., Kim, S., Barry, R. A., & Philibert, R. A. (2011). Children's genotypes interact with maternal responsive care in predicting children's competence: Diathesis-stress or differential susceptibility? *Development and Psychopathology, 23,* 605–616.

Kochanska, G., Murray, K. T., & Harlan, E. T. (2000). Effortful control in early childhood: Continuity and change, antecedents, and implications for social development. *Developmental Psychology, 36*(2), 220–232.

Kolak, A. M., & Volling, B. L. (2013). Coparenting moderates the association between firstborn children's temperament and problem behavior across the transition to siblinghood. *Journal of Family Psychology, 27,* 355–364.

Ladd, G. W., & Pettit, G. S. (2002). Parenting and the development of children's peer relationships. In M. H. Bornstein (Ed.), *Handbook of parenting: Vol. 5. Practical issues in parenting* (2nd ed., pp. 269–310). Mahwah, NJ: Erlbaum.

Lahey, B. B., Van Hulle, C. A., Keenan, K., Rathouz, P. J., D'Onofrio, B. M., Rodgers, J. L., et al. (2008). Temperament and parenting during the first year predict future child conduct problems. *Journal of Abnormal Child Psychology, 36,* 1139–1158.

Lee, C. L., & Bates, J. E. (1985). Mother–child interaction at age two years and perceived difficult temperament. *Child Development, 56,* 1314–1325.

Lee, E. H., Zhou, Q., Eisenberg, N., & Wang, Y. (2013). Bidirectional relations between temperament and parenting styles in Chinese children. *International Journal of Behavioral Development, 37,* 57–67.

Lengua, L. J. (2006). Growth in temperament and parenting as predictors of adjustment during children's transition to adolescence. *Developmental Psychology, 42*(5), 819–832.

Lengua, L. J. (2008). Anxiousness, frustration, and effortful control as moderators of the relation between parenting and adjustment in middle childhood. *Social Development, 17,* 554–577.

Lengua, L. J., & Kovacs, E. A. (2005). Bidirectional associations between temperament and parenting and the prediction of adjustment problems in middle childhood. *Journal of Applied Developmental Psychology, 26*(1), 21–38.

Lengua, L. J., & Wachs, T. D. (2012). Temperament and risk: Resilient and vulnerable responses to adversity. In M. Zentner & R. L. Shiner (Eds.), *Handbook of temperament* (pp. 519–540). New York: Guilford Press.

Leve, L. D., Kim, H. K., & Pears, K. C. (2005). Childhood temperament and family environment as predictors of internalizing and externalizing trajectories from ages 5 to 17. *Journal of Abnormal Child Psychology, 33,* 505–520.

Lewis-Morrarty, E., Degnan, K. A., Chronis-Tuscano, A., Rubin, K. H., Cheah, C. S. L., Pine, D. S., et al. (2012). Maternal over-control moderates the association between early childhood behavioral inhibition and adolescent social anxiety symptoms. *Journal of Abnormal Child Psychology, 40,* 1363–1373.

Lindhout, I. E., Markus, M. T., Hoogendijk, T. H. G., & Boer, F. (2009). Temperament and parental child-rearing style: Unique contributions to clinical anxiety disorders in childhood. *European Child and Adolescent Psychiatry, 18*, 439–446.

Maccoby, E. E. (1992). The role of parents in the socialization of children: An historical overview. *Developmental Psychology, 28*(6), 1006–1017.

Maccoby, E. E., & Martin, J. A. (1983). Socialization in the context of the family: Parent–child interaction. In P. H. Mussen & E. M. Hetherington (Eds.), *Handbook of child psychology: Vol. 4. Socialization, personality, and social development* (4th ed., pp. 1–101). New York: Wiley.

Mize, J., & Pettit, G. S. (1997). Mothers' social coaching, mother–child relationship style, and children's peer competence: Is the medium the message? *Child Development, 68*(2), 312–332.

Moffitt, T. E., & Caspi, A. (2007) Evidence from behavioral genetics for environmental contributions to antisocial conduct. In J. E. Grusec & P. D. Hastings (Eds.), *Handbook of socialization theory and research* (pp. 96–123). New York: Guilford Press.

Molfese, V. J., Rudasill, K. M., & Molfese D. L. (2013). Sleep in preschoolers: School readiness, academics, temperament, and behavior. In A. Wolfson & H. Montgomery-Downs (Eds.), *The Oxford handbook of infant, child and adolescent sleep and behavior* (pp. 397–413). New York: Oxford University Press.

Natsuaki, M. N., Leve, L. D., Harold, G. T., Neiderhiser, J. M., Shaw, D. S., Ganiban, J., et al. (2013). Transactions between child social wariness and observed structured parenting: Evidence from a prospective adoption study. *Child Development, 84*, 1750–1765.

Neyer, F. J., & Lehnart, J. (2007). Relationships matter in personality development: Evidence from an 8-year longitudinal study across young adulthood. *Journal of Personality, 75*, 535–568.

Park, S.-Y., Belsky, J., Putnam, S., & Crnic, K. (1997). Infant emotionality, parenting, and 3-year inhibition: Exploring stability and lawful discontinuity in a male sample. *Developmental Psychology, 33*, 218–227.

Pauli-Pott, U., Mertesacker, B., & Beckmann, D. (2004). Predicting the development of infant emotionality from maternal characteristics. *Development and Psychopathology, 16*(1), 19–42.

Paulussen-Hoogeboom, M. C., Stams, G. J. J. M., Hermanns, J. M. A., & Peetsma, T. T. D. (2007). Child negative emotionality and parenting from infancy to preschool: A meta-analytic review. *Developmental Psychology, 43*, 438–453.

Pettit, G. S., & Bates, J. E. (1989). Family interaction patterns and children's behavior problems from infancy to age 4 years. *Developmental Psychology, 25*, 413–420.

Pluess, M., & Belsky, J. (2010). Differential susceptibility to parenting and quality child care. *Developmental Psychology, 46*, 379–390.

Poehlmann, J., Schwichtenberg, A. J. M., Shlafer, R. J., Hahn, E., Bianchi, J.-P., & Warner, R. (2011). Emerging self-regulation in toddlers born preterm or low birth weight: Differential susceptibility to parenting. *Development and Psychopathology, 23*, 177–193.

Rapee, R. M., Kennedy, S. J., Ingram, M., Edwards, S. L., & Sweeney, L. (2010). Altering the trajectory of anxiety in at-risk young children. *American Journal of Psychiatry, 167*, 1518–1525.

Rapee, R. M., Schniering, C. A., & Hudson, J. L. (2009). Anxiety disorders during childhood and adolescence: Origins and treatment. *Annual Review of Clinical Psychology, 5*, 311–341.

Raver, C. C., Blair, C., Willoughby, M., & the Family Life Project Key Investigators. (2013). Poverty as a predictor of 4-year-olds' executive function: New perspectives on models of differential susceptibility. *Developmental Psychology, 49*, 292–304.

Roisman, G. I., Newman, D. A., Fraley, R. C., Haltigan, J. D., Groh, A. M., & Haydon, K. C. (2012). Distinguishing differential susceptibility from diathesis-stress: Recommendations for evaluating interaction effects. *Development and Psychopathology, 24*, 389–409.

Rothbart, M. K. (2011). *Becoming who we are: Temperament and personality in development.* New York: Guilford Press.

Rothbart, M. K., & Bates, J. E. (1998). Temperament. In W. Damon (Editor-in-Chief) & N.

Eisenberg (Vol. Ed.), *Handbook of child psychology: Vol. 3. Social, emotional, and personality development* (5th ed., pp. 105–176). Hoboken, NJ: Wiley.

Rothbart, M. K., & Bates, J. E. (2006). Temperament. In N. Eisenberg, W. Damon, & R. M. Lerner (Eds.), *Handbook of child psychology: Social, emotional, and personality development* (6th ed., Vol. 4, pp. 99–166). Hoboken, NJ: Wiley.

Rubin, K. H., Burgess, K. B., Dwyer, K. M., & Hastings, P. D. (2003). Predicting preschoolers' externalizing behaviors from toddler temperament, conflict, and maternal negativity. *Developmental Psychology, 19*, 164–176.

Rubin, K. H., & Mills, R. S. L. (1991). Conceptualizing developmental pathways to internalizing disorders in childhood. *Canadian Journal of Behavioural Science, 23*(3), 300–317.

Rubin, K. H., Nelson, L. J., Hastings, P., & Asendorpf, J. (1999). The transaction between parents' perceptions of their children's shyness and their parenting styles. *International Journal of Behavioral Development, 23*(4), 937–957.

Sameroff, A. J. (2009). Conceptual issues in studying the development of self-regulation. In S. L. Olson & A. J. Sameroff (Eds.), *Biopsychosocial regulatory processes in the development of childhood behavioral problems* (pp. 1–18). New York: Cambridge University Press.

Scaramella, L. V., Sohr-Preston, S. L., Mirabile, S. P., Robison, S. D., & Callahan, K. L. (2008). Parenting and children's distress reactivity during toddlerhood: An examination of direction of effects. *Social Development, 17*, 578–595.

Schermerhorn, A. C., Bates, J. E., Goodnight, J. A., Lansford, J. E., Dodge, K. A., & Pettit, G. S. (2013). Temperament moderates associations between exposure to stress and children's externalizing problems. *Child Development, 84*(5), 1579–1593.

Sheeber, L. (1995). Empirical dissociations between temperament and behavior problems: A response to the Sanson, Prior and Kyrios study. *Merrill–Palmer Quarterly, 41*, 554–561.

Smith, H. J., Sheikh, H. I., Dyson, M. W., Olino, T. M., Laptook, R. S., Durbin, C. E., et al. (2012). Parenting and child DRD4 genotype interact to predict children's early emerging effortful control. *Child Development, 83*, 1932–1944.

Sroufe, L. A., & Rutter, M. (1984). The domain of developmental psychopathology. *Development and Psychopathology, 55*, 17–29.

Taylor, Z. E., Eisenberg, N., Spinrad, T. L., & Widaman, K. F. (2013). Longitudinal relations of intrusive parenting and effortful control to ego-resiliency during early childhood. *Child Development, 84*, 1145–1151.

Thomas, A., Chess, S., Birch, H. G., Herzig, M. E., & Korn, S. (1963). *Behavioral individuality in early childhood*. New York: New York University Press.

Ursache, A., Blair, C., Stifter, C., & Voegtline, K. (2013). Emotional reactivity and regulation in infancy interact to predict executive functioning in early childhood. *Developmental Psychology, 49*, 127–137.

Wachs, T. D., & Bates, J. E. (2010). Temperament. In J. G. Bremner & T. D. Wachs (Eds.), *Wiley-Blackwell handbook of infant development: Vol. 1. Basic research* (2nd ed., pp. 592–622). Malden, MA: Wiley-Blackwell.

Willams, L. R., Degnan, K. A., Perez-Edgar, K. E., Henderson, H. A., Rubin, K. H., Pine, D. S., et al. (2009). Impact of behavioral inhibition and parenting style on internalizing and externalizing problems from early childhood through adolescence. *Journal of Abnormal Child Psychology, 37*(8), 1063–1075.

Zuckerman, M. (1991). *Psychobiology of personality*. New York: Cambridge University Press.

CHAPTER 17

Biological and Psychological Processes Linking Chronic Family Stress to Substance Abuse and Obesity

Rena L. Repetti
Theodore F. Robles
Bridget M. Reynolds

The socialization that children receive at home helps lay the foundation for their long-term health and well-being. Although connections between early rearing experiences and future health are complex and multilayered, there are promising advances in our understanding of how the family's shaping of emotional, behavioral, and biological processes—and the linkages between them—contributes to health outcomes (Repetti, Taylor, & Seeman, 2002). Our chapter focuses on obesity and substance abuse, two significant public health challenges that result from dysfunctional behavior and share common mechanisms that link them to family environments.

Adolescent alcohol and drug use, described as an epidemic, has consequences that place enormous burdens on health care, criminal justice, education, and social service systems (see, e.g., National Center on Addiction and Substance Abuse [CASA], 2011). Increased rates of obese and overweight children, also described as an epidemic, are especially worrisome because of the physical and psychosocial consequences that continue into adulthood, including reduced life expectancy (Garasky, Stewart, Gundersen, Lohman, & Eisenmann, 2009; Reilly et al., 2003).

An obvious risk factor for substance use problems is a household in which parents, siblings, and other members regularly misuse alcohol and other substances (Bowles, DeHart, & Webb, 2012). The family is likewise key to understanding how children and adolescents develop obesity. Routines around eating, sleeping, physical activity, screen time, as well as the "food environment" in the home (which includes access to fresh fruits and vegetables, and parent knowledge, attitudes, and preferences regarding food, eating, and meal preparation) can modify risk for obesity in offspring (Fiese, Hammons, Bost, & Wiley, 2013). However, family practices specifically related to the use of substances or to eating and exercise are not the primary foci of this chapter. Our analysis highlights a different type of socialization experience: chronic stress in a child's emotional and social environment that leads to difficulties with self-regulation, which, we argue, comprise a common pathway that connects stressful family environments to both the abuse of substances and unhealthy patterns of eating.

Our chapter integrates these research findings with several biological processes that may play a role in both obesity and substance abuse, and whose functions have been directly or indirectly linked with chronic family stress. Given that adolescence is a critical period for the development of both obesity and substance abuse, the first biological factor we discuss is pubertal maturation. We next review evidence suggesting that the development of the hypothalamic–pituitary–adrenal (HPA) stress response system and inflammatory responses are influenced by chronic family stress. Those biological processes are then tied to the functioning of the dopaminergic reward system in the brain, the neuronal circuits that are associated with the "wanting" that motivates behaviors such as overeating and substance use.

Figure 17.1 presents a schematic diagram depicting the key family, biological, psychological, behavioral, and health variables that are discussed in this chapter.

The Roles of Chronic Stressors in the Family and Problems with Self-Regulation in Substance Abuse and Obesity

In the next two sections, we review research linking substance abuse and obesity to childhood family environments and problems with self-regulation. We then highlight negative and positive urgency, patterns of rash action in the face of strong emotion, as elements of emotion dysregulation that translate into problems with substance use and eating.

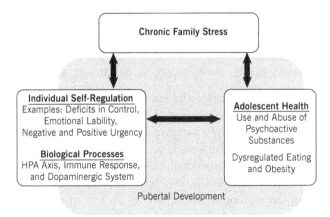

FIGURE 17.1. Psychological and biological processes linking chronic family stress to substance abuse and obesity in adolescence.

Substance Use and Abuse

Family Risk Factors for Substance Use and Abuse

Individual traits, social context, and genetic factors combine to shape vulnerability to substance use problems in adolescence. Developmental psychologists have described a dynamic cascade model in which early experiences interact with individual characteristics to set in motion a chain of events that magnify over time (Dodge et al., 2009). Social ecologies of the peer group, neighborhood, and school can each play a role, but the family environment is a primary contributor early in the cascade. In addition to socialization specific to substance use in the home (Bowles et al., 2012), certain chronic stressors in the family also increase the likelihood of substance abuse in adolescence. Sexual, physical, or emotional abuse, as well as other adversities during childhood, including the death of a loved one, and the emotional or physical absence of a parent, increase vulnerability (Bowles et al., 2012). A lack of stability at home, such as frequent maternal partner change, when coupled with lower maternal control, predicts problematic drinking later in adolescence (Alati et al., 2010).

In addition to exposure to abuse, loss, and instability in the home, deficient parenting and a negative emotional climate during childhood can also act as chronic stressors and, most importantly, as training grounds for self-regulation and coping strategies that ultimately increase attraction to substances during the teenage years. Harsh discipline tactics, ineffective control, and poor supervision and monitoring in adolescence are risk factors for substance abuse (Dodge et al., 2009). Poor management—reflected in parents' lack of knowledge about children's whereabouts, a lack of clear family rules, less time spent discussing important issues, and a failure to acknowledge children's achievements and positive behavior—also predicts substance use disorders in adulthood (Herrenkohl, Lee, Kosterman, & Hawkins, 2012). Many studies point to conflict and a lack of support at home as increasing risk for the problematic use of alcohol and other substances (Repetti et al., 2002). In a large longitudinal study, family conflict in childhood was the strongest and most consistent predictor of substance use disorders in adulthood (Herrenkohl et al., 2012). Although these experiences may be more or less pertinent at different developmental stages (Dodge et al., 2009), they all contribute to self-regulation deficits in children, such as problems with delay of gratification and emotional lability (Crossley & Buckner, 2012), that are also observed in substance abusers.

Problems with Self-Regulation as Risk Factors for Substance Abuse

Difficulties with cognitive, behavioral, and emotional self-regulation, which are associated with growing up in a chronically stressful family environment, predict an increased risk for future substance abuse. For example, deficits in cognitive functioning, encompassing executive control mechanisms such as working memory and mental planning, have been identified in stimulant-dependent individuals and their siblings (Ersche et al., 2012). *Effortful control*, which is considered to be central to the regulation of emotion and behavior, involves the conscious, voluntary regulation of attention and persistence, and the ability to suppress a more pressing or dominant response in favor of behavior that may have long-term value to the individual. Either alone, or in conjunction with a substance use lifestyle (e.g., friends who abuse substances), deficits in effortful control during adolescence predict progressions to problematic tobacco, marijuana, and alcohol use in early adulthood (Piehler, Véronneau, & Dishion, 2012).

Severe affective and behavioral dysregulation in childhood (including anxiety and depression, attention problems, and aggressive behavior) predict a higher likelihood of substance use disorder in young adulthood, and poorer overall functioning (Holtmann et al., 2011). Dodge and colleagues (2009) highlight the presence of externalizing symptoms in general, and conduct problems in particular, as risk factors for the later development of substance use disorders. Underlying these behavior problems may be an unusually strong tendency for novelty, or sensation seeking, and a generally uncontrolled temperament, as seen in children who are impulsive, restless, negativistic, distractible, and labile in their emotional responses (Dodge et al., 2009; Holtmann et al., 2011).

Figure 17.1 depicts self-regulation as a link between chronic stressors in the family and risk for adolescent substance abuse. We suggest that a chaotic and stressful childhood home marked by conflict and a lack of support impedes the development of good self-regulation skills. The fact that the same family characteristics are associated with such a wide array of adverse outcomes suggests that interactions with preexisting risks represent the primary mechanism of family influence. Some child vulnerabilities based on temperament and genetic predispositions may modulate the effects of chronic stressors in the family, and the expression of those vulnerabilities may also be exacerbated in risky families (Repetti et al., 2002).

Unhealthy Eating and Obesity

Family Risk Factors for Unhealthy Eating and Obesity

Like substance abuse, obesity is complex and multidetermined. The risk factors that contribute to overweight children cut across different levels, encompassing genes, personality, and a child's larger social context, including socioeconomic status, and peer and neighborhood characteristics; chief among the social environmental factors is the family (Schreier & Chen, 2012). Among other mechanisms, the association between poverty and obesity is thought to be partially mediated by behaviors related to acquiring, providing, and distributing food at home, which can lead to a sense of food insecurity in some children and the unhealthy eating patterns often found in overweight children (McCurdy, Gorman, & Metallinos-Katsaras, 2010). Parents' knowledge, attitudes, and behaviors related to eating and physical activity all play a role (Hendrie, Coveney, & Cox, 2012; Puder & Munsch, 2010; Schreier & Chen, 2012).

Other aspects of the family social environment, besides the socialization of habits that revolve around diet and physical activity, are also relevant. Rates of overweight and obesity in childhood are higher in single-parent households and those not headed by stable two-married-parent families (Garasky et al., 2009; Schmeer, 2012). Certain styles of parenting are risk factors, including parenting that is harsh and punitive (K. E. Grant et al., 2003; Schreier & Chen, 2012), authoritarian (Garasky et al., 2009), or controlling, although other evidence points to more indulgent or permissive parenting (Hoerr et al., 2009; Olvera & Power, 2010; Schreier & Chen, 2012). Lack of emotional support, parental neglect, and difficult communication with parents are also risk factors (Garasky et al., 2009; Schreier & Chen, 2012; Vander Wal, 2012; Wen, Simpson, Baur, Rissel, & Flood, 2011). Rates of obesity are greater among children exposed to ineffective parenting (Brotman et al., 2012) and a broad array of indicators of unhealthy family functioning, including a negative emotional climate, avoidance of open discussion of concerns or fears, and difficulty making decisions and planning family activities (Wen et al., 2011). The parenting and family social climate variables described here are consistent with research indicating that chronic stress in the family is associated with increased risk for overweight and obesity in children (Evans, Fuller-Rowell & Doan, 2012; Puder & Munsch, 2010; Schreier & Chen, 2012; Stenhammar et al., 2010).

Problems with Self-Regulation as Risk Factors for Obesity

Several emotional and behavioral characteristics that are overrepresented in obese children and teens are also associated with chronically stressful family environments, such as poor self-awareness, and higher rates of internalizing and externalizing symptoms (Brotman et al., 2012; Harrist et al., 2012; Puder & Munsch, 2010; Schreier & Chen, 2012). Other evidence suggests increased risk taking both in obese adolescents (Ratcliff, Jenkins, Reiter-Purtill, Noll, & Zeller, 2011) and teens from risky families (Repetti et al., 2002). Although emotional problems may result from the social obstacles that obese children face, emotional and behavioral factors also contribute to unhealthy eating patterns.

One of the vulnerabilities observed in many obese children and adolescents is increased reactivity to stress and poor self-regulation (Harrist et al., 2012; Schreier & Chen, 2012). As depicted in Figure 17.1, research evidence is consistent with the idea that one pathway to obesity and overweight begins in a childhood family environment that is harsh, neglectful, and chronically stressful, one that does not facilitate developing effective means for regulating emotions and behavior, perhaps through interactions with child temperament or other preexisting risk factors. When children face social and emotional challenges in daily life, unhealthy eating behaviors may represent a way of coping (Evans, Fuller-Rowell, & Doan, 2012; Schreier & Chen, 2012). For example, researchers have identified a pattern of "emotional" eating (Harrist et al., 2012), or an increase in food consumption, particularly high sucrose and fatty foods, in response to stress (Evans et al., 2012). Both state and trait anxiety are associated with episodes of emotional eating in obese individuals (Schneider, Appelhans, Whited, Oleski, & Pagoto, 2010) and with binge eating in female college students (Fitzsimmons-Craft, Bardone-Cone, Brownstone, & Harney, 2012).

Negative and Positive Urgency in Substance Abuse and Obesity

The research literatures on precursors of substance abuse and obesity contain at least two common threads: chronic stress in the early family environment and problems with self-regulation. We focus here on positive and negative urgency, the tendency to engage in rash, ill-considered action when experiencing intense emotion, as one pattern of self-regulation that may help to explain individual differences in adolescents' risky behavior (Cyders & Smith, 2008). *Negative urgency* is impulsive behavior in response to distress that can lead to coping through escape and self-medication. Although self-regulation deficits are common to many emotional and behavioral problems, the inclination to act rashly when distressed, rather than the experience of distress alone, may be specifically associated with engaging in risky behaviors (Settles et al., 2012). *Positive urgency* is a tendency to act rashly in response to positive mood.

Alcohol consumption can provide escape from distress for some individuals and is reinforced by distraction. Other individuals misuse alcohol in an intense positive mood state. In fact, both negative urgency and positive urgency predict increases in alcohol use and alcohol dependence symptoms in college students (Cyders, Flory, Rainer, & Smith, 2009; Settles et al., 2012; Stojek & Fisher, 2013). With respect to dysregulated eating, negative urgency increases the odds of future binge eating in female college students (Fischer, Peterson, & McCarthy, 2013), and the two are associated through negative reinforcement; the binge distracts from the original source of distress and provides a short-term positive experience (Fischer, Smith, & Cyders, 2008).

Although negative and positive urgency have been conceptualized as personality traits and are therefore generally not studied within a family socialization or stress framework, they are associated with experiences in the family. Negative urgency underlies "emotional eating" as a response to stress, and both emotional eating by parents and parental punishment without justification or explanation have been linked to emotional eating in children (Snoek, Engels, Janssens, & van Strien, 2007; Topham et al., 2011). In adolescent girls, less closeness to fathers was associated with higher positive urgency scores (Rostad, 2012). The connection from chronic family stress to problems regulating emotions and behavior (Repetti et al., 2002) suggests that researchers should explore how urgent reactions to intense emotion may be influenced by the kinds of family socialization experiences highlighted here.

Adolescence is a critical period for understanding how individual and family patterns included in Figure 17.1 combine to shape risk for substance abuse and obesity. Next, we highlight how pubertal maturation may contribute to these processes.

Adolescence and Puberty as Key Developmental Contexts

Often described as a sensitive period in development, adolescence sees a dramatic rise in morbidity and mortality, ushers in heightened risk for psychiatric disorder and deviant behavior, and further solidifies many patterns of behavior and regulation that play a role in the onset of health problems into adulthood. Given its far-reaching impacts on emotion, behavior, and physiology, pubertal maturation (the shaded area in the Figure 17.1) represents a key developmental context in which the regulatory processes described earlier become increasingly stable, forming the groundwork for later health problems.

Youth from harsh and controlling or cold and neglectful homes manifest maladjustment across a broad spectrum of functioning. With this adjustment profile as a backdrop, the challenges associated with pubertal maturation can prove especially difficult. Children reared in stressful home environments not only encounter puberty with low levels of parental supportiveness, but they also lack adequate regulatory resources to cope with its associated stressors.

Experiencing puberty at a younger than normal age can be particularly stressful, due to not only the social challenges associated with being the first among peers to develop, but also because early maturing youth have less time to acquire and strengthen cognitive and emotion regulation skills prior to confronting pubertal changes (Susman & Dorn, 2009). A large body of research has linked early pubertal development with a range of psychological, behavioral, and social adjustment difficulties (Graber, Lewinsohn, Seeley, & Brooks-Gunn, 1997; Mendle, Turkheimer, & Emery, 2007), including substance use and obesity (e.g., Biehl, Natsuaki, & Ge, 2007; Prentice & Viner, 2012; Westling, Andrews, & Peterson, 2012). We also know that early maturation is itself associated with stressful family environments (e.g., Ellis & Essex, 2007; Saxbe & Repetti, 2009). Below, we provide a brief overview of research linking early family experiences with the timing and pace of pubertal development. We then review literature linking early pubertal maturation with risk for substance use and obesity, and describe the interplay between family environment and pubertal development in predicting these negative adolescent health outcomes.

Chronic Family Stress and Pubertal Development

Numerous factors play a role in the timing and tempo of pubertal development, including environmental conditions. Much of the research on this topic has focused on females, in part because menarche allows for a relatively concrete assessment of pubertal maturation. Recent work prospectively links family conflict and parent marital behavior with daughters' earlier pubertal development. Specifically, parents who reported greater levels of marital conflict had daughters whose physical development was more advanced when assessed 2 years later in sixth grade (Saxbe & Repetti, 2009). A composite measure of "family nonsupportiveness" during the preschool years was associated with earlier adrenarche in first grade among children of both sexes, and more advanced development of secondary sexual characteristics among daughters in fifth grade (Ellis & Essex, 2007). Similarly, maternal reports of a harsh and cold parenting style prior to age 5 prospectively predicted daughters' early pubertal maturation (Belsky et al., 2007). Childhood maltreatment (physical or sexual abuse, neglect) was also linked with earlier physical development among girls (Costello, Sung, Worthman, & Angold, 2007), and family disruptions, particularly father absence, predicted earlier age of menarche (Bogaert, 2005; Quinlan, 2003).

Although isolating specific biological mediators of the timing and tempo of pubertal development is challenging, research is illuminating a complex interplay among genetics, stress physiology, and environmental factors (e.g., Ellis, Shirtcliff, Boyce, Deardorff, & Essex, 2011; Graber, Sontag, & Brooks-Gunn, 2009; Susman & Dorn, 2009; Walker, Sabuwalla, & Huout, 2004). Neuroendocrine axes (including the HPA axis) regulate pubertal development and may be implicated in linking family stress with early physical maturation. For example, low family supportiveness in preschool predicted faster initial pubertal tempo and more advanced pubertal maturation by age 12.5 years, but only among children with heightened cardiovascular and cortisol reactivity to stress (Ellis et al., 2011). Overall, research on whether stress response systems might explain links between early family characteristics and pubertal development remains inconclusive, in part because genetic and body composition factors that influence pubertal timing are also associated with family stress and HPA axis functioning (Susman & Dorn, 2009). In addition, cortisol reactivity to acute stressors normatively increases across the pubertal transition, even after researchers control for the chronological age at which puberty is experienced (Gunnar, Wewerka, Frenn, Long, & Griggs, 2009; Stroud et al., 2009; Walker et al., 2004).

On a broader level, some researchers have evoked evolutionary theory to explain environmental or psychosocial influences on pubertal development (see Bugental, Corpuz, & Beaulieu, Chapter 14, this volume). Specifically, early life experiences are thought to provide cues regarding the availability and predictability of resources in one's environment, particularly those related to close relationships. By signaling a lack of parental investment and limited opportunity for reproductive success, lack of support in family relationships and stressors such as father absence and marital conflict may contribute to more rapid pubertal development (Belsky, Steinberg, & Draper, 1991). Thus, among children living in chronically stressful home environments, resources that would otherwise be invested in a prolonged period of growth and development are instead devoted to accelerated reproductive maturity.

Pubertal Timing and Substance Use

Earlier pubertal maturation is associated with increased illicit substance use and abuse (Hayatbakhsh, Najman, McGee, Bor, & O'Callaghan, 2009), and with elevated alcohol use, heavy drinking, and drunkenness in adolescence and early adulthood (e.g., Biehl et al., 2007; Costello et al., 2007; Dick, Rose, Viken, & Kaprio, 2000; Wichstrom, 2001). Some work has linked late pubertal timing with increased alcohol and substance use problems among boys (Andersson & Magnusson, 1990; Graber et al., 1997; Shelton & van den Bree, 2010); however, a recent population-based prospective study found no consistent evidence supporting this effect (Biehl et al., 2007). Rather, among both males and females, early pubertal timing predicted elevated alcohol use and heavy drinking trajectories from adolescence into young adulthood. Finally, early pubertal timing is a risk factor for cigarette use among both girls and boys (Dick et al., 2000; Shelton & van den Bree, 2010; Westling, Andrews, Hampson, & Peterson, 2008). Early maturing adolescents are more likely to smoke at the start of high school, and show a steeper increase in smoking across the high school years compared to their peers (Westling et al., 2012).

Because both early maturation and family stress are associated with adolescent substance use, when combined they may amplify risk. According to the *contextual amplification hypothesis* (Ge & Natsuaki, 2009), puberty-related challenges, especially when encountered at a young age, can interact with stressors in one's social environment to predict increased risk for maladjustment. In support of this hypothesis, research has shown that early pubertal timing is more strongly associated with behavior problems and emotional maladjustment among adolescents exposed to harsh, inconsistent parenting (Ge, Brody, Conger, Simons, & McBride, 2002) and low levels of parental nurturance and communication (Mrug, Loosier, & Windle, 2008).

Risk for substance use in particular appears to be amplified in the context of overly lax parental supervision. Prospective studies have shown that early maturing boys and girls who are poorly monitored by parents are more likely to start drinking at a young age compared to early maturing adolescents exposed to better parental monitoring and greater supervision (Costello et al., 2007; Westling et al., 2008). These findings are important inasmuch as early alcohol use initiation has negative consequences for substance use and abuse trajectories across the life span (B. F. Grant & Dawson, 1997). While external forms of regulation (i.e., parental supervision) might attenuate risks for substance use, we also know that internal self-regulatory characteristics are linked with substance use among early maturing individuals. For example, adolescents with early pubertal onset reported higher levels of positive and negative urgency, as well as more positive drinking expectations, which in turn predicted early onset of alcohol use (Gunn & Smith, 2010). Thus, early maturing adolescents are at increased risk for substance use problems that may be partially attributable to self-regulatory deficits that arise within the context of stressful family environments. The risk may be even greater when combined with lax parental supervision.

Pubertal Timing and Obesity

A growing body of literature has linked early pubertal timing with elevated fat mass and risk for obesity, especially among females. In population-based studies, the prevalence of overweight/obesity is nearly twice as high among early compared to non-early maturing girls (Adair & Gordon-Larsen, 2001; Wang, 2002). Although less consistent, some evidence suggests a similar association among boys (Ribeiro, Santos, Duarte, & Mota, 2006; Sørensen, Aksglaede, Petersen, & Juul, 2010). Early maturing adolescents accumulate more subcutaneous adipose tissue on the lower trunk than do later maturing peers (Koziel & Malina, 2005; Lassek & Gaulin, 2007), a notable finding given the health risks associated with a more central distribution of fat (Freedman, Serdula, Srinivasan, & Berenson, 1999). Earlier pubertal timing has also been linked with elevated cardiovascular and metabolic risk factors (higher triglycerides and total cholesterol, lower high-density lipoprotein [HDL] cholesterol) in a population-based sample of young adult women (Allsworth, Weitzen, & Boardman, 2005). In a longitudinal study, early pubertal maturation predicted greater sedentary behavior among male and female adolescents, suggesting one pathway to overweight and associated health risks (Van Jaarsveld, Fidler, Simon, & Wardle, 2007).

Childhood overnutrition and fat mass contribute to early pubertal maturation, particularly among females (Kaplowitz, 2008). For instance, elevated body mass index (BMI) and greater BMI change across childhood prospectively predict earlier pubertal timing in girls (Davison, Susman, & Birch, 2003; Lee et al., 2007; Ventura, Loken, & Birch, 2009). Although the underlying mechanisms require further examination, the permissive effects of leptin on neural circuits that regulate gonadotropin secretion might help explain the link between body fat stores and pubertal timing (Kaplowitz, 2008). Leptin, a hormone secreted by adipose (fat) tissue, signals the body's level of energy stores to the brain. Obese children have higher leptin levels compared to children with normal BMI (Hassink et al., 1996), and higher leptin levels are associated with earlier pubertal development (Matkovic et al., 1997). Mice injected with leptin show earlier pubertal onset compared to control mice, providing further evidence of leptin's role in early maturation (see Shalitin & Phillip, 2003).

The question of whether early puberty might also place adolescents at risk for subsequent increases in overweight and obesity has yet to be resolved. In some studies, the association between early pubertal timing and higher adult BMI is at least partially independent of childhood BMI (Freedman et al., 2003; Lobstein, Baur, & Uauy, 2004; Prentice & Viner, 2012). Thus, while childhood family environment and its impact on nutrition and body fat likely contribute to early pubertal development (Ellis & Essex, 2007), early puberty might in turn accentuate these preexisting vulnerabilities to overweight and obesity.

Youth with emotion regulation vulnerabilities arising in the context of a stressful family setting might attempt to cope with the stressors of early puberty in ways that further contribute to weight gain, such as unhealthy eating. For example, early pubertal onset was linked with increased negative urgency across the transition to middle school, which in turn predicted increased expectancies that eating will help manage negative mood states (Pearson, Combs, Zapolski & Smith, 2012). In the same study, early pubertal onset predicted increased binge eating across the middle school transition. Thus, early pubertal maturation is associated with unhealthy eating behavior and expectancies that may be partially attributable to self-regulatory patterns characteristic of children growing up in stressful family environments. The stressors of early puberty might contribute to accelerated weight gain inasmuch as unhealthy eating is used as a form of escape or self-medication.

Summary

Youth with preexisting vulnerabilities arising in the context of a chronically stressful family confront the challenges of early puberty with less adequate coping resources and therefore face greater susceptibility to substance use and obesity. Despite complexities associated with unraveling directions of causation, pubertal maturation is clearly a key developmental context in our model. As depicted in Figure 17.1, puberty represents a backdrop against which the regulatory processes associated with chronic family stress become increasingly solidified, laying the groundwork for the emergence of serious health consequences during adolescence.

The next sections introduce several biological mechanisms in our conceptual model: Over the course of childhood, chronic stress influences the function of the HPA axis and the immune system (Repetti, Robles, & Reynolds, 2011). Their subsequent impact on risk for substance abuse and obesity in adolescence may be tied to activity in the dopaminergic reward system in the brain.

Chronic Stressors in the Family and Biological Mechanisms

Chronic Stress and HPA Axis Activity

The HPA axis regulates the production of the hormone cortisol, which has numerous effects on most cells and systems within the body (Sapolsky, Romero, & Munck, 2000). Importantly, the HPA axis is under direct influence of neural regions implicated in cognitive and emotional responses to stressful events (Dedovic, Duchesne, Andrews, Engert, & Pruessner, 2009). Adolescence is a key developmental transition, ushering in substantial changes in HPA activity (see Romeo, 2010). Cortisol reactivity to acute stress increases from childhood to adolescence, and some evidence suggests these changes coincide with pubertal maturation independently of chronological age (Gunnar, Wewerka, et al., 2009; Stroud et al., 2009; Walker et al., 2004).

Cortisol reactivity measures typically involve measuring short-term responses to psychological stressors. Early life stress (Gunnar, Frenn, Wewerka, & Van Ryzin, 2009), parental psychopathology (Hardie, Moss, Vanyukov, Yao, & Kirillovac, 2002), and maltreatment (Gordis, Granger, Susman, & Trickett, 2008) have been associated with lower cortisol reactivity to laboratory stressors (cf. Gump et al., 2009). Similarly, adolescents and young adults characterized by negative relationships with the family of origin show lower cortisol reactivity (Luecken, Kraft, & Hagan, 2009). Thus, cumulative exposure to early life stressors appears to "blunt" cortisol responses to acute stressors, when the normative response should be a robust reactivity to and recovery from acute stress (Lovallo, 2011).

Resting (basal) cortisol also shows a regular daily rhythm, with levels highest upon waking and decreasing during the day. To assess basal HPA activity, cortisol is sampled several times a day, primarily in saliva or urine (Lovallo & Thomas, 2000). Superimposed upon normative age- and puberty-related increases in basal cortisol levels across the adolescent transition (Gunnar & Vazquez, 2006; Gunnar, Wewerka, et al., 2009), the pattern for basal measures of HPA function in middle childhood and adolescence suggests that average cortisol levels are higher and slopes of change are flatter in children exposed to parents with lower marital functioning (Pendry & Adam, 2007) or to early physical and/or sexual abuse (Cicchetti & Rogosch, 2001; Cicchetti, Rogosch, Gunnar, & Toth, 2010). Additionally, elevated evening cortisol levels have been associated with exposure to crowding, noise, and family turmoil (Evans, 2003; Evans & Kim, 2007), and low marital functioning (Pendry & Adam, 2007), but not parental depression (Schreiber et al., 2006).

Chronic Stress and Immune Function

The immune system recognizes and eliminates "nonself" threats, including viruses and bacteria (Rabin, 2005). We focus on *innate immunity*, which generates *inflammation*—a cascade of physiological changes that eradicate infectious threats. Stressful family environments may increase molecular signals (e.g., gene expression) that initiate the inflammatory response (Miller & Chen, 2006; Miller, Rohleder, & Cole, 2009). Cortisol typically suppresses inflammation, but with repeated exposure to elevated levels, immune cells can become insensitive to the hormone's signal, further increasing inflammation. Adolescents who reported exposure to adverse family environments showed larger stimulated production of the proinflammatory cytokine interleukin-6 over 18-month follow-up, and showed greater resistance to cortisol's anti-inflammatory effects (Miller & Chen, 2010). In the short term, by contributing to enhanced inflammation during infections, chronic family stress may promote faster clearing of infection, but over the long term, accumulating inflammation may increase risk for chronic illness (Miller, Chen, & Parker, 2011). Fortunately, the reverse effect may also be true: Adults who grew up in a low socioeconomic status environment but reported high maternal warmth during childhood showed lower inflammation-related gene expression (Chen, Miller, Kobor, & Cole, 2011). A key unanswered question is whether such responses have implications for adolescent health, before the onset of chronic illness in adulthood.

Overall, the same chronically stressful family environments implicated as risk factors for substance abuse and obesity also influence HPA axis functioning and inflammatory processes. Next, we suggest that the brain's dopaminergic reward system acts as a pathway that connects HPA axis activity and inflammation to the behaviors that underlie substance abuse and obesity.

A "Central" Role for Dopamine System Functioning in Substance Abuse and Obesity

Substance use problems and obesity result from the motivated pursuit of reinforcing substances or food. Motivated behaviors are driven by experiencing pleasure while consuming the desired substance, described as "liking," and those behaviors persist through nonconsciously attaching reward value to consumption and cues that predict consumption (e.g., smells from cigarette smoke or cooking), described as "wanting" (Berridge, 2009). Both liking and wanting are necessary for motivated behavior, and researchers have focused considerable effort on identifying their underlying brain circuitry.

Much like cities are connected via roads, brain circuits are clusters of neurons interconnected by neuronal projections. The physical connections between neural regions are characterized by specific neurochemical signals, such as serotonin or dopamine. In substance use and obesity, a key circuit of interest is the *mesolimbic dopaminergic system*, formed by cells in the midbrain (ventral tegmental area, substantia nigra) that project to and release dopamine into the ventral striatum and prefrontal cortex (Alcaro, Huber, & Panksepp, 2007). Mesolimbic dopaminergic system activity is specifically implicated in wanting (Berridge, 2009; Kenny, 2011; Volkow, Wang, Tomasi, & Baler, 2013). All drugs of abuse lead to large dopamine increases in the ventral striatum from midbrain cells, and food rewards may have similar effects. Over time, repeated consumption leads to changes within the mesolimbic dopaminergic system that increase wanting.

Our discussion centers on how the HPA axis and immune system modulate wanting. Other developmental changes occur that increase compulsive behaviors, impulsivity (i.e., negative and positive urgency), and the negative reinforcement value of rewarding stimuli. Indeed, the mesolimbic dopaminergic system appears to mature at a faster rate than the ability of prefrontal regions to exert inhibition on reward circuits (known as *cognitive control*; Casey & Jones, 2010). Thus, changes to dopamine reward circuitry attributable to the HPA axis and immune system must be considered within the larger context of neural changes that occur during adolescence, a time when dopaminergic system hyperresponsiveness to rewarding stimuli is normative (Galvan, 2010).

HPA Axis and Dopaminergic Activity

HPA axis activation can increase dopamine release under acute exposure to stress or inhibit dopamine production with chronic exposure (Sinha, 2008). Moreover, animal studies suggest that corticosterone (equivalent to cortisol) may partially mediate the association between injecting drugs of abuse and increased dopamine levels in the ventral striatum (Goeders, 2002; Marinelli, Aouizerate, Barrot, Le Moal, & Piazza, 1998). Similarly, in humans, greater cortisol reactivity to acute stress is associated with increased dopamine release in ventral striatum (Oswald et al., 2005; Pruessner, Champagne, Meaney, & Dagher, 2004).

When substance use is initiated and transitions to increased frequency of use, a particular problem is *cross-sensitization*, in which stress exposure and subsequent HPA axis dysregulation increase dopaminergic responses to substances. For example, maternal separation in rats early in development leads to HPA axis hyperactivation during stress and increased sensitivity to stimulant effects (Meaney, Brake, & Gratton, 2002). Less is known about such links in children, but sensitization through HPA axis activation during stressors may increase wanting, thus hastening dependence.

Regarding obesity, stressful events can contribute to increased food intake (Block, He, Zaslavsky, Ding, & Ayanian, 2009; Torres & Nowson, 2007). Additionally, our prior discussion of HPA axis activation and wanting suggests similar effects for food. Moreover, during stress, both animals and humans prefer "comfort foods" with higher fat and sugar content, which have a potentially self-medicating effect that can actually dampen HPA axis activation but contribute to abdominal fat deposition and obesity (Dallman et al., 2003; Dallman, Pecoraro, & la Fleur, 2005; Tomiyama, Dallman, & Epel, 2011). Thus, chronic stress in adverse family environments may contribute to increasing the wanting of certain foods, particularly comfort foods, and increased ingestion of those foods, which may inhibit HPA axis activation but increase abdominal fat deposition.

Immune Function and Dopaminergic Activity

Inflammation also has effects on the mesolimbic dopaminergic system. Inducing increased proinflammatory cytokine production contributes to anhedonia-like behavior in which previously pleasurable stimuli lose their reward value (Borowski, Kokkinidis, Merali, & Anisman, 1998), accompanied by increased dopamine levels in the brain. Substance abuse research suggests that, paradoxically over time, acute dopamine release in the dopaminergic pathway may actually result in decreased neural activity (Volkow, Fowler, Wang, & Swanson, 2004). Interestingly, individuals receiving a low dose of endotoxin (which induces inflammation) showed reduced ventral striatum activity when presented with monetary reward cues, as well as greater depressed mood (Eisenberger et al., 2010). Thus, heightened inflammation may decrease the reward value of stimuli through reduced dopaminergic activity.

By making normally pleasurable activities (e.g., social interaction) less pleasurable, anhedonia may lead adolescents to seek out more stimulating activities. Similar to cross-sensitization, described earlier, inflammation may also increase "wanting" of drugs. While this has not been explored in children, in adults with major depression but no history of amphetamine dependence, greater depression severity (strongly correlated with anhedonia) was associated with more positive feelings following amphetamine ingestion (Tremblay, Naranjo, Cardenas, Herrmann, & Busto, 2002), as well as greater mesolimbic dopaminergic circuit activation (Tremblay et al., 2005). In cross-sectional population data, higher anhedonia is associated with greater lifetime prevalence of stimulant use and dependence (Leventhal et al., 2010).

Research on inflammation and obesity has primarily focused on how increasing adiposity contributes to increased inflammation and metabolic dysregulation (Gregor & Hotamisligil, 2011), rather than modifications to the mesolimbic dopaminergic system. However, given the role of the dopaminergic reward systems in substance use and obesity, connections between inflammation and reward processing are quite plausible. Thus, cumulative exposure to inflammation may contribute to anhedonia and heightened wanting of certain types of foods via modification of dopaminergic reward systems.

Taken together, the effects of the HPA axis and inflammation on the mesolimbic dopaminergic system may help explain how family environments contribute to substance use and obesity. Puberty appears to be a particularly sensitive period in terms of physiological stress response systems, but much more research is needed to clarify how neuroendocrine and immune dysregulation during the pubertal transition might modulate links among family environment, emotion regulation, and adolescent health. Our chapter highlights neural mechanisms related to wanting substances and food. The HPA axis may modulate wanting via alterations in the mesolimbic dopaminergic system, and inflammation may play a similar role in terms of contributing to anhedonia and the reward value of substances and food.

Future Directions for Research

Some family environments effectively operate as chronic stressors in children's lives, with implications for the way that emotions, behavior, and biology are regulated. There has been rapid progress in our understanding of how multiple biological systems—endocrine, neuroendocrine, immune, and central nervous system (CNS)—operate, interact, and develop. Psychologists should continue to pursue interdisciplinary approaches that mesh those advances with research on family social processes and psychological development. The time is right for prospective longitudinal studies that include assessments of the family social environment, individual self-regulation and biological variables, and health outcomes to disentangle the complex causal relations and feedback loops among the variables discussed here. For example, a growing body of research suggests that early pubertal timing is more strongly associated with emotional and behavioral problems among adolescents in stressful family environments: Future work should examine the interplay between pubertal development and family environment factors in predicting the stress response processes we have identified as intermediary components linking family socialization with later health consequences. Some evidence suggests that early puberty is associated with greater emotional reactivity and use of less constructive coping strategies in response to stress (Rudolph & Troop-Gordon, 2010; Sontag, Graber, Brooks-Gunn, & Warren, 2008). It also appears that pubertal maturation is an important moderator of physiological reactivity to stress (Gunnar, Frenn, et al., 2009; Stroud et al., 2009). Further investigation is needed to elucidate the role of the family environment in such processes. We know that adolescence is a critical period for the development of obesity and substance use problems, and such work may prove beneficial in identifying concrete points of intervention.

Together with the availability of substances (e.g., prescription drugs, nicotine) and high-fat, high-energy-dense foods (i.e., comfort foods and "junk" foods) in the environment, the influences of family socialization on HPA and immune activity may increase risk for future health problems. Establishing these mechanistic pathways in children and adolescents is a key direction for future basic and translational research. For example, the contributions of the HPA axis and immune system to increasing the reward value of certain foods and substances may exacerbate and direct the effects of positive and negative urgency. The response that the individual turns to when experiencing intense emotion may be a function both of the reward value of that particular behavior and behavior-specific expectancies for reinforcement (Fischer, Settles, Collins, Gunn, & Smith, 2012). Beliefs about the benefits of substance use and eating are based in direct experience, as well as vicarious learning, including socialization that takes place in the family.

Finally, although not a focus of this chapter, genes have been mentioned throughout because they are essential to every variable and every link depicted in Figure 17.1. Genetically sensitive research designs will help to tease apart the roles that genes play in the biological and psychological processes that link chronic stressors in the family to substance abuse and obesity.

REFERENCES

Adair, L. S., & Gordon-Larsen, P. (2001). Maturational timing and overweight prevalence in US adolescent girls. *American Journal of Public Health, 91,* 642–644.

Alati, R., Maloney, E., Hutchinson, D. M., Najman, J. M., Mattick, R. P., Bor, W., et al. (2010). Do maternal parenting practices predict problematic patterns of adolescent alcohol consumption? *Addiction, 105*(5), 872–880.

Alcaro, A., Huber, R., & Panksepp, J. (2007). Behavioral functions of the mesolimbic dopaminergic system: An affective neuroethological perspective. *Brain Research Reviews, 56,* 283–321.

Allsworth, J. E., Weitzen, S., & Boardman, L. A. (2005). Early age at menarche and allostatic load: Data from the Third National Health and Nutrition Examination Survey. *Annals of Epidemiology, 15*(6), 438–444.

Andersson, T., & Magnusson, D. (1990). Biological maturation in adolescence and the development of drinking habits and alcohol abuse among young males: A prospective longitudinal study. *Journal of Youth and Adolescence, 19*(1), 33–41.

Belsky, J., Steinberg, L., & Draper, P. (1991). Childhood experience, interpersonal development and reproductive strategy: An evolutionary theory of socialization. *Child Development, 62,* 647–670.

Belsky, J., Steinberg, L., Houts, R. M., Friedman, S. L., DeHart, G., Cauffman, E., et al. (2007). Family rearing antecedents of pubertal timing. *Child Development, 78,* 1302–1321.

Berridge, K. C. (2009). "Liking" and "wanting" food rewards: Brain substrates and roles in eating disorders. *Physiology and Behavior, 97,* 537–550.

Biehl, M. C., Natsuaki, M. N., & Ge, X. (2007). The influence of pubertal timing on alcohol use and heavy drinking trajectories. *Journal of Youth and Adolescence, 36,* 153–167.

Block, J. P., He, Y. L., Zaslavsky, A. M., Ding, L., & Ayanian, J. Z. (2009). Psychosocial stress and change in weight among US adults. *American Journal of Epidemiology, 170,* 181–192.

Bogaert, A. F. (2005). Age at puberty and father absence in a national probability sample. *Journal of Adolescence, 28,* 541–546.

Borowski, T., Kokkinidis, E., Merali, Z., & Anisman, H. (1998). Lipopolysaccharide, central *in vivo* biogenic amine variations, and anhedonia. *NeuroReport, 9,* 3797–3802.

Bowles, M. A., DeHart, D., & Webb, J. R. (2012). Family influences on female offenders' substance use: The role of adverse childhood events among incarcerated women. *Journal of Family Violence, 27,* 681–686.

Brotman, L. M., Dawson-McClure, S., Huang, K. Y., Theise, R., Kamboukos, D., Wang, J., et al. (2012). Early childhood family intervention and long-term obesity prevention among high-risk minority youth. *Pediatrics, 129,* e621–e628.

CASA (National Center on Addiction and Substance Abuse). (2011, June). *Adolescent substance use: America's #1 public health problem* [Report]. New York: Columbia University, CASA. Retrieved April 23, 2013, from *www.casacolumbia.org.*

Casey, B. J., & Jones, R. M. (2010). Neurobiology of the adolescent brain and behavior: Implications for substance use disorders. *Journal of the American Academy of Child and Adolescent Psychiatry, 49,* 1189–1201.

Chen, E., Miller, G. E., Kobor, M. S., & Cole, S. W. (2011). Maternal warmth buffers the effects of low early-life socioeconomic status on pro-inflammatory signaling in adulthood. *Molecular Psychiatry, 16,* 729–737.

Cicchetti, D., & Rogosch, F. A. (2001). Diverse patterns of neuroendocrine activity in maltreated children. *Development and Psychopathology, 13,* 677–693.

Cicchetti, D., Rogosch, F. A., Gunnar, M. R., & Toth, S. L. (2010). The differential impacts of early physical and sexual abuse and internalizing problems on daytime cortisol rhythm in school-aged children. *Child Development, 81,* 252–269.

Costello, E. J., Sung, M., Worthman, C., & Angold, A. (2007). Pubertal maturation and the development of alcohol use and abuse. *Drug and Alcohol Dependence, 88,* 50–59.

Crossley, I. A., & Buckner, J. C. (2012). Maternal-related predictors of self-regulation among low-income youth. *Journal of Child and Family Studies, 21*(2), 217–227.

Cyders, M. A., Flory, K., Rainer, S., & Smith, G. T. (2009). The role of personality dispositions to risky behavior in predicting first-year college drinking. *Addiction, 104,* 193–202.

Cyders, M. A., & Smith, G. T. (2008). Emotion-based dispositions to rash action: Positive and negative urgency. *Psychological Bulletin, 134,* 807–828.

Dallman, M. F., Pecoraro, N., Akana, S. F., la Fleur, S. E., Gomez, F., Houshyar, H., et al. (2003). Chronic stress and obesity: A new view of "comfort food." *Proceedings of the National Academy of Sciences USA, 100,* 11696–11701.

Dallman, M. F., Pecoraro, N. C., & la Fleur, S. E. (2005). Chronic stress and comfort foods: Self-medication and abdominal obesity. *Brain Behavior and Immunity, 19,* 275–280.

Davison, K. K., Susman, E. J., & Birch, L. L. (2003). Percent body fat at age 5 predicts earlier pubertal development among girls at age 9. *Pediatrics, 111,* 815–821.

Dedovic, K., Duchesne, A., Andrews, J., Engert, V., & Pruessner, J. C. (2009). The brain and the stress axis: The neural correlates of cortisol regulation in response to stress. *NeuroImage, 47,* 864–871.

Dick, D. M., Rose, R. J., Viken, R. J., & Kaprio, J. (2000). Pubertal timing and substance use: Associations between and within families across late adolescence. *Developmental Psychology, 36*(2), 180–189.

Dodge, K. A., Malone, P. S., Lansford, J. E., Miller, S., Pettit, G. S., & Bates, J. E. (2009). A dynamic cascade model of the development of substance-use onset. *Monographs of the Society for Research in Child Development, 74*(3), vii–119.

Eisenberger, N. I., Berkman, E. T., Inagaki, T. K., Rameson, L. T., Mashal, N. M., & Irwin, M. R. (2010). Inflammation-induced anhedonia: Endotoxin reduces ventral striatum responses to reward. *Biological Psychiatry, 68,* 748–754.

Ellis, B. J., & Essex, M. J. (2007). Family environments, adrenarche, and sexual maturation: A longitudinal test of a life history model. *Child Development, 78,* 1799–1817.

Ellis, B. J., Shirtcliff, E. A., Boyce, W. T., Deardorff, J., & Essex, M. J. (2011). Quality of early family relationships and the timing and tempo of puberty: Effects depend on biological sensitivity to context. *Development and Psychopathology, 23,* 85–99.

Ersche, K. D., Turton, A. J., Chamberlain, S. R., Muller, U., Bullmore, E. T., & Robbins, T. W. (2012). Cognitive dysfunction and anxious-impulsive personality traits are endophenotypes for drug dependence. *American Journal of Psychiatry, 169*(9), 926–936.

Evans, G. W. (2003). A multimethodological analysis of cumulative risk and allostatic load among rural children. *Developmental Psychology, 39,* 924–933.

Evans, G. W., Fuller-Rowell, T. E., & Doan, S. N. (2012). Childhood cumulative risk and obesity: The mediating role of self-regulatory ability. *Pediatrics, 129*(1), e68–e73.

Evans, G. W., & Kim, P. (2007). Childhood poverty and health: Cumulative risk exposure and stress dysregulation. *Psychological Science, 18,* 953–957.

Fiese, B., Hammons, A. J., Bost, K. K., & Wiley, A. (2013, April). Household routines and nutrition in early childhood: An entry way to building family strengths. In K. Purtell (Chair), *Unhealthy eating among children: Understanding predictors, consequences, and targets for intervention.* Symposium conducted at the SRCD biennial meeting, Seattle, WA.

Fischer, S., Peterson, C. M., & McCarthy, D. (2013). A prospective test of the influence of negative urgency and expectancies on binge eating and purging. *Psychology of Addictive Behaviors, 27,* 294–300.

Fischer, S., Settles, R., Collins, B., Gunn, R., & Smith, G. T. (2012). The role of negative urgency and expectancies in problem drinking and disordered eating: Testing a model of comorbidity in pathological and at-risk samples. *Psychology of Addictive Behaviors, 26,* 112–123.

Fischer, S., Smith, G. T., & Cyders, M. A. (2008). Another look at impulsivity: A meta-analytic review comparing specific dispositions to rash action in their relationship to bulimic symptoms. *Clinical Psychology Review, 28,* 1413–1425.

Fitzsimmons-Craft, E. E., Bardone-Cone, A. M., Brownstone, L. M., & Harney, M. B. (2012). Evaluating the roles of anxiety and dimensions of perfectionism is dieting and binge eating using weekly diary methodology. *Eating Behaviors, 13,* 418–422.

Freedman, D. S., Khan, L. K,. Serdula, M. K., Dietz, W. H., Srinivasan, S. R., & Berenson, G. S. (2003). The relation of menarcheal age to obesity in childhood and adulthood: The Bogalusa Heart Study. *BMC Pediatrics, 3,* 3.

Freedman, D. S., Serdula, M. K., Srinivasan, S. R., & Berenson, G. S. (1999). Relation of circumferences and skinfold thicknesses to lipid and insulin concentrations in children and adolescents: The Bogalusa Heart Study. *American Journal of Clinical Nutrition, 69,* 308–317.

Galvan, A. (2010). Adolescent development of the reward system. *Frontiers in Human Neuroscience, 4,* 1–9.

Garasky, S., Stewart, S. D., Gundersen, C., Lohman, B. J., & Eisenmann, J. C. (2009). Family stressors and child obesity. *Social Science Research, 38,* 755–766.

Ge, X., Brody, G. H., Conger, R. D., Simons, R. L., & McBride, V. M. (2002). Contextual amplification of pubertal transition effects on deviant peer affiliation and externalizing behavior among African American children. *Developmental Psychology, 38,* 42–54.

Ge, X., & Natsuaki, M. N. (2009). In search of explanations for early pubertal timing effects on developmental psychopathology. *Current Directions in Psychological Science, 18*(6), 327–331.

Goeders, N. E. (2002). Stress and cocaine addiction. *Journal of Pharmacology and Experimental Therapeutics, 301,* 785–789.

Gordis, E. B., Granger, D. A., Susman, E. J., & Trickett, P. K. (2008). Salivary alpha amylase–cortisol asymmetry in maltreated youth. *Hormones and Behavior, 53,* 96–103.

Graber, J. A., Lewinsohn, P. M., Seeley, J. R., & Brooks-Gunn, J. (1997). Is psychopathology associated with the timing of pubertal development? *Journal of the American Academy of Child and Adolescent Psychiatry, 36,* 1768–1776.

Graber, J. A., Sontag, L. M., & Brooks-Gunn, J. (2009, April). *The moderating role of physiological and contextual factors on timing-adjustment associations during the entry into puberty.* Paper presented at the biennial meeting of the Society for Research in Child Development, Denver, CO.

Grant, B. F., & Dawson, D. A. (1997). Age at onset of alcohol use and its association with DSM–IV alcohol abuse and dependence: Results from the National Longitudinal Alcohol Epidemiologic Survey. *Journal of Substance Abuse, 9,* 103–110.

Grant, K. E., Compas, B. E., Stuhlmacher, A. F., Thurm, A. E., McMahon, S. D., & Halpert, J. A. (2003). Stressors and child and adolescent psychopathology: Moving from markers to mechanisms of risk. *Psychological Bulletin, 129,* 447–466.

Gregor, M. F., & Hotamisligil, G. S. (2011). Inflammatory mechanisms in obesity. *Annual Review of Immunology, 29,* 415–445.

Gump, B. B., Reihman, J., Stewart, P., Lonky, E., Darvill, T., Granger, D. A., et al. (2009). Trajectories of maternal depressive symptoms over her child's life span: Relation to adrenocortical, cardiovascular, and emotional functioning in children. *Development and Psychopathology, 21,* 207–225.

Gunn, R. L., & Smith, G. T. (2010). Risk factors for elementary school drinking: Pubertal status, personality, and alcohol expectancies concurrently predict 5th grade alcohol consumption. *Psychology of Addictive Behavior, 24*(4), 617–627.

Gunnar, M. R., Frenn, K., Wewerka, S. S., & Van Ryzin, M. J. (2009). Moderate versus severe early life stress: Associations with stress reactivity and regulation in 10–12-year-old children. *Psychoneuroendocrinology, 34*(1), 62–75.

Gunnar, M. R., & Vazquez, D. (2006). Stress neurobiology and developmental psychopathology. In D. Cicchetti & D. Cohen (Eds.), *Developmental psychopathology: Vol. 2. Developmental neuroscience* (2nd ed., pp. 533–577). New York: Wiley.

Gunnar, M. R., Wewerka, S., Frenn, K., Long, J. D., & Griggs, C. (2009). Developmental changes in hypothalamus–pituitary–adrenal activity over the transition to adolescence: Normative changes and associations with puberty. *Development and Psychopathology, 21,* 69–85.

Hardie, T. L., Moss, H. B., Vanyukov, M. M., Yao, J. K., & Kirillovac, G. P. (2002). Does adverse family environment or sex matter in the salivary cortisol responses to anticipatory stress? *Psychiatry Research, 112,* 121–131.

Harrist, A. W., Topham, G. L., Hubbs-Tait, L., Page, M. C., Kennedy, T. S., & Shriver, L. H. (2012). What developmental science can contribute to a transdisciplinary understanding of childhood obesity: An interpersonal and intrapersonal risk model. *Child Development Perspectives, 6*(4), 445–455.

Hassink, S. G., Sheslow, D. V., de Lancey, E., Opentanova, I., Considine, R. V., & Caro, J. F. (1996). Serum leptin in children with obesity: Relationship to gender and development. *Pediatrics, 98*(2), 201–203.

Hayatbakhsh, M. R., Najman, J. M., McGee, T. R., Bor, W., & O'Callaghan, M. J. (2009). Early pubertal maturation in the prediction of early adult substance use: A prospective study. *Addiction, 104*(1), 59–66.

Hendrie, G. A., Coveney, J., & Cox, D. N. (2012). Defining the complexity of childhood obesity and related behaviours within the family environment using structural equation modelling. *Public Health Nutrition, 15*(1), 48–57.

Herrenkohl, T. I., Lee, J. O., Kosterman, R., & Hawkins, J. D. (2012). Family influences related to adult substance use and mental health problems: A developmental analysis of child and adolescent predictors. *Journal of Adolescent Health, 51*, 129–135.

Hoerr, S. L., Hughes, S. O., Fisher, J. O., Nicklas, T. A., Liu, Y., & Shewchuk, R. M. (2009). Associations among parental feeding style and children's food intake in families with limited incomes. *International Journal of Behavioral Nutrition and Physical Activity, 6*, 55.

Holtmann, M., Buchmann, A. F., Esser, G., Schmidt, M. H., Banaschewski, T., & Laucht, M. (2011). The Child Behavior Checklist–Dysregulation profile predicts substance use, suicidality, and functional impairment: A longitudinal analysis. *Journal of Child Psychology and Psychiatry, 52*(2), 139–147.

Kaplowitz, P. B. (2008). Link between body fat and the timing of puberty. *Pediatrics, 121*, S208–S217.

Kenny, P. J. (2011). Reward mechanisms in obesity: New insights and future directions. *Neuron, 69*, 664–679.

Koziel, S., & Malina, R. M. (2005). Variation in relative fat distribution associated with maturational timing: The Wrocbaw Growth study. *Annals of Human Biology, 32*(6), 691–701.

Lassek, W. D., & Gaulin, J. C. (2007). Menarche is related to fat distribution. *American Journal of Physical Anthropology, 133*, 1147–1151.

Lee, J. M., Appugliese, D., Kaciroti, N., Corwyn, R. F., Bradley, R. H., & Lumeng, J. C. (2007). Weight status in young girls and the onset of puberty. *Pediatrics, 119*, e624–e630.

Leventhal, A. M., Brightman, M., Ameringer, K. J., Greenberg, J., Mickens, L., Ray, L. A., et al. (2010). Anhedonia associated with stimulant use and dependence in a population-based sample of American adults. *Experimental and Clinical Psychopharmacology, 18*, 562–569.

Lobstein, T., Baur, L., & Uauy, R. (2004). Obesity in children and young people: A crisis in public health. *Obesity Review, 5*(Suppl. 1), 4–104.

Lovallo, W. R. (2011). Do low levels of stress reactivity signal poor states of health? *Biological Psychology, 86*, 121–128.

Lovallo, W. R., & Thomas, T. L. (2000). Stress hormones in psychophysiological research: Emotional, behavioral, and cognitive implications. In J. T. Cacioppo, L. G. Tassinary, & G. G. Berntson (Eds.), *Handbook of psychophysiology* (2nd ed., pp. 342–367). New York: Cambridge University Press.

Luecken, L. J., Kraft, A., & Hagan, M. J. (2009). Negative relationships in the family-of-origin predict attenuated cortisol in emerging adults. *Hormones and Behavior, 55*, 412–417.

Marinelli, M., Aouizerate, B., Barrot, M., Le Moal, M., & Piazza, P. V. (1998). Dopamine-dependent responses to morphine depend on glucocorticoid receptors. *Proceedings of the National Academy of Sciences USA, 95*, 7742–7747.

Matkovic, V., Ilich, J. Z., Skugor, M., Badenhop, N. E., Goel, P., Clairmont, A., et al. (1997). Leptin is inversely related to age at menarche in human females. *Journal of Clinical Endocrinology and Metabolism, 82*(9), 3239–3245.

McCurdy, K., Gorman, K. S., & Metallinos-Katsaras, E. (2010). From poverty to food insecurity and child overweight: A family stress approach. *Child Development Perspectives, 4*(2), 144–151.

Meaney, M. J., Brake, W., & Gratton, A. (2002). Environmental regulation of the development of mesolimbic dopamine systems: A neurobiological mechanism for vulnerability to drug abuse? *Psychoneuroendocrinology, 27*, 127–138.

Mendle, J., Turkheimer, E., & Emery, R. E. (2007). Detrimental psychological outcomes associated with early pubertal timing in adolescent girls. *Developmental Review, 27*, 151–171.

Miller, G. E., & Chen, E. (2006). Life stress and diminished expression of genes encoding glucocorticoid receptor and ß2-adrenergic receptor in children with asthma. *Proceedings of the National Academy of Sciences USA, 103*, 5496–5501.

Miller, G. E., & Chen, E. (2010). Harsh family climate in early life presages the emergence of a proinflammatory phenotype in adolescence. *Psychological Science, 21*, 848–856.

Miller, G. E., Chen, E., & Parker, K. J. (2011). Psychological stress in childhood and susceptibility to the chronic diseases of aging: Moving toward a model of behavioral and biological mechanisms. *Psychological Bulletin, 137*, 959–997.

Miller, G. E., Rohleder, N., & Cole, S. W. (2009). Chronic interpersonal stress predicts activation of pro- and anti-inflammatory signaling pathways 6 months later. *Psychosomatic Medicine, 71*, 57–62.

Mrug, S., Loosier, P. S., & Windle, M. (2008). Violence exposure across multiple contexts: Individual and joint effects on adjustment. *American Journal of Orthopsychiatry, 78*(1), 70–84.

Olvera, N., & Power, T. G. (2010). Brief report: Parenting styles and obesity in Mexican American children: A longitudinal study. *Journal of Pediatric Psychology, 35*, 243–249.

Oswald, L. M., Wong, D. F., McCaul, M., Zhou, Y., Kuwabara, H., Choi, L., et al. (2005). Relationships among ventral striatal dopamine release, cortisol secretion, and subjective responses to amphetamine. *Neuropsychopharmacology, 30*, 821–832.

Pearson, C. M., Combs, J. L., Zapolski, T. C. B., & Smith, G. T. (2012). A longitudinal transactional risk model for early eating disorder onset. *Journal of Abnormal Psychology, 121*(3), 707–718.

Pendry, P., & Adam, E. K. (2007). Associations between parents' marital functioning, maternal parenting quality, maternal emotion and child cortisol levels. *International Journal of Behavioral Development, 31*, 218–231.

Piehler, T. F., Véronneau, M., & Dishion, T. J. (2012). Substance use progression from adolescence to early adulthood: Effortful control in the context of friendship influence and early-onset. *Journal of Abnormal Child Psychology, 40*, 1045–1058.

Prentice, P., & Viner, R. M. (2012). Pubertal timing and adult obesity and cardiometabolic risk in women and men: A systematic review and meta-analysis. *International Journal of Obesity, 37*, 1036–1043.

Pruessner, J. C., Champagne, F., Meaney, M. J., & Dagher, A. (2004). Dopamine release in response to a psychological stress in humans and its relationship to early life maternal care: A positron emission tomography study using (11)C raclopride. *Journal of Neuroscience, 24*, 2825–2831.

Puder, J. J., & Munsch, S. (2010). Psychological correlates of childhood obesity. *International Journal of Obesity, 34*, S37–S43.

Quinlan, R. J. (2003). Father absence, parental care, and female reproductive development. *Evolution and Human Behavior, 24*, 376–390.

Rabin, B. S. (2005). Introduction to immunology and immune-endocrine interactions. In K. Vedhara & M. R. Irwin (Eds.), *Human psychoneuroimmunology* (pp. 1–24). New York: Oxford University Press.

Ratcliff, M. B., Jenkins, T. M., Reiter-Purtill, J., Noll, J. G., & Zeller, M. H. (2011). Risk-taking behaviors of adolescents with extreme obesity: Normative or not? *Pediatrics, 127*, 827–834.

Reilly, J. J., Methven, E., McDowell, Z. C., Hacking, B., Alexander, D., Stewart, L., et al. (2003). Health consequences of obesity. *Archives of Disease in Childhood, 88*, 748–752.

Repetti, R. L., Robles, T. F., & Reynolds, B. (2011). Allostatic processes in the family. *Development and Psychopathology, 23*, 921–938.

Repetti, R. L., Taylor, S. E., & Seeman, T. (2002). Risky families: Family social environments and the mental and physical health of offspring. *Psychological Bulletin, 128*, 330–366.

Ribeiro, J., Santos, P., Duarte, J., & Mota, J. (2006). Association between overweight and early sexual maturation in Portuguese boys and girls. *Annals of Human Biology, 33*(1), 55–63.

Romeo, R. D. (2010). Adolescence: A central event in shaping stress reactivity. *Developmental Psychobiology, 52*(3), 244–253.

Rostad, W. L. (2012). *The influence of dad: An investigation of adolescent females' perceived closeness with fathers and risky behaviors.* Unpublished master's thesis, University of Montana, Missoula.

Rudolph, K. D., & Troop-Gordon, W. (2010). Personal-accentuation and contextual-amplification models of pubertal timing: Predicting youth depression. *Development and Psychopathology, 22*(2), 433–451.

Sapolsky, R. M., Romero, M., & Munck, A. U. (2000). How do glucocorticoids influence stress responses?: Integrating permissive, suppressive, stimulatory, and preparative actions. *Endocrine Reviews, 21,* 55–89.

Saxbe, D., & Repetti, R. L. (2009). Fathers' and mothers' marital relationship predicts daughters' pubertal development two years later. *Journal of Adolescence, 32,* 415–423.

Schmeer, K. K. (2012). Family structure and obesity in early childhood. *Social Science Research, 41*(4), 820–832.

Schneider, K. L., Appelhans, B. M., Whited, M. C., Oleski, J., & Pagoto, S. L. (2010). Trait anxiety, but not trait anger, predisposes obese individuals to emotional eating. *Appetite, 55,* 701–706.

Schreiber, J. E., Shirtcliff, E., Van Hulle, C., Lemery-Chatfant, K., Klein, M. H., Kalin, N. H., et al. (2006). Environmental influences on family similarity in afternoon cortisol levels: Twin and parent-offspring designs. *Psychoneuroendocrinology, 31,* 1131–1137.

Schreier, H. M., & Chen, E. (2012). Socioeconomic status and health of youth: A multilevel, multidomain approach to conceptualizing pathways. *Psychological Bulletin, 139,* 606–654.

Settles, R. E., Fischer, S., Cyders, M. A., Combs, J. L., Gunn, R. L., & Smith, G. T. (2012). Negative urgency: A personality predictor of externalizing behavior characterized by neuroticism, low conscientiousness, and disagreeableness. *Journal of Abnormal Psychology, 121,* 160–172.

Shalitin, S., & Phillip, M. (2003). Role of obesity and leptin in the pubertal process and pubertal growth—a review. *International Journal of Obesity, 27,* 869–874.

Shelton, K. H., & van den Bree, M. B. M. (2010). The moderating effects of pubertal timing on the longitudinal associations between parent–child relationship quality and adolescent substance use. *Journal of Research on Adolescence, 20*(4), 1044–1064.

Sinha, R. (2008). Chronic stress, drug use, and vulnerability to addiction. *Addiction Reviews, 1141,* 105–130.

Snoek, H. M., Engels, R. C. M. E., Janssens, J. M. A. M., & van Strien, T. (2007). Parental behavior and adolescents' emotional eating. *Appetite, 49,* 223–230.

Sontag, L., Graber, J., Brooks-Gunn, J., & Warren, M. (2008). Coping with social stress: Implications for psychopathology in young adolescent girls. *Journal of Abnormal Child Psychology, 36*(8), 1159–1174.

Sørensen, K., Aksglaede, L., Petersen, J. H., & Juul, A. (2010). Recent changes in pubertal timing in healthy Danish boys: Associations with body mass index. *Journal of Clinical Endocrinology and Metabolism, 95*(1), 263–270.

Stenhammar, C., Olsson, G. M., Bahmanyar, S., Hulting, A.-L., Wettergren, B., Edlund, B., et al. (2010). Family stress and BMI in young children. *Acta Paediatrica, 99*(8), 1205–1212.

Stojek, M., & Fisher, S. (2013). Impulsivity and motivations to consume alcohol: A prospective study on risk of dependence in young adult women. *Alcoholism: Clinical and Experimental Research, 37,* 292–299.

Stroud, L. R., Foster, E., Papandonatos, G. D., Handwerger, K., Granger, D. A., Kivlighan, K. T., et al. (2009). Stress response and the adolescent transition: Performance versus peer rejection stressors. *Development and Psychopathology, 21*(1), 47–68.

Susman, E. J., & Dorn, L. D. (2009). Puberty: Its role in development. In R. M. Lerner & L. Steinberg (Eds.), *Handbook of adolescent psychology* (pp. 116–151). New York: Wiley.

Tomiyama, A. J., Dallman, M. F., & Epel, E. S. (2011). Comfort food is comforting to those most stressed: Evidence of the chronic stress response network in high stress women. *Psychoneuroendocrinology, 36,* 1513–1519.

Topham, G. L., Hubbs-Tait, L., Rutledge, J. M., Page, M. C., Kennedy, T. S., Shriver, L. H., et al. (2011). Parenting styles, parental response to child emotion, and family emotional responsiveness are related to child emotional eating. *Appetite, 56,* 261–264.

Torres, S. J., & Nowson, C. A. (2007). Relationship between stress, eating behavior, and obesity. *Nutrition, 23*, 887–894.

Tremblay, L. K., Naranjo, C. A., Cardenas, L., Herrmann, N., & Busto, U. E. (2002). Probing brain reward system function in major depressive disorder: Altered response to dextroamphetamine. *Archives of General Psychiatry, 59*, 409–416.

Tremblay, L. K., Naranjo, C. A., Graham, S. J., Herrmann, N., Mayberg, H. S., Hevenor, S., et al. (2005). Functional neuroanatomical substrates of altered reward processing in major depressive disorder revealed by a dopaminergic probe. *Archives of General Psychiatry, 62*, 1228–1236.

Vander Wal, J. S. (2012). The relationship between body mass index and unhealthy weight control behaviors among adolescents: The role of family and peer social support. *Economics and Human Biology, 10*, 395–404.

Van Jaarsveld, C. H. M., Fidler, J. A., Simon, A. E. P., & Wardle, J. (2007). Persistent impact of pubertal timing on trends in smoking, food choice, activity, and stress in adolescence. *Psychosomatic Medicine, 69*, 798–806.

Ventura, A. K., Loken, E., & Birch, L. L. (2009). Developmental trajectories of girls' BMI across childhood and adolescence. *Obesity, 17*, 2067–2074.

Volkow, N. D., Fowler, J. S., Wang, G. J., & Swanson, J. M. (2004). Dopamine in drug abuse and addiction: Results from imaging studies and treatment implications. *Molecular Psychiatry, 9*, 557–569.

Volkow, N. D., Wang, G. J., Tomasi, D., & Baler, R. D. (2013). Obesity and addiction: Neurobiological overlaps. *Obesity Reviews, 14*, 2–18.

Walker, E. F., Sabuwalla, Z., & Huout, R. (2004). Pubertal neuromaturation, stress sensitivity, and psychopathology. *Development and Psychopathology, 16*, 807–824.

Wang, Y. (2002). Is obesity associated with early sexual maturation?: A comparison of the association in American boys versus girls. *Pediatrics, 110*(5), 903–910.

Wen, L., Simpson, J. M., Baur, L. A., Rissel, C., & Flood, V. M. (2011). Family functioning and obesity risk behaviors: Implications for early obesity intervention. *Obesity, 19*(6), 1252–1258.

Westling, E., Andrews, J. A., Hampson, S. E., & Peterson, M. (2008). Pubertal timing and substance use: The effect of gender, parental monitoring and deviant peers. *Journal of Adolescent Health, 42*, 555–563.

Westling, E., Andrews, J. A., & Peterson, M. (2012). Gender differences in pubertal timing, social competence, and cigarette use: A test of the early maturation hypothesis. *Journal of Adolescent Health, 51*, 150–155.

Wichstrom, L. (2001). The impact of pubertal timing on adolescents' alcohol use. *Journal of Research on Adolescence, 11*(2), 131–150.

CHAPTER 18

Caregiver Socialization Factors Influencing Socioemotional Development in Infancy and Childhood

A Neuroscience Perspective

Tahl I. Frenkel
Nathan A. Fox

The topic of socialization is broad, encompassing a wide range of contextual influences (from caregiving to culture) across different developmental periods (infancy, preschool, school, adolescence). Our focus in this chapter is on the influence of caregiving on two domains of socialization during early development that lay the foundation for key socioemotional capacities: (1) the formation of attachment relationships and (2) the emergent abilities of emotion regulation that allow one to display–inhibit–modulate experienced and expressed emotions in an adaptive and culturally appropriate manner. We first briefly describe the functional importance of each of these domains, then examine the relevant neuroscience research. We focus primarily on electrophysiological methodologies, including electroencephalography (EEG) and event-related potentials (ERPs), as well as functional magnetic resonance imaging (fMRI). EEG is used for the continuous recording of electrical brain activity along the scalp, whereas ERPs and fMRI both are used in an attempt to link specific external events and their consequent cognitive-emotional processes with underlying neural activity. By examining the electrical brain activity that is time-locked to a specific event of interest, ERPs allow for a detailed delineation of the time course of neural processing at the resolution of milliseconds. Synchronous time-locked neural activity gives rise to various ERP waveforms, a series of positive and negative peaks that vary in polarity, amplitude, and duration as the waveform unfolds over time (Kappenman & Luck, 2012). Within these waveforms, ERP researchers have identified specific components, namely, scalp-recorded voltage changes that reflect specific neurocognitive processes. Components relevant to the domains of attachment or emotion regulation include, for instance, the negative central (Nc) component related to allocation of attention, as well as recognition memory, the attention-related N100 component, the N170 component that is specific to face processing, the error-related negativity (ERN) component associated with self-monitoring, the N2 component related to inhibitory control, and the late positive potential (LPP) component related to sustained attention and emotion regulation. Individual variations in the amplitudes and/or latencies of these components are thought to reflect meaningful differences in neurocognitive processing. Below we review some of the relevant ERP findings relative to these and additional ERP components of interests and their functional significance.

Functional neuroimaging procedures such as fMRI measure brain activity by detecting associated changes in blood flow (i.e., hemodynamic responses). fMRI data provide detailed mapping of the neural circuitry involved in specific neurocognitive processes at a very high spatial resolution. In the sections below, we review some of the relevant imaging results, while pointing out particular neural structures and circuits that have been found to be involved in attachment or socialization of emotion. These regions include, for instance, the orbitofrontal cortex (OFC), which is particularly involved in reward processing, the amygdala and insula, which are particularly reactive to emotion in general and threat in particular, as well as the prefrontal cortex (PFC) and the anterior cingulate cortex (ACC), which are involved in cognitive control, the modulation of emotion, and down-regulation. Finally, we provide examples of potential negative outcomes of perturbed functioning within each domain.

Socialization Processes and the Development of the Attachment System

The Functional Importance of Attachment in the Context of Socialization

The attachment system serves as a foundation and medium for the occurrence of key socialization processes early in child development. Security in the caregiver–child relationship is thought to moderate the relations between the child and the environment by providing a base from which the child may explore the wider world with confidence and independence (Sroufe, 2005), thereby creating interrelational contexts in which socialization may occur. Furthermore, attachment security has been shown to increase child susceptibility to caregiver socialization influences (for review, see Laible, Thompson, & Froimson, Chapter 2, this volume).

Both human adults and infants have emergent skills that set the context for reciprocal interactions between caregivers and infants. Adults selectively attend to infant faces and recognize cues of distress (see Parsons, Young, Murray, Stein, & Kringelbach, 2010, for a review). Infants display enhanced orientation and preference for social stimuli such as face-like forms (Johnson, Dziurawiec, Ellis, & Morton, 1991) and speech (Vouloumanos & Werker, 2004). Very young infants display clear preferences for their mothers' face (e.g., Bushnell, 2001), voice (e.g., DeCasper & Fifer, 1980), and even the smell of breast milk (e.g., Porter & Winberg, 1999). Importantly, specialization of the infant face-processing system develops as a function of experience and exposure and is not unique only to the mother's face (e.g., Pascalis, de Haan, & Nelson, 2002). Thus, an infant develops the ability to discriminate between faces to which it has been exposed to and is less able to discriminate between faces with which it has had less experience (Nelson, 2001).

Attachment from a Neuroscience Perspective

Over the past 15 years, a diverse spectrum of research has begun to explore the neural basis of attachment. While there has been a substantial focus on delineation of neural circuits supporting attachment responses in adults who are parents, less is known about the development of the relevant circuits within the infant (see Parsons et al., 2010, for review). We begin with a description of related neural circuits in the infant, then we provide an illustrative review of literature delineating neural circuits in the parent.

Neural Correlates of Attachment in the Infant

During the first years of life, remarkable synaptic plasticity increases the extent to which the brain is susceptible to environmental influences (Bourgeois, 2005). Maternal behaviors and subsequent emergence of mother–infant attachment are initially elicited by exchange of sensory cues. Functional activity indexed by glucose uptake reveals enhanced neural activity in the sensorimotor cortex (Chugani & Phelps, 1986), underlying neural control over the face muscles that allows newborns to signal to the caregiver in the form of facial expressions and vocalizations (Parsons et al., 2010). Over the first months of life, brain activity gradually becomes more distributed to include primary sensory cortices in response to other sensory stimuli modalities (e.g., Taga, Asakawa, Maki, Konishi, & Koizumi, 2003). Together, these developing neural activities appear to underlie infants' increasing capabilities to process complex social stimuli and to support fundamental orienting behaviors (Parsons et al., 2010). Furthermore, the early predisposition to orient toward faces increases visual exposure to faces, thereby facilitating interaction with caregivers and biasing the developing neural circuitry to achieve increasing specialization in face processing (Parsons et al., 2010). While face processing in young infants appears to be guided by both subcortical (e.g., Johnson, 2005) and cortical regions (e.g., Grossmann & Johnson, 2007), face processing in adults is more specialized, guided primarily by the fusiform gyrus and superior temporal sulcus (e.g., de Haan, Pascalis, & Johnson, 2002). This greater specialization is related to increased neural efficacy supporting increased ability to process complex facial cues rapidly and accurately.

Very early on infants begin to demonstrate specific neural activity in response to their mother' faces versus unknown faces (for reviews, see Parsons et al., 2010; Rilling, 2013) indexing increased salience of the primary caregiver to the infant. For instance, relative to unknown faces, maternal facial recognition elicits increased infant activity in the right frontotemporal cortex (Carlsson, Lagercrantz, Olson, Printz, & Bartocci, 2008). Additionally, 6-month-old infants have demonstrated increased Nc components in response to the face of the mother versus unknown faces (de Haan & Nelson, 1997). In a study of toddlers between ages 18 and 24 months, participants showed greater Nc in response to a mother's face stimulus than to a stranger's face stimulus, whereas participants between ages 45 and 54 months showed the reverse pattern. The authors propose that these findings reflect age-related differences in the perceived salience of the face of the primary caregiver versus strangers (Carver et al., 2003). At very young ages of high dependency primarily on caregivers, infants and toddlers perceive their own mothers' faces as having the highest salience. As they get older, preschoolers appear to be attracted to orienting toward strangers, perhaps facilitating broader socialization and achievement of developmentally appropriate goals. Nevertheless, while some argue that the Nc may indeed reflect these infants' greater allocation of attention to their mother's faces, indicating greater salience, a series of studies supports the notion the Nc may in fact reflect differences in infants' recognition memory of their mothers' faces (de Haan & Nelson, 1997). The Nc amplitude has also been found to be associated with age-appropriate infant proximity seeking, such that infants who showed more proximity seeking had larger Nc waves in response to a stranger's face stimulus than to a mother's face stimulus (Swingler, Sweet, & Carver, 2007). Finally, using auditory ERPs, 4-month-old infants' early ERP components were elicited at significantly shorter latency in response to their own mothers' voices relative to an unfamiliar voice, whereas later ERP components were significantly delayed and attenuated in response to their own mothers' versus an unfamiliar voice (Purhonen, Kilpeläinen-Lees, Valkonen-Korhonen, Karhu, & Lehtonen, 2005). Early ERP components are typically considered to be "obligatory" potentials that mainly are influenced by the physical characteristics of the eliciting stimulus. In this instance, the shorter ERP latencies for the early ERP components in response to the mother's voice is thought to reflect quicker involuntary orienting of attention toward the mother's voice because of its special salience and importance of these signals to the infant. The later ERP potentials are thought to be influenced by more endogenous cognitive processes, such as memory. The authors suggest that the delayed latency and attenuation of the later ERPs in response to the mother's voice may be interpreted as a sign of already existing memory for her voice. Taken together, the findings are thought to reflect enhanced arousal alongside an infant's already existing memory template for its own mother's voice.

Neural Correlates of Attachment in the Caregiver

Viewed from an evolutionary perspective, it seems that behavioral repertoires associated with adaptive caregiving skills that facilitate the development of attachment security would be subject to intense selective pressure (Clutton-Brock, 1991), and that underlying these may be neural circuits that support the expression of these caregiving capacities. Specifically, parent sensitivity, namely, adults' capacity to perceive infant cues and to respond to these promptly and appropriately (Ainsworth, Blehar, Waters, & Wall, 1978), has been identified as an important precursor of infant attachment security (De Wolff & van IJzendoorn, 1997). Neuroscience has attempted to elucidate the neural correlates of this caregiver responsiveness by adopting two main approaches:

1. Delineating electrophysiological (EEG/ERP) and hemodynamic (fMRI) activity of the caregiver's brain in response to auditory and visual infant cues.
2. Assessing neuroendocrine changes around pregnancy in mothers and fathers, primarily focusing on the roles of oxytocin, cortisol, prolactin, and testosterone.

NEURAL CORRELATES OF CAREGIVER RESPONSE TO INFANT CRIES

Infant vocalizations are pertinent in communicating information about the infant's current behavioral, physiological, and affective state. From the first day postpartum, mothers and fathers become increasingly capable of reliably recognizing their own infant's cry

(Cismaresco & Montagner, 1990). Building on the thalamocingulate theory of maternal behavior in animals developed by MacLean (1990), Lorberbaum and colleagues (2002) found evidence for a role of thalamocingulate circuitry in maternal responsivity to infant cries. They reported increased activity in response to infant cries in a wide range of areas that comprise what they call the *thalamocingulate circuitry.*

The region of neural response to infant cries appears to change as the parent–infant relationship evolves over time. In the initial weeks postpartum, first-time mothers' responses to their own infants' cries are guided by "alarm" circuits indexed by activity in the amygdala and the insula. Such an "alarm" response may serve to facilitate immediate action in response to the infant's distress. Interestingly, the level of right amygdala activation was associated with parents' measures of obsessive symptoms, such as anxious or intrusive thoughts and harm-avoidant behaviors (Swain, Leckman, Mayes, Feldman, & Schultz, 2005), and the activated regions resemble those activated in humans with obsessive–compulsive disorder (OCD) (Abramowitz, Taylor, & McKay, 2009). Later on, at 3–4 months postpartum, the pattern of neural response appears to shift to be more indicative of social engagement indexed by activation of areas in the hypothalamus and the ventral tegmental area. Further underscoring the experience-related shift in caregiver neural response, neural responses in experienced parents at 2 weeks closely resembled neural responses at 3–4 months in first-time parents (Swain et al., 2004). Finally, demonstrating the notion that parental status enhances sensitivity specific to infant distress, an additional study revealed that while parents showed increased activity in the amygdala and bilateral insula in response to crying but not to infant laughter, nonparents showed increased activity in response to laughter but not to crying (Seifritz et al., 2003). Studies have also examined mothers' sensitive responsiveness and neural response to their own infant's distress (cry sound), revealing an association between sensitive responses and activation of the right superior frontal gyrus and amygdala (Kim et al., 2011), as well as right frontopolar and inferior frontal activation (Musser, Kaiser-Laurent, & Ablow, 2012). These studies implicate the role of these regions in guiding maternal response to infant distress. Though somewhat inconsistent, gender differences are also evident, with some studies revealing that, relative to men, women display decreased activity in response to baby cries in the subgenual ACC (e.g., Seifritz et al., 2003), whereas others report to the contrary (e.g., Swain et al., 2004, 2005). The ACC ventral to the genu of the corpus callosum has been implicated in the modulation of emotional behavior, and research indicates that gray-matter volume of the subgenual ACC is reduced in individuals with significant mood disorders (Drevets, Savitz, & Trimble, 2008).

Finally, electrophysiological correlates of maternal sensitivity to infant cries have also been reported. For instance, one study revealed augmented auditory N100 responses in mothers relative to nonmothers. The authors take this neural augmentation of the attention-related N100 component to reflect an increase in maternal alertness that promotes prompt response to infant needs (Purhonen et al., 2001).

NEURAL CORRELATES OF CAREGIVER RESPONSE TO INFANT VISUAL STIMULI

Behavioral research underscores the biological salience of infant schemata, revealing that these are prioritized by the adult attention system (Brosch, Sander, & Scherer, 2007). Infant facial expressions are key in signaling affective states in preverbal stages of communication. The neuroscience literature reveals that, similar to adult faces, infant faces elicit activity in the brain's fusiform face area. Yet unlike adult faces, infant faces elicit activity in additional brain regions as well. Activation that appears to be specific to infant (and not adult) facial stimuli is thought possibly to reflect the neural basis for adult caregiving behaviors (Mayes, Swain, & Leckman, 2005).

Relative to nonmothers, mothers show increased activation of the right PFC when discriminating infant facial emotions. However, no such difference was elicited when mothers and nonmothers viewed adult facial expressions. Nishitani and colleagues (2011) propose that these results underscore the involvement of the frontal cortex in human maternal behavior related to infant facial emotion discrimination (Nishitani, Doi, Koyama, & Shinohara, 2011). Specifically, one of the most consistent findings in neural responses to infant facial images is increased activity in the OFC (e.g., Bartels & Zeki, 2004; Nitschke et al., 2004; Noriuchi, Kikuchi, & Senoo, 2008; Ranote et al., 2004), elicited as early as 130 milliseconds (ms) poststimulus presentation (Kringelbach et al., 2008). Research has implicated the OFC in reward-related processing (Kringelbach, 2005) of pleasant sensory stimuli. Increased activity in the OFC has indeed been found to correlate with self-reported increases in positive mood when a mother views a picture of her infant, compared to an unfamiliar infant (Nitschke et al., 2004). One study revealed that whereas activity in the left OFC was related to joyful feelings, activity in the right OFC was related to anxious feelings in response to infants (Noriuchi et al., 2008).

In addition to the OFC, infant facial stimuli have been found to elicit activity in a widely distributed network of brain regions (for reviews, see Parsons et al., 2010; Swain, 2008; Swain et al., 2004; Swain, Lorberbaum, Kose, & Strathearn, 2007). These include regions involved in emotion processing (medial PFC, ACC, and insula cortex), cognition (dorsolateral PFC), and motor/behavioral outputs (primary motor area). Together, these allow for the integration of affective and cognitive information toward motor/behavioral outputs (Strathearn, Li, Fonagy, & Montague, 2008).

Interestingly, different neural circuits appear to be activated as a function of type of stimulus emotion. For instance, specifically in response to a mother's own infant's distress but not for other emotions, maternal brain activation was found in a widely distributed network, including the dorsal region of OFC, caudate nucleus, right inferior frontal gyrus, dorsomedial PFC, ACC, posterior cingulate, thalamus, substantia nigra, and posterior superior temporal sulcus (Noriuchi et al., 2008). Another study revealed activation of dopaminergic reward-related brain regions specifically in response to happy, but not sad, infant faces (Strathearn et al., 2008). Integrating these findings, Bartels and Zeki (2004) suggest a "push–pull" mechanism for maternal behavior that selectively activates motivation and reward systems on the one hand (via activations in the ACC, insula, basal ganglia–striatum, and midbrain periaqueductal gray regions of the brain), while on the other hand suppressing circuits responsible for negative emotions, avoidance behavior, and negative social assessment.

Finally, using ERPs, several studies examined the time course and electrophysiological correlates of maternal processing of infant facial cues. In one study, birth and foster/adoptive mothers viewed pictures of their own children, and of familiar and unfamiliar children and adults. All mothers, regardless of type, showed ERP patterns suggestive of increased attention allocation to their own children's faces compared to other child and adult faces, beginning as early as 100–150 ms after stimulus onset. Additionally, late positive potentials associated with greater allocation of attention predicted mothers' perceptions of the parent–child relationship as positive and influential to their children's psychological development (Grasso, Moser, Dozier, & Simons, 2009). In another study, ERPs in response to infant stimuli were examined among new parents, new lovers, and romantically unattached singles. Parents exhibited attenuated amplitudes in the parietal P300 component (implicated in controlled attention) toward the unfamiliar infant but increased P300 amplitude in response to their own infant. When viewing unfamiliar infants, both parents and lovers exhibited greater activation compared to singles at occipital–lateral (N170) and central–frontal (P3a) sites, indicating greater initial attention to infant cues (Weisman, Feldman, & Goldstein, 2012). Taken together, these findings demonstrate that it is not necessarily the biological status of maternity that drives specified neural systems; rather, it is the formation of the attachment relationships (whether it be between a foster parent and infant or between two lovers) that activates caregiving brain reactivity to infant cues.

Neural Activity in Relation to Attachment Styles

In the attempt to identify some of the neural processes underlying the relation between adult attachment styles and emotion regulation, several studies have examined neural activity in response to attachment-relevant stimuli and assessed attachment styles of the participants. For instance, studies reveal that women with insecure, disorganized attachment patterns showed increased activation of medial temporal regions, including the amygdala, a region that is highly reactive to emotional stimuli (Vrticka, Andersson, Grandjean, Sander, & Vuilleumier, 2008), as well as the hippocampus, particularly in response to attachment-related distressing stimuli (Buchheim et al., 2006). Another study revealed that adult activity within the bilateral amygdala was positively associated with attachment insecurity and autonomic response during performance in a stress condition but not in a neutral prime condition (Lemche et al., 2006). Taken together, these studies implicate the key role that perturbed sensitivity of the amygdala may have in mediating emotional dysregulation and autonomic activity associated with attachment insecurity, particularly when individuals are threatened with social rejection or relationship loss.

In addition to increased reactivity of emotion-related areas of the brain (e.g., the amygdala), studies reveal that adults with anxious attachment representations may simultaneously have difficulty down-regulating negative emotion via OFC activity due to nonsufficient activation of the OFC (Gillath, Bunge, Shaver, Wendelken, & Mikulincer, 2005). Furthermore, mothers who report having had a better history of parental care when they themselves were children (possibly indicating a history of secure attachment) display enhanced activation in the OFC and temporal cortex, as well as occipital, parietal, and cerebellar circuits in response to infant cues (Kim et al., 2010).

Unlike attachment-related anxiety which is associated with increased emotional arousal, attachment-related avoidance is characterized by tendencies to withdraw from close relationships and emotional situations. Attachment-related avoidance appears to be related to diminished activation of both reward-related (Vrticka et al., 2008) and negative emotion cues (Suslow et al., 2009) in regions generating an emotional response on the one hand, and less efficient suppression indexed by exaggerated activation of cognitive and affective control circuits in the face of distressing stimuli on the other (Gillath et al., 2005).

Finally, Laurent and Ablow (2012b) examined "the missing link" between parent neural circuitry and infant attachment style indexed by infant behavior. Findings revealed altered processing of infant distress cues in mothers as a function of specific infant attachment-related behaviors. Specifically, in response to their infants' cries, mothers of infants with lower continuous attachment security scores displayed exaggerated activation (failure to deactivate) in neural circuits involved in painful or emotionally charged memories. The authors suggested that these findings support the notion of transmission of attachment insecurity due to the priming of negative schematic memories within the mother. Additionally, mothers of infants demonstrating behaviors characteristic of both attachment anxiety (i.e., contact maintenance) and avoidance (i.e., avoidance) responded less to infants' cries in prefrontal regions previously implicated in successful emotion regulation. The authors suggested that a problematic attachment history inhibits the development of prefrontal regulatory capacities that, in turn, make it difficult for a parent to down-regulate activation adequately in responding to his or her own infant's distress and thereby foster secure attachment.

Examples of Perturbed Attachment-Related Networks

In line with Bowlby's (1978) assertion more than 4 decades ago that attachment theory can be used to frame the etiology of psychiatric disorders, longitudinal research demonstrates the detrimental effects of perturbed attachment on child socioemotional development. As demonstrated in earlier sections of this chapter, infant cues enhance maternal care in a reciprocal fashion. In the same vein, when interaction is reduced (e.g., due to mother–infant separation, maternal depression, or neglect) or dysregulated (e.g., due to temperamental predispositions, extreme prematurity, or birth defects), there may be an increased risk for disturbed attachment or maltreatment (e.g., Sanson & Rothbart, 1995; Weinfield, Stroufe, & Egeland, 2000). From a neuroscience perspective, research has typically focused on examining the effects of perturbed parenting on brain responses to infant cues. For instance, ERP studies have shown perturbations in the N170 component, typically associated with the perceptual processing of faces, in response to infant distress in both neglectful mothers (Rodrigo et al., 2011) and depressed mothers (Noll, Mayes, & Rutherford, 2012). Additionally, neglectful mothers displayed an overall attenuated LPP, a component associated with elaborate stages of processing and emotion regulation, that was related to their higher scores in social anhedonia. Finally, a neuroimaging study revealed that in response to their own infants' cries, nondepressed mothers showed activation of a distributed network of both paralimbic ("emotional" regions of the brain) and prefrontal (down-regulatory regions of the brain), whereas depressed mothers failed to show such activation (Laurent & Ablow, 2012a).

Together, these studies suggest that perturbed neurophysiological responsiveness to infant cues may interfere with parental perceptual coding that is necessary for attuned contingent responsiveness. Such contingent interactions mirror the infant's affective states and are thought to promote understanding of the infant's emotions and subsequent ability to regulate these emotional experiences and expressions in a socially adaptive manner. Viewed as a regulatory system, attachment plays a fundamental role in the dyadic regulation of emotion (Schore, 2000). In fact, self-regulation is thought to be acquired by virtue of coregulation between the infant and the attachment figures. We dedicate the following sections to key processes underlying the development of emotion regulation and the socialization of these regulatory capacities.

Socializing Emotional Regulatory Capacities

The Functional Importance of Emotion Regulation in the Context of Socialization

Emotions have a key evolutionary function in facilitating necessary behavioral responses and interpersonal interactions. Emotion regulation is aimed at eliciting changes in "emotion dynamics" to manage in a socially adaptive manner the latency, rise time, magnitude, duration, and offset of emotional responses in behavioral, experiential, or physiological domains (Gross & Thompson, 2007). Research reveals that children and adults who are more competent at emotion regulation are more successful in social interaction, more capable of focused problem solving, better at prioritizing delayed rewards over immediate ones, and have a higher probability of achieving overall emotional well-being. Transactions between infants and caregivers provide the context in which infants begin to understand and regulate emotional experience and expression (for reviews, see Thompson & Meyer, 2007; Thompson, Virmani, Waters, Raikes, & Meyer, 2013). While research in the adult literature typically focuses on *intrinsic processes* of emotion regulation, whereby an individual regulates his or her own emotions (Gross & Thompson, 2007), developmental literature focuses more on *extrinsic processes* of emotion regulation, whereby one individual (i.e., the parent) regulates the emotions of another (i.e., the infant). This relative focus is reflective of the salience of extrinsic processes in early development (e.g., Cole, Martin, & Dennis, 2004; Fox & Calkins, 2003). Through these extrinsic processes, children's emotions are socialized, and children learn to regulate their own emotions. Caregivers socialize infant emotionality by scaffolding the development of control processes, allowing for the gradual and eventual shift from extrinsic dyadic coregulation to intrinsic self-regulation of emotion.

Decades of research support the notion that caregivers are the most important socializers of emotion regulation in early childhood, and several mechanisms of parent socialization have been identified (for reviews, see Eisenberg, Cumberland, & Spinrad, 1998; Thompson & Meyer, 2007). Research using rodents indicates that maternal care during infancy may in fact "program" regulatory responses to stress in the offspring (Caldji et al., 1998). In the following sections, we describe the main mechanisms through which caregiver socialization of emotion regulation occurs and note the emotion regulation strategies that are acquired through these mechanisms.

Mechanisms of Parent Socialization of Emotion and Emotion Regulation

There are numerous ways that caregivers can influence how children understand and respond to emotionally charged situations (see Eisenberg et al., 1998, for review; Denham, Bassett, & Wyatt, Chapter 25, this volume). Much of the existing research on mechanisms of parent socialization of emotion during the preverbal stages of development can be categorized into three topics: contingent synchronous face-to-face interactions, caregiver reactions to children's emotions, and parental expression of emotion.

CONTINGENT SYNCHRONOUS FACE-TO-FACE INTERACTIONS

Consistent with social learning theory (Bandura, 1977), the most direct method of caregiver socialization of emotion regulation occurs when a caregiver responds contingently to the infant's affective behavior. Infants have the ability to detect social contingencies very early on. Infants as young as 1 month of age display increased ability to learn social relative to nonsocial contingencies; this suggests the existence of a mechanism that specifically facilitates learning about the social world very early in life (Reeb-Sutherland, Levitt, & Fox, 2011). While some data suggest a developmental shift in the sensitivity to social contingencies between ages 1 and 3 months (Striano, Henning, & Stahl, 2005) others demonstrate these abilities in infants as young as 5 weeks of age, but only in infants of *highly attuned mothers* (defined as mothers whom maintain attention and display warm sensitivity and social responsiveness toward their infants), not in infants of nonattuned mothers (Markova & Legerstee, 2006). Furthermore, underscoring the role that contingency learning plays in the ontogeny of social behaviors, individual differences in the rate of contingency learning at 1 month of age have been found to be an enduring predictor of social, imitative, and discriminative social behaviors at 5, 9, and 12 months of age, as well as face-evoked discriminative neural activity at 9 months of age (Reeb-Sutherland et al., 2012). The fact that there are individual differences in the rate of associative learning at 1 month of age may, of course, be a result of inborn differences in sensitivity or alertness, and the fact that these differences influence the rate of learning and in turn predict adaptive social behavior suggests the importance of these processes early in life.

Socioemotional processing rapidly develops over the first months of life (see Parsons et al., 2010, for review). Newborn infants are capable of imitating simple facial gestures (Meltzoff & Moore, 1983). By age 3 months, they are able to discriminate between smiling and frowning facial expressions (Barrera & Maurer, 1981), and fearful and angry expressions by 5 months (Schwartz, Izard, & Ansul, 1985). By 7 months of age, infants recognize the same facial expression across individuals (Kotsoni, de Haan, & Johnson, 2001).

Taken together, the capacity for contingency learning, along with the perceptual ability to process and discriminate socioemotional stimuli, allows the infant to partake in mutually responsive, conversation-like interactions with the caregiver, which provide the context in which the infant begins to understand and organize its own affective experience and shape the neural architecture underlying emotion regulation. The young infant naturally reaches out for nonverbal interactions, and the adult responds by mirroring contingent vocalizations and gestures. Through these contingent interactions the caregiver attempts to maintain the infant's positive arousal at an optimal level and decrease negative arousal. Fogel (1993) termed this interactive regulation in parent–infant dyads *coregulation*. Both the caregiver and the infant are remarkably paced and attuned to each other's cues (for reviews, see Beebe, 2000; Papousek, 2007), and symmetrical coregulation patterns between the caregiver and the infant increase over time (Evans & Porter, 2009). The caregiver interprets the infant's behavior and mirrors the ascribed meaning back to the infant in a developmentally appropriate manner, thereby facilitating infant ability to partake in expansive communicative dialogues. Interestingly, the infant displays extreme dysregulation when normal contingent responsiveness is perturbed experimentally, for instance, when the mother is instructed to adopt a "still face" expression in response to infant expression of emotion (Tronick, Als, & Adamson, 1978). In early postpartum stages, prompt responses serve to modulate infant arousal and function as learning experiences for the infant (e.g., Eisenberg et al., 1998). Consistent with this view, and contrary to reinforcement theory, mothers' immediate responsiveness to infant signals has been linked to a gradual decrease in the level of the infant crying over the first year of life (Bell & Ainsworth, 1972). As time passes, the caregiver begins gradually to increase progressively the time lag between the infant's demands and their satisfaction, allowing the infant to acquire a growing capacity to tolerate delay and develop self-soothing behaviors. This development perhaps demonstrates the gradual shift from extrinsic to intrinsic emotion regulation.

Importantly, through infant–caregiver face-to-face interactions, infants acquire increasing control over intentional attentional deployment, one of the first emotion regulatory strategies to appear in development (Rothbart, Ziaie, & O'Boyle, 1992). *Attentional deployment* refers to how individuals shift, direct, and control their attention within a given situation in order to influence their emotions. Infants spontaneously shift their gaze away from aversive events and toward pleasant ones in order to regulate sympathetic arousal (Field, 1981). Caregivers may promote the development of these capacities by allowing their infants to shift their gaze back and forth spontaneously as needed, without intrusively attempting to maintain infant gaze despite overstimulation. Additionally, in the early postpartum period, infants demonstrate the ability to comprehend the communicative function of eye gaze in redirecting attention to specific targets, allowing parents to use *referential gaze* to distract infant attention from distress and redirect allocation of attention for purposes of emotion management. In toddlerhood, maternal negative and controlling behavior was found to be negatively related to the use of distraction techniques in a frustrating situation (Fox & Calkins, 2003), underscoring the importance of nonintrusive parenting strategies in facilitating the development of these capacities.

CAREGIVER REACTIONS TO CHILDREN'S EMOTIONS

Caregiver reactions, particularly during exchanges that involve child expressions of negative emotions, provide important opportunities for emotion socialization. A distressed child may elicit a variety of emotions from the parent, ranging from helplessness, anger, and anxiety to sympathy, caring, and protectiveness. As parents regulate their own experience in coping with these emotions, they model their emotion management style to their observing child. The caregiver's own regulatory strategies may give rise to a wide variety of socialization behaviors, including avoidance, expression of negative affect, punitive actions, and minimization of infant emotion or, alternatively, validation and attempts to comfort and teach the child ways to understand, manage, and regulate emotional experiences (e.g., Eisenberg & Fabes, 1994). These socialization behaviors give rise to an emotion regulation strategy termed *response modulation*, the process through which the caregiver directly influences the physiological, experiential, and behavioral responses of the child. Interestingly, encouraging suppression of emotion-expressive behavior seems to effect emotional experience differentially, decreasing positive but not negative emotion experience and actually increasing sympathetic activation in adults (e.g., Gross & Levenson, 1997). Similarly, suppression of negative but not positive emotion has been found to increase sympathetic activation in children (Musser et al., 2011). Thus, although learning emotional display rules is an important part of socialization of emotion regulation, suppression of negative emotion may not always be an effective emotion regulation strategy, both experientially and sympathetically. Behavioral evidence suggests that helping a child to find alternative adaptive ways of expression may be more effective in facilitating emotion regulation (Thompson & Meyer, 2007). Finally, supportive sympathetic parental reactions extrinsically alter the emotional impact of a potentially stressful situation by helping the child to cope with potentially distressing situations, an emotion regulation strategy referred to as *situation modification*.

CAREGIVER EXPRESSION OF EMOTION

Caregiver expression of emotion is linked to children's socioemotional competence, both directly and indirectly. Direct links occur through processes whereby children directly imitate the caregiver's expression of emotion. Indirect links occur whereby the caregiver's expression of emotion provides information about the emotional significance of a given situation, which influences the way infants interpret and experience that context. This indirect emotion regulation strategy is termed *cognitive change*. Caregiver expression of emotion has evolutionary importance, particularly in the context of threat (Cook & Mineka, 1989). Caregivers' affective signals have been found to alter infants' interpretation of ambiguity, fostering either inhibition- or approach-related behaviors (e.g., Gunnar & Stone, 1984). Such processes raise the possibility of perturbed socialization via the transmission of nonwarranted biases. Finally, a vast literature has examined maternal expressed emotion (EE), namely, the mother's affective tone, level of criticism, and level of emotional involvement, typically coded from a 5-minute speech sample. The literature indicates that maternal EE is an important environmental risk or protective factor for the development of adaptive or maladaptive child regulation (e.g., McCarty & Weisz, 2002), even after researchers control for genetic influences (Caspi et al., 2004).

Emotion Regulation from a Neuroscience Perspective

Caregiver–infant relationships are the context in which early socialization of emotion regulation occurs. Emotion socialization processes not only modify behavior but also alter physiological, hormonal, and even genetic expressions, as well as neural networks within the brain. In the following sections we first describe changes in physiological, neuroendocrine, and genetic activity, and their relation to early socialization of emotion regulation. We then provide an illustrative review of both neuroimaging and electrophysiological data regarding emotion regulation. Within this section, we (1) describe the neural circuitry underlying emotion regulation, (2) describe the development of this neural circuitry, and (3) review the small but important neuroscience literature that demonstrates the susceptibility of this neural circuitry to influences of parent socialization.

Physiological Changes and Early Socialization of Emotion Regulation

Physiological correlates of regulatory behavior such as heart rate and vagal tone have been suggested as mechanisms that may mediate the relations between caregiver influence and developmental changes in infant emotional reactivity and regulation (see Propper & Moore, 2006, for review). Findings reveal that interactions between caregivers and infants directly influence infants' physiological reactivity and regulation.

Vagal tone, namely, parasympathetic control over cardiac functioning, is measured as the amplitude of respiratory sinus arrhythmia (RSA), and is considered to be an index of underlying regulatory abilities in mammals (Porges, 1996). The vagal system has been suggested as a possible biological substrate for regulation of arousal and reactivity underlying individual differences in temperament (e.g., Fox, 1989; Fox & Stifter, 1989), and it appears to be susceptible to extrinsic socialization influences. For instance, in a series of studies, relative to nonreactive infants, infants at age 5 months who were emotionally reactive to mildly stressful stimuli (i.e., an arm restraint procedure) and displayed high vagal tone responses, were found to be more sociable and positively reactive to a series of novel events several months later at age 14 months. Those who displayed appropriately distressed reactivity in response to a stressful stimulus at age 5 months were more likely to exhibit reduced negative affect in the face of novelty several months later (Calkins & Fox, 1992). The mechanism by which individual differences in vagal control and reactivity are linked to later emotion regulation may reside in the caregiver–infant interaction (Propper & Moore, 2006). Young infants with a greater parasympathetic response may be more expressive in a distressing context and better at signaling to their caregivers that assistance is needed. In turn, the caregiver can then effectively attend to and soothe the infant, thereby regulating negative emotions. This pattern of effective signaling may facilitate the development of subsequent regulatory capacities.

Links between child vagal tone and early caregiver–infant communicative patterns underscore the importance of synchronous contingent interactions in shaping infants' emerging patterns of regulation (for reviews, see Feldman, 2012; Propper & Moore, 2006). There is evidence of an association between synchronized contingent mother–infant exchanges and regulation, as indexed by vagal tone in general (Porter, 2003), and in the context of the still-face paradigm in particular (e.g., Moore & Calkins, 2004). Moreover, greater maternal sensitivity in the context of distress has been shown to moderate infant vagal tone above and beyond maternal sensitivity during neutral play episodes, thus underscoring the specific importance of external regulation in the context of infant distress (Conradt & Ablow, 2010; Moore et al., 2009).

Interestingly, both mothers' and infants' physiological responses appear to be a function of synchronized mutual responsiveness (Moore et al., 2009). During social interactions, mothers' and infants' heart rhythms synchronize within lags of less than 1 second. Moreover, the level of mother–infant heart rate concordance is significantly higher during episodes of behavioral synchrony relative to nonsynchrony (Feldman, 2012). Finally, increasing mother–infant biological synchrony has been displayed developmentally, with concordance between mother–infant vagal withdrawal significantly increasing over the first 6 months of life (Bornstein & Suess, 2000). Vagal tone is a measure of respiratory sinus arrhythmia, the variability in heart rate due to respiratory activity. Vagal tone and the decrease in vagal tone as a function of stimulus challenge (known as *vagal withdrawal*) has been used as an index of physiological reactivity related to risk. For example, Calkins, Graziano, and Keane (2007) found less vagal withdrawal in children at risk for externalizing problems.

Neuroendocrine Changes and Early Socialization of Emotion Regulation

The hypothalamic–pituitary–adrenal (HPA) axis is a complex set of direct influences and feedback interactions among three endocrine glands: the hypothalamus, the pituitary gland, and the adrenal glands. It serves as the primary stress response system and regulates many body processes, including mood and emotions. The HPA axis's product, a steroid hormone called cortisol (CORT), is the key stress hormone that acts in all parts of the body, with the brain being a primary target for its actions (Gunnar, Doom, & Esposito, in press). Neuroendocrine findings reveal evidence for early socialization of emotion regulation during the neonatal period via coregulation within the caregiver–infant relationship. For instance, the more time the parent and infant spend in physical contact with one another, the smaller the infant CORT elevations in response to everyday stressors (for review, see Hostinar & Gunnar, 2012). Additionally, sensitive maternal responses to infant distress have been shown to regulate the HPA axis, returning CORT levels more promptly to baseline (Albers, Riksen-Walraven, Sweep, & De Weerth, 2008). Increased stability of the diurnal CORT rhythm achieved by the age of 4 months is thought to reflect early development of regulatory mechanisms (Gunnar et al., in press). Over the first year of life, the attachment figure appears to become increasingly potent in buffering stress in the context of distress. While stressful situations elicit increases in child CORT despite the parent's presence at 2, 4, and 6 months of age, from 12 to 18 months, these elevations were no longer present (Gunnar et al., in press). The authors note that this developmental shift occurs when the child begins actively to organize security-seeking behavior around attachment figures. Finally, between ages 3 and 6 months, findings reveal a decrease in concordance between mother–infant adrenocortical responses to stress during a stress-eliciting situation, perhaps reflecting a gradual transition from extrinsic to intrinsic regulation of emotion as the infant gains increasing psychophysiological independence (Thompson & Trevathan, 2009).

Gene Expression and Early Socialization of Emotion Regulation

Recent approaches encourage the study of development as a bidirectional process in which the relation between genes and behavior examines not only the impact of genes on environment but also environmental influences on genetic expression in normal and abnormal development (e.g., Avinun & Knafo-Noam, Chapter 15, this volume; Rutter, Moffitt, & Caspi, 2006). Research from molecular genetics clearly points toward the fact that social experience, especially quality of caregiving and family environments, influences gene expression. With regard to reactivity and regulatory behaviors, evidence to date suggests that the short allele of the serotonin transporter gene and the long allele of the DRD4 dopamine receptor gene may be related to distinct patterns of infant emotionality and to later problems with depression, impulse control, and externalizing/antisocial behaviors. Importantly, the greatest risk appears to be when genetic predisposition is paired with insensitive or abusive parenting (e.g., Rutter et al., 2006).

Recent research has also examined epigenetic changes to the glucocorticoid receptor (GR) system as underlying stress-related psychopathology. A recent study found increased GR NR3C1 methylation in the promoter region of the gene in maltreated compared to nonmaltreated children (Romens, Svaren, & Pollak, in press). The authors suggest that increased methylation contributes to fewer GRs in the brain and blood, impairing the physiology of stress regulation and thereby pointing toward a molecular mechanism linking childhood stress with biological changes and potential maladaptive outcomes.

The Neural Circuitry Underlying Emotion Regulation

Adaptive emotion regulation is one of the key outcomes of successful socialization of emotion. Researchers have seldom studied the direct mechanisms through which socialization facilitates the development of the neural underpinnings of emotion regulation. Developmental accounts of emotion regulation propose that it is shaped both separately and interactively by emotional reactivity and inhibitory cognitive control processes (e.g., Derryberry & Rothbart, 1997). Neuroscience literature indicates that emotional reactions and subsequent regulation of these are supported by a widely distributed neural network that specifically distinguishes between two complementary but highly interconnected neural systems: the ventral system and the dorsal system (see Dennis, O'Toole, & DeCicco, 2013, for review). The ventral system underlies emotional arousal by rapidly and relatively automatically evaluating emotional significance of stimuli. It includes lower emotion centers, such as the amygdala, hypothalamus, brain stem, insula, striatum, and the medial OFC. The dorsal network is a higher cortical system that underlies cognitive control, namely, relatively effortful, executive control functions (e.g., Critchley, 2005; Dolan, 2002) and supports the ability to regulate arousal in more deliberate ways. The cognitive control processes supported by the dorsal network serve to modulate emotional experiences and exert top-down cortical control over lower emotion centers. This system includes four key areas of the PFC, that have been implicated in the use of cognitive emotion regulation strategies: the lateral prefrontal cortex (LPFC), the medial prefrontal cortex (MPFC), the lateral orbitofrontal cortex (LOFC), and the ACC (Dennis et al., 2013). Recent research provides evidence that emotion regulation occurs through mutual activity of higher and lower brain regions (for reviews, see Dennis et al., 2013; Thompson et al., 2013). Structurally, the ventral and dorsal systems are strongly interconnected via corticolimbic circuitry, and neuroimaging studies indicate a pattern in which downregulation of the ventral system and up-regulation of the dorsal system are associated with adaptive emotion regulation. Up-regulatory influences of the limbic systems alter perceptual sensitivity of the cortical regions to affective cues, whereas down-regulatory influences of the amygdala alter ACC functioning in subsequent emotional appraisal and regulatory processes (see Dennis et al., 2013, for review).

Development of the Neural Circuitry Underlying Emotion Regulation

Socialization influences are thought to impact both the degree of arousal and reactivity of the ventral system (the "emotional brain") and scaffold the development of the dorsal system (the "cognitive regulatory brain"). Nevertheless, direct socialization influences on the development of these systems have not been empirically examined.

NEUROIMAGING STUDIES

Neuroimaging studies suggest that structural and functional brain changes across childhood underlie the development of emotion regulatory capacities (see Dennis et al., 2013, for review). Performance on behavioral tasks related to cognitive control (i.e., effortful control, attentional control, and executive functions) gradually improve from early childhood through adolescence (e.g., Kochanska, Coy, & Murray, 2001). Developmental neuroimaging studies point toward gradual maturation and increasing neural efficiency of the dorsal system with age (e.g., Durston et al., 2002) and specifically the ACC (Casey, Giedd, & Thomas, 2000), underscoring the specific significance of the PFC in underlying the increasing efficiency with which higher-order cognitive control processes are engaged.

Nevertheless, recent findings indicate the need to move away from discussing specific functional regions toward considering functional circuitry. Network modeling techniques reveal that from childhood to adulthood, the functional interactions between regions show lessening of short-range functional connections with neighboring regions and strengthening of long-distance connections between distal regions (Fair et al., 2009). These network-level findings support the claim that cognitive maturation occurs not in unitary structures but in the connectivity and interactions between structures. In line with this notion, Somerville and Casey (2010) present a model in which development of top-down prefrontal regions interacts with a ∩-shaped function development of bottom-up striatal regions to determine changes in the regulatory capacities over the course of childhood and adolescence. In this model, in adolescence, bottom-up striatal influences involved in the detection of salient environmental stimuli tend to override top-down cognition, whereas in both children and adults, top-down cognitive control is better able to override bottom-up striatal influences. Thus, the interaction between the relative influences of both regions explains the enhanced risk taking and sensitivity to emotional rewards that characterizes adolescence. In the context of socialization, the peer group appears to be one of the most salient socialization influences in adolescence. Inclusion and approval (vs. rejection) by the peer group, for instance, may be a very salient reward that overrides higher-level cognitive control influences in decision-making processes (e.g., in the context in which an adolescent needs to decide whether to take part in a risky behavior). Similarly, a functional connectivity perspective also underlies the "triadic model" (Ernst & Fudge, 2009), which proposes that motivated behavior is governed not by the separate functioning of one region or another but by the complex interaction among approach, avoidance, and regulatory systems whose neural representatives are roughly represented by the striatum, the amygdala, and the MPFC.

In line with a functional connectivity perspective of emotion regulation, a study in typically developing 5- to 11-year-olds revealed that the connectivity between ACC and amygdala increased as a function of increase in emotion regulation demands and age (Perlman & Pelphrey, 2011). Interestingly, developmental imaging studies have revealed links between voluntary, deliberate use of emotion regulation strategies in childhood and patterns of functional connectivity. For instance, one study revealed that deliberate use of reappraisal and suppression strategies in children (ages 8–12) was associated with a similar but more widely distributed neural network than that found in adults. The relatively wider distribution of neural activation found in children is thought to reflect immaturity of the functional connectivity between the prefrontal and the limbic regions, which are more specialized in adults (Lévesque et al., 2004). In the context of socialization, caregiver reactions to children's emotions (e.g., response modulation or situation modification) that specifically encourage the recurrent use of these regulatory strategies may facilitate the specialization of this neural circuitry to enhance connectivity within these underlying networks.

ERP LITERATURE

ERP literature has focused mainly on delineating changes in the amplitudes of responses of electrophysiological components related to cognitive control, which underlie deliberate regulation of emotion. These cognitive control functions include action monitoring and inhibitory control, which are typically examined in speeded tasks that assess the participant's ability to suppress/inhibit responses that are inappropriate in a particular context. ERP analyses focus on three components thought to be generated in the ACC. The inhibitory N2, peaking 200–350 ms poststimulus, reflects successful inhibition of pre-potent responses. The ERN peaks 50–100 ms after an erroneous response and is thought to reflect a process involved in evaluating the need for, or implementation of, control due to either early automatic error detection (Falkenstein, Hoormann, Christ, & Hohnbein, 2000) or *conflict* monitoring (i.e., concurrent activation of multiple competing responses; van Veen & Carter, 2002). The error positivity (Pe) follows the ERN and typically peaks around 200–400 ms after an erroneous response. Pe may reflect an affective response to the error, may be involved in awareness of the error, or may be involved in adapting response strategies following an error (Gehring, Liu, Orr, & Carp, 2012).

Recent developmental studies have demonstrated these cognitive control compo-nents in very young children. Clear ERNs have been demonstrated in children age 10 (Friedman, Nessler, Cycowicz, & Horton, 2009), the age of 7 (Lahat et al., 2014), ages 5–7 (Torpey, Hajcak, Kim, Kujawa, & Klein, 2012), and even in preschool 4-year-old children (Brooker, Buss, & Dennis, 2011). Similarly, the inhibitory N2 has also been displayed in children at the age of 7 (e.g., Lamm, Zelazo, & Lewis, 2006; Lamm et al., in press) and even at ages 5–6 (Lewis, Lamm, Segalowitz, Stieben, & Zelazo, 2006). The PE has been demonstrated in children ages 5–7 (Torpey et al., 2012).

Because these cognitive control capacities are thought to be important outcomes of successful socialization processes, one might expect these ERP amplitudes to be related to behavioral indices of socialization. Indeed, one study reported in 10-year-old children an association between ERN amplitude and level of socialization (as indexed by subscales on the Junior Eysenck Personality Questionnaire). Though personality is greatly influ-enced by innate biological dispositions (e.g., temperament), it is generally considered to be shaped over time by the interaction between these dispositions and the environment (i.e., socialization influences). Specifically, according to the authors, low socialization influences may be indexed by high scores on the Psychoticism scale and low scores on the Lie scale. Interestingly, these were found to be related to smaller ERNs (Santesso, Segalowitz, & Schmidt, 2005). In line with these findings, ERN amplitude has generally been shown to increase with age (e.g., Davies, Segalowitz, & Gavin, 2004; Torpey et al., 2012). Developmental changes have also been reported for the PE and N2 components. PE amplitudes have been shown to increase with age (Torpey et al., 2012), whereas N2 amplitudes and latencies have been shown to decrease with age, possibly due to gradually increasing neural efficiency (e.g., Lamm et al., 2006; Lewis et al., 2006). In the context of socialization, one might expect that these neural developmental changes would be susceptible to those socialization influences that specifically scaffold the development of cognitive control and emotion regulation over time.

Some researchers have examined the direct link between neural correlates of cog-nitive control and behavioral indices of child emotional dysregulation. Decreased ERP amplitudes have been shown to be associated with externalizing symptoms (e.g., Pliszka, Liotti, & Woldorff, 2000), while increased amplitudes have been demonstrated in indi-viduals with internalizing problems, including clinical (Gehring, Himle, & Nisenson, 2000) and subclinical levels of OCD (Hajcak & Simons, 2002), as well as children with anxiety disorders (Ladouceur, Dahl, Birmaher, Axelson, & Ryan, 2006). Individual dif-ferences in temperament have also been shown to be associated with ERP amplitudes in children. For instance, behavioral inhibition in children at the age of 7 has been found to relate to increased N2 negativity (Lamm et al., in press) and increased ERN (Lahat et al., 2014). However, another study of younger children revealed greater N2 amplitudes in children with lower temperamental effortful control (Buss, Dennis, Brooker, & Sippel, 2011). These mixed results may be explained by the fact that some children display simultaneous (i.e., comorbid) internalizing and externalizing symptoms, each of which is associated with different neural correlates. For instance, in a study that investigated children with subtypes of aggression, Stieben and colleagues (2007) revealed that aggressive children with comorbid internalizing problems displayed greater N2 amplitudes than children with only externalizing problems. In the context of socialization, it appears that whereas positive socialization outcomes (expected to be associated with adaptive development of cognitive control) yield relatively consistent ERP findings, neural correlates of maladaptive dysregulation are mixed.

As described in earlier sections, caregiver socialization of emotion regulation is key, particularly in the context of child distress. Several studies have examined the ability of children to recruit cognitive control under emotionally distressing contexts. Findings reveal augmented ERPs to be indicative of a child's attempt to recruit increased cognitive resources in the face of emotional demands (Lewis et al., 2006; Pérez-Edgar & Fox, 2005). Additional studies revealed greater ERP amplitudes in children in response to negatively charged relative to happy (e.g., Lewis, Todd, & Honsberger, 2007) or neutral pictures (Lamm, White, McDermott, & Fox, 2012), underscoring the impact of affective stimuli on recruitment of brain regions involved in cognitive control. To our knowledge, no studies have directly linked these findings to specific mechanisms of caregiver socialization influences, making this an important avenue for future research.

The examination of neural correlates of deliberate use of emotion regulation strategies has focused on an ERP component, the LPP, a broad superior–posterior component that becomes evident approximately 300 ms following stimulus onset and lasts up to 2,000 ms. The LPP is particularly appropriate for capturing dynamic changes in level of arousal when emotion regulation strategies are used (for reviews, see Dennis et al., 2013; Hajcak, MacNamara, & Olvet, 2010). During a directed reappraisal task, Dennis and Hajcak (2009) found evidence of a developmental shift in the efficacy of reappraisal in modulating LPP amplitudes in children between ages 5 and 9 years.

Finally, frontal EEG asymmetry has been found to reflect important patterns of emotional and behavioral reactivity, and subsequent emotion regulation via either approach or avoidance behaviors. Research with adults suggests that individuals exhibiting right frontal EEG asymmetry may be more vulnerable to stress, and tend to respond to mild stress with avoidance and negative affect (Fox & Calkins, 2003). Studies with infants and children indicate right frontal EEG asymmetry as a marker for temperamental negative reactivity and a predictor of continuity of fearful temperament over the first 4 years of life (Fox, Henderson, Rubin, Calkins, & Schmidt, 2001).

Neural Correlates of Caregiver Socialization of Emotion Regulation

NEURAL CORRELATES WITHIN THE CHILD

Despite the established notion that parenting plays a key role in shaping emotion regulation outcomes in offspring, research that directly addresses the neural underpinnings of caregiver socialization of emotion regulation is relatively scarce. Supporting the idea we discussed earlier, that referential gazing allows for redirection of infant attention, ERP studies reveal that as early as 3–4 months of age, infants demonstrate augmented neural responses to objects cued by the direct gaze of an adult or the averted gaze of an adult portraying a fearful compared to neutral expression (Hoehl, Wiese, & Striano, 2008). By the age of 9 months, infants appear to process referential information of gaze in a manner that is comparable that of adults, as reflected by similar ERP patterns elicited in both age groups (Senju, Johnson, & Csibra, 2006).

In a directly demonstration of the effect of parent socialization of emotion on infant neural and behavioral response to emotional stimuli, infants with mothers who displayed increased levels of positive EE tended to look longer at fearful rather than happy faces, and those infants rated as having a positive, exuberant temperament demonstrated a larger Nc component, suggesting enhanced attention and memory for fearful faces (de Haan, Belsky, Reid, Volein, & Johnson, 2004). Finally, one study revealed that children who displayed larger LPP amplitudes in response to unpleasant versus neutral stimuli were more fearful during an emotional challenge, but only when parents showed low levels of "promoting" parenting, which involved focusing their children on approach-related behaviors. The findings underscore the interactive influence of parent socialization of emotion and children's neural regulatory response in predicting child behavior (Kessel, Huselid, DeCicco, & Dennis, 2013).

NEURAL CORRELATES WITHIN THE CAREGIVER

As detailed in earlier sections, contingent and accurate mirroring of emotion is a key mechanism through which infants begin to organize their affective experience. Caregiver ability to mirror affective states accurately largely relies on parental empathy and mentalizing capacity, namely, understanding and predicting the infant's mental states underlying its behaviors and experiencing appropriate corresponding emotions. Neuroimaging studies of adults indicate a consistent set of cortical regions associated with thinking about other people's thoughts or *theory of mind*: the bilateral temporoparietal junction, the MPFC, and the posterior cingulate cortex (see Parsons et al., 2010, for review). Nevertheless, research regarding the direct relation between neural indices of parental mentalizing and behavioral and neural indices of child socioemotional outcome is lacking.

Importantly, several additional caregiver characteristics that have been shown to influence the way in which parents socialize the regulation of emotion have failed to receive sufficient neuroscience attention. These include parent "meta-emotion philosophies" (i.e., parental beliefs regarding emotional expression; Gottman, Katz, & Hooven, 1997) and the parent's own emotion regulation abilities. In addition, caregiver scaffolding of the emotion regulation strategies described in earlier sections particularly necessitate efficient levels of caregiver executive functioning. For instance, attention deployment heavily relies on attention-shifting capacities, and caregiver ability to choose adaptive responses over impulsive ones in the face of child distress heavily relies on successful inhibitory control and self-monitoring. Interestingly, despite all of this, researchers have yet to examine the neural mechanisms underlying the relation among parent executive functions, caregiver socialization of emotion regulation, and consequent neural correlates of child outcome.

Maladaptive Outcomes Related to Perturbed Socialization of Emotion Regulation

Developmental psychologists characterize affective psychopathology as a problem of emotion dysregulation, often deriving from an interaction of innate predispositions with aversive family environments (e.g., Fox, Henderson, Marshall, Nichols, & Ghera, 2005). High-risk parenting is related to either maternal behavior, characterized by intrusive or overcontrolling behavior that overrides the infant's signals, or the absence of the caregiver, as in instances of neglect that minimize the opportunity for a synchronous exchange. Excessive maternal behavior is typically associated with maternal anxiety, whereas maternal lack of engagement is typically associated with maternal depression, as reflected by a temporal pattern of inactivity, flat affect, minimal contact, and few social episodes in face-to-face mother–infant interactions (Feldman, 2012). Parents' behavior is also influenced by level of infant social responsiveness. Findings support the notion that infant temperament (e.g., irritability, intensity, soothability) or emotional reactivity predicts subsequent attachment behaviors and attachment classification (e.g., Calkins & Fox, 1992). Moreover, individual differences in infant temperament appear to interact with attachment status in predicting children's distress-related CORT reactions to novel events (Nachmias, Gunnar, Mangelsdorf, Parritz, & Buss, 1996). Specifically, elevated CORT responses were found only for toddlers who were both inhibited in their temperament and in insecure attachment relationships. Longitudinal research indicates that temperamental inhibition interacts with parenting to predict continuity–discontinuity of inhibition over time and subsequent risk for anxiety disorders (Degnan & Fox, 2007; Lewis-Morrarty et al., 2012). In this regard, it is important to recognize potential conflicts between multiple goals underlying emotion regulatory efforts. Particularly, although inhibited children may reveal innate avoidant tendencies that allow them to accomplish the immediate short-term goal of avoiding contact with anxiety-provoking situations, these may in fact enhance their long-term risk for anxiety. Studies reveal that temperamentally inhibited children are more likely to elicit overprotection and solicitous caregiving than are noninhibited children, and that such a parenting style is associated with greater internalizing problems in the child (Rubin, Cheah, & Fox, 2001). With such high-risk populations, the socialization goal of the environment may be in fact to direct these children in a way that facilitates exposure and not protective avoidance, underscoring the importance of "goodness of fit" between caregiver and child. Different family environments and styles may be a better fit for some children than others depending on the child's neural patterns related to emotion regulation.

Finally, regardless of temperamental risk, context shapes the way in which children process and experience cues in their environment. Research on maltreated children reveals altered functioning of the HPA axis and behavioral profiles of stress hyperreactivity (see Gunnar et al., in press, for review). In addition, maltreated children demonstrate biased processing of emotional cues, including hypersensitivity to and difficulty disengaging from adult expressions of anger (for review, see Pollak, 2012). Furthermore, physically abused school-age children reveal enhanced attentional allocation and enhanced attentional ERP responses specifically to their own mothers' facial anger cues, and these were associated with severity of physical maltreatment (Shackman, Shackman, & Pollak, 2007). Together, these findings highlight the key role that responsive caregiving plays in the shaping of the neural architecture underlying adaptive emotion understanding and emotion regulation.

Conclusions

This chapter underscores the prominent role that caregivers play in early socialization of infant key socioemotional capacities. An extensive body of research has examined the influence of parenting on behavioral expressions of infant attachment and emotionality, and recent research has made great progress in delineating the neural underpinnings of these processes in both the parent and the child. Nevertheless, research that directly addresses the influence of neural underpinnings of caregiver socialization particularly on the neural and behavioral development of child emotion regulation is relatively scarce. Existing evidence points toward this area as an important and promising avenue for future research.

Within behavioral research, there has been a shift over time from a focus on the actions of each individual to a focus on the coaction of members of the dyad and the nature of the relationship between them. Modern family systems perspectives view the parent–infant dyad as a subsystem within a higher-level system. Moreover, the systems perspective views these systems as having self-equilibrating properties of their own, over and above the properties of the individuals making them up. It appears that, to date, current behavioral research is primarily still focusing on the dyadic level of functioning, whereas neuroscience research is still at the level of delineating neural underpinnings of each individual member of the dyad. Interestingly, within the neuroscience literature, research has gone from examining activation patterns of individual structures to examining connectivity between different structures. Supporting this research are the increasing computational capacities that allow for systems analyses within the human individual. In order to achieve a complete understanding of socialization processes, namely, how individuals develop and interact within an ever-changing environment, systems thinking is required. It appears that future neuroscience research in this domain may benefit from moving beyond the individual level of research and applying current methodologies to study interacting neural systems between people.

REFERENCES

Abramowitz, J. S., Taylor, S., & McKay, D. (2009). Obsessive–compulsive disorder. *Lancet, 374,* 491–99.

Ainsworth, M. D. S., Blehar, M., Waters, E., & Wall, S. (1978). *Patterns of attachment.* Hillsdale, NJ: Erlbaum.

Albers, E. M., Riksen-Walraven, J. M., Sweep, F. C., & De Weerth, C. (2008). Maternal behavior predicts infant cortisol recovery from a mild everyday stressor. *Journal of Child Psychology and Psychiatry, 49,* 97–103.

Bandura, A. (1977). *Social learning theory.* Oxford, UK: Prentice-Hall.

Barrera, M. E., & Maurer, D. (1981). The perception of facial expressions by the three-month-old. *Child Development, 52,* 203–206.

Bartels, A., & Zeki, S. (2004). The neural correlates of maternal and romantic love. *NeuroImage, 21,* 1155–1166.

Beebe, B. (2000). Constructing mother–infant distress: The microsynchrony of maternal impinge-ment and infant avoidance in the face-to-face encounter. *Psychoanalytic Inquiry: A Topical Journal for Mental Health Professionals, 20*(3), 421–440.

Bell, S. M., & Ainsworth, M. D. S. (1972). Infant crying and maternal responsiveness. *Child Development, 43*, 1171–1190.

Bornstein, M. H., & Suess, P. E. (2000). Physiological self-regulation and information processing in infancy: Cardiac vagal tone and habituation. *Child Development, 2*, 273–287.

Bourgeois, J. P. (2005). Brain synaptogenesis and epigenesis. *Medecine Sciences (Paris), 21*, 428–433.

Bowlby, J. (1978). Attachment theory and its therapeutic implications. *Adolescent Psychiatry, 6*, 5–33.

Brooker, R., Buss, K. A., & Dennis, T. A. (2011). Associations between error-monitoring ERPs and temperamental shyness in children. *Developmental Cognitive Neuroscience, 1*, 141–152.

Brosch, T., Sander, D., & Scherer, K. R. (2007). That baby caught my eye: Attention capture by infant faces. *Emotion, 7*(3), 685–689.

Buchheim, A., Erk, S., George, C., Kachele, H., Ruchsow, M., Spitzer, M., et al. (2006). Mea-suring attachment representation in an fMRI environment: A pilot study. *Psychopathology, 39*,144–152.

Bushnell, I. W. R. (2001). Mother's face recognition in newborn infants: Learning and memory. *Infant and Child Development, 10*, 67–74.

Buss, K. A., Dennis, T. A., Brooker, R., & Sippel, L. M. (2011). An ERP study of conflict moni-toring in 4–8-year-old children: Associations with temperament. *Developmental Cognitive Neuroscience, 1*(2), 131–140.

Caldji, C., Tannenbaum, B., Sharma, S., Francis, D., Plotsky, P. M., & Meaney, M. J. (1998). Maternal care during infancy regulates the development of neural systems mediating the expression of fearfulness in the rat. *Proceedings of the National Academy of Sciences USA, 95*, 5335–5340.

Calkins, S. D., & Fox, N. A. (1992). The relations among infant temperament, security of attach-ment, and behavioral inhibition at 24 months. *Child Development, 63*, 1456–1472.

Calkins, S. D., Graziano, P. A., & Keane, S. P. (2007). Cardiac vagal regulation among children at risk for behavior problems. *Biological Psychology, 74*, 144–153.

Carlsson, J., Lagercrantz, H., Olson, L., Printz, G., & Bartocci, M. (2008). Activation of the right fronto-temporal cortex during maternal facial recognition in young infants. *Acta Paediat-rica, 97*, 1221–1225.

Carver, L. J., Dawson, G., Panagiotides, H., Meltzoff, A. N., McPartland, J., Gray, J., et al. (2003). Age-related differences in neural correlates of face recognition during the toddler and preschool years. *Developmental Psychobiology, 42*, 148–159.

Casey, B. J., Giedd, J. N., & Thomas, K. M. (2000). Structural and functional brain development and its relation to cognitive development. *Biological Psychology, 54*(1–3), 241–257.

Caspi, A., Moffitt, T. E., Morgan, J., Rutter, M., Taylor, A., Kim-Cohen, J., et al. (2004). Mater-nal expressed emotion predicts children's antisocial behavior problems: Using monozygotic-twin differences to identify environmental effects on behavioral development. *Developmen-tal Psychology, 40*(2), 149–161.

Chugani, H. T., & Phelps, M. E. (1986). Maturational changes in cerebral function in infants determined by 18FDG positron emission tomography. *Science, 231*, 840–843.

Cismaresco, A., & Montagner, H. (1990). Mothers' discrimination of their neonates' cry in rela-tion to cry acoustics: The first week of life. *Early Child Development and Care, 65*, 3–11.

Clutton-Brock, T. H. (1991). *The evolution of parental care.* Princeton, NJ: Princeton University Press.

Cole, P., Martin, S., & Dennis, T. (2004). Emotion regulation as a scientific construct: Method-ological challenges and directions for child development research. *Child Development, 75*, 317–333.

Conradt, E., & Ablow, J. (2010). Infant physiological response to the still-face paradigm: Contributions of maternal sensitivity and infants' early regulatory behavior. *Infant Behavior and Development, 33*(3), 251–265.

Cook, M., & Mineka, S. (1989). Observational condition of fear to fear-relevant versus fear-irrelevant stimuli in rhesus monkeys. *Journal of Abnormal Psychology, 98*(4), 448–459.

Critchley, H. D. (2005). Neural mechanisms of autonomic, affective, and cognitive integration. *Journal of Comparative Neurology, 493*(1), 154–166.

Davies, P. L., Segalowitz, S. J., & Gavin, W. J. (2004). Development of response-monitoring ERPs in 7–25-year-olds. *Developmental Neuropsychology, 25*, 355–376.

de Haan, M., Belsky, J., Reid, V., Volein, A., & Johnson, M. H. (2004). Maternal personality and infants' neural and visual responsivity to facial expressions of emotion. *Journal of Child Psychology and Psychiatry, 45*, 1209–1218.

de Haan, M., & Nelson, C. A. (1997). Recognition of the mother's face by six-month-old infants: A neurobehavioral study. *Child Development, 68*, 187–210.

de Haan, M., Pascalis, O., & Johnson, M. H. (2002). Specialization of neural mechanisms underlying face recognition in human infants. *Journal of Cognitive Neuroscience, 14*, 199–209.

De Wolff, M. S., & van IJzendoorn, M. H. (1997). Sensitivity and attachment: A metaanalysis on parental antecedents of infant attachment. *Child Development, 68*, 571–591.

DeCasper, A. J., & Fifer, W. P. (1980). Of human bonding: Newborns prefer their mothers' voices. *Science, 208*, 1174–1176.

Degnan, K. A., & Fox N. A. (2007). Behavioral inhibition and anxiety disorders: Multiple levels of a resilience process. *Development and Psychopathology, 19*, 729–746

Dennis, T. A., & Hajcak, G. (2009). The late positive potential: A neurophysiological maker for emotion regulation in children. *Journal of Child Psychology and Psychiatry, 50*(11), 1373–1383.

Dennis, T. A., O'Toole, L. J., & DeCicco, M. (2013). Emotion regulation from the perspective of developmental neuroscience: What, where, when and why. In K. C. Barrett, N. A. Fox, G. A. Morgan, D. J. Fidler, & L. A. Daunhauer (Eds.), *Handbook of self-regulatory processes in development: New directions and international perspectives* (pp. 135–172). New York: Psychology Press.

Derryberry, D., & Rothbart, M. K. (1997). Reactive and effortful processes in the organization of temperament. *Development and Psychopathology, 9*, 633–652.

Dolan, R. J. (2002). Emotion, cognition, and behavior. *Science, 298*, 1191–1194.

Drevets, W. C., Savitz, J., & Trimble, M. (2008). The subgenual anterior cingulate cortex in mood disorders. *CNS Spectrums, 13*(8), 663–681.

Durston, S., Thomas, K. M., Yang, Y., Uluğ, A. M., Zimmerman, R. D., & Casey, B. J. (2002). A neural basis for the development of inhibitory control. *Developmental Science, 5*(4), 9–16.

Eisenberg, N., Cumberland, A., & Spinrad, T. L. (1998). Parental socialization of emotion. *Psychological Inquiry, 9*, 241–273.

Eisenberg, N., & Fabes, R. A. (1994). Mothers' reactions to children's negative emotions: Relations to children's temperament and anger behavior. *Merrill–Palmer Quarterly, 40*, 138–156.

Ernst, M., & Fudge, J. L. (2009). A developmental neurobiological model of motivated behavior: Anatomy, connectivity and ontogeny of the triadic nodes. *Neuroscience and Biobehavioral Reviews, 33*, 367–382.

Evans, C. A., & Porter, C. L. (2009). The emergence of mother–infant co-regulation during the first year: Links to infants' developmental status and attachment. *Infant Behavior and Development, 32*(2), 147–158.

Fair, D. A., Cohen, A. L., Power, J. D., Dosenbach, N. U., Church, J. A., Miezin F. M., et al. (2009). Functional brain networks develop from a "local to distributed" organization. *PLoS Computational Biology, 5*, 1–14.

Falkenstein, M., Hoormann, J., Christ, S., & Hohnbein, J. (2000). ERP components on reaction time errors and their functional significance: A tutorial. *Biological Psychology, 51*(2), 87–107.

Feldman, R. (2012). Bio-behavioral synchrony: A model for integrating biological and microsocial behavioral processes in the study of parenting. *Parenting: Science and Practice, 12*, 154–164.

Field, T. (1981). Infant gaze aversion and heart rate during face-to-face interactions. *Infant Behavior and Development, 4*, 307–315.

Fogel, A. (1993). *Developing through relationships.* Chicago: University of Chicago Press.

Fox, N. A. (1989). Psychophysiological correlates of emotional reactivity during the first year of life. *Developmental Psychology, 25*, 364–372.

Fox, N. A. (l989). Heart rate variability and behavioral reactivity: Individual differences in autonomic patterning and their relation to infant and child temperament. In J. S. Reznick (Ed.), *Perspectives on behavioral inhibition* (pp. 177–196). Chicago: University of Chicago Press.

Fox, N. A., & Calkins, S. D. (2003). The development of self-control of emotion: Intrinsic and extrinsic influences. *Motivation and Emotion, 27*, 7–26.

Fox, N. A., Henderson, H. A., Marshall, P. J., Nichols, K. E., & Ghera, M. M. (2005). Behavioral inhibition: Linking biology and behavior within a developmental framework. *Annual Review of Psychology, 56*, 235–262.

Fox, N. A., Henderson, H. A., Rubin, K. H., Calkins, S. D., & Schmidt, L. A. (2001). Continuity and discontinuity of behavioral inhibition and exuberance: Psychophysiological and behavioral influences across the first four years of life. *Child Development, 72*(1), 1–21.

Fox, N. A., & Stifter, C. A. (1989). Biological and behavioral differences in infant reactivity and regulations. In G. Kohnstamm, J. Bates, & M. Rothbart (Eds.), *Handbook of temperament in childhood* (pp. 169–183). Oxford, UK: Wiley.

Friedman, D., Nessler, D., Cycowicz, Y. M., & Horton, C. (2009). Development of and change in cognitive control: A comparison of children, young and older adults. *Cognitive, Affective, and Behavioral Neuroscience, 9*(1), 91–102.

Gehring, W. J., Himle, J., & Nisenson, L. G. (2000). Action-monitoring dysfunction in obsessive–compulsive disorder. *Psychological Science, 11*(1), 1–6.

Gehring, W. J., Liu, Y., Orr, J. M., & Carp, J. (2012). The error-related negativity (ERN/Ne). In S. J. Luck & E. S. Kappenman (Eds.), *The Oxford handbook of event-related potential components* (pp. 231–291). Oxford, UK: Oxford University Press.

Gillath, O., Bunge, S. A., Shaver, P. R., Wendelken, C., & Mikulincer, M. (2005). Attachment-style differences in the ability to suppress negative thoughts: Exploring the neural correlates. *NeuroImage, 28*, 835–847.

Gottman, J. M., Katz, L. F., & Hooven, C. (1997). *Meta-emotion: How families communicate emotionally.* Mahwah, NJ: Erlbaum.

Grasso, D. J., Moser, J. S., Dozier, M., & Simons, R. (2009). ERP correlates of attention allocation in mothers processing faces of their children. *Biological Psychology, 81*(2), 95–102.

Gross, J. J., & Levenson, R. W. (1997). Hiding feelings: The acute effects of inhibiting positive and negative emotions. *Journal of Abnormal Psychology, 106*, 95–103.

Gross, J. J., & Thompson, R. A. (2007). Emotion regulation: Conceptual foundations. In J. J. Gross (Ed.), *Handbook of emotion regulation* (pp. 3–24). New York: Guilford Press.

Grossmann, T., & Johnson, M. H. (2007). The development of the social brain in human infancy. *European Journal of Neuroscience, 25*, 909–919.

Gunnar, M. R., Doom, J., & Esposito, E. (in press). Psychoneuroendocrinology of stress: Normative development and individual differences. In R. Lerner, M. Lamb, & C. Garcia Coll (Eds.), *Handbook of child psychology and developmental science* (7th ed., Vol. 3). New York: Wiley.

Gunnar, M. R., & Stone, C. (1984). The effects of positive maternal affect on infant responses to pleasant, ambiguous, and fear-provoking toys. *Child Development, 55*, 1231–1236.

Hajcak, G., MacNamara, A., & Olvet, D. M. (2010). Event-related potentials, emotion, and emotion regulation: An integrative review. *Developmental Neuropsychology, 35*(2), 129–155.

Hajcak, G., & Simons, R. F. (2002). Error-related brain activity in obsessive–compulsive undergraduates. *Psychiatry Research, 110*(1), 63–72.

Hoehl, S., Wiese, L., & Striano, T. (2008). Young infants' neural processing of objects is affected by eye gaze direction and emotional expression. *PLoS ONE, 3*(6), e2389.

Hostinar, C. E., & Gunnar, M. R. (2012). The developmental psychobiology of stress and emotion in childhood. In R. M. Lerner, M. A. Esterbrooks, & J. Mistry (Eds.), *Developmental psychology* (Vol. 6, pp. 121–141). Hoboken, NJ: Wiley.

Johnson, M. H. (2005). Subcortical face processing. *Nature Reviews Neuroscience, 6,* 766–774.

Johnson, M. H., Dziurawiec, S., Ellis, H., & Morton, J. (1991). Newborns' preferential tracking of face-like stimuli and its subsequent decline. *Cognition, 40,* 1–19.

Kappenman, E. S., & Luck, S. J. (2012). ERP components: The ups and downs of brainwave recordings. In S. J. Luck & E. S. Kappenman (Eds.), *The Oxford handbook of event-related potential components.* Oxford, UK: Oxford University Press.

Kessel, E. M., Huselid, R. F., DeCicco, J. M., & Dennis, T. A. (2013). Neurophysiological processing of emotion and parenting interact to predict inhibited behavior: An affective–motivational framework. *Frontiers in Human Neuroscience, 7,* 326.

Kim, P., Feldman, R., Mayes, L. C., Eicher, V., Thompson, N., Leckman, J. F., et al. (2011). Breastfeeding, brain activation to own infant cry, and maternal sensitivity. *Journal of Child Psychology and Psychiatry, 52*(8), 907–915.

Kim, P., Leckman, J. F., Mayes, L. C., Newman, M., Feldman, R., & Swain, J. E. (2010). Perceived quality of maternal care in childhood and structure and function of mothers' brain. *Developmental Science, 13,* 662–673.

Kochanska, G., Coy, K. C., & Murray, K. T. (2001). The development of self-regulation in the first four years of life. *Child Development, 72*(4), 1091–1111.

Kotsoni, E., de Haan, M., & Johnson, M. H. (2001). Categorical perception of facial expressions by 7-month-old infants. *Perception, 30,* 1115–1125.

Kringelbach, M. L. (2005). The orbitofrontal cortex: Linking reward to hedonic experience. *Nature Reviews Neuroscience, 6,* 691–702.

Kringelbach, M. L., Lehtonen, A., Squire, S., Harvey, A. G., Craske, M. G., Holliday, I. E., et al. (2008). A specific and rapid neural signature for parental instinct. *PLoS ONE, 3,* e1664.

Ladouceur, C. D., Dahl, R. E., Birmaher, B., Axelson, D. A., & Ryan, N. D. (2006). Increased error-related negativity (ERN) in childhood anxiety disorders: ERP and source localization. *Journal of Child Psychology and Psychiatry, 47*(10), 1073–1082.

Lahat, A., Lamm, C., Chronis-Tuscano, A., Pine, D. S., Henderson, H. A., & Fox, N. A. (2014). Early behavioral inhibition and increased error monitoring predict later social phobia symptoms in childhood. *Journal of the American Academy of Child and Adolescent Psychiatry, 53*(4), 447–455.

Lamm, C., Walker, O. L., Degnan, K. A., Henderson, H. A., Pine, D. S., McDermott, J. M., et al. (in press). Cognitive control moderates early childhood temperament in predicting social behavior in seven year old children: An ERP study. *Developmental Science.*

Lamm, C., White, L. K., McDermott, J. M., & Fox, N. A. (2012). Neural activation underlying cognitive control in the context of neutral and affectively charged pictures in children. *Brain and Cognition, 79,* 181–187.

Lamm, C., Zelazo, P. D., & Lewis, M. D. (2006). Neural correlates of cognitive control in childhood and adolescence: Disentangling the contributions of age and executive function. *Neuropsychologia, 44*(11), 2139–2148.

Laurent, H. K., & Ablow, J. C. (2012a). A cry in the dark: Depressed mothers show reduced neural activation to their own infant's cry. *Social Cognitive and Affective Neuroscience, 7*(2), 125–134.

Laurent, H. K., & Ablow, J. C. (2012b). The missing link: Mothers' neural response to infant cry related to infant attachment behaviors. *Infant Behavior and Development, 35,* 761–772.

Lemche, E., Giampietro, V. P., Surguladze, S. A., Amaro, E. J., Andrew, C. M., Williams, S. C. R., et al. (2006). Human attachment security is mediated by the amygdala: Evidence from combined fMRI and psychophysiological measures. *Human Brain Mapping, 27,* 623–635.

Lévesque, J., Joanette, Y., Mensour, B., Beaudoin, G., Leroux, J. M., Bourgouin, P., et al. (2004). Neural basis of emotional self-regulation in childhood. *Neuroscience, 129*(2), 361–369.

Lewis, M. D., Lamm, C., Segalowitz, S. J., Stieben, J., & Zelazo, P. D. (2006). Neurophysiological correlates of emotion regulation in children and adolescents. *Journal of Cognitive Neuroscience, 18*(3), 430–443.

Lewis, M. D., Todd, R. M., & Honsberger, M. (2007). Event-related potential measures of emotion regulation in early childhood. *NeuroReport, 18*, 61–65.

Lewis-Morrarty, E., Degnan, K. A., Chronis-Tuscano, A., Rubin, K. H., Cheah, C. S. L., Pine, D. S., et al. (2012). Maternal over-control moderates the association between early childhood behavioral inhibition and adolescent social anxiety symptoms. *Journal of Abnormal Child Psychology, 40*(8), 1363–1373.

Lorberbaum, J. P., Newman, J. D., Horwitz, A. R., Dubno, J. R., Lydiard, R. B., Hamner, M. B., et al. (2002). A potential role for thalamocingulate circuitry in human maternal behavior. *Biological Psychiatry, 51*(6), 431–455.

MacLean, P. D. (1990). *The triune brain in evolution: Role in pleocerebral functions.* New York: Plenum Press.

Markova, G., & Legerstee, M. (2006). Contingency, imitation and affect sharing: Foundations of infants' social awareness. *Developmental Psychology, 42*, 132–141.

Mayes, L. C., Swain, J. E., & Leckman, J. F. (2005). Parental attachment systems: Neural circuits, genes, and experiential contributions to parental engagement. *Clinical Neuroscience Reserves, 4*, 301–313.

McCarty, C. A., & Weisz, J. R. (2002). Correlates of expressed emotion in mothers of clinically-referred youth: An examination of the five-minute speech sample. *Journal of Child Psychology and Psychiatry and Allied Disciplines, 43*, 759–768.

Meltzoff, A. N., & Moore, M. K. (1983). Newborn infants imitate adult facial gestures. *Child Development, 54*, 702–709.

Moore, G. A., & Calkins, S. D. (2004). Infants' vagal regulation in the still-face paradigm is related to dyadic coordination of mother–infant interaction. *Developmental Psychology, 40*, 1068–1080.

Moore, G. A., Hill-Soderlund, A. L., Propper, C. B., Calkins, S. D., Mills-Koonce, W. R., & Cox, M. J. (2009). Mother–infant vagal regulation in the face-to-face still-face paradigm is moderated by maternal sensitivity. *Child Development, 80*, 209–223.

Musser, E., Kaiser-Laurent, H., & Ablow, J. C. (2012). Neural correlates of maternal sensitivity, intrusiveness, and mother–infant dyadic harmony: An fMRI study. *Developmental Cognitive Neuroscience, 2*(4), 428–436.

Musser, E. D., Backs, R. W., Schmitt, C. F., Ablow, J. C., Measelle, J. R., & Nigg, J. T. (2011). Emotion regulation via the autonomic nervous system in children with attention-deficit/hyperactivity disorder (ADHD). *Journal of Abnormal Child Psychology, 39*(6), 841–852.

Nachmias, M., Gunnar, M., Mangelsdorf, S., Parritz, R. H., & Buss, K. (1996). Behavioral inhibition and stress reactivity: The moderating role of attachment security. *Child Development, 67*, 508–522.

Nelson, C. A. (2001). The development and neural bases of face recognition. *Infant and Child Development, 10*, 3–18.

Nishitani, S., Doi, H., Koyama, A., & Shinohara, K. (2011). Differential prefrontal response to infant facial emotions in mothers compared with non-mothers. *Neuroscience Research, 70*(2), 183–188.

Nitschke, J. B., Nelson, E. E., Rusch, B. D., Fox, A. S., Oakes, T. R., & Davidson, R. J. (2004). Orbitofrontal cortex tracks positive mood in mothers viewing pictures of their newborn infants. *NeuroImage, 21*, 583–592.

Noll, L. K., Mayes, L. C., & Rutherford, H. J. V. (2012). Investigating the impact of parental status and depression symptoms on the early perceptual coding of infant faces: An event-related potential study. *Social Neuroscience, 7*(5), 525–536.

Noriuchi, M., Kikuchi, Y., & Senoo, A. (2008). The functional neuroanatomy of maternal love: Mother's response to infant's attachment behaviors. *Biological Psychiatry, 63*, 415–423.

Papousek, M. (2007). Communication in early infancy: An arena of intersubjective learning. *Infant Behavior and Development, 30*, 258–266.

Parsons, C. E., Young, K. S., Murray, L., Stein, A., & Kringelbach, M. L. (2010). The functional neuroanatomy of the evolving parent–infant relationship. *Progress in Neurobiology, 91*, 220–241.

Pascalis, O., de Haan, M., & Nelson, C. A. (2002). Is face processing species-specific during the first year of life? *Science, 296*, 1321–1323.

Pérez-Edgar, K., & Fox, N. A. (2005). A behavioral and electrophysiological study of children's selective attention under neutral and affective conditions. *Journal of Cognition and Development, 6*(1), 89–118.

Perlman, S. B., & Pelphrey, K. A. (2011). Developing connections for affective regulation: Age-related changes in emotional brain connectivity. *Journal of Experimental Child Psychology, 108*, 607–620.

Pliszka, S. R., Liotti, M., & Woldorff, M. G. (2000). Inhibitory control in children with attention deficit/hyperactivity disorder: Event related potentials identify the processing component and timing of an impaired right frontal response inhibition mechanism. *Biological Psychiatry, 48*(3), 238–246.

Pollak, S. D. (2012). The role of parenting in the emergence of human emotion: New approaches to the old nature-nurture debate. *Parenting: Science and Practice, 12*, 232–242.

Porges, S. W. (1996). Physiological regulation in high-risk infants: A model for assessment and potential intervention. *Development and Psychopathology, 8*, 43–58.

Porter, C. L. (2003). Corregulation in mother–infant dyads: Links to infants' cardiac vagal tone. *Psychological Reports, 92*, 307–319.

Porter, R. H., & Winberg, J. (1999). Unique salience of maternal breast odors for newborn infants. *Neuroscience and Biobehavioral Reviews, 23*, 439–449.

Propper, C., & Moore, G. A. (2006). The influence of parenting on infant emotionality: A multilevel psychobiological perspective. *Developmental Review, 26*, 427–460.

Purhonen, M., Kilpeläinen-Lees, R., Pääkkönen, A., Yppärilä, H., Lehtonen, J., & Karhu, J. (2001). Effects of maternity on auditory event-related potentials to human sound. *NeuroReport, 12*(13), 2975–2979.

Purhonen, M., Kilpeläinen-Lees, R., Valkonen-Korhonen, M., Karhu, J., & Lehtonen, J. (2005). Four-month-old infants process own mother's voice faster than unfamiliar voices—electrical signs of sensitization in infant brain. *Cognitive Brain Research, 24*, 627–633.

Ranote, S., Elliott, R., Abel, K. M., Mitchell, R., Deakin, J. F. W., & Appleby, L. (2004). The neural basis of maternal responsiveness to infants: An fMRI study. *NeuroReport, 15*, 1825–1829.

Reeb-Sutherland, B. C., Fifer, W. P., Byrd, D. L., Hammock, E. A. D., Levitt, P., & Fox, N. A. (2011). One-month-old human infants learn about the social world while they sleep. *Developmental Science, 14*(5), 1134–1141.

Reeb-Sutherland, B. C., Levitt, P., & Fox, N. A. (2012). The predictive nature of individual differences in early associative learning and emerging social behavior. *PLoS ONE, 7*(1), e30511.

Rilling, J. K. (2013). The neural and hormonal bases of human parental care. *Neuropsychologia, 51*, 731–747.

Rodrigo, M. J., Leon, I., Quinones, I., Lage, A., Byrne, S., & Bobes, M. A. (2011). Brain and personality bases of insensitivity to infant cues in neglectful mothers: An event-related potential study. *Development and Psychopathology, 23*, 163–176.

Romens, S. E., Svaren, J., & Pollak, S. D. (in press). Associations between early life stress and gene methylation in children. *Child Development*.

Rothbart, M. K., Ziaie, H., & O'Boyle, C. G. (1992). Self-regulation and emotion in infancy. In N. Eisenberg & R. A. Fabes (Eds.), *Emotion and its regulation in early development* (pp. 7–23). San Francisco: Jossey-Bass.

Rubin, K. H., Cheah, C. S. L., & Fox, N. A. (2001). Emotion regulation, parenting, and display of social reticence in preschoolers. *Early Education and Development, 12*, 97–115.

Rutter, M., Moffitt, T. E., & Caspi, A. (2006). Gene–environment interplay and psychopathology: Multiple varieties but real effects. *Journal of Child Psychology and Psychiatry, 47*, 226–261.

Sanson, A. V., & Rothbart, M. K. (1995). Child temperament and parenting. In M. H. Bornstein (Ed.), *Handbook of parenting* (pp. 299–321). Hillsdale, NJ: Erlbaum.

Santesso, D. L., Segalowitz, S. J., & Schmidt, L. A. (2005). ERP correlates of error monitoring in 10-year olds are related to socialization. *Biological Psychology, 70*(2), 79–87.

Schore, A. N. (2000). Attachment and the regulation of the right brain. *Attachment and Human Development, 2*(1), 23–47.

Schwartz, G. M., Izard, C. E., & Ansul, S. E. (1985). The 5-month-old's ability to discriminate facial expressions of emotion. *Infant Behavior and Development, 8*, 65–77.

Seifritz, E., Esposito, F., Neuhoff, J. G., Luthi, A., Mustovic, H., Dammann, G., et al. (2003). Differential sex-independent amygdala response to infant crying and laughing in parents versus nonparents. *Biological Psychiatry, 54*(12), 1367–1375.

Senju, A., Johnson, M. H., & Csibra, G. (2006). The development and neural basis of referential gaze perception. *Social Neuroscience, 1*, 220–234.

Shackman, J. E., Shackman, A. J., & Pollak, S. D. (2007). Physical abuse amplifies attention to threat and increases anxiety in children. *Emotion, 7*, 838–852.

Somerville, L. H., & Casey, B. J. (2010). Developmental neurobiology of cognitive control and motivational systems. *Current Opinion in Neurobiology, 20*, 236–241.

Sroufe, L. A. (2005). Attachment and development: A prospective, longitudinal study from birth to adulthood. *Attachment and Human Development, 7*, 349–367.

Stieben, J., Lewis, M. D., Granic, I., Zelazo, P. D., Segalowitz, S., & Pepler, D. (2007). Neurophysiological mechanisms of emotion regulation for subtypes of externalizing children. *Development and Psychopathology, 19*(2), 455–480.

Strathearn, L., Li, J., Fonagy, P., & Montague, P. R. (2008). What's in a smile?: Maternal brain responses to infant facial cues. *Pediatrics, 122*, 40–51.

Striano, T., Henning, A., & Stahl, D. (2005). Sensitivity to social contingencies between 1 and 3 months of age. *Developmental Science, 8*(6), 509–518.

Suslow, T., Kugel, H., Rauch, A. V., Dannlowski, U., Bauer, J., Konrad, C., et al. (2009). Attachment avoidance modulates neural response to masked facial emotion. *Human Brain Mapping, 30*, 3553–3562.

Swain, J. E. (2008). Baby stimuli and the parent brain: Functional neuroimaging of the neural substrates of parent–infant attachment. *Psychiatry, 5*(8), 28–36.

Swain, J. E., Leckman, J. F., Mayes, L. C., Feldman, R., Constable, R. T., & Schultz, R. T. (2004). Neural substrates and psychology of human parent–infant attachment in the postpartum. *Biological Psychiatry, 55*(8), 153S.

Swain, J. E., Leckman, J. F., Mayes, L. C., Feldman, R., & Schultz, R. T. (2005). Early human parent–infant bond development: fMRI, thoughts and behaviors. *Biological Psychiatry, 57*(8), 112S.

Swain, J. E., Lorberbaum, J. P., Kose, S., & Strathearn, L. (2007). Brain basis of early parent–infant interactions: Psychology, physiology, and *in vivo* functional neuroimaging studies. *Journal of Child Psychology and Psychiatry, 48*(3–4), 262–287.

Swingler, M. M., Sweet, M. A., & Carver, L. J. (2007). Relations between mother–child interaction and the neural correlates of face processing in 6-month-olds. *Infancy, 11*, 63–86.

Taga, G., Asakawa, K., Maki, A., Konishi, Y., & Koizumi, H. (2003). Brain imaging in awake infants by near-infrared optical topography. *Proceedings of the National Academy of Sciences USA, 100*, 10722–10727.

Thompson, L. A., & Trevathan, W. R. (2009). Cortisol reactivity, maternal sensitivity, and infant preference for mother's familiar face and rhyme in 6-month-old infants. *Journal of Reproductive and Infant Psychology, 27*, 143–167.

Thompson, R. A., & Meyer, S. (2007). The socialization of emotion regulation in the family. In J. J. Gross (Ed.), *Handbook of emotion regulation* (pp. 249–268). New York: Guilford Press.

Thompson, R. A., Virmani, E. A., Waters, S. F., Raikes, H. A., & Meyer, S. (2013). The development of emotion self-regulation: The whole and the sum of the parts. In K. C. Barrett, N. A. Fox, G. A. Morgan, D. J. Fidler, & L. A. Daunhauer (Eds.), *Handbook of self-regulatory processes in development: New directions and international perspectives* (pp. 5–26). New York: Psychology Press.

Torpey, D. C., Hajcak, G., Kim, J., Kujawa, A., & Klein, D. N. (2012). Electrocortical and behavioral measures of response monitoring in young children during a go/no-go task. *Developmental Psychobiology, 54,* 139–150.

Tronick, E., Als, H., & Adamson, L. (1978). The infant's response to entrapment between contradictory messages in face-to-face interaction. *Journal of the American Academy of Child Psychiatry, 17,* 1–13.

van Veen, V., & Carter, C. S. (2002). The anterior cingulate as a conflict monitor: fMRI and ERP studies. *Physiology and Behavior, 77,* 477–482.

Vouloumanos, A., & Werker, J. F. (2004). Tuned to the signal: The privileged status of speech for young infants. *Developmental Science, 7,* 270–276.

Vrticka, P., Andersson, F., Grandjean, D., Sander, D., & Vuilleumier, P. (2008). Individual attachment style modulates human amygdala and striatum activation during social appraisal. *PLoS ONE, 3,* e2868.

Weinfield, N. S., Stroufe, L. A., & Egeland, B. (2000). Attachment from infancy to early adulthood in a high-risk sample: Continuity, discontinuity, and their correlates. *Child Development, 71*(3), 695–702.

Weisman O., Feldman, R., & Goldstein A. (2012). Parental and romantic attachment shape brain processing of infant cues. *Biological Psychology, 89*(3), 533–538.

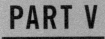

PART V

CULTURAL PERSPECTIVES ON SOCIALIZATION

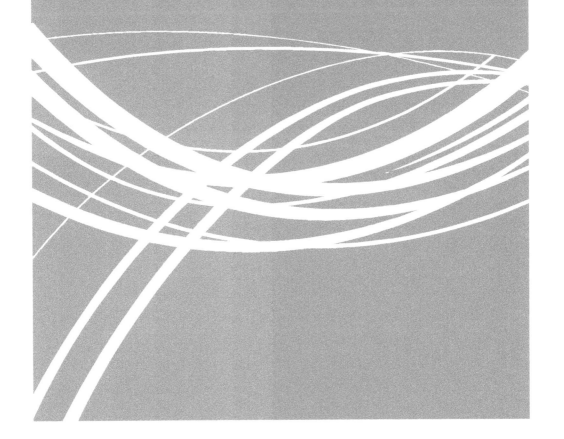

CHAPTER 19

Culture and Socialization

Xinyin Chen
Rui Fu
Siman Zhao

Human beings across cultures may differ in various aspects of socioemotional and cognitive functioning. For example, compared with their Western counterparts, children and adolescents in some African and Asian societies are less extraverted and more introverted (e.g., Lee, Okazaki, & Yoo, 2006; Oakland, Pretorius, & Lee, 2008). African and Asian children appear to be less expressive of emotions in social situations and to engage in fewer sociodramatic activities in social interactions than North American children (e.g., Camras et al., 1998; Edwards, 2000; Farver, Kim, & Lee, 1995; Gartstein et al., 2006). Chinese and Korean toddlers exhibit more fearful and anxious reactions than Italian and Australian toddlers in novel situations (Rubin, Hemphill, et al., 2006). Chinese and Korean preschoolers also tend to perform more competently than their U.S. counterparts on executive function tasks assessing self-control abilities (X. Chen et al., 2003; Oh & Lewis, 2008; Sabbagh, Xu, Carlson, Moses, & Lee, 2006). In addition, researchers have noticed that children in traditional, subsistence-based societies within which extended families live together display more cooperative behaviors toward people they know than children in economically complex societies with class structures and occupational divisions of labor (Edwards, 2000).

Given this background, it would appear essential to ask what factors are responsible for cultural variations in children's and adolescents' socioemotional and cognitive functions, and more importantly, what the processes are in which culture is involved in individual development. Obviously, socialization plays an important role in mediating the links between sociocultural conditions and human development. In the study of socialization factors, researchers have traditionally paid much attention to the family and the peer group (e.g., Rogoff, 2003). In this chapter, we first discuss some conceptual and methodological issues and major theoretical perspectives in the study of culture and socialization. Then, we review cross-cultural research on parental socialization beliefs

451

and practices. In the next section, we discuss cultural values and social processes, including evaluation and regulation in peer socialization. We conclude the chapter with a discussion of future directions in the field.

Some Conceptual and Methodological Issues

The concept of culture was initially considered mainly sociological rather than psychological by many scholars (e.g., Hofstede, 1994). Like political and economic systems, culture was discussed mainly as a contextual phenomenon in characterizing different societies rather than individuals. Largely due to the work of Triandis (1995) and other social and cultural psychologists, researchers have examined culture as a personal trait and to "measure" culture at the individual level. It makes sense to conceptualize culture as contextual, as well as personal, given that culture clearly influences societal- or community-level activities and structures (e.g., political and economic policies) and, at the same time, individual beliefs, emotions, and behaviors. *Culture* has been defined as a wide range of phenomena, from the "man-made part of the environment" to the meaning system that individuals use to understand the world (e.g., Cole & Cagigas, 2010). However, most theorists and researchers agree that even as a belief and value system, culture is concerned with the aspects that are shared and commonly endorsed by most people within the society.

The feature of culture concerning "shared" beliefs and values in a society does not seem to be an issue for cross-cultural researchers, who focus on comparing groups of individuals in different cultural communities on culture-related attitudes and behavioral reactions, because group-level scores may indicate the predominant cultural orientation. For example, a generally high tendency of authoritarian parenting in Asian parents, as assessed by parental reports or behavioral observations, may reflect cultural values of parental authority and hierarchical parent–child relationships in Asian societies. However, the notion of shared culture creates considerable challenges for developmental researchers, who are interested in how culture affects socialization and development at the individual level. The impact of societal cultural values on individual development is a complicated issue because there are no easy ways to establish logical and empirical links between the collective endorsement of cultural values (e.g., parental authority) and the behaviors that are displayed by individuals.

Several approaches have been taken to address the issue in developmental research. First, culture in a given society is considered relatively distinct, so that differences across societies in individual socialization experiences or behaviors, or their relations, are *assumed* to be contributed by culture. For example, researchers have found that Chinese children tend to be more compliant in parent–child interactions than North American children (Ho, 1986). It seems reasonable to argue that the Confucian values of filial piety that emphasize child obedience to adults may play a significant role in family socialization, which in turn leads to child compliance. A major concern with this approach is that societies and communities may differ in many social, economic, and ecological aspects in addition to culture, and the assumption that cultural effects are represented by differences in country, nation, or ethnicity group membership may therefore not be tenable.

As a second way of addressing the issue, researchers have examined individual cultural experiences or processes such as acculturation and their relations with social and cognitive functions. However, acculturation or other cultural experiences are not culture per se and may tap into only a part of it. In a study of social and psychological adjustment of immigrant Chinese children in Canada, X. Chen and Tse (2010) found that participation in Chinese cultural activities (e.g., listening to Chinese music, celebrating Chinese festivals, interactions with Chinese friends), an index of acculturation, was positively associated with social competence and negatively associated with adjustment problems. However, participation in Chinese culture-related activities or other measures of acculturation, such as proficiency in the Chinese language, provides little information about what specific aspects of Chinese culture help children develop their social competence and control their problems.

Third, culture is viewed as an individual-level construct such as a specific personal trait, which ignores the shared aspect of culture. In this approach, each individual is believed to have a unique "culture." Using this approach, researchers may measure "culture" using self-report questionnaires such as those about collectivism versus individualism or independent and interdependent self-construals (Triandis, 1995), then use the scores to analyze their relations with parenting, peer relationships, or other psychological or behavioral characteristics. Despite its popularity in cross-cultural psychology, this approach raises some concerns. It is unclear to what extent culture at the contextual level is reflected in a personal trait and whether it is appropriate to treat culture as a personal trait. Also, developmental researchers are interested in culture as a context mainly because it may serve to guide socialization processes and therefore may affect developmental patterns (e.g., Hinde, 1987). It would appear less interesting to examine an individual cultural trait, as one of possibly many individual traits, and its relations with other psychological attributes or behaviors. In addition, individual cultural traits, such as "collectivism" and "individualism," often conceptually and empirically overlap with personal attitudes and behaviors, such as sociability, communality, social assertiveness, and independence. It is difficult to distinguish cultural and noncultural traits and to maintain conceptual and methodological clarity in research. Finally, a number of measures have been developed to assess individual cultural traits (e.g., Singelis, 1994). Whereas they may show adequate psychometric qualities, such as satisfactory internal reliabilities and clear factor structures, researchers are still uncertain about whether they are appropriate for cross-cultural comparisons. Issues such as the *group-reference biases* (i.e., what group individuals refer to as a norm when they answer questions or rate items) and culturally related *response biases* (e.g., individuals in certain cultures tend to select extreme vs. moderate responses) may be confounding factors that undermine meaningful cross-cultural comparisons (e.g., Schneider, French, & Chen, 2006).

Culture, Socialization, and Human Development: Major Perspectives

The role of socialization in mediating relations between culture and child development has been recognized in two major developmental theories: Bronfenbrenner's socioecological theory (Bronfenbrenner & Morris, 2006) and Vygotsky's (1978) sociocultural theory. According to Bronfenbrenner and Morris (2006), cultural beliefs and practices are a part of the socioecological environment that affects socialization settings and parent–child and other social interactions. Although culture was considered a distal influence in the outmost layer of the environment in the early version of the theory (e.g., Bronfenbrenner,

1979), recent conceptualizations have integrated culture with proximal socialization forces such as the family and peer groups (Tietjen, 2006). In a developmental niche model, which is largely consistent with the socioecological perspective, Super and Harkness (1986) proposed that the "developmental niche" includes three interacting subsystems: the physical and social settings; the historically constituted customs and practices of child care and childrearing; and the psychology of the caretakers, particularly parental ethnotheories shared within the community. Culturally prescribed socialization conditions, beliefs, and practices are important components in the model.

Vygotsky's (1978) sociocultural theory highlights the role of socialization in the internalization of cultural systems such as language and symbols. Vygotsky asserted that, in addition to direct collaborative or guided learning in which more experienced individuals act as representatives of the culture and assist children in understanding and solving problems, broad socialization experiences—participation in social and cultural practices—affect the processes of individual development. Transformations in sociocultural structures often result in changes in social practices, which in turn lead to the reorganization of mental systems and the creation of new psychological functions (Luria, 1976). Consistent with the Vygotskian perspective, researchers who studied the effects of social and cultural transitions, from traditional rural villages to communities with more complex and planned social activities in Africa, Asia, and Central and South America, found that youth who participated in formal education and urbanized activities might display new ways of thinking (e.g., Beach, 1995; Luria, 1976; Rogoff, 2003). The cognitive processes of individuals in these societies became more decontextualized and less constrained by the specific features of the environment as they engaged in more social activities and formal school learning.

Based on socioecological and sociocultural theories, X. Chen (2012; X. Chen & French, 2008) proposed a contextual–developmental perspective that stresses social interaction as a context for human development. This perspective indicates that parents and other socialization agents, particularly peers from middle childhood onward, evaluate and respond to children's behaviors in interactions according to culturally based social expectations and standards. Adults' and peers' evaluations and responses during interaction in turn serve to regulate the development of behaviors. The evaluation and regulation processes during social interaction constitute a major mechanism of cultural influence on development.

The central theme in the contextual–developmental perspective is elaborated in several major arguments. First, the need for social acceptance, intimate affect within social relationships, and a sense of belonging (Sullivan, 1953) is the main force that directs children to participate in interactions, to attend to social evaluations, and to adjust their reactions. Second, the social interaction context elicits children's attention to feedback from others, which promotes children's awareness of social expectations and standards, and discrepancies between their behaviors and these expectations and standards. Third, whereas social approval informs children that their behaviors are regarded as appropriate, negative social evaluations create a pressure on them to modify their behaviors. The regulation of social interaction occurs as children attempt to maintain or change their behaviors or behavioral styles according to social evaluations. Fourth, interpersonal or group activities such as the establishment and modification of group norms and acceptance-based social evaluations of children's behaviors are the main mediators of links between culture and individual development, although individual characteristics such as sensitivity to social expectations may facilitate or weaken group influence. Finally, as children develop their social cognitive abilities, they play an increasingly active role in the social processes by displaying their reactions (e.g., compliance, resistance) to social influence and participating in construction of new cultures to direct social evaluations and other interaction activities. Thus, the social processes are transactional in nature (see X. Chen, 2012).

Cultural Values and Parental Childrearing Attitudes and Practices

Researchers have found cross-cultural similarities and differences in parental childrearing attitudes and practices (e.g., Dornbusch, Ritter, Leiderman, Roberts, & Fraleigh, 1987). To understand the similarities and differences, it is necessary to consider cultural values, particularly those concerning socialization goals, in societies. As required by the demands of specific social, economic, historical, and ecological circumstances, people in different societies may place different values on different aspects of children's behaviors such as emotion expressivity, obedience, and independence (García Coll, Akerman, & Cicchetti, 2000; Rogoff, 2003). X. Chen and French (2008) have argued that two basic dimensions of socioemotional functioning, social initiative and self-control, are reflected in most of these values. *Social initiative* refers to the tendency to lead and maintain social participation, especially in challenging situations; reactivity to social novelty or perceived social evaluation may impede spontaneous engagement in social participation. *Self-control*, which is often indicated by cooperative–responsive or defiant–aggressive behaviors, is concerned with the ability to modulate reactivity in interactions to maintain social appropriateness.

In Western, self-oriented societies in which the development of personal assertiveness and independence is regarded as an important socialization goal, social initiative is highly valued and encouraged. On the other hand, although self-control is viewed as conducive to achieving personal goals, children are encouraged to maintain a balance between the needs of the self and those of others; undercontrol and overcontrol are both considered maladaptive in social and psychological adjustment. In many group-oriented societies, social initiative is not highly appreciated because it may interfere with interpersonal cooperation and group harmony. However, controlling personal desires is considered important for group functioning and is therefore strongly emphasized. Different cultural values of social initiative and self-control may affect parental attitudes and practices during socialization of specific behaviors such as sociability (active social initiative with effective control), defiance–aggression (high social initiative and low control), and shyness–inhibition (low social initiative and adequate control to constrain behaviors and emotions toward self) (X. Chen & French, 2008).

Parental Childrearing Attitudes and Practices in Socialization of Social Initiative and Related Behaviors

Research has shown cross-cultural differences on major dimensions of parental childrearing attitudes and practices such as warmth, sensitivity, and emotion expressiveness. For example, Harkness and colleagues (2007) reported that, compared with mothers in Korea, the Netherlands, Spain, and the United States, Italian mothers had the highest scores on socioemotional closeness, which indicates parental sensitivity to infants' need for social interaction and parental effort to stimulate and promote infants' sociability and liveliness. Moreover, Italian mothers used a variety of practices to provide a rich environment for infants to engage in social contact (e.g., taking the baby to social places, talking to the baby, just being with the baby). Similarly, other researchers (e.g., Bornstein et al., 2012; Hsu & Lavelli, 2005) found that, relative to their counterparts in North America, Italian mothers were more sensitive and displayed greater affection in childrearing and valued more socially oriented interactions with their children.

Relative to parents in Italy and some other Western countries, Asian parents tend to be less affectionate and sensitive, and less likely to engage in affective communication with their children (e.g., Chao, 1994; X. Chen, Hastings, et al., 1998; Dornbusch et al., 1987; Jose, Huntsinger, Huntsinger, & Liaw, 2000; Porter et al., 2005), which is believed to be related to the low motivation to socialize children in sociability and social initiative in traditional Asian cultures (Chao, 1995; X. Chen, 2010). Wörmann, Holodynski, Kärtner, and Keller (2012) compared maternal parenting behaviors in German middle-class families and Nso families in rural communities in Cameroon. Unlike German middle-class families that value individuality and autonomy, Nso families have a predominantly interdependent sociocultural orientation. Consistent with the hypotheses, German mothers displayed more positive emotions such as smiles to infants and were more likely to respond to and reinforce infants' smiles. According to Keller (2007) and Wörmann and colleagues (2012), the expression of positive emotions in parent–child interactions is more encouraged in independent cultures than in interdependent cultures because it promotes children's development of sociable and autonomous behaviors.

In addition to cultural differences in parental warmth and affect expression, parents in different societies may differ on another major dimension of parenting—parental control and power assertion. Compared with North American parents, for example, Asian parents have been found to be more controlling, power assertive, and punishment-oriented, and less likely to use "child-centered" parenting methods, such as inductive reasoning (e.g., Dornbusch et al., 1987; Jose et al., 2000; Lin & Fu, 1990; Porter et al., 2005; Rudy & Grusec, 2006). Researchers have also found that Latino parents who value familism emphasize child obedience and respect for adults (e.g., Dornbusch et al., 1987; Livingston & McAdoo, 2007). Latino mothers are more likely than European American mothers to use directive and controlling practices in childrearing (Bornstein et al., 1992; Carlson & Harwood, 2003; Chaudhuri, Easterbrooks, & Davis, 2009). As indicated by X. Chen (2010), high-power parenting in Asian and other societies may be due to traditional cultural endorsement of parental authority. This parenting style may lead to the development of restrained and inhibited behavior and low levels of social initiative, which are thought of as less problematic in group-oriented than in self-oriented societies.

As argued by Greenfield (2009), sociodemographic trends during urbanization and modernization have altered socialization environments for children. Indeed, researchers found that as people in traditional rural societies adapted to more commercial lifestyles and received more formal education, children were encouraged to learn more independent and initiative-taking skills (Greenfield, Maynard, & Childs, 2003; Rogoff, 2003). Similarly, as many countries such as Brazil, China, India, and Vietnam are experiencing rapid social and economic transformations during globalization, significant changes are occurring in parental socialization goals and values. For example, China has changed dramatically in recent years from a society with a centrally planned command economy toward a market-oriented society, particularly in urban regions. Behavioral qualities, such as assertiveness, competitiveness, and self-reliance, that have traditionally been neglected are required for adaptation and success in the new environment. Consequently, these qualities are increasingly appreciated and positively evaluated. In contrast, behaviors and characteristics such as inhibition and shyness that impede self-expression and initiative taking are perceived to be incompetent and maladaptive (X. Chen, Cen, Li, & He, 2005; X. Chen, Wang, & Wang, 2009).

Kagitçibaşi and Ataca (2005) found that urbanization in Turkey over the past three decades has led to increased approval of child autonomy. Compared with their counterparts in 1975, Turkish parents in 2003 were more likely to appreciate affective parent–child interactions and to encourage their children to display independent behaviors. X. Chen and Chen (2010) examined similarities and differences in parental childrearing attitudes between parents of elementary school children in two cohorts (1998 and 2002) in urban China. The results showed that both mothers and fathers in the 2002 cohorts reported higher levels of parental warmth (e.g., "My child and I have warm, good times together," "I comfort my child when he or she is upset or afraid," "I like to play with my child") and lower levels of power assertion (e.g., "I do not allow my child to question my decisions," "I believe physical punishment to be the best way of discipline," "I believe that scolding and criticism make my child improve") than those in the 1998 cohort. Mothers in the 2002 cohort also reported higher autonomy support (e.g., "I let my child make many decisions for him- or herself," "When my child gets into trouble, I expect him or her to handle the problem mostly by him- or herself," "I encourage my child to be independent of me") than mothers in the 1998 cohort. The cohort differences in parental childrearing attitudes clearly reflected the rapid social and cultural changes during that period in the country.

Researchers have conducted urban–rural comparisons to examine the effects of culture and its change on socialization beliefs and practices because rural societies tend to hold more traditional values. For example, Bornstein and colleagues (2012) compared mother–child interactions between rural and urban families in Argentina, Italy, and the United States. The analyses revealed that, across the samples, rural mothers were more directive and intrusive than urban mothers. According to the authors, intrusiveness in rural mothers reflected parental perceptions of the need to "teach" their children to handle a more demanding and challenging environment, since rural families possess fewer external health, educational, and financial resources.

In China, comprehensive economic reform such as the opening of stock markets has been mainly limited to urban centers and cities, and rural children and adults do not have as much exposure as their urban counterparts to the influence of the free-market economy. Researchers found that rural parents were less likely to display warmth toward children, were less engaged in play activities, and used more power-assertive practices in childrearing (X. Chen & Chen, 2010). X. Chen and Li (2012) studied the impact of urbanization on parental attitudes such as parental encouragement of initiative taking in social activities (e.g., "I encourage my child to take the lead in initiating activities," "I encourage my child to express his or her opinions in school and other public places," "I encourage my child to actively participate in social activities"). In this study, due to the expansion of a city into its surrounding rural areas, the government changed the status of families in the areas from rural to urban (urbanized families) about 5 years before the data collection. The results showed that parents in the urbanized families became similar to urban parents, with significantly higher scores than parents in rural families on encouragement of initiative taking.

Parental Childrearing Attitudes and Practices in Socialization of Self-Control

In most societies, an important socialization goal is to help children develop self-control abilities in order to behave according to social standards and requirements (Maccoby & Martin, 1983; Whiting & Edwards, 1988). Parents start to help children learn self-control in the first or second year of life, when children demonstrate an awareness of social demands and the ability to direct their behaviors (Kopp, 1982). Nevertheless, cultures differ in their values of self-control, which affects parental socialization efforts. In general, parents in cultures with greater emphasis on group harmony and social responsibility tend to be more motivated to promote self-control in childrearing (e.g., Edwards, 2000; Whiting & Edwards, 1988).

In the Chinese society, self-control is emphasized in socialization consistently from early childhood to adolescence (Chao, 1995; Ho, 1986). According to the Confucian ideologies, cultivating and strengthening innate virtues require individuals to follow a set of rules for actions called *li*, or propriety. The doctrine of *filial piety* dictates that children pledge obedience and reverence to parents (Ho, 1986). Children are expected to comply with parental demands and, more importantly, to understand more general social standards and expectations, which is believed to facilitate the development of self-control at a higher level. The socialization of self-control in Chinese and some other Asian societies is also supported by the belief that human behavior is malleable and controllable (Stevenson, Chen, & Uttal, 1990). The poor control of one's own behavior is considered incompetent and unacceptable because it may lead to personal and group failures due to the lack of effort.

Research findings have supported the argument about cultural values of self-control in parental socialization attitudes and practices. For example, compared with Canadian parents, Chinese parents expected their toddlers to maintain a higher level of behavioral control. When children failed to do so, Chinese parents expressed more negative attitudes, such as dissatisfaction, disappointment, and concern (X. Chen et al., 2003). Kohnstamm, Halverson, Mervielde, and Havill (1998) found that in the description of their children, relative to parents in many Western countries, Chinese parents provided much higher proportions of descriptors about child conscientiousness or diligence and were more concerned about the lack of control in their children. The expectation of high control in children was also observed in daily life parent–child activities. X. Chen and colleagues (2003) noted that that whereas most Canadian children, particularly boys, wore diapers at 2 years of age, virtually all the children at this age in the Chinese sample had finished toilet training. Many Chinese parents indicated that they started toilet training when their children were less than 1 year old.

A high tendency to socialize self-control has also been found among parents in non-Asian cultures. For example, Keller and colleagues (2004) examined parent–child interactions in Nso families in rural Cameroon, Costa Rican families, and middle-class Greek families. The results showed that Cameroonian Nso mothers displayed toward their children more of the body contact and body stimulation believed to facilitate child obedience and regulation than did Costa Rican mothers, who in turn displayed more of such behavior than Greek mothers. As argued by Keller and colleagues, whereas behavioral control is often viewed as interfering with the child's freedom in individualistic cultures, self-control is viewed as a duty, indicating social maturity and competence, in group-oriented cultures.

Researchers have investigated parental attitudes toward control-based behaviors such as aggression and defiance. Hackett and Hackett (1993), for example, interviewed Gujarati and English parents of 4- to 7-year-old children in Manchester, England. The Gujarati community comprised three largely endogamous groups from India and East Africa who had emigrated during 1970s. They found that Gujarati parents were less tolerant of their children's undercontrolled behavior than English parents. In response to a hypothetical situation in which a peer hit their child or grabbed a toy from their child, significantly more Gujarati parents than English parents said that they would encourage their children to exert self-control and that they disapproved of hitting back or getting the toy back by force. When their child had a fight with a peer, more Gujarati parents would stop the fight immediately and punish their child, whereas more English parents would ignore the fight and allow it to subside.

In summary, cultural beliefs and values may be reflected directly in parental socialization attitudes and practices. Through organizing the family socialization environment, culture influences children's and adolescents' behavioral characteristics, such as those related to social initiative and self-control (e.g., sociability–cooperation, aggression–defiance, shyness). As a result, children and adolescents in different societies may differ in developmental outcomes (e.g., Edwards, 2000; Farver et al., 1995; Oakland et al., 2008; Rubin, Hemphill, et al., 2006).

Cultural Values and Peer Attitudes and Regulation

The role of peers in children's social, behavioral, and cognitive development has been well recognized in developmental science (e.g., Hartup, 1992; Piaget, 1932; Rubin, Bukowski, & Parker, 2006). Peer interactions provide opportunities for children to learn social and problem-solving skills such as cooperation and negotiation from each other. The experiences of activities with peers helps children understand rules for appropriate behaviors in social settings. Peer group affiliations also provide a sense of belonging, which is important for the development of psychological well-being (e.g., Sullivan, 1953). Moreover, while parental influence becomes more distal as children develop greater autonomy with age and engage in more activities outside the home, peers become increasingly salient in shaping children's attitudes and behaviors. Failure to form constructive peer relationships and to obtain peer group acceptance may have an enduring impact on child development in various domains (Dodge, Greenberg, & Malone, 2008; Kiesner, Poulin, & Nicotra, 2003; Ladd & Troop-Gordon, 2003).

Cultural norms and values affect the nature and features of peer interactions and relationships (X. Chen, 2012; Edwards, de Guzman, Brown, & Kumru, 2006; Hinde, 1987). In Western, individualistic cultures, children are encouraged to participate in peer interactions to develop a sense of autonomy from the family (Rothbaum, Pott, Azuma, Miyake, & Weisz, 2000). During peer interactions, children are further encouraged to learn independence and acquire self-identity, while maintaining positive relationships with others. Thus, peer interactions provide opportunities for children to understand themselves in relation to others and experience self-validation (Sullivan, 1953).

Group-oriented cultures emphasize conformity to the group and commitment to social relationships (Sharabany, 2006). In these cultures, children need to learn skills to sustain strong social affiliations. Different cultural expectations regarding individual independence and group commitment may determine, in part, peer socialization practices, including (1) the features of dyadic relationships and groups, (2) peer interaction processes such as social evaluations and responses, and (3) the peer regulatory function in development. We discuss each of these in turn.

Features of Friendships and Peer Groups across Cultures

The majority of school-age children (over 70%) in most societies have mutual friends or group networks (e.g., Attili, Vermigli, & Schneider, 1997; X. Chen, Chang, Liu, & He, 2008; French, Jansen, Riansari, & Setiono, 2003; Salmivalli, Huttunen, & Lagerspetz, 1997). In general, boys' friendships are less stable over time than girls' friendships (e.g., Benenson, Apostoleris, & Parnass, 1997; Schneider, Fonzi, Tani, & Tomada, 1997). Boys are more likely than girls to form group networks, and boys' groups tend to be larger in size than girls' groups (e.g., Benenson et al., 1997; Deković, Engels, Shirai, De Kort, & Anker, 2002; Salmivalli et al., 1997). Research indicates that children and adolescents may hang around together and develop relationships and groups on the basis of social, behavioral, and other attributes (e.g., prosocial or antisocial orientation, learning problems) that are significant in the culture. Once formed, peer relationships, particularly peer groups, serve as an important socialization force for both boys and girls in the development of socioemotional functioning, personality, and academic competence (Cairns & Cairns, 1994; X. Chen et al., 2008; Kindermann, McCollam, & Gibson, 1996).

Cross-cultural differences have been found in the features of friendships and peer groups such as exclusivity and conflict. In a series of studies by, French, Bae, Pidada, and Lee (2006), South Korean children displayed exclusivity and duration of friendships to a greater extent than their counterparts in Indonesia and the United States. Driven by a Confucian belief about social relationships, children in South Korea value exclusivity and intimacy between friends as interpersonal necessities. Arab school-age children reported their peer groups as more intimate than did Jewish children, which is believed to be consistent with the fact that Arab society is more collectivistic than Jewish society (Scharf & Hertz-Lazarowitz, 2003). In addition, Latino and black youth in the United States rated their friendships as more intimate and closer than did their counterparts with a European background (González, Moreno, & Schneider, 2004; Way, 2006).

Sharabany (2006) reported some interesting results about peer relationships of children in Israeli kibbutzim. Although the Israeli kibbutz is a communal society that emphasizes shared responsibilities, kibbutz children reported low exclusivity and intimacy in dyadic friendships. Compared with city children in Israel, children in Israeli kibbutzim reported that they engaged in more activities with their best friends. However, they were less open and communicative with their friends, and reported less trust and exclusiveness in the relationships. According to Josselson, Lieblich, Sharabany, and Wiseman (1997), limited involvement of kibbutz children with friends may be due to the belief that closeness and intimacy with specific persons may be an indication of rejection of others in the larger group and a potential source of jealousy and conflict.

Studies of functions of peer relationships have revealed that youth are more likely to report enhancement of self-worth in Western societies than in societies that value interdependence, such as China (X. Chen, Kaspar, Zhang, Wang, & Zheng, 2004), Japan (Kitayama, Markus, Matsumoto, & Norasakkunkit, 1997), and Indonesia (French, Pidada, & Victor, 2005). For example, one of the major reasons for friendship among North American children is that friends make them feel good about themselves. However, children in many other cultures perceive self-validation as less important in friendship (e.g., X. Chen et al., 2004; Cho, Sandel, Miller, & Wang, 2005; Dayan, Doyle, & Markiewicz, 2001; French, Pidada, & Victor, 2005). In contrast to enhancement of self-worth, children in Asian and Latino group-oriented cultures tend to value instrumental assistance, such as sharing of money, protecting friends from harm, and helping with problem solving, to a greater extent than children in self-oriented cultures (French et al., 2006; González et al., 2004; Way, 2006). A salient theme that emerged from interviews with Chinese adolescents, for example, is the appreciation of mutual assistance of friends in learning and school achievement (X. Chen et al., 2004; Way, 2006).

Remarkable cross-cultural differences have been observed in the occurrence and solution of conflict in friendships. Researchers found that relative to North American and Western European children, children in Indonesia, southern Spain, and Taiwan engaged in fewer peer conflicts that were considered detrimental to their relationships (Benjamin, Schneider, Greenman, & Hum, 2001; French, Pidada, Denoma, McDonald, & Lawton, 2005; Martínez Lozano, 2003). Moreover, across cultures, children use different strategies to handle peer conflicts. For example, whereas children in the United States tend to display assertiveness and negotiation, Indonesian children often use disengagement and avoidance in conflict situations (French, Pidada, Denoma, et al., 2005). Andalusian children in southern Spain, where conflicts were considered disruptive to the maintenance of peer relationships, used more indirect tactics during conflicts than did Dutch children (Martínez Lozano, 2003).

Finally, cultural norms and values may affect the features of children's and adolescents' peer groups. Individualistic values in Western societies are reflected in the diversity of peer groups, such as those labeled as jocks, populars, partyers, druggies, nerds, and burnouts (e.g., Brown, 1990). Children and adolescents typically form groups based on their particular individual interests, even though affiliation with deviant groups may lead to individual adjustment problems, including school dropout, substance use, and antisocial behavior (e.g., Cairns & Cairns, 1994; Espelage, Holt, & Henkel, 2003; Kiesner et al., 2003). In addition, consistent with values of individual autonomy, intensive interaction within the group appears to decline with increasing age, especially during late adolescence, in Western societies. The development of social and cognitive abilities allows adolescents to form affiliations with multiple groups and larger crowds (e.g., Brown, 1990). At the same time, adolescents increasingly seek independence and attempt to avoid group restrictions, which leads to a loosening of group ties and weakened sense of belonging (Rubin, Bukowski, et al., 2006).

In collectivistic societies, due to the cultural emphasis on their role in helping children learn social standards and develop socially valued behaviors, peer groups may not be as diverse as those based mainly on personal interests in individualistic societies. In Chinese schools, for example, peer groups vary mostly in terms of academic and social orientations (X. Chen et al., 2008). The academic orientation is indicated by the extent to which the group values academic achievement as a major norm and is organized on the basis of academic activities. Members of academically oriented groups are more motivated to learn, help each other on school tasks, and obtain higher achievement than members of nonacademically oriented groups. Group variations in social orientations are characterized by engagement in prosocial–cooperative and antisocial–destructive activities. Whereas prosocial–cooperative groups are represented by the tendency of group members to display socially acceptable and responsible behaviors, children in antisocial–destructive groups tend to display disruptive, hostile, and rebellious behaviors (X. Chen et al., 2004). The emphasis on the socialization function of peer groups in the development of socially desired behaviors in collectivistic societies places a great pressure on children and adolescents to follow group norms in peer activities. Youth in these societies often describe group activities in terms of whether they are guided by the "right" goals and fulfill adults' requirements (X. Chen et al., 2004; Sharabany, 2006). Groups that engage in activities without the "right" goals are viewed by adults and peers as deviant and antisocial.

Culture and Peer Evaluations

In peer interactions, children interpret and evaluate behaviors of one another based on group norms. Moreover, peers make responses to others' behaviors accordingly and express particular attitudes (e.g., acceptance, rejection) toward children who display behaviors that are more or less consistent with those group norms. In a study of peer interactions among Chinese and Canadian preschool-age children, X. Chen, DeSouza, Chen, and Wang (2006) examined peer attitudes toward children who displayed shy and reticent behaviors. The results indicated that peers in Canada were likely to show overt refusal and disagreement, and intentionally ignore the initiations made by shy children. In contrast, peers in China tended to respond in a more positive manner by exhibiting support and approval, and by controlling their negative actions.

Peers across cultures also display different attitudes toward shyness in middle to late childhood. X. Chen and colleagues found that whereas shyness was associated with negative peer experiences in Canadian children, it was associated with peer acceptance in urban Chinese children in the early 1990s and rural Chinese children in recent years (X. Chen, Rubin, & Sun, 1992; X. Chen, Wang, & Cao, 2011). Positive relations between shyness and peer acceptance were also found in other Asian countries such as Indonesia, Japan, and Korea (Eisenberg, Pidada, & Liew, 2001; Heinrichs et al., 2006). Moreover, as the society becomes more urbanized, with endorsement of more individualistic values in social interactions, peer attitudes toward shyness may change. Along with the transformation of urban China toward a market-oriented society, for example, children's shyness is associated with more negative peer attitudes. By the early part of the 21st century, urban shy children, unlike their urban counterparts in the early 1990s and rural counterparts in recent years, were rejected by peers (X. Chen et al., 2005, 2009).

Compared with shy and anxious behaviors, control-based behaviors such as aggression and disruption seem to be associated with negative peer evaluations more consistently across cultures (e.g., X. Chen et al., 2005; X. Chen & French, 2008). Nevertheless, cultural variations have been found, at least in the extent to which these behaviors are perceived and evaluated by peers. Chagnon (1983) noted that in Yanoamo Indians, who considered violent behaviors to be socially acceptable or desirable, children, especially boys, who displayed these behaviors might be regarded as "heroes" by their peers. Researchers also found that in some central and southern Italian communities, due to social and historical circumstances, aggressive and defiant behaviors might be perceived by children as an indication of assertiveness (Casiglia, LoCoco, & Zappulla, 1998; Schneider & Fonzi, 1996). In the United States, although aggression is generally discouraged, being able to fight and display aggressive behaviors is related to peer support and the attainment of personal "honor" and status in certain youth groups (e.g., Bernburg & Thorlindsson, 2005; Cairns & Cairns, 1994; Graham & Wells, 2003; Rodkin, Farmer, Pearl, & van Acker, 2000).

Greenberger and colleagues (e.g., C. Chen, Greenberger, Lester, Dong, & Guo, 1998; Greenberger, Chen, Tally, & Dong, 2000) examined peer approval and disapproval of externalizing behaviors in Chinese, Korean, and North American adolescents. They found that Chinese and Korean adolescents had lower scores on peer approval and higher scores on peer disapproval for externalizing behaviors than did European American adolescents. Moreover, peers in China and Korea were more likely than peers in the United States to show negative emotional reactions, such as upset, in response to physical aggression and other externalizing behaviors. These results suggest that undercontrolled, externalizing behaviors may elicit relatively more unfavorable peer evaluations and responses (e.g., disapproval and criticism) in Asian than in North American societies.

Culturally Directed Peer Regulatory Function in Development

The contextual–developmental perspective (X. Chen, 2012) asserts that culturally guided social evaluations and responses in peer interactions may regulate children's behaviors and their development. The regulation of peer interaction is an integral part of the process that mediates the impact of cultural influence on human development. The peer regulatory role in socialization has been shown in a number of studies.

In a study of the impact of adolescent crowds on individual shy and anxious behavior in Sweden, Van Zalk, Van Zalk, and Kerr (2011) examined radical crowds (Punks and Goths) of adolescents who were believed to create an unusual appearance (e.g., wearing white face paint, faked bloodstains around the eyes or mouth, or half-shaved, long black hair) to limit their own anxiety-arousing social contacts. The researchers found that adolescents in these crowds were more susceptible than individuals in other groups to within-group peer influence. Members in these crowds tended to promote and reinforce one another's socially anxious behavior by providing approval in situations that provoke social fear.

Dishion and his colleagues (Dishion, McCord, & Poulin, 1999; Piehler & Dishion, 2007) investigated how delinquent and nondelinquent adolescents engaged in the discussion of social problems in American culture. The researchers first found that delinquent youth engaged in four times more talk about rule breaking than nondelinquent youth. Delinquent youth were also likely to display contingent positive reactions, such as laughter and expression of attention and interest, to deviant talk, whereas nondelinquent youth often ignored deviant talk. More importantly, interactions among youth with behavioral problems led to the escalation of problems through "deviancy training" or "peer contagion" processes. For example, engagement in peer talk about rule breaking predicted increases in substance use, delinquency, violence, and high-risk sexual behavior in subsequent years (e.g., Patterson, Dishion, & Yoerger, 2000; Piehler & Dishion, 2007). Thus, the interaction of adolescents with behavioral problems provides a context that elicits and reinforces their deviant behaviors. The salience of the group norm, the homogeneity of the group, and the quality of relationships among members may moderate the influence on individual behaviors (Dishion et al., 1999; Laursen, Hafen, Kerr, & Stattin, 2012). Thus, the cultural socialization of the peer group is constrained by its structural and organizational features.

The peer regulatory function may be more evident in East Asian cultures, in which the view of others is regarded as more important than the view of one's self. Relative to children in Western cultures, who are encouraged to display autonomy and independence in social interactions (e.g., Greenfield, Suzuki, & Rothstein-Fisch, 2006), children in East Asian cultures are more inclined to attend to others' perceptions of themselves and to be more sensitive to social evaluations (X. Chen, 2012). As a result, peer interactions may be more influential in shaping individual behavior and development in East Asian cultures. Consistent with this argument, Deković and colleagues (2002) found that experiences in peer activities were associated more strongly with developmental outcomes, such as emotional well-being, in Japanese than in Dutch adolescents. In the Greenberger and colleagues study (2000), perceptions of friends' negative attitudes toward externalizing behaviors were negatively associated with adolescents' display of aggressive and antisocial behaviors and misconduct in the U.S., Korean, and Chinese samples, but the association was stronger in Korean and Chinese adolescents than in the U.S. adolescents.

In summary, children's experiences in peer interactions are culturally bound, as argued by Stevenson-Hinde (2011). Cultural beliefs and values provide a basis for peer socialization by guiding the social evaluation and regulation processes. Along with parenting practices, peer interactions constitute an important cultural socialization context in which children and adolescents develop their socioemotional characteristics and cognitive abilities.

Conclusions and Future Directions

Findings from a variety of research programs have indicated considerable cross-cultural differences in children's and adolescents' attitudes, emotions, and behaviors. Socialization plays an important role in mediating cultural influence on human development, particularly in areas characterized by social initiative and self-control. Cultural norms and values guide the social interaction processes in the family, the peer group, and other socialization settings, which in turn affect the patterns and outcomes of individual development.

In this chapter, we have focused mainly on culture and two major socialization factors, parenting and peer influence. Although they represent important proximal forces that directly affect child development, other socialization factors, such as community services, school practices, and teacher–student relationships, are likely to be associated with culture and, at the same time, exert a significant impact on children's behaviors. It will be important to investigate the mediating role of these factors in the influence of culture on child development. It will also be interesting to explore how culture is involved in socialization processes at macro levels such as child-, family-, and school-related policies, social and economic conditions of the society or community, and the mass media.

It has been argued that children play an active role in socialization and development (e.g., X. Chen, 2012; Corsaro & Nelson, 2003; Edwards et al., 2006). Children may display their active role through their choices of activities and playmates, and their reactions to socialization influence. Moreover, children may actively participate in socialization by adoption of existing cultures and construction of new cultures for social evaluations, especially in peer group activities. Despite the argument, little research has been conducted on this issue, especially in non-Western societies. Researchers need to pay greater attention to the active role of children in cross-cultural research.

Finally, research on culture and human development often relies on comparisons between individuals in Western, self-oriented societies and those in collectivist or group-oriented societies. The rapid increase in cross-border trade, integration of political and economic systems, development of new technologies, and large-scale movements of populations over the past few decades have led to comprehensive cultural changes in both Western and non-Western societies. The heightened exchanges and interactions among cultures have resulted in the merging and coexistence of diverse value systems (Tamis-LeMonda et al., 2008). As a result of globalization, for example, individualistic values have been introduced into many non-Western societies and exerted influence on socialization attitudes and practices in these societies. However, Western values are unlikely to be accepted completely; instead, they may be integrated with the cultural traditions. According to Kagitçibaşi (2012), social change during urbanization in group-oriented societies may allow for greater individual autonomy, but they may not necessarily weaken interpersonal socioemotional support and interdependence. Similarly, Yang (1986) argues that group harmony and social connectedness represent the core of the Confucian value system in East Asian cultures. The system has guided individual behaviors and social interactions for thousands of years and is robust in spite of social change. It will be interesting to investigate socialization and human development in culturally integrated and sophisticated settings.

REFERENCES

Attili, G., Vermigli, P., & Schneider, B. H. (1997). Peer acceptance and friendship patterns among Italian schoolchildren within a cross-cultural perspective. *International Journal of Behavioral Development, 21*, 277–288.

Beach, K. (1995). Activity as a mediator of sociocultural change and individual development: The case of schoolwork transition in Nepal. *Mind, Culture, and Activity, 2*, 285–302.

Benenson, J. F., Apostoleris, N. H., & Parnass, J. (1997). Age and sex differences in dyadic and group interaction. *Developmental Psychology, 33*, 538–543.

Benjamin, W. J., Schneider, B. H., Greenman, P. S., & Hum, M. (2001). Conflict and childhood friendship in Taiwan and Canada. *Canadian Journal of Behavioural Science, 33*, 203–211.

Bernburg, J. G., & Thorlindsson, T. (2005). Violent values, conduct norms, and youth aggression: A multilevel study in Iceland. *Sociological Quarterly, 46*, 457–478.

Bornstein, M. H., Tal, J., Rahn, C., Galperin, C. Z., Pecheux, M.-G., Lamour, M., et al. (1992). Functional analysis of the contents of maternal speech to infants of 5 and 13 months in four cultures: Argentina, France, Japan, and the United States. *Developmental Psychology, 28*, 593–603.

Bornstein, M. H., Putnick, D. L., Suwalsky, J. T. D., Venuti, P., de Falco, S., de Galperín, C. Z., et al. (2012). Emotional relationships in mothers and infants: Culture-common and community-specific characteristics of dyads from rural and metropolitan settings in Argentina, Italy, and the United States. *Journal of Cross-Cultural Psychology, 43*, 171–197.

Bronfenbrenner, U. (1979). *The ecology of human development: Experiments in nature and design.* Cambridge, MA: Harvard University Press.

Bronfenbrenner, U., & Morris, P. A. (2006). The bioecological model of human development. In

W. Damon & R. M. Lerner (Eds.), *Handbook of child psychology: Vol. 1. Theoretical models of human development* (6th ed., pp. 793–828). New York: Wiley.

Brown, B. B. (1990). Peer groups and peer culture. In S. S. Feldman & G. R. Elliott (Eds.), *At the threshold: The developing adolescent* (pp. 171–196). Cambridge, MA: Harvard University Press.

Cairns, R. B., & Cairns, B. D. (1994). *Lifelines and risks: Pathways of youth in our time.* New York: Cambridge University Press.

Camras, L. A., Oster, H., Campos, J., Campos, R., Ujiie, T., Miyake, K., et al. (1998). Production of emotional facial expressions in European American, Japanese, and Chinese infants. *Developmental Psychology, 34,* 616–628.

Carlson, V. J., & Harwood, R. L. (2003). Attachment, culture, and the caregiving system: The cultural patterning of everyday experiences among Anglo and Puerto Rican mother–infant pairs. *Infant Mental Health Journal, 24,* 53–73.

Casiglia, A. C., LoCoco, A., & Zappulla, C. (1998). Aspects of social reputation and peer relationships in Italian children: A cross-cultural perspective. *Developmental Psychology, 34,* 723–730.

Chagnon, N. (1983). *Yanomamo: The fierce people.* New York: Holt, Rinehart & Winston.

Chao, R. K. (1994). Beyond parental control and authoritarian parenting style: Understanding Chinese parenting through the cultural notion of training. *Child Development, 65,* 1111–1119.

Chao, R. K. (1995). Chinese and European American cultural models of the self-reflected in mothers' childrearing beliefs. *Ethos, 23,* 328–354.

Chaudhuri, J. H., Easterbrooks, M. A., & Davis, C. R. (2009). The relation between emotional availability and parenting style: Cultural and economic factors in a diverse sample of young mothers. *Parenting: Science and Practice, 9,* 277–299.

Chen, C., Greenberger, E., Lester, J., Dong, Q., & Guo, M. (1998). A cross-cultural study of family and peer correlates of adolescent misconduct. *Developmental Psychology, 34,* 770–781.

Chen, X. (2010). Socioemotional development in Chinese children. In M. H. Bond (Ed.), *Handbook of Chinese psychology* (pp. 37–52). Oxford, UK: Oxford University Press.

Chen, X. (2012). Culture, peer interaction, and socio-emotional development. *Child Development Perspectives, 6,* 27–34.

Chen, X., Cen, G., Li, D., & He, Y. (2005). Social functioning and adjustment in Chinese children: The imprint of historical time. *Child Development, 76,* 182–195.

Chen, X., Chang, L., Liu, H., & He, Y. (2008). Effects of the peer group on the development of social functioning and academic achievement: A longitudinal study in Chinese children. *Child Development, 79,* 235–251.

Chen, X., & Chen, H. (2010). Children's social functioning and adjustment in the changing Chinese society. In R. K. Silbereisen & X. Chen (Eds.), *Social change and human development: Concepts and results* (pp. 209–226). Thousand Oaks, CA: Sage.

Chen, X., DeSouza, A. T., Chen, H., & Wang, L. (2006). Reticent behavior and experiences in peer interactions in Chinese and Canadian children. *Developmental Psychology, 42,* 656–665.

Chen, X., & French, D. C. (2008). Children's social competence in cultural context. *Annual Review of Psychology, 59,* 591–616.

Chen, X., Hastings, P. D., Rubin, K. H., Chen, H., Cen, G., & Stewart, S. L. (1998). Child-rearing attitudes and behavioral inhibition in Chinese and Canadian toddlers: A cross-cultural study. *Developmental Psychology, 34,* 677–686.

Chen, X., Kaspar, V., Zhang, Y., Wang, L., & Zheng, S. (2004). Peer relationships among Chinese boys: A cross-cultural perspective. In X. Chen (Eds.), *Adolescent boys: Exploring diverse cultures of boyhood* (pp. 197–218). New York: New York University Press.

Chen, X., & Li, D. (2012). Parental encouragement of initiative-taking and adjustment in Chinese children from rural, urban, and urbanized families. *Journal of Family Psychology, 26,* 927–936.

Chen, X., Rubin, K. H., Liu, M., Chen, H., Wang, L., Li, D., et al. (2003). Compliance in Chinese and Canadian toddlers: A cross-cultural study. *International Journal of Behavioral Development, 27,* 428–436.

Chen, X., Rubin, K. H., & Sun, Y. (1992). Social reputation and peer relationships in Chinese and Canadian children: A cross-cultural study. *Child Development, 63,* 1336–1343.

Chen, X., & Tse, H. C. (2010). Social and psychological adjustment of Chinese Canadian children. *International Journal of Behavioral Development, 34,* 330–338.

Chen, X., Wang, L., & Cao, R. (2011). Shyness–sensitivity and unsociability in rural Chinese children: Relations with social, school, and psychological adjustment. *Child Development, 82,* 1531–1543.

Chen, X., Wang, L., & Wang, Z. (2009). Shyness–sensitivity and social, school, and psychological adjustment in rural migrant and urban children in China. *Child Development, 80,* 1499–1513.

Cho, G. E., Sandel, T. L., Miller, P. J., & Wang, S. (2005). What do grandmothers think about self-esteem?: American and Taiwanese folk theories revisited. *Social Development, 14,* 701–721.

Cole, M., & Cagigas, X. E. (2010). Cognition. In M. H. Bornstein (Ed.), *Handbook of cultural developmental science* (pp. 127–142). New York: Psychology Press.

Corsaro, W. A., & Nelson, E. (2003). Children's collective activities and peer culture in early literacy in American and Italian preschools. *Sociology of Education, 76,* 209–227.

Dayan, J., Doyle, A., & Markiewicz, D. (2001). Social support networks and self-esteem of idiocentric and allocentric children and adolescents. *Journal of Social and Personal Relationships, 18,* 767–784.

Deković, M., Engels, R. C. M. E., Shirai, T., De Kort, G., & Anker, A. L. (2002). The role of peer relations in adolescent development in two cultures: The Netherlands and Japan. *Journal of Cross-Cultural Psychology, 33,* 577–595.

Dishion, T. J., McCord, J., & Poulin, F. (1999). When interventions harm: Peer groups and problem behavior. *American Psychologist, 54,* 755–764.

Dodge, K. A., Greenberg, M. T., & Malone, P. S. (2008). Testing an idealized dynamic cascade model of the development of serious violence in adolescence. *Child Development, 79,* 1907–1927.

Dornbusch, S. M., Ritter, P. L., Leiderman, P. H., Roberts, D. F., & Fraleigh, M. J. (1987). The relation of parenting style to adolescent school performance. *Child Development, 58,* 1244–1257.

Edwards, C. P. (2000). Children's play in cross-cultural perspective: A new look at the six cultures study. *Cross-Cultural Research: Journal of Comparative Social Science, 34,* 318–338.

Edwards, C. P., de Guzman, M. R., Brown, J., & Kumru, A. (2006). Children's social behaviors and peer interactions in diverse cultures. In X. Chen, B. Schneider, & D. French (Eds.), *Peer relationships in cultural context* (pp. 23–51). New York: Cambridge University Press.

Eisenberg, N., Pidada, S., & Liew, J. (2001). The relations of regulation and negative emotionality to Indonesian children's social functioning. *Child Development, 72,* 1747–1763.

Espelage, D. L., Holt, M. K., & Henkel, R. R. (2003). Examination of peer-group contextual effects on aggression during early adolescence. *Child Development, 74,* 205–220.

Farver, J. A. M., Kim, Y. K., & Lee, Y. (1995). Cultural differences in Korean- and Anglo-American preschoolers' social interaction and play behaviors. *Child Development, 66,* 1088–1099.

French, D. C., Bae, A., Pidada, S., & Lee, O. (2006). Friendships of Indonesian, South Korean, and U.S. college students. *Personal Relationships, 13,* 69–81.

French, D. C., Jansen, E. A., Riansari, M., & Setiono, K. (2003). Friendships of Indonesian children: Adjustment of children who differ in friendship presence and similarity between mutual friends. *Social Development, 12,* 606–621.

French, D. C., Pidada, S., Denoma, J., McDonald, K., & Lawton, A. (2005). Reported peer conflicts of children in the United States and Indonesia. *Social Development, 14,* 458–472.

French, D. C., Pidada, S., & Victor, A. (2005). Friendships of Indonesian and United states youth. *International Journal of Behavioral Development, 29,* 304–313.

García Coll, C. G., Akerman, A., & Cicchetti, D. (2000). Cultural influences on developmental processes and outcomes: Implications for the study of development and psychopathology. *Development and Psychopathology, 12*, 333–356.

Gartstein, M. A., Gonzalez, C., Carranza, J. A., Ahadi, S. A., Ye, R., Rothbart, M. K., et al. (2006). Studying cross-cultural differences in the development of infant temperament: People's Republic of China, the United States of America, and Spain. *Child Psychiatry and Human Development, 37*, 145–161.

González, Y. S., Moreno, D. S., & Schneider, B. H. (2004). Friendship expectations of early adolescents in Cuba and Canada. *Journal of Cross-Cultural Psychology, 35*, 436–445.

Graham, K., & Wells, S. (2003). "Somebody's gonna get their head kicked in tonight!": Aggression among young males in bars—a question of values? *British Journal of Criminology, 43*, 546–566.

Greenberger, E., Chen, C., Tally, S. R., & Dong, Q. (2000). Family, peer, and individual correlates of depressive symptomatology among U.S. and Chinese adolescents. *Journal of Consulting and Clinical Psychology, 68*, 209–219.

Greenfield, P. M. (2009). Linking social change and developmental change: Shifting pathways of human development. *Developmental Psychology, 4*, 401–418.

Greenfield, P. M., Maynard, A. E., & Childs, C. P. (2003). Historical change, cultural learning, and cognitive representation in Zinacantec Maya children. *Cognitive Development, 18*, 455–487.

Greenfield, P. M., Suzuki, L. K., & Rothstein-Fisch, C. (2006). Cultural pathways through human development. In K. A. Renninger & I. E. Sigel (Eds.), *Handbook of child psychology: Vol. 4. Child psychology in practice* (pp. 655–699). New York: Wiley.

Hackett, L., & Hackett, R. J. (1993). Parental ideas of normal and deviant child behaviour: A comparison of two ethnic groups. *British Journal of Psychiatry, 162*, 353–357.

Harkness, S., Super, C. M., Moscardino, U., Rha, J.-H., Blom, M. J. M., Huitrón, B., et al. (2007). Cultural models and developmental agendas: Implications for arousal and self-regulation in early infancy. *Journal of Developmental Processes, 1*, 5–39.

Hartup, W. W. (1992). Friendships and their developmental significance. In H. McGurk (Ed.), *Childhood social development* (pp. 175–205). Hove, UK: Erlbaum.

Heinrichs, N., Rapee, R. M., Alden, L. A., Bögels, S., Hofmann, S. G., Oh, K. J., et al. (2006). Cultural differences in perceived social norms and social anxiety. *Behaviour Research and Therapy, 44*, 1187–1197.

Hinde, R. A. (1987). *Individuals, relationships and culture.* Cambridge, UK: Cambridge University Press.

Ho, D. Y. F. (1986). Chinese pattern of socialization: A critical review. In M. H. Bond (Ed.), *The psychology of the Chinese people* (pp. 1–37). New York: Oxford University Press.

Hofstede, G. (1994). Foreword. In U. Kim, H. C. Triandis, Ç. Kagitçibaşi, S.-C. Choi, & G. Yoon (Eds.), *Individualism and collectivism: Theory, method, and applications* (pp. ix–xiii). Thousand Oaks, CA: Sage.

Hsu, H., & Lavelli, M. (2005). Perceived and observed parenting behavior in American and Italian first-time mothers across the first 3 months. *Infant Behavior and Development, 28*, 503–518.

Jose, P. E., Huntsinger, C. S., Huntsinger, P. R., & Liaw, F. (2000). Parental values and practices relevant to young children's social development in Taiwan and the United States. *Journal of Cross-Cultural Psychology, 31*, 677–702.

Josselson, R., Lieblich, A., Sharabany, R., & Wiseman, H. (1997). *Conversation as method: Analyzing the relational world of people who were raised communally.* Thousand Oaks, CA: Sage.

Kagitçibaşi, C. (2012). Sociocultural change and integrative syntheses in human development: Autonomous-related self and social-cognitive competence. *Child Development Perspectives, 6*, 5–11.

Kagitçibaşi, C., & Ataca, B. (2005). Value of children and family change: A three-decade portrait from Turkey. *Applied Psychology: An International Review, 54*, 317–337.

Keller, H. (2007). *Cultures of infancy.* Mahwah, NJ: Erlbaum.

Keller, H., Yovsi, R., Borke, J., Kärtner, J., Jensen, H., & Papaligoura, Z. (2004). Developmental consequences of early parenting experiences: Self-recognition and self-regulation in three cultural communities. *Child Development, 75*, 1745–1760.

Kiesner, J., Poulin, F., & Nicotra, E. (2003). Peer relations across contexts: Individual-network homophily and network inclusion in and after school. *Child Development, 74*, 1328–1343.

Kindermann, T. A., McCollam, T. L., & Gibson, E. (1996). Peer networks and students' classroom engagement during childhood and adolescence. In T. A. Kinderman, T. L. McCollam, & E. Gibson (Eds.), *Social motivation: Understanding children's school adjustment* (pp. 279–312). New York: Cambridge University Press.

Kitayama, S., Markus, H. R., Matsumoto, H., & Norasakkunkit, V. (1997). Individual and collective processes in the construction of the self: Self-enhancement in the United States and self-criticism in Japan. *Journal of Personality and Social Psychology, 72*, 1245–1267.

Kohnstamm, G. A., Halverson, C. F., Mervielde, I., & Havill, V. L. (1998). Analyzing parental free descriptions of child personality. In G. A. Kohnstamm (Ed.), *Parental descriptions of child personality: Developmental antecedents of the Big Five?* (pp. 1–19). Mahwah, NJ: Erlbaum.

Kopp, C. B. (1982). Antecedents of self-regulation: A developmental perspective. *Developmental Psychology, 18*, 199–214.

Ladd, G. W., & Troop-Gordon, W. (2003). The role of chronic peer difficulties in the development of children's psychological adjustment problems. *Child Development, 74*, 1344–1367.

Laursen, B., Hafen, C. A., Kerr, M., & Stattin, H. (2012). Friend influence over adolescent problem behaviors as a function of relative peer acceptance: To be liked is to be emulated. *Journal of Abnormal Psychology, 121*, 88–94.

Lee, M. R., Okazaki, S., & Yoo, H. C. (2006). Frequency and intensity of social anxiety in Asian Americans and European Americans. *Cultural Diversity and Ethnic Minority Psychology, 12*, 291–305.

Lin, C. C., & Fu, V. R. (1990). A comparison of child-rearing practices among Chinese, immigrant Chinese, and Caucasian-American parents. *Child Development, 61*, 429–433.

Livingston, J., & McAdoo, H. (2007). The roles of African American fathers in the socialization their children. In H. McAdoo (Ed.), *Black families* (pp. 219–237). Thousand Oaks, CA: Sage.

Luria, A. R. (1976). *Cognitive development: Its cultural and social foundations.* Cambridge, MA: Harvard University Press.

Maccoby, E. E., & Martin, J. A. (1983). Socialization in the context of the family: Parent–child interaction. In P. H. Mussen (Series Ed.) & E. M. Hetherington (Vol. Ed.), *Handbook of child psychology: Vol. 4. Socialization, personality, and social development* (4th ed., pp. 1–101). New York: Wiley.

Martínez Lozano, V. (2003). *Cultura, socializacíon e interaccíon entre iguales: Un estudio del conflicto en preescolares andaluces y holandeses* [Culture, socialization, and peer interaction: A study of conflicts in Andalusian and Dutch preschoolers]. Unpublished doctoral dissertation, Universidad Pablo de Olavide, Sevilla, Spain.

Oakland, T., Pretorius, J. D., & Lee, D. H. (2008). Temperament styles of children from South Africa and the United States. *School Psychology International, 29*, 627–639.

Oh, S., & Lewis, C. (2008). Korean preschoolers' advanced inhibitory control and its relation to other executive skills and mental state understanding. *Child Development, 79*, 80–99.

Patterson, G. R., Dishion, T. J., & Yoerger, K. (2000). Adolescent growth in new forms of problem behavior: Macro- and micro-peer dynamics. *Prevention Science, 1*, 3–13.

Piaget, J. (1932). *The moral judgment of the child.* London: Routledge & Kegan Paul.

Piehler, T. F., & Dishion, T. J. (2007). Interpersonal dynamics within adolescent friendships: Dyadic mutuality, deviant talk, and patterns of antisocial behavior. *Child Development, 78*, 1611–1624.

Porter, C. L., Hart, C. H., Yang, C., Robinson, C. C., Olsen, S. F., Zeng, Q., et al. (2005). A comparative study of child temperament and parenting in Beijing, China and the western United States. *International Journal of Behavioral Development, 29*, 541–551.

Rodkin, P. C., Farmer, T. W., Pearl, R., & Van Acker, R. (2000). Heterogeneity of popular boys: Antisocial and prosocial configurations. *Developmental Psychology, 36*(1), 14–24.

Rogoff, B. (2003). *The cultural nature of human development.* New York: Oxford University Press.

Rothbaum, F., Pott, M., Azuma, H., Miyake, K., & Weisz, J. (2000). The development of close relationships in Japan and the United States: Paths of symbiotic harmony and generative tension. *Child Development, 71,* 1121–1142.

Rubin, K. H., Bukowski, W., & Parker, J. (2006). Peer interactions, relationships, and groups. In N. Eisenberg (Ed.), *Handbook of child psychology: Social, emotional, and personality development* (6th ed., pp. 571–645). New York: Wiley.

Rubin, K. H., Hemphill, S. A., Chen, X., Hastings, P., Sanson, A., Coco, A. L., et al. (2006). A cross-cultural study of behavioral inhibition in toddlers: East–west–north–south. *International Journal of Behavioral Development, 30,* 219–226.

Rudy, D., & Grusec, J. E. (2006). Authoritarian parenting in individualist and collectivist groups: Associations with maternal emotion and cognition and children's self-esteem. *Journal of Family Psychology, 20,* 68–78.

Sabbagh, M. A., Xu, F., Carlson, S. M., Moses, L. J., & Lee, K. (2006). The development of executive functioning and theory of mind: A comparison of Chinese and U.S. preschoolers. *Psychological Science, 17,* 74–81.

Salmivalli, C., Huttunen, A., & Lagerspetz, K. M. J. (1997). Peer networks and bullying in schools. *Scandinavian Journal of Psychology, 38,* 305–312.

Scharf, M., & Hertz-Lazarowitz, R. (2003). Social networks in the school context: Effects of culture and gender. *Journal of Social and Personal Relationships, 20,* 843–858.

Schneider, B. H., & Fonzi, A. (1996). La stabilita deH'amicizia: Uno studio cross-culturale Italia–Canada [Friendship stability: A cross-cultural study in Italy–Canada]. *Eta Evolutiva, 3,* 73–79.

Schneider, B. H., Fonzi, A., Tani, F., & Tomada, G. (1997). A cross-cultural exploration of the stability of children's friendships and predictors of their continuation. *Social Development, 6,* 322–339.

Schneider, B. H., French, D., & Chen, X. (2006). Peer relationship in cultural perspective: Methodological reflections. In X. Chen, D. French, & B. Schneider (Eds.), *Peer relationships in cultural context* (pp. 489–500). New York: Cambridge University Press.

Sharabany, R. (2006). The cultural context of children and adolescents: Peer relationships and intimate friendships among Arab and Jewish children in Israel. In X. Chen, B. Schneider, & D. French (Eds.), *Peer relationships in cultural context* (pp. 452–478). New York: Cambridge University Press.

Singelis, T. M. (1994). The measurement of independent and interdependent self-construals. *Personality and Social Psychology Bulletin, 20,* 580–591.

Stevenson, H. W., Chen, C., & Uttal, D. H. (1990). Beliefs and achievement: A study of black, white, and Hispanic children. *Child Development, 61,* 508–523.

Stevenson-Hinde, J. (2011). Culture and socioemotional development, with a focus on fearfulness and attachment. In X. Chen & K. H. Rubin (Eds.), *Socioemotional development in cultural context* (pp. 11–28). New York: Guilford Press.

Sullivan, H. S. (1953). *The interpersonal theory of psychiatry.* New York: Norton.

Super, C. M., & Harkness, S. (1986). The developmental niche: A conceptualization at the interface of child and culture. *International Journal of Behavioral Development, 9,* 545–569.

Tamis-LeMonda, C., Way, N., Hughes, D., Yoshikawa, H., Kalman, R. K., & Niwa, E. Y. (2008). Parents' goals for children: The dynamic coexistence of individualism and collectivism in cultures and individuals. *Social Development, 17,* 183–209.

Tietjen, H. C. (2006). Cultural influences on peer relations: An ecological perspective. In X. Chen, D. French, & B. Schneider (Eds.), *Peer relationships in cultural context* (pp. 52–74). New York: Cambridge University Press.

Triandis, H. C. (1995). *Individualism and collectivism*. Boulder, CO: Westview Press.

Van Zalk, N., Van Zalk, M., & Kerr, M. (2011). Socialization of social anxiety in adolescent crowds. *Journal of Abnormal Child Psychology, 39*, 1239–1249.

Vygotsky, L. S. (1978). Interaction between learning and development (M. Lopez-Morillas, Trans.). In M. Cole, V. John-Steiner, S. Scribner, & E. Souberman (Eds.), *Mind in society: The development of higher psychological processes* (pp. 79–91). Cambridge, MA: Harvard University Press.

Way, N. (2006). The cultural practice of close friendships among urban adolescents in the United States. In X. Chen, B. Schneider, & D. French (Eds.), *Peer relationships in cultural context* (pp. 403–425). New York: Cambridge University Press.

Whiting, B., & Edwards, C. P. (1988). A cross-cultural analysis of sex differences in the behavior of children aged 3 through 11. In G. Handel (Ed.), *Childhood socialization* (pp. 281–297). New York: Hawthorne.

Wörmann, V., Holodynski, M., Kärtner, J., & Keller, H. (2012). A cross-cultural comparison of the development of the social smile: A longitudinal study of maternal and infant imitation in 6- and 12-week-old infants. *Infant Behavior and Development, 35*, 335–347.

Yang, K. S. (1986). Chinese personality and its change. In M. H. Bond (Ed.), *The psychology of the Chinese people* (pp. 106–170). Hong Kong: Oxford University Press.

CHAPTER 20

Children Develop Cultural Repertoires through Engaging in Everyday Routines and Practices

Barbara Rogoff
Leslie C. Moore
Maricela Correa-Chávez
Amy L. Dexter

Culturally rooted community routines and practices are crucial contributors to human development that are often overlooked. Throughout everyday life, people build on the routines and practices of previous generations that provide them with standing patterns of engagement, and they often do so without reflecting on them.

Our interest is in understanding the *cultural practices*—ways of living—with which children become facile, based on engagement in cultural traditions and institutions created by previous generations as well as their own generation. We stress the dynamic nature of both individuals' active participation and the guiding role of cultural traditions. People actively develop their individual histories, identifications, and resulting interests and familiarity with multiple cultural traditions, and the traditions themselves change as successive generations adapt them to current circumstances. Investigating distinct ways of organizing children's participation in routine activities offers a way to address the dynamic nature of *repertoires* of cultural practices—the formats of (inter)action that individuals experience and that they may take up, resist, or transform (Gutiérrez & Rogoff, 2003).

Our focus on cultural practices differs from research that equates culture with race or ethnicity (Rogoff, 2003, 2011). Clearly, cultural practices may be associated more with some racial or ethnic groups than with others, based on previous generations' histories, as well as imposed structural limitations. But our approach focuses on ways of living rather than on ancestry.

To elaborate on the organization of children's participation in the culturally and historically developed routines and practices of their communities, we first emphasize the frequently tacit nature of children's everyday routines and practices. This chapter examines the range of formats available in everyday life, from broad societal institutions to momentary interactions, and children's fluency and agency within the traditions of their communities. We then mention several complementary approaches to culture that similarly focus on the ways of life in which children participate. Next we build on ways that scholars across several disciplines have conceptualized the organization of people's participation in cultural practices, providing tools for examining cultural variation. We illustrate these points with three distinct cultural traditions, involving routine cultural practices that often organize children's learning in different ways: Learning by Observing and Pitching In, Assembly-Line Instruction, and Guided Repetition of Text.

We conclude the chapter by discussing several key features of the concept of repertoires of practice:

1. Individuals' engagement in several cultural communities may well involve conflict among the practices within their repertoires.
2. Although certain practices are more common in some cultural communities than in others, it is important not to assume that they necessarily characterize individuals from those communities (so as to avoid static, essentialist racial or ethnic characterizations).
3. Both individuals' and communities' repertoires of practice change in dynamic ways, at the same time as maintaining some continuities.
4. Individual agency is key in people's repertoires of practice, especially as individuals determine how to engage with the everyday routines and practices of their circumstances.

Routines and Practices Organize Development, Often in Tacit Ways

The organization of practices and routines in which children participate and the ways their participation is supported by others are often "invisible." That is, they are often not made explicit by community members. Few researchers, policymakers, or parents take note of their community's routine institutional, societal organizers of childhood. However, these organizers play a powerful role in creating the settings that children frequent, their roles, and the routine activities in which they engage. For example, the lives of current-day North American children are routinely channeled by the usual segregation of children from opportunities to observe or participate in their community's range of mature work, and by compulsory involvement in schooling. Some other communities provide children with much more extensive opportunities to learn through observing and contributing to ongoing community endeavors (Correa-Chávez, Roberts, & Martínez Pérez, 2011; Morelli, Rogoff, & Angelillo, 2003; Paradise & Rogoff, 2009; Rogoff, 2003, 2011).

On a more intimate scale, many cultural practices that organize the life experience of children may also be taken for granted. For middle-class North American children, for example, these often include routine involvement in bedtime stories, sleeping in a separate room, following local gender role expectations, and being encouraged to structure show-and-tell narratives in a particular manner and regulate peer access to possessions by taking turns (Rogoff, 2003).

Tacit, routine expectations of everyday life are likely to be among the most powerful cultural experiences—especially *because* they are expected and often unexamined (Rogoff, 2003). As Bourdieu (1977) suggested, through experience with one's environment and routine performances, strong dispositions develop that may be beyond the grasp of consciousness. These dispositions may be relatively impervious to efforts to change them or even to articulate them.

Tacit lessons from participation in everyday life—about who may participate, how, and when—are a key part of how people organize their interactions. Through participation in these interactions, children have the opportunity to learn, often without noticing, their community's unspoken expectations and values. As Rheingold argued, development is a process of becoming familiar with the environment and with one's interactions with the worlds it involves; each new skill becomes "submerged in consciousness" (1985, p. 5), and the effort to achieve it is forgotten as it becomes familiar.

Macro and Micro in the Cultural Infrastructures of Everyday Life

Social scientists have examined practices that range in "grain size" from the broad institutional organization of a lifetime (such as years of involvement in Western schooling) to daily routines (such as bedtime) and the organization of specific activities (such as doing a seminar or preparing onions for market) to moment-by-moment interactions (such as attentional practices). Broad traditions that organize children's opportunities to learn in generally recognizable formats (such as in formal Western schooling, in catechism, or Qur'anic schooling) are themselves routinely composed of particular formats that organize a particular activity or moment-by-moment interaction. For example, Western schooling frequently employs a format in which the teacher asks questions to which he or she already knows the answer, a student or the class responds briefly, and the teacher evaluates the response and goes on to another question that has an answer that he or she already knows (Mehan, 1979). As we describe later, this format is seldom used outside school in communities in which schooling is not prevalent, but it is usually part of the repertoire of children whose families have participated in Western schooling for generations.

The formats organizing children's participation in cultural activities provide standing patterns of engagement that form macro- and microcultural infrastructures of everyday life. Such formats are key among the resources on which humans draw to coordinate social encounters.

Children's Agency and Fluency in Community Traditions

As children move across settings that involve different formats for participation, they actively engage and become fluent in multiple forms of participation; these multiple forms of participation can be described as their own *repertoire of practice* (Gutiérrez & Rogoff, 2003).The concept of *repertoires of practice* helps us to focus on children's own agency in selecting, rejecting, and transforming multiple ways of engaging in the world. In the process, children in turn contribute to the formation of the routines and practices available to the next generation.

Attention to the organization of participation brings together a focus on individual agency and a focus on community traditions, in a mutually constituting process (Rogoff, 2003, 2011). Individuals play an active role as they engage in and make use of community traditions—or buck or change them. At the same time, the formats available to organize individuals' roles and connect them with community traditions contribute to the ongoing organization of individuals' participation. The focus on standing patterns of action and interaction helps to underline the dynamic nature of both individual and community processes.

Complementary Approaches
Examining Cultural Aspects of Children's Everyday Settings

Our interest in children's repertoires of practice relates to complementary approaches that focus on the cultural organization of children's everyday lives by examining their niches and activity settings. These approaches, and our own, have been heavily influenced by the work of Beatrice Whiting, who focused on the role of children's settings and the company they keep:

> Whether it is caring for an infant sibling, working around the house in the company of adult females, working on the farm with adults and siblings, playing outside with neighborhood children, hunting with adult males, or attending school with age mates, the daily assignment of a child to one or another of these settings has important consequences on the development of habits of interpersonal behavior, consequences that may not be recognized by the socializers who make the assignments. (1980, p. 111)

Children's settings and cast of characters are closely related to the propensities that they develop. For example, Whiting and Whiting (1975) found that six cultural communities differed greatly in the frequency with which children inhabited settings involving agemates (e.g., in school) versus younger children (e.g., in communities where child caregiving was routine). Heavy involvement with agemates was associated with children's aggressiveness and egoism, whereas extensive involvement with younger children was associated with nurturance.

Subsequent work by other scholars has elaborated these ecological ideas (along with other ecological approaches; e.g., those of Barker & Wright, 1954) to examine societal arrangements of children's opportunities to learn. Several scholars who use the idea of *activity settings* or *ecocultural niches* focus on the identity and motivations of the personnel who engage with children; cultural scripts that guide their conduct and routine activities; and cultural goals and beliefs (Tharp & Gallimore, 1988; Weisner, 1984; Weisner, Gallimore, & Jordan, 1988). Relatedly, scholars referring to *developmental niches* focus on physical and social settings in which children develop; the customs of childrearing that parents negotiate; and scripts, routines, and tools that are used to achieve cultural goals and values in socially organized ways (Gauvain, 1995; Harkness & Super, 1992, 2002).

The focus on scripts in these approaches, which connects with our emphasis on the organization of children's participation, builds on Bartlett's (1932) notion of scripts as cultural expectations of how events are organized. Similarly, Schank and Abelson (1977) referred to scripts as a shared understanding of a sequence of events in a specific situation, such as at dinner or at a bank. Use and understanding of such scripts for cultural routines appear in early childhood (Nelson & Gruendel, 1988). Children's learning from particular experiences is strengthened by redundancy that is "largely rooted in culture" (Gauvain, 2004, p. 13).

Scripts are closely related to cultural goals that guide parents' childrearing practices and children's experiences (Goodnow, 1992; Harkness & Super, 1992, 2002). For example, LeVine (1980) proposed that parents in different circumstances prioritize distinct goals, ranging from the physical survival and health of their children, to their economic security, to achieving locally valued goals such as social status, religious piety, and self-actualization. For example, Gusii (Kenyan) mothers engaged routinely in intensive protective infant care, reflecting their goal of ensuring survival where infant mortality was high, whereas mothers in London, with far less reason to be worried about infant survival, were concerned with preparing their infants for school and engaged extensively in pedagogical games and lessons (LeVine et al., 1994).

Although parents' goals and practices transform with changing circumstances, such as immigration (Rosenthal & Roer-Strier, 2001), they often do not change as rapidly as the circumstances do. LeVine (1980) suggested that childrearing practices are solutions to problems of rearing children that parents inherit from the previous generation, whose immediate circumstances are likely to have differed in some ways. Thus, cultural variations in childrearing practices and children's routines are intimately tied to the histories of communities in which families participate (Lancy, Gaskins, & Bock, 2010; Rogoff, 2003, 2011). Before we discuss three ways of organizing cultural practices to promote learning, we consider how the organization of participation has been conceptualized.

Ideas on The Organization of Participation

Anthropologists, sociologists, and linguists have provided valuable approaches to the study of social organization of peoples' participation in cultural activities. Sociologist Erving Goffman (1979, 1981) inspired several related lines of scholarship that address how humans organize social interaction, including Marjorie Goodwin's (1990) concept of *participant framework*. Our work is especially informed by the concepts and research provided by Susan Philips and Fred Erickson.

Philips (1983, 2001) introduced the concept of *participant structure*—a particular type of encounter or structural arrangement of interaction—and employed it in her pathbreaking research in a Native American community and the school attended by its children. Philips noted mismatches between the participant structures prevalent in the children's homes and their school, especially those having to do with how children's attention is organized and how talking turns are allocated and regulated. As a result of the unfamiliarity of classroom participant structures, the Native American children were less willing than their Anglo peers to speak alone in front of the class or to speak at moments determined by the teacher, both of which were key classroom practices. They were accustomed to a high degree of autonomy in determining when or if they spoke and to peer-group activities in which individuals were rarely singled out.

Building on work by Goffman and Philips, Fred Erickson (1982) analyzed interactional/communicative norms of the *social participation structure*. This is the allocation of interactional rights and obligations of participants that shape discourse; that is, the speaking and listening behaviors required or allowed for different participants, and the canonical patterns of turn taking.

Such concepts have facilitated empirical work on cultural variation in how adults and children structure and coordinate their participation in shared endeavors. For example, in some communities, learning through third-party attention is especially important, whereas in other communities, verbal explanations take precedence; teasing exchanges are valued tools of socialization in some communities, whereas in others they are regarded as hostile; some communities favor multiparty engagements over dyadic or solo ones, and vice versa (Rogoff, 2003). The unspoken "rules" or "grammars" of interaction vary across cultural communities in somewhat systematic ways (C. Heath, 1986; Hutchins & Palen, 1997; Kendon, 1990). After examining three distinct historical traditions organizing learning, we discuss how children develop repertoires of multiple practices with which they are relatively familiar and fluent.

Three Traditions of Learning

In this section, we argue that children's participation in one cultural tradition or another (or several) contributes to the development of distinct repertoires of practice. Human development research needs to investigate the repertoires of practice associated with children's participation in the varied traditions organizing the routines and familiar practices of their daily lives. Here we examine three widely used multidimensional cultural learning traditions to illustrate distinct ways of organizing learning: *Learning by Observing and Pitching In*, in which children have access to learning by observing and contributing to ongoing endeavors of their community; *Assembly-Line Instruction*, in which teaching is organized by experts around specialized exercises to introduce children to the skills and practices of their community without actual productive involvement; and *Guided Repetition of Text*, in which novices learn text by observing, imitating, and rehearsing models presented by experts. The three traditions differ markedly in both macro and micro forms of organization. They each have an internal "logic" or "grammar" (usually not articulated, or perhaps not even noticed by those involved in the practice) that make them coherent fields of practice.

Articles published over more than a decade have attempted to hone in on the defining features of Learning by Observing and Pitching In and Assembly-Line Instruction (Paradise & Rogoff, 2009; Rogoff, 2014; Rogoff et al., in the 2007 version of this chapter; Rogoff, Paradise, Mejía-Arauz, Correa-Chávez, & Angelillo, 2003). (Learning by Observing and Pitching In has undergone a name change: in earlier versions, it was called *intent community participation* or *intent participation*.) In this chapter, we discuss the latest account of each of these learning traditions (Rogoff, 2014) and update the description of Guided Repetition of Text, from the version presented in the previous edition of this handbook.

The prisms defining each of these learning traditions emphasize the integration and coherence of their multidimensional features, which are displayed on the facets of the prisms. The facets form a coherent set of features to be considered as a whole. Taken singly, a particular facet/feature is likely to fit with a number of distinct learning traditions; it does not define a learning tradition. For example, one feature of Learning by Observing and Pitching In involves learning through wide attention, but by itself, attentiveness does not necessarily indicate that what is going on fits with Learning by Observing and Pitching In. The other facets also need to be present for what is going on to fit the whole pattern comprising this learning tradition.

Hence, the prisms and their facets are not coding schemes for examining brief moments of interaction; rather, they are conceptual guides. To investigate a learning tradition, a global analysis of an event is required to determine whether all the facets of a learning tradition are present. (For a global coding scheme examining 20- to 40-minute interactions for their fit with a coherent multidimensional pattern, see Matusov & Rogoff's [2002] study of philosophies-in-action of adults interacting with groups of children.)

The prisms represent "pure" forms that define the pattern of features that, we argue, fit together as whole cultural traditions. In life, however, there are often mixtures or resemblances among different traditions, not just pure forms. Even in efforts to follow a "pure" tradition, everyday activity involves "seepage" in practice. (Indeed, this seepage may be a strength allowing for adaptation of the tradition to circumstances or supporting transformation.) In addition, the generic forms portrayed in the prisms vary in specific characteristics when instantiated within a particular community or institution.

Learning by Observing and Pitching In

Learning by Observing and Pitching In (LOPI) is a widely practiced and long-standing tradition in which people learn by actively observing (and "listening in") and contributing during ongoing community activities. This way of learning is effective in activities as varied as using statistics, weaving, conversing, reading, or programming computers. Figure 20.1 shows key facets of this cultural tradition.

LOPI is especially prevalent in some communities in which children are routinely included in the range of mature endeavors of daily community life. In other communities, being excluded from many mature settings makes it difficult for children to be attentive to and participate in the full range of economic and social activities (Morelli et al., 2003; Rogoff, Mistry, Göncü, & Mosier, 1993; Whiting & Whiting, 1975).

If children are integrated in a wide range of community settings, they are able to observe and listen in on ongoing activities as *legitimate peripheral participants* (Lave & Wenger, 1991). For example, toddlers in an African American community participated in daily community events and spent hours quietly listening to adults converse (Ward, 1971). Inuit men of Quebec reported that as boys, they learned to hunt from just watching the men, and they learned vocabulary and many other things by listening to stories that were not intended for them (Crago, 1992).

In communities in which children have access to observe and listen in on ongoing community events, they can begin to "pitch in," contributing to their families' social and economic lives from a young age (Alcalá, Rogoff, Mejía-Arauz, Coppens, & Dexter, 2014; Coppens, Alcalá, Mejía-Arauz, & Rogoff, 2014; López et al., 2012; Orellana, 2001, 2009; Rogoff, 2003). For example, in an East African farming community, 3- to 4-year-old children spent 25–35% of their time doing work, compared with 0–1% for middle-class U.S. children of the same age (Harkness & Super, 1992; also see Kramer, 2005).

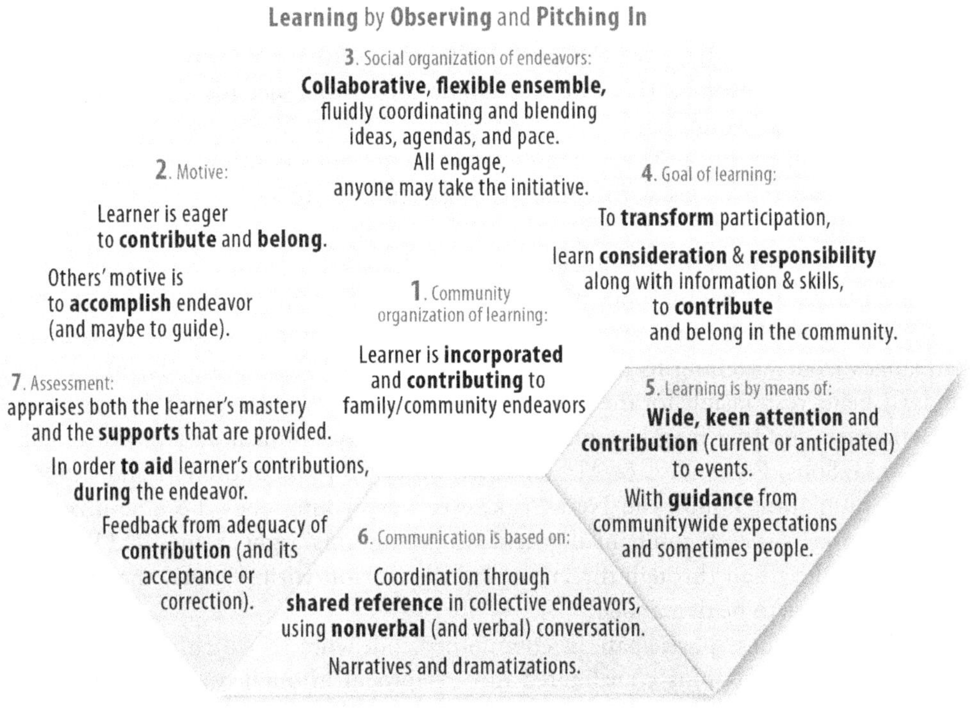

Learning by **Observing** and **Pitching In**

3. Social organization of endeavors:
Collaborative, flexible ensemble,
fluidly coordinating and blending
ideas, agendas, and pace.
All engage,
anyone may take the initiative.

2. Motive:
Learner is eager
to **contribute** and **belong**.

Others' motive is
to **accomplish** endeavor
(and maybe to guide).

4. Goal of learning:
To **transform** participation,
learn **consideration** & **responsibility**
along with information & skills,
to **contribute**
and belong in the community.

1. Community
organization of learning:
Learner is **incorporated**
and **contributing** to
family/community endeavors

7. Assessment:
appraises both the learner's mastery
and the **supports** that are provided.

In order **to aid** learner's contributions,
during the endeavor.
Feedback from adequacy of
contribution (and its
acceptance or
correction).

6. Communication is based on:
Coordination through
shared reference in collective endeavors,
using **nonverbal** (and verbal) conversation.
Narratives and dramatizations.

5. Learning is by means of:
Wide, keen attention and
contribution (current or anticipated)
to events.
With **guidance** from
communitywide expectations
and sometimes people.

FIGURE 20.1. Prism showing key facets (features) of the prism defining the cultural tradition of Learning by Observing and Pitching In. Copyright 2014 by Barbara Rogoff.

Jordan (1989) described how Yucatecan Mayan girls whose mothers and grandmothers are midwives absorb the essence of midwifery practice, as well as specific knowledge. As they grow up, they are surrounded by the routines and practices of this profession and pitch in as they become able to assist.

> They know what the life of a midwife is like (for example, that she needs to go out at all hours of the day or night), what kinds of stories the women and men who come to consult her tell, what kinds of herbs and other remedies need to be collected, and the like. As young children they might be sitting quietly in a corner as their mother administers a prenatal massage; they would hear stories of difficult cases, of miraculous outcomes, and the like. As they grow older, they may be passing messages, running errands, getting needed supplies. A young girl might be present as her mother stops for a postpartum visit after the daily shopping trip to the market. (p. 932)

Although the range of opportunities for children to be involved in ongoing mature activities tends to be limited in middle-class cultural settings, where Western schooling is prevalent (Morelli et al., 2003), LOPI also occurs in such communities. For example, children's impressive learning of their first language occurs through opportunities to observe and listen in (Akhtar, 2005; Akhtar, Jipson, & Callanan, 2001), and they begin to pitch in to shared communicative endeavors in which the aim is getting things accomplished with words. (In addition, some children receive language lessons.) Likewise, young children in general are interested in engaging in the activities of those around them (Eckerman, Whatley, & McGhee, 1979; Hay, Murray, Cecire, & Nash, 1985; Meltzoff & Williamson, 2013; Nielsen, Moore, & Mohamedally, 2012; Rheingold, 1982). LOPI brings young children worldwide—including middle-class children—into the practices and routines of their families and communities, although extent of use of this way of learning varies with children's opportunities to be present and contribute (see Figure 20.2).

Central to the pattern of cultural practices related to LOPI is "being there" during valued activities and having opportunities to contribute. Children in the United States whose parents work at home are often involved in their parents' work, in a progression that ranges from watching to carrying out simple tasks to giving regular assistance to regularly being responsible for the work (Beach, 1988). Likewise, if given the opportunity to participate, children may become part of community political action. For example, Solís (2003; Solís, Fernández, & Alcalá, 2013) observed that children in undocumented Mexican immigrant families in New York, even very young ones, became involved in political action as they accompanied parents to immigrants' rights rallies and learned by observing (rather than through direct, explicit discussion with parents) that rights and fair treatment are to be demanded.

In LOPI, learners participate in community endeavors in which engagement with more experienced people is coordinated in a reciprocal (though usually asymmetrical) manner, with mutual responsibility and respect for each other's contributions (Rogoff, 2014; Ruvalcaba, Rogoff, López, Correa-Chávez, & Gutiérrez, 2014). Roles are taken up with flexibility, such that people play varying roles in the activity at different times (Paradise & de Haan, 2009). Participants have some room to maneuver within their role. They are expected to contribute as they are able and tend not to be micromanaged in specific actions (Paradise et al., 2014). Even small children contribute and coordinate around shared family and community endeavors (Coppens et al., 2014).

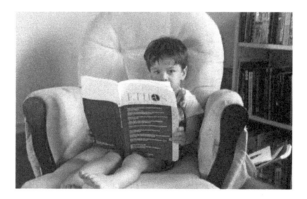

FIGURE 20.2. Two-year-old Solomon reading a journal in which his anthropologist mother's article appears. This illustrates the involvement of young children in the ongoing activities that surround them (note also all the books behind him), consistent with Learning by Observing and Pitching In. Photo copyright 2013 by David Magarian.

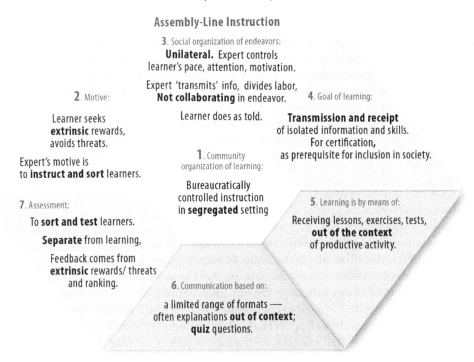

FIGURE 20.3. Prism showing key facets (features) of the cultural tradition of Assembly-Line Instruction. Copyright 2014 by Barbara Rogoff.

Assembly-Line Instruction

Assembly-Line Instruction involves "transmission" of information from experts, in specialized exercises outside the context of productive, purposive activity (see Figure 20.3). It is common in many schools and middle-class families, in communities where children are routinely segregated from many mature settings (Rogoff, 2003). Of course, Assembly-Line Instruction is not the only way that schooling and middle-class parent–child interactions are organized. For example, some schools operate according to philosophies related to LOPI in the community (Rogoff, Goodman Turkanis, & Bartlett, 2001; Sato, 1996).

However, assumptions and practices regarding learning in middle-class communities (both at home and at school, and among developmental psychologists) are heavily influenced by the centrality of particular school formats that became prevalent when mass, compulsory schooling became widespread, about a century ago (Rogoff, 2003). School-based Assembly-Line Instruction was explicitly modeled on the organization of factories, with learners (and teachers, too) treated as part of a mechanism designed by administrators or consultants for bureaucratic efficiency (Callahan, 1962). This tradition is based on a mechanical metaphor, with experts inserting information into children, as raw materials, and sorting the children in terms of their quality and the extent to which they have received the information.

An example of bureaucratic control of learners is the common "switchboard participant structure" (Philips, 1983), in which teachers take a speaking turn between each child turn and determine which children may or have to speak. Adults with extensive schooling experience may have difficulty avoiding attempts to control children's attention, pace, and behavior in informal settings (Paradise et al., 2014). Echoes of Assembly-Line Instruction can also be seen in dinner conversations of European American families in Hawaii, where children raised their hand for a turn and parents managed the children's turns to talk and the structure of the children's accounts of their day in a style that resembles school forms of reporting (Martini, 1995).

Middle-class families have extensive experience with the formats of formal schooling, usually over several generations in the United States, and they often engage young children in a variety of practices related to school formats. For example, they frequently engage their children in lessons and school-like discourse formats, including questions with known answers (Rogoff et al., 1993). Rather than children joining adults in work and social activities, in middle-class communities, adults often engage in children's play and child-focused exercises, in which they manage young children's attention and help them practice school-relevant skills in play (Haight, 1991; Harkness, 1977; Lareau, 2011; Martini, 1995; Morelli et al., 2003; Ochs & Kramer-Sadlik, 2013).

For example, middle-class mothers in the United States and Turkey more often engaged their toddlers in language lessons and school-like quizzes about properties of objects than did mothers in a tribal community in India and a Mayan community in which schooling was not prevalent (Rogoff et al., 1993). Similarly, middle-class European American 3-year-olds more often engaged with adults in scholastic play (like the alphabet song) and in free-standing conversations with adults on child-related topics than did 3-year-olds in a foraging community in the Democratic Republic of Congo and an agricultural Mayan community in Guatemala, where children had more opportunity to observe adult work and frequently emulated these themes in their play (Morelli et al., 2003).

The specialized child-focused formats that young middle-class children experience can be seen as attempts to aid them in assembling skills for later entry into mature activities from which they are often excluded as children. The social organization of Assembly-Line Instruction involves experts managing learners in a unilateral manner, without participating, in exercises designed to induce transmission of information and that seldom yield a useful product or outcome for the larger community. The learners' involvement is managed with extrinsic inducements (such as praise, grades, and threats), with assessments aiming to determine the quality of both the raw materials (in assessments of IQ or scholastic "aptitude") and the receipt of the curriculum "delivered." Communication in Assembly-Line Instruction is heavily reliant on extensive explanations and specialized formats, such as quiz questions with known answers, outside of shared productive endeavors.

The contrast between Assembly-Line Instruction and Learning by Observing and Pitching In is particularly clear in de Haan's (2001) study of Mazahua (Indigenous Mexican) children engaged in a building task with either their parent or a non-Mazahua teacher. The parents treated the children as responsible contributors to a shared endeavor, in which children sometimes led the effort. Children were expected to learn by watching the parents' contribution while they participated, and to take on more responsibility as the joint activity proceeded, but they were not forced to do so. In contrast, when the children worked with a non-Mazahua teacher, the teacher held the initiative and expected the child to perform the task under the teacher's directions. If the child made suggestions, these were evaluated by the teacher as a test of the child's knowledge, not treated as a contribution to a task that needed to be done.

Guided Repetition of Text

In communities around the globe, guided repetition is used to teach and learn a wide range of skills, including music, athletics, and crafts. Perhaps the most common use of Guided Repetition is in the teaching of oral or written texts. Guided Repetition of Text (or "recitation") is a tradition of teaching and learning that involves modeling by an expert, imitation of the model by a novice, rehearsal by the novice until he or she has mastered the skill or task, and performance by the novice so that his or her mastery may be assessed by an expert (Moore, 2006a, 2012). In each phase, the expert supervises the novice and may provide assistance, evaluation, and/or correction as the novice works toward mastery (see Figure 20.4).

Guided Repetition of Text has been disparaged and dismissed by most Western educators and researchers since it fell out of favor in the late 19th and early 20th centuries with the advance of the progressive education movement (Hori, 1996). It is now widely believed—but not proven—to have a negative influence on children's cognitive abilities, fostering the development of memory skills at the expense of so-called "higher cognitive skills," such as logical and creative thinking (Wagner, 1983). However, this approach continues to be part of the educational experience of millions of children around the world.

Guided Repetition of Text is historically rooted in the teaching of sacred texts. In the religions that have promoted literacy—including Judaism, Christianity, Islam, Hinduism, Buddhism, and Confucianism—traditional pedagogy places "a strong emphasis on verbatim oral mastery of a body of essential written teachings and ritual" (Wagner, 1983, p. 112). In many communities, learning sacred texts by heart is the path into literacy and verbatim recitation the preferred way to attain and display knowledge, as well as a

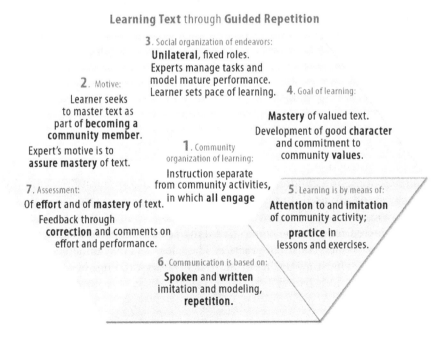

FIGURE 20.4. Prism showing key facets (features) of the cultural tradition of learning through Guided Repetition of Text. Copyright 2014 by Leslie Moore.

means to preserve texts of great importance to the community (e.g., S. B. Heath, 1983; Tambiah, 1968). Common to all of these traditional pedagogies is the ideology that the achievement of verbatim oral mastery of sacred texts through rote learning is an appropriate and effective way to instill religious commitment and good moral character.

Built on the foundations of religious education, secular schooling often uses Guided Repetition of Text. Repetition and memorization figure prominently in descriptions of East Asian educational practice and the learning styles of Asian students (Jin, 2012; On, 1996). Western education has long emphasized memorization, too. For centuries, the recitation and memorization of Greek and Latin texts constituted a large part of curricula in European schools (Carruthers, 1992; Nash, 1968). Until the late 1800s, European and North American pedagogical practices emphasized textbook memorization (Cubberley, 1922). Currently in the United States, there is growing interest in classical (Christian) education, which emphasizes memorization of a body of knowledge in the early years of education, leaving analysis and discussion to later stages (e.g., Wise Bauer & Wise, 2009).

The memorization of a fixed body of knowledge may serve as the basis for application to *new* contexts and materials and the development of new understanding. For example, some Fulbe who have memorized the Qur'an build on this foundation, developing a high degree of competence in Arabic as a second language (Moore, 2013). Hori (1996) argued that the formalism of rote learning in a Zen monastery is an important route to insight. He argued that this process resembles the process of learning propositional logic in a university philosophy class. He noticed that the students who could solve logic problems had memorized the basic transformation formulas and, as a result, they could "just see" common factors to cancel out in the equations or "just see" logical equivalences. The students who had not memorized the formulas were mystified by the problems, trying to reason their way through them without the logical insight that the others had developed through rote memorization.

As in Assembly-Line Instruction, roles within Guided Repetition of Text are generally unilateral and fixed. The expert's responsibilities are to model the text, task, or skill correctly and in suitable increments, and to monitor, correct, and evaluate the learner as he or she attempts to imitate, rehearse, and master it. The novice is expected to pay close attention to the expert and to be focused and diligent during all phases of the activity. In addition to tests for mastery, assessment is often ongoing; errors are corrected immediately or soon after they are committed in order to support learning.

Guided Repetition of Text involves specialized learner-focused lessons, but unlike Assembly-Line Instruction, it does not necessarily occur in settings that are removed from adult activities, and children have regular access to community activities in which the texts they study are used. In many communities, religious instruction takes place at the temple or mosque, where learners may observe more competent community members as they recite sacred texts in the context of daily ritual. Moreover, learners may apply lessons in their own emergent ritual practice. Thus, learners may understand the purpose and importance of what they are learning. (Such understanding, however, may not be regarded as necessary to learning.)

Dynamic Practices and Repertoires

The use of particular cultural traditions to organize learning is dynamic, not fixed and stable. People who have been raised mostly within one tradition of learning may switch their approach to another when they have experience in a tradition that is new to them (or they may blend or otherwise revise the traditions, or resist them). For example, schooled mothers from communities that are newly adopting Western schooling more often interact with children in some Assembly-Line ways—including praise, lessons, and assignment of divided tasks—than do mothers with little or no schooling from the same communities (Chavajay & Rogoff, 2002; Rabain-Jamin, 1989; Richman, Miller, & LeVine, 1992; Rogoff et al., 1993). Similarly, experienced middle-class parent volunteers in a collaborative school were more likely to engage with children in ways that fit with Learning by Observing and Pitching In than parents with less such experience, even though the prior schooling of almost all the parents was likely to have been similar to Assembly-Line Instruction (Matusov & Rogoff, 2002; Rogoff et al., 2001).

The use of Guided Repetition of Text is similarly dynamic. For example, in the Qur'anic schools of an urban Fulbe community in northern Cameroon, children have long been taught one-on-one to recite, read, and write the Qur'an (Moore, 2006a, 2010). As Fulbe participation in public schooling has increased, however, the public school practice of collective instruction (in addition to individual instruction) has come to be used in a growing number of Qur'anic schools. Guided Repetition of Text has also seeped from school into homes. Whereas Fulbe children once learned folktales only through Observing and Pitching In, many now learn through Guided Repetition of Text (Moore, 2006b). A similar shift has occurred in the Kaska community in the Yukon, where children's opportunities to learn Kaska through Learning by Observing and Pitching In had become so restricted that the community adopted a government-supplied language curriculum for language revitalization that emphasized repetition and memorization (Meek, 2013).

Not Limited by Type of Learning or Context

The processes of Learning by Observing and Pitching In and Assembly-Line Instruction are not specific to particular types of activities or "subject" matter (such as practical vs. theoretical endeavors, or "concrete" vs. "abstract" information). For example, people may master statistics through observing and pitching in as they carry out research to contribute to their field, or they may be involved in Assembly-Line Instruction in a class in which the material is studied in isolation from using it for research. Likewise, LOPI was very effective for traditional Maori (New Zealand) children's learning of both abstract spiritual knowledge and practical skills (Metge, 1984).

Although certain traditions and practices may be more prevalent in a given community or context, people generally participate in a variety of traditions and practices as they engage in the different activities of their daily lives. Institutions and individuals develop repertoires of practices that may be culturally and contextually distinct in their roots but spread with contact among communities and individuals.

Repertoires of Practice

According to Webster's dictionary, a *repertoire* is the set of operas, songs, and parts that can readily be performed by members of a company because they have practiced or performed them many times. In sociolinguistics, the term *repertoire* refers to the range of languages or varieties of a language available for use by a speaker, each of which enables him or her to perform a particular social role or purpose. We use the term *repertoire* to describe the variety of practices with which individuals are familiar, yielding a disposition to apply different formats under distinct circumstances. The idea of *repertoires of practice* addresses the fact that people engage in multiple traditions (Gutiérrez & Rogoff, 2003; Rogoff, 2003, 2011; Zentella, 1998). Through their lives and the different endeavors in which they engage, people develop fluency with a variety of formats for participation.

Figure 20.5 depicts Jean Piaget's attempt to expand his repertoire to include skills in a practice new to him, during a visit to Kyoto, Japan. (Note the keen attention he employs to try to learn from Bärbel Inhelder's approach.)

A number of scholars have made use of the concept of *repertoire* (e.g., Davies & Harré, 1990; Erickson, 2004). This concept in some ways resembles Bourdieu's concept of *habitus*—"systems of durable, transposable *dispositions*" (1977, p. 72, original emphasis). Gutiérrez, Baquedano-López, and Tejeda (1999) pointed out that the linguistic repertoires of students are tools for their participation and meaning making in the classroom. Gutiérrez and Rogoff noted that children with differing experience with distinct cultural traditions vary in their repertoires

> for engaging in discussions with authority figures, answering known-answer questions, analyzing word problems on the basis of counterfactual premises, seeking or avoiding being singled out for praise, spontaneously helping classmates, observing ongoing events without adult management, responding quickly or pondering ideas before volunteering their contributions, and many other approaches. (2003, p. 22)

People's repertoires of practice describe the formats they are likely to employ in upcoming situations, based on their own prior experience in similar settings. Repertoires of practice are highly constrained by people's opportunities and access to participate

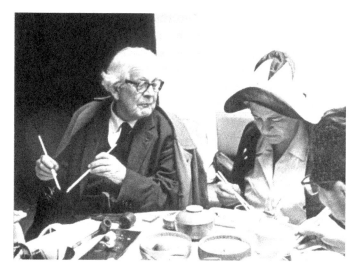

FIGURE 20.5. Jean Piaget attempting to expand his repertoire to include skill in a practice new to him. Photograph courtesy Matsui Kimio.

directly or vicariously in settings and activities in which particular formats are employed. For example, children who are newcomers to classroom organization are less skilled in aligning their participation with the structure of lessons and the conversational formats employed in their classroom; at the end of the school year, they are much more effective in following and using the structure of classroom formats, including instruction–response–evaluation sequences (Mehan, 1979). We could say that their repertoire comes to include some dexterity in participating in instruction–response–evaluation sequences, among other classroom formats. And in the next school year, they may be more likely to engage in this manner in another teacher's classroom.

Although people's readiness, efficiency, fluency, and dexterity in engaging in a particular practice depend on familiarity with the specific practice or similar ones, at the same time, the agency of individuals is key. Individuals choose (with or without reflection) among the formats with which they are familiar, and they may actively transform or reject engagement in particular formats as they navigate the different settings of their lives.

In Figure 20.6, which was taken right after the photograph shown in Figure 20.5, Jean Piaget illustrates the idea that individuals' agency and familiarity with particular practices play a role in their engagement with particular practices.

An example of children determining which approach to use from their repertoires can be seen in research on Pima Indian children's ways of speaking. In grades 1–3, their dialect was fairly similar to their teacher's standard dialect, but by grade 4, the children's way of speaking became increasingly similar to the local native dialect, despite the children's growing competence in expressing themselves with the standard dialect (Nelson-Barber, 1982). Nelson-Barber speculated that the children's shift to use of the local dialect over the standard dialect may have been an affirmation of their community membership, in response to the school's negative attitude toward their community.

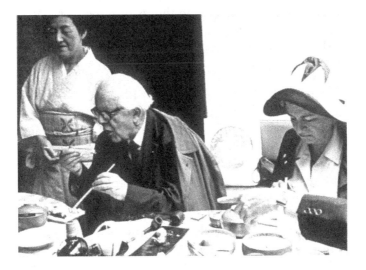

FIGURE 20.6. Jean Piaget's attempt to expand his repertoire to include an unfamiliar skill shows his agency in adapting the practice of eating with chopsticks to a form he can manage. Photograph courtesy Matsui Kimio.

Although people can reflect on occasion about the ways in which they engage with others, this does not imply that they draw on their repertoires as stored menus to be called up; repertoires are a description for the sake of analysis. Thus, repertoires are not possessions of individuals (or communities) themselves; rather, they are analytical tools to describe often-implicit patterns, for the sake of reflection by researchers, practitioners, and other analysts (including individuals themselves at times).

The idea of repertoires of practice offers several benefits for the analysis of individual and group cultural patterns, which we discuss in the remainder of this chapter:

- It assists understanding of conflict among different communities' learning traditions.
- It helps to get beyond treating cultural variation in terms of ethnic stereotypes.
- It accommodates the fact that cultural routines and practices transform dynamically, as individuals and communities expand, prune, hybridize, and adapt their repertoires.
- It aids in understanding the role of individual agency along with affordances and constraints supplied by prevalent cultural practices.

Possible Conflicts between Distinct Community Traditions for Supporting Learning

Participants in an activity may vary in what they consider preferable or acceptable, based on differing repertoires of practice associated with their histories of involvement in distinct traditions of learning and the social identities or stances they associate with a given practice. The juxtaposition of conflicting practices is a common source of many minority students' difficulties in formal schooling. For example, when a Warm Springs Indian child turns her gaze down from her teacher's face in order to show respectful listening, her Anglo teacher is likely to read this as disrespect or inattentiveness (Philips, 1983).

In discussing the juxtaposition of differently valued ways of learning, Jordan (1989) described the limited uptake of training efforts by Western medical personnel among Yucatecan (Mexican) Mayan midwives. The trainers' efforts resembled Assembly-Line Instruction, with didactic lectures emphasizing definitions and quizzes, whereas the midwives' lifetime experience of learning involved the kind of Learning by Observing and Pitching In that Jordan (quoted earlier) described for girls learning midwifery by participating in the practices and skills in everyday life. Much of the training sessions provided by the Western medical personnel involved rhetorical questions about definitions. For example, a nurse asked a group of traditional midwives, "What is a family?" and proceeded to give a definition that she wrote on the blackboard; the midwives barely responded—most of them stared vacantly. The nurse looked at them expectantly, waiting for them to copy the definition (although most of the midwives could neither read nor write) and telling them that the definition would be on the final test.

Jordan pointed out that in the midwives' familiar way of learning, talk is used to extend communication that occurs in shared activity, rather than being the sole means of instruction. Talk has an important role *in the context of practice*, as midwives and birth assistants discuss diagnoses and consider different courses of action, drawing on their accounts of previous cases and collaboratively considering their applicability to the current case.

> Talk in such situations is always closely tied to, and supportive of, action. In the traditional system, to know something is to know *how to do it*, and only derivatively to know *how to talk about it*. . . . [With the nurses, the midwives] learned new ways of talking, new ways of legitimizing themselves, new ways of presenting themselves as being in league with the powerful [Western medical establishment], which, however, had little impact on their daily practice. (Jordan, 1989, p. 928)

When asked by the Western medical personnel whether they used traditional birthing practices (such as external cephalic version or cauterizing the umbilical stump—disdained by Western medicine until recently), the midwives did not admit to using them. They could all give answers promoted by Western medicine (e.g., to treat the umbilical stump with alcohol and merthiolate).

> But when we were alone, swinging in our hammocks at night in the dormitory, and I intimated that I actually knew how to do those things [having learned them from a Mayan midwife] and thought they were good for mother and baby, every one of them admitted that she engaged in those practices routinely. As a matter of fact, a lively discussion and exchange of information about specific techniques ensued. I would suggest, then that current teaching methods produce only minimal changes in the behavior of trainees, while, at the same time, providing new resources for *talking about* what they do. (Jordan, 1989, pp. 928–929, original emphasis)

These distinctions drawn by Jordan in her participant observation of the midwives' training courses may well apply when individuals whose repertoires are based on one tradition for learning (such as LOPI) are thrown into settings based on another (such as Assembly-Line Instruction).

The unilateral nature of Assembly-Line Instruction is part of the problem that prevented the medical personnel from detecting that their means of instruction was not connecting with the backgrounds of the trainees. This is problematic even for many students who function well within it. For example, in the natural sciences, often top students who finish a course are able to answer exam questions fluently but maintain their initial ideas about the phenomena, without their professors noticing ("misconceptions" from the instructors' perspective; National Research Council, 2012).

A rigid form of instruction is particularly problematic for students who are unfamiliar with its rules and how to "play the game." The emphasis in Assembly-Line Instruction is on learning subject-matter information and skills, but to do well in this way of organizing learning requires also learning the values and forms of social interaction that it involves. Ironically, students are likely to learn how to participate in Assembly-Line Instruction through LOPI—by observing and attempting to make contributions as they enter institutions (schools, museums, families) that use Assembly-Line Instruction!

Although our focus in this chapter has been on how individuals change their repertoires, it is important to note that institutions can also (and should) be flexible in the traditions of learning that they employ. School reform efforts generally attempt to move away from Assembly-Line Instruction toward ways of learning that involve active student involvement and sensitivity to students' background knowledge (Bransford, Brown, Cocking, & Committee on Developments in the Science of Learning, 1999; Committee on Conceptual Framework for the New K–12 Science Education Standards, 2012).

However, schooled adults' familiarity with the routines and practices of Assembly-Line Instruction make it difficult to improve schools. For the most part, traditions of learning are unreflectively used by practitioners, based on their own familiarity with particular traditions and practices (Matusov & Rogoff, 2002; Paradise et al., 2014). School reform efforts seldom pay sufficient attention to the need to address the repertoires of adults themselves, which often require opportunities to *participate* in the new practices in order to make the paradigm shift they require in order to develop new ways of assisting others' learning (Rogoff et al., 2001).

Adults and children alike may expand their repertoires of practice to include conflicting cultural practices, to be employed in appropriate circumstances. Often this process involves Learning by Observing and Pitching In, when people have the opportunity to be included in cultural ways that are new to them. People who have conflicting cultural practices in their repertoire may feel internal conflict, especially if some practices challenge allegiance to a particular community or require difficult choices at times when there are negative consequences to choosing one over another (e.g., Rogoff, 2011). The connection of different cultural practices with ethnic or racial or class-based groups is an important feature of everyone's repertoire of practices. Awareness of this connection helps to distinguish an approach focused on repertoires of practice from ethnic or racial characterizations.

Getting Beyond Ethnic Stereotypes

The idea of repertoires of practice helps to make sense of the distinct, customary ways of acting of people from distinct backgrounds, without assuming that these ways of acting are an inherent characteristic of the individuals or backgrounds. In social science research (and in national censuses), individuals' cultural heritage has often been treated as a single social address. In contrast, we argue that conceptions of individuals' cultural backgrounds should be tied to the cultural practices in which they have participated (Gutiérrez & Rogoff, 2003; Rogoff, 2011; Rogoff & Angelillo, 2002). National or ethnic labels such as "French" or "Mexican" or hybrid forms such as "African American" or "European American" are useful, but we suggest that they be treated as indices of likely common experience with particular cultural/historical practices rather than simply as a marker of ancestry.

A focus on repertoires of practice addresses the fact that most people have some history of participation (in varied forms, including resistance) in the practices of several cultural communities and institutions. This concept contrasts with a common approach in which a person identified with a given ethnic group is *assumed* to have certain "traits" that are considered typical of that group, homogenous, and stable across time and circumstances. As Gutiérrez and Rogoff (2003) suggested, the concept of repertoires of practice enables us to talk about probable patterns of engagement based on historical and life experience, rather than to stereotype members of a group in a timeless, uniform fashion.

Our aim is to contribute to shifting the field from a concept of culture as a stable, singular characteristic of individuals to focusing on people's *experience* with cultural practices, through their life history and community history. These histories contribute to individuals' (and communities') proclivities to do things in certain ways—ways that are dynamic, potentially changing with generations and contact with different ways.

Repertoires Often Change in Dynamic Ways, for Both Individuals and Communities

Our dynamic approach also differs from the idea that socialization provides inputs that yield outcomes. As people actively participate in distinct cultural practices, they develop their repertoires of distinct ways of treating the situations of their lives—but in a dynamic, agentic way. Individuals (and communities) may expand, refine, prune, and transform their repertoires of practices, and they may hybridize conflicting practices (Rogoff, 2003). Gutiérrez and Rogoff noted:

> Of course, there are regularities in the ways that cultural groups participate in everyday practices of their respective communities. However, the relatively stable characteristics of these environments are in constant tension with the emergent goals and practices participants construct, which stretch and change over time and with other constraints. This conflict and tension contribute to the variation and ongoing change in an individual's and a community's practices. (2003, p. 21)

Hybridization can be viewed as a process of using particular interactional formats as cultural tools for accomplishing participants' current purposes. For example, faced with home–school discontinuities, children (and parents) often adjust their ways of participating to fit with school ways, or they may develop hybrid forms that allow children to engage in the classroom in ways that are new for both the children and the school (Baquedano-López, Solís, & Kattan, 2005; Gutiérrez et al., 1999).

The process of hybridization is an important contributor to the continually changing repertoires of individuals and communities, especially when individuals and communities with different traditions interact. Over generations, Guatemalan Mayan mothers with extensive exposure to schooling seem to carry over their experience with school formats to their interactions with their own children, which come to resemble the interactions of highly schooled, middle-class European American mothers (Chavajay & Rogoff, 2002; Correa-Chávez & Rogoff, 2009; Rogoff et al., 1993). Conversely, teachers from Native American communities sometimes make use of local ways of organizing social interaction (Erickson & Mohatt, 1982; Lipka, 1991; Van Ness, 1981).

Immigrant Latino parents in the United States modified their ideas about literacy and adjusted their reading practices with their children through contact with models of literacy embodied in their children's school routines (Reese & Gallimore, 2000).

> "Hybrid language practices" enable linguistically and ethnically diverse children and teachers to reorganize classroom functioning, creating a learning context where "no single language or register is privileged, and the larger linguistic repertoires of participants become tools for participating and making meaning in [a] new collaborative activity." (Gutiérrez et al., 1999, p. 293)

Accompanying such processes of cultural change are continuities, also involving individual agency, as individuals and their generations choose to maintain or even to revitalize cultural practices of prior generations (Rogoff, 2011).

The Role of Individual Agency: Fitting Approaches to Circumstances

The idea of repertoires of practice helps relate individual agency to contextual processes and how people navigate between different situations. Children (and adults) determine when to apply what approach, as they choose and modify standing patterns of engagement. For example, the children of undocumented Mexican immigrant families in New York City who became involved in political protests needed to determine whether to distinguish or generalize such public protests from "protests" against unfair decisions by a teacher or a parent (Solís, 2003; Solís et al., 2013). If children automatically transfer one mode of learning to other settings, this may have negative consequences, such as when Indigenous American children attempt to collaborate with each other in classrooms that treat helping as cheating (López et al., 2012).

Rather than assuming that skills should generalize broadly, an important goal of development is appropriate generalization—learning "which strategies are helpful in what circumstances" Rogoff (2003, p. 253). Learning to fit approaches flexibly to the circumstances is an important feature of what Hatano (1982) called *adaptive expertise.*

Although particular practices are associated with specific social identities, activities, and places, there may be a range of practices one may use in a given situation, in addition to the possibility of developing new approaches. Lave and Wenger (1991) argued that integral to participation is an individual's sense of belonging to a web of social relationships and, accordingly, the meanings the activity holds for him or her.

An example of children distinguishing distinct purposes for different approaches in their repertoires is provided by a study that revealed contextual differences in how African American children narrated stories concerning conflict resolution, within a school-based violence prevention program (Daiute, Buteau, & Rawlins, 2002). The third- and fifth-grade children were asked to respond to two narrative prompts: One asked for an ending to a fictional story, and the other asked for an autobiographical story concerning social conflict. The children used more extensive and elaborated resolution strategies in their autobiographical narratives and more school-like resolutions in the fictional narratives, suggesting that they interpreted each task as signifying a particular narrative mode of discourse, each with different interpretive strategies.

In some communities, children are provided with support in determining whether the purposes or goals of given approaches are the same or different across settings. For example, Japanese mother–child and teacher–child interaction may often provide children with explicit "boundary training," marking the differences in behavior expected in different contexts and providing strategies to handle new contexts (Lebra, 1994). Likewise, adults in African American working-class communities provide encouragement to children to use their own experiences in flexibly determining roles and relationships as these shift across situations (S. B. Heath, 1983).

Individuals may choose how to engage in an activity with some deliberateness, or they may adapt or select an approach from their repertoires with little or no reflection. When people experience points of disruption regarding their own and others' expectations about how to engage in a particular activity, the issue of repertoires may become salient, especially as people traverse settings that are disparate in the goals and meanings assigned to particular actions. In those moments of disruption, people may reflect on their own ways of acting that are not in accord with modes of participation in other settings (Roberts & Rogoff, 2012).

Although adjustment and modification of repertoires is often not accompanied by such reflection, determining which approach to take nonetheless involves an individual's agency, attending at some level to the affordances and cues in a particular situation and how they relate to familiar practices. Determining which approach in one's repertoire to apply or to build on requires attentiveness to the structure of situations and how they fit with one's goals, in order to align with the direction of ongoing events, to invent new approaches when old ones do not work, to revamp an original way of participating by combining with other forms, to determine whose approach to align with in a politically charged or divisive situation, and to decide which goals to prioritize in a given situation (e.g., resisting involvement in a distasteful event, showing solidarity with a peer, competing with others, or avoiding being noticed).

Courses of action are therefore a matter that involves both the active roles of individuals and the dynamic structures of situations. The determination of an action is *in the process of participation* itself—of the individual involved in the activity—not within the individual or the context separately.

The idea of repertoires as cultural tools that change as people use them is consistent with Erickson's (2004) examination of the relation of social "structure" and individual agency in the everyday interactions of social life. These interactions take place in real time, with improvisation by participants who make use of the affordances and deal with the constraints of historically developed practices that precede the particular interaction.

As such, the everyday lives of individuals are agentic, as people engage in continual opportunistic history-in-the-making, usually on a small scale, building on as well as building longer-term historical processes (Rogoff, 2011). People's opportunism often requires innovation, as participants make use of what is available in cultural practices to address their current needs and intentions. Human life simultaneously involves changes *and* continuities—innovations using cultural repertoires to build current approaches.

In summary, we have argued that understanding the routine formats and activities in which children engage aids in understanding human development. It is a fruitful way to understand all children's cultural experience and preparation to engage in particular settings with specific cultural practices. Attention to the social organization of routine events (such as bedtime storytelling, or language games, or helping around the house) reveals reasons for certain children's ease or confusion, or even resistance, when they enter new settings that are organized in ways that may relate to, differ from, or conflict with settings with which they have experience.

Noticing the cultural organization of everyday practices and even of whole learning traditions (such as Learning by Observing and Pitching In, Assembly-Line Instruction, and Guided Repetition of Text) can help researchers understand all people's development as cultural beings. Such understanding can also help practitioners ease the entry of newcomers to a specific tradition, such as that commonly employed in traditional schooling, innovative schooling, or in collaborative teams in classroom or work settings. In addition, understanding the routines and practices of children's lives can help develop ways to revise the structure and practices of such institutions to better serve people with varying cultural experience, if the institutions' practitioners are themselves given the opportunity and time to expand or adjust their own repertoires.

ACKNOWLEDGMENTS

Writing of this chapter was supported by the UCSC Foundation Chair in Psychology and the UC Presidential Chair (to Barbara Rogoff), National Science Foundation support from the Center for Informal Learning and Schools (to Barbara Rogoff, Leslie C. Moore, and Amy L. Dexter), National Institutes of Health traineeship (Grant No. T32-MH20025, to Jocelyn Solís), and a Ford Foundation Fellowship (to Maricela Correa-Chávez).

In the development of the prisms representing Learning by Observing and Pitching In and Assembly-Line Instruction, we are extremely grateful for the critique and suggestions of colleagues who attended a series of University of California Presidential Workshops on this topic, especially Rebeca Mejía-Arauz and Ruth Paradise. Although two authors of the original handbook chapter (2007), Behnosh Najafi and Jocelyn Solís, were not involved in this revision of our chapter, their earlier contributions to the original chapter are still important in the current version.

REFERENCES

Akhtar, N. (2005). The robustness of learning through overhearing. *Developmental Science, 8*, 199–209.

Akhtar, N., Jipson, J., & Callanan, M. (2001). Learning words through overhearing. *Child Development, 72*, 416–430.

Alcalá, L., Rogoff, B., Mejía-Arauz, R., Coppens, A. D., & Dexter, A. L. (2014). Children's initiative in contributions to family work in Indigenous-heritage and cosmopolitan communities in Mexico. *Human Development, 57*, 96–115.

Baquedano-López, P., Solís, J. L., & Kattan, S. (2005). Adaptation: The language of classroom learning. *Linguistics and Education, 16*, 1–26.

Barker, R. G., & Wright, H. F. (1954). *Midwest and its children.* New York: Row, Peterson.

Bartlett, F. C. (1932). *Remembering.* Cambridge, UK: Cambridge University Press.

Beach, B. A. (1988). Children at work: The home workplace. *Early Childhood Research Quarterly, 3*, 209–221.

Bourdieu, P. (1977). *Outline of a theory of practice* (R. Nice, Trans.). Cambridge, UK: Cambridge University Press.

Bransford, J., Brown, A. L., Cocking, R., & Committee on Developments in the Science of Learning. (1999). *How people learn: A report of the National Research Council of the National Academy of Science.* Washington, DC: National Academy Press.

Callahan, R. E. (1962). *Education and the cult of efficiency.* Chicago: University of Chicago Press.

Carruthers, M. (1992). *Book of memory* (2nd ed.). Cambridge, UK: Cambridge University Press.

Chavajay, P., & Rogoff, B. (2002). Schooling and traditional collaborative social organization of problem solving by Mayan mothers and children. *Developmental Psychology, 38*, 55–66.

Committee on Conceptual Framework for the New K–12 Science Education Standards, National Research Council. (2012). *Framework for K–12 science education: Practices, crosscutting concepts, and core ideas.* Washington, DC: National Academies Press.

Coppens, A. D., Alcalá, L., Mejía-Arauz, R., & Rogoff, B. (2014). Children's initiative in family household work in Mexico. *Human Development, 57*, 116–130.

Correa-Chávez, M., Roberts, A. L. D., & Martínez Pérez, M. (2011). Cultural patterns in children's learning through keen observation and participation in their communities. In J. B. Benson (Ed.), *Advances in child development and behavior* (pp. 209–241). Philadelphia: Elsevier.

Correa-Chávez, M., & Rogoff, B. (2009). Children's attention to interactions directed to others: Guatemalan Mayan and European-American patterns. *Developmental Psychology, 45*, 630–641.

Crago, M. B. (1992). Communicative interaction and second language acquisition: An Inuit example. *TESOL Quarterly, 26*, 487–505.

Cubberley, E. P. (1922). *A brief history of education*. Boston: Houghton Mifflin.

Daiute, C., Buteau, E., & Rawlins, C. (2002). Social relational wisdom: Developmental diversity in children's written narratives about social conflict. *Narrative Inquiry, 11*, 277–306.

Davies, B., & Harré, R. (1990). Positioning: The discursive production of selves. *Journal for the Theory of Social Behavior, 20*, 43–63.

de Haan, M. (2001). Intersubjectivity in models of learning and teaching. In S. Chaiklin (Ed.), *The theory and practice of cultural–historical psychology* (pp. 174–199). Aarhus, Denmark: Aarhus University Press.

Eckerman, C. O., Whatley, J. L., & McGhee, L. J. (1979) Approaching and contacting the object another manipulates. *Developmental Psychology, 15*, 585–593.

Erickson, F. (1982). Classroom discourse as improvisation. In L. C. Wilkinson (Ed.), *Communication in the classroom* (pp. 153–181). New York: Academic Press.

Erickson, F. (2004). *Talk and social theory*. Cambridge, UK: Polity Press.

Erickson, F., & Mohatt, G. (1982). Cultural organization of participation structures in two classrooms of Indian students. In G. Spindler (Ed.), *Doing the ethnography of schooling* (pp. 132–174) New York: Holt, Rinehart & Winston.

Gauvain, M. (1995). Thinking in niches. *Human Development, 38*, 25–45.

Gauvain, M. (2004). Sociocultural contexts of learning. In A. Maynard & M. Martini (Eds.), *The psychology of learning in context* (pp. 11–40). New York: Kluwer Academic/Plenum Press.

Goffman, E. (1979). Footing. *Semiotica, 25*, 1–29.

Goffman, E. (1981). *Forms of talk*. Philadelphia: University of Pennsylvania Press.

Goodnow, J. J. (1992). Parents' ideas, children's ideas. In I. E. Sigel, A. V. McGillicuddy-DeLisi, & J. J. Goodnow (Eds.), *Parental belief systems* (pp. 293–318). Hillsdale, NJ: Erlbaum.

Goodwin, M. H. (1990). *He-said-she-said: Talk as social organization among black children*. Bloomington: Indiana University Press.

Gutiérrez, K. D., Baquedano-López, P., & Tejeda, C. (1999). Rethinking diversity: Hybridity and hybrid language practices in the third space. *Mind, Culture, and Activity, 6*, 286–303.

Gutiérrez, K., & Rogoff, B. (2003). Cultural ways of learning: Individual traits or repertoires of practice. *Educational Researcher, 32*, 19–25.

Haight, W. (1991, April). *Belief systems that frame and inform parental participation in their children's pretend play*. Paper presented at the annual meeting of the Society for Research in Child Development, Seattle, WA.

Harkness, S. (1977). Aspects of social environment and first language acquisition in rural Africa. In C. Ferguson & C. Snow (Eds.), *Talking to children* (pp. 309–316). New York: Cambridge University Press.

Harkness, S., & Super, C. M. (1992). Parental ethnotheories in action. In I. E. Sigel, A. V. McGillicuddy-DeLisi, & J. J. Goodnow (Eds.), *Parental belief systems: The psychological consequences for children* (2nd ed., pp. 373–392). Hillsdale, NJ: Erlbaum.

Harkness, S., & Super, C. M. (2002). Culture and parenting. In M. H. Bornstein (Ed.), *Handbook of parenting* (Vol. 1, pp. 253–280). Mahwah, NJ: Erlbaum.

Hatano, G. (1982). Cognitive consequences of practice in culture specific procedural skills. *Quarterly Newsletter of the Laboratory of Comparative Human Cognition, 4*, 15–17.

Hay, D. F., Murray, P., Cecire, S., & Nash, A. (1985). Social learning of social behavior in early life. *Child Development, 56*, 43–57.

Heath, C. (1986). *Body movement and speech in medical interaction*. Cambridge, UK: Cambridge University Press.

Heath, S. B. (1983). *Ways with words*. Cambridge, UK: Cambridge University Press.

Hori, G. V. S. (1996). Teaching and learning in the Rinzai Zen monastery. In T. Rohlen & G. LeTendre (Eds.), *Teaching and learning in Japan* (pp. 20–49). Cambridge, UK: Cambridge University Press.

Hutchins, E., & Palen, L. (1997). Constructing meaning from space, gesture, and speech. In L. Resnick, R. Saljo, C. Pontecorvo, & B. Burge (Eds.), *Discourse, tools, and reasoning: Essays on situated cognition* (pp. 23–40). Berlin: Springer.

Jin, L. (2012). *Cultural foundations of learning.* Cambridge, UK: Cambridge University Press.

Jordan, B. (1989). Cosmopolitical obstetrics. *Social Science and Medicine, 28*, 925–944.

Kendon, A. (1990). *Conducting interaction.* Cambridge, UK: Cambridge University Press.

Kramer, K. L. (2005). *Maya children: Helpers on the farm.* Cambridge, MA: Harvard University Press.

Lancy, D. F., Gaskins, S., & Bock, J. (Eds.). (2010). *The anthropology of learning in childhood.* Lanham, MD: AltaMira Press.

Lareau, A. (2011). *Unequal childhoods* (2nd ed.). Berkeley: University of California Press.

Lave, J., & Wenger, E. (1991). *Situated learning.* Cambridge, UK: Cambridge University Press.

Lebra, T. S. (1994). Mother and child in Japanese socialization: A Japan–U.S. comparison. In P. M. Greenfield & R. R. Cocking (Eds.), *Cross-cultural roots of minority child development* (pp. 259–274). Hillsdale, NJ: Erlbaum.

LeVine, R. A. (1980). A cross-cultural perspective on parenting. In M. D. Fantini & R. Cardenas (Eds.), *Parenting in a multicultural society* (pp. 17–26). New York: Longman.

LeVine, R. A., LeVine, S., Leiderman, P. H., Brazelton, T. B., Dixon, S., Richman, A., et al. (1994). *Child care and culture.* Cambridge, UK: Cambridge University Press.

Lipka, J. (1991). Toward a culturally based pedagogy: A case study of one Yup'ik Eskimo teacher. *Anthropology and Education Quarterly, 22*, 203–223.

López, A., Najafi, B., Mejía-Arauz, R. M., & Rogoff, B. (2012). Collaboration and helping as cultural practices. In J. Valsiner (Ed.), *The Oxford handbook of culture and psychology* (pp. 869–884). New York: Oxford University Press.

Martini, M. (1995). Features of home environments associated with children's school success. *Early Child Development and Care, 111*, 49–68.

Matusov, E., & Rogoff, B. (2002). Newcomers and oldtimers. *Anthropology and Education Quarterly, 33*, 415–440.

Meek, B. A. (2013). *We are our language.* Tucson: University of Arizona Press.

Mehan, H. (1979). *Learning lessons.* Cambridge, MA: Harvard University Press.

Meltzoff, A. N., & Williamson, R. A. (2013). Imitation: Social, cognitive, and theoretical perspectives. In P. R. Zelazo (Ed.), *The Oxford handbook of developmental psychology: Vol. 1. Mind and body* (pp. 651–682). New York: Oxford University Press.

Metge, R. (1984). *Learning and teaching: He tikanga Maori.* Wellington: New Zealand Ministry of Education.

Moore, L. C. (2006a). Changes in folktale socialization in a Fulbe community. *Studies in African Linguistics, Supplement 11*, 176–187.

Moore, L. C. (2006b). Learning by heart in public and Qur'anic schools in Maroua, Cameroon. *Social Analysis: International Journal of Cultural and Social Practice, 50*, 109–126.

Moore, L. C. (2010). Learning in schools. In D. F. Lancy, J. Bock, & S. Gaskins (Eds.), *The anthropology of learning in childhood* (pp. 207–232). Lanham, MD: AltaMira Press.

Moore, L. C. (2012). Language socialization and repetition. In A. Duranti, E. Ochs, & B. Schieffelin (Eds.), *The handbook of language socialization* (pp. 209–226). Malden, MA: Blackwell.

Moore, L. C. (2013). Qur'anic school sermons as a site for sacred and second language socialisation. *Journal of Multilingual and Multicultural Development, 34*(5), 445–458.

Morelli, G., Rogoff, B., & Angelillo, C. (2003). Cultural variation in children's access to work or involvement in specialized child-focused activities. *International Journal of Behavioral Development, 27*, 264–274.

Nash, P. (1968). *Models of man: Explorations in the Western educational tradition.* New York: Wiley.

National Research Council. (2012). *A framework for K–12 science education.* Washington, DC: National Academies Press.

Nelson, K., & Gruendel, J. M. (1988). At morning it's lunchtime. In M. B. Franklin & S. S. Barten (Eds.), *Child language* (pp. 263–277). London: Oxford University Press.

Nelson-Barber, S. (1982). Phonologic variations of Pima English. In R. St. Clair & W. Leap (Eds.),

Language renewal among American Indian tribes (pp. 115–132). Rosslyn, VA: National Clearinghouse for Bilingual Education.

Nielsen, M., Moore, C., & Mohamedally, J. (2012). Young children overimitate in third-party contexts. *Journal of Experimental Child Psychology, 112*, 73–83.

Ochs, E., & Kramer-Sadlik, T. (Eds.). (2013). *Fast-forward family: Home, work, and relationships in middle-class America*. Berkeley: University of California Press.

On, L. W. (1996). The cultural context for Chinese learners. In D. Watkins & J. B. Biggs (Eds.), *The Chinese learner* (pp. 29–41). Hong Kong: Comparative Education Research Centre; Melbourne: Australian Council for Educational Research.

Orellana, M. F. (2001). The work kids do. *Harvard Educational Review, 71*, 366–389.

Orellana, M. F. (2009). *Translating childhoods*. Chicago: University of Chicago Press.

Paradise, R., & de Haan, M. (2009). Responsibility and reciprocity: Social organization of Mazahua learning practices. *Anthropology and Education Quarterly, 4*, 187–204.

Paradise, R., Mejía-Arauz, R., Silva, K., Dexter, A. L., & Rogoff, B. (2014). One, two, three, eyes on me!: Adults attempting control versus guiding in support of initiative. *Human Development, 57*, 131–149.

Paradise, R., & Rogoff, B. (2009). Side by side. *Ethos, 37*, 102–138.

Philips, S. U. (1983). *The invisible culture*. New York: Longman.

Philips, S. U. (2001). Participant structures and communicative competence. In A. Duranti (Ed.), *Linguistic anthropology: A reader* (pp. 302–318). Oxford, UK: Blackwell.

Rabain-Jamin, J. (1989). Culture and early social interactions. *European Journal of Psychology of Education, 4*, 295–305.

Reese, L., & Gallimore, R. (2000). Immigrant Latinos' cultural model of literacy development. *American Journal of Education, 108*, 103–134.

Rheingold, H. L. (1982). Little children's participation in the work of adults: A nascent prosocial behavior. *Child Development, 53*, 114–125.

Rheingold, H. L. (1985). Development as the acquisition of familiarity. *Annual Review of Psychology, 36*, 1–17.

Richman, A., Miller, P., & LeVine, R. (1992). Cultural and educational variations in maternal responsiveness. *Developmental Psychology, 28*, 614–621.

Roberts, A. L. D., & Rogoff, B. (2012). Children's reflections on two cultural ways of working together: "Talking with hands and eyes" or requiring words. *International Journal of Educational Psychology, 1*, 73–99.

Rogoff, B. (2003). *The cultural nature of human development*. New York: Oxford University Press.

Rogoff, B. (2011). *Developing destinies*. New York: Oxford University Press.

Rogoff, B. (2014). Learning by Observing and Pitching In to family and community endeavors: An orientation. *Human Development, 57*, 69–81.

Rogoff, B., & Angelillo, C. (2002). Investigating the coordinated functioning of multifaceted cultural practices in human development. *Human Development, 45*, 211–225.

Rogoff, B., Goodman Turkanis, C., & Bartlett, L. (2001). *Learning together: Children and adults in a school community*. New York: Oxford University Press.

Rogoff, B., Mistry, J., Göncü, A., & Mosier, C. (1993). Guided participation in cultural activity by toddlers and caregivers. *Monographs of the Society for Research in Child Development, 58*, 1–179.

Rogoff, B., Paradise, R., Mejía-Arauz, R., Correa-Chávez, M., & Angelillo, C. (2003). Firsthand learning through intent participation. *Annual Review of Psychology, 54*, 175–203.

Rosenthal, M., & Roer-Strier, D. (2001). Cultural differences in mothers' developmental goals and ethnotheories. *International Journal of Psychology, 36*, 20–31.

Ruvalcaba, O., Rogoff, B., López, A., Correa-Chávez, M., & Gutiérrez, K. (2014). *Children's consideration of others' activities: Respeto in requests for help in Mexican- and European-heritage children*. Manuscript submitted for publication.

Sato, N. (1996). Honoring the individual. In T. Rohlen & G. LeTendre (Eds.), *Teaching and learning in Japan* (pp. 119–153). Cambridge, UK: Cambridge University Press.

Schank, R., & Abelson, R. (1977). *Scripts, plans, goals, and understanding.* Hillsdale, NJ: Erlbaum.

Solís, J. (2003). Re-thinking illegality as a violence against, not by Mexican immigrants, children, and youth. *Journal of Social Issues, 59,* 15–31.

Solís, J., Fernández, J. S., & Alcalá, L. (2013). Mexican immigrant children's contributions to a community organization. *Sociological Studies of Children and Youth, 16,* 177–200.

Tambiah, S. J. (1968). The magical power of words. *Man, 3,* 175–208.

Tharp, R. G., & Gallimore, R. (1988). *Rousing minds to life: Teaching, learning and schooling in social context.* Cambridge, UK: Cambridge University Press.

Van Ness, H. (1981). Social control and social organization in an Alaskan Athabaskan classroom. In H. T. Trueba, G. P. Guthrie, & K. H. Au (Eds.), *Culture and the bilingual classroom* (pp. 120–138). Rowley, MA: Newbury House.

Wagner, D. A. (1983). Learning to read by "rote." *International Journal of the Sociology of Language, 42,* 111–121.

Ward, M. C. (1971). *Them children.* New York: Holt, Rinehart & Winston.

Weisner, T. S. (1984). A cross-cultural perspective. In A. Collins (Ed.), *The elementary school years* (pp. 335–369). Washington, DC: National Academy Press.

Weisner, T. S., Gallimore, R., & Jordan, C. (1988). Unpackaging cultural effects on classroom learning. *Anthropology and Education Quarterly, 19,* 327–352.

Whiting, B. B. (1980). Culture and social behavior. *Ethos, 8,* 95–116.

Whiting, B. B., & Whiting, J. W. M. (1975). *Children of six cultures.* Cambridge, MA: Harvard University Press.

Wise Bauer, S., & Wise, J. (2009). *The well-trained mind* (3rd ed.). New York: Norton.

Zentella, A. C. (1998). Multiple codes, multiple ethnicities. In S. M. Hoyle & C. T. Adger (Eds.), *Kids talk* (pp. 95–107). Oxford, UK: Oxford Studies in Sociolinguistics.

CHAPTER 21

Emotion Socialization from a Cultural Perspective

Pamela M. Cole
Patricia Z. Tan

The capacity for emotion is biologically prepared, affording very rapid processing of and responding to environmental changes in the interest of an individual's survival. Although emotions were often conceived of as occasional feelings or behavioral expressions, contemporary models of emotion have moved toward understanding that this capacity operates continuously and largely out of conscious awareness. In addition to this basic, highly automatic processing and readiness to act to preserve or regain well-being, humans also have the capacity to anticipate, reflect on, and regulate emotion. This allows for behavioral flexibility—we are able not only to act immediately to protect well-being but also to modulate responses so that they conform to social standards for behavior. Thus, a universal capacity—emotion—comes under social influence, through the process of socialization. Social standards, however, appear to vary from locale to locale in terms of shared practices that are transmitted from generation to generation (i.e., culture). Our chapter addresses how culture contributes to the differential socialization of the universal capacity for emotion.

Developmental science is dominated by evidence based on relatively advantaged children and families in Western industrialized nations, mainly of Northern European heritage, who represent a fraction of the world's population. An increasing call for a broader knowledge base reflects an appreciation that seems related to historical changes. In 1969, for example, astronauts gave us a view of the planet from the moon, catalyzing awareness of the world as a community. In addition, worldwide immigration trends, economic globalization, and information technology have furthered our exposure to and discourse with other cultures and have revealed the power of macro-level shifts in cultural values. These changes have penetrated the field of developmental science, as evidenced by research that involves international collaborations and employs more sophisticated conceptualizations of culture and research designs that go beyond indexing culture solely on the basis of nationality. In the process, we are ever more aware of the complexity of studying culture and human development. Demographic trends reveal marked increases in the number of children in communities that have been underrepresented in developmental science, making a cultural framework all the more essential. In this chapter, we first discuss how we conceptualize emotion, culture, and socialization. We next summarize research on culture and infant temperament, infant attachment, and parental socialization of children's emotions. We conclude with suggestions for future research directions.

Emotional, Cultural, and Socialization Processes

Emotion, Culture, and Socialization

All human beings are equipped with a capacity to be emotional, but it is also clear that culture influences emotion processes. There is intense debate, however, about whether cultural research can employ a universal construct of "emotion" or set of basic emotion categories. Historically, studies debating the universality of emotion focused on adults in different nations rather than on developmental processes that might illustrate *how* a universal capacity comes to be influenced by culture. In addition, cross-cultural studies tended to compare nations (e.g., the United States and China), settings that vary in so many ways that one cannot determine *why* participants differ. A developmental, ecological approach to examining how and why culture influences emotional processes could offer a more promising solution.

We assume that the capacity for emotions is universal and critical to infant survival. Infants signal information about their states via emotional expressions, and these elicit care that helps infants regain or maintain well-being. These expressions seem to reflect universal prototypes (Ekman, 1992; Elfenbein & Ambady, 2002). The emotion-eliciting circumstances of infancy and early childhood also share commonalities across societies (e.g., being physically uncomfortable, seeing an unfamiliar face, or having something desirable taken away), suggesting some ecological commonalities. Furthermore, caregivers worldwide share the goals of raising healthy children to become competent adults (LeVine et al., 1994; Whiting & Edwards, 1988). Among these commonalities, culture plays a role. It influences how infant caregivers and others conceive of internal states and expressions, what they define as personal and group well-being, how they appraise situations, how they communicate emotionally to members of their own and other groups, and how they believe one should act in the interest of personal or group well-being (Markus & Kitayama, 1991; Mesquita & Frijda, 1992).

As parents share the goal of raising competent children, and today we must consider competence within one's heritage and in a global society, it is unclear how salient emotional competence is to parents. Emotional competence is viewed as an integral feature of child competence (Halberstadt, Denham, & Dunsmore, 2001; Saarni, 1999), but it may not be foremost in maternal conceptions of child competence. German, Indian, Nepalese, South Korean, and U.S. mothers' open-ended descriptions of first-graders' competence do not mention emotional competence frequently. They focus on social and cognitive competencies such as getting along with others, being obedient, and doing well in school, although they vary in the behaviors they use to describe these skills (Wood et al., 2014). Yet when probed about how competent children *misbehave*, they refer to poorly regulated emotion. Emotion socialization may be embedded in practices aimed at guiding children toward culturally defined competencies (Keller, 2007; LeVine & Norman, 2001). In summary, community standards and the means by which they are achieved vary culturally, implicitly involving the enculturation of emotions (Berry, Poortinga, Segall, & Dasen, 2002), as early as infancy.

The Nature of Culture

Socialization occurs in cultural context (Bornstein, 2002; Bronfenbrenner, 1977; Keller, 2003; Super & Harkness, 1986), but what is culture? Definitions vary widely, but a common element is shared practices transmitted from generation to generation. Food preparation and eating customs, styles of music and dress, and the rearing of children are examples of domains in which shared practices are passed across generations. To the new arrival in a community, such as an infant or an immigrant, these practices are the leading edge of cultural socialization (Rogoff, 2003; Weisner, 2002). Shared practices are often linked to beliefs about acceptable conduct and to caregivers' goals for socializing acceptable conduct, and their intuitive theories about how to achieve such socialization (Harkness & Super, 1996).

These shared practices are best understood locally, situated in a particular ecology, with particular resources and pressures, and at a particular time in a community's history (LeVine, 1969; Super & Harkness, 1986). Thus, understanding cultural influences requires appreciation of the conditions in which shared practices and associated beliefs evolved and are evolving. For this reason, comparative studies that index culture by nation of origin, race, or ethnicity are imprecise, overlooking many dynamic social factors that may be the potent factors in cultural variations (García Coll et al., 1996; Gjerde, 2004; McLoyd, 2004). Studies of urban families in China and Turkey demonstrate the dynamic nature of culture as they transition from traditional to modern circumstances. Societal changes offer opportunity to interact and compete in the global community, both of which alter parental socialization practices and goals, and their relations to child outcomes (Kağıtçıbaşı & Ataca, 2005).

Another important issue in the study of cultural influences is within-culture variation. Although shared values guide common practices, individuals within any group embrace these to varying degrees, perhaps even more so in periods of rapid change. Indeed, the rapid pace of technology and globalization throughout the world is affecting how culture can be defined and measured (Bohr, 2010). Exposure to different cultures has created a "context of diverse values" for emotional development (Chen, 2012, p. 321). As families grapple with clashes between different cultural values (e.g., personal ambition and filial piety), socialization traditions are confronted with new problems, and caregivers vary in how they resolve potential culture clashes they encounter in raising their children.

Given these complexities, how should we classify cultural differences? Nations have been viewed as being oriented toward the good of the collective or of the individual (Hofstede, 1984; Triandis, 1989) and selves as being oriented toward their interdependence or independence (Markus & Kitayama, 1991). These models generated considerable research that has led to more nuanced views of cultural variations that assert that individuals balance their needs to belong and to individuate (Rothbaum, Pott, Azuma, Miyake & Weisz, 2000) or to achieve agency and social distance (Kağıtçıbaşi, 1996). A more recent trend is to appreciate cultures in terms of types and rates of social change

(Greenfield, 2009; Kağitçibaşi, 2007; Keller & Lamm, 2005; Rogoff, 2003). All of these invoke the distinction between self and others, a distinction that is at the nexus of socialization. The socialization of the individual child into a community of others at particular periods in the community's evolution, which influences the degree to which practices are stable or fluid and the degree to which they are shared.

A Framework for Conceptualizing Emotion Socialization from a Cultural Perspective

Contemporary views on the socialization of emotion (Denham, Bassett, & Wyatt, Chapter 25, this volume; N. Eisenberg, Cumberland, & Spinrad, 1998) focus on social processes that occur in parent–child interactions. These interactions can be understood within the broader dynamic ecological and social pressures that influence human development (Bronfenbrenner, 1977; Greenfield, 2009; LeVine et al., 1994; Super & Harkness, 1986). In our discussion we try to maintain recognition of this dynamic, ecological perspective, appreciating that macro-level processes and changes intersect with more proximal experiences of parent–child interactions as a child becomes a competent member of the family, the community, and the society. An infant is born into a family in a community with standards for social interaction that influence and are influenced by the standards of a larger community. An infant born in the United States, for example, is affected by the political history of the nation. At its inception, the United States was founded on a standard that personal liberty is as important as life. Individuals banded together against a common enemy, Britain. Laws codified social practices that guaranteed individual rights; these laws were created, protected, and sometimes changed by collections of individual votes, not bestowed by a monarch. Thus, a community of individuals worked together to generate community solutions to changing resources and challenges, nonetheless keeping the individual's rights to life, liberty, and pursuit of happiness at center stage. These historical events represent powerful influences on how parents interacted with their children, as they established a context for a strong sense of individuality in the American definition of *competence*.

Although the United States is often characterized as highly individualistic, functional and evolutionary perspectives maintain that, across cultures, emotions reflect the *individual's* goals to maintain well-being. Culture influences the definition of well-being, which is often regarded as the degree to which personal well-being is more or less relative to the group's well-being. But in any group, to create and maintain social order, individual goals must be coordinated with community goals. The community—family members, schools, peers, media, and the societal structure of intergroup relations—all influence the socialization of emotion. Research on emotion socialization has tended to focus on parental practices with young children who are establishing a sense of self and developing the ability to assert the self, all of which provide foundations for the socialization of emotion. Parents communicate standards as young children try to achieve their individual goals. When children encounter obstacles or unachievable goals, parents may socialize their emotions directly (e.g., "Big boys don't cry," "I know you are mad but it's not nice to hit your sister"). However, it is generally agreed that children's emotions are more often influenced by subtle, indirect means. These include observations of others' emotional exchanges, others' reactions to a child's emotions, and opportunities to experience varied emotions (Denham, 1998; N. Eisenberg et al., 1998). In this way, cultural factors influence how individuals achieve personal goals for well-being within the community's standards via socialization. As noted, these processes begin early in a child's life. How often an infant is held, how quickly a fussy infant is soothed, and who soothes an infant all contribute to emotion socialization. Infants from the African Afa foraging community appear to be more trusting of their environment than infants in African farming or American industrial communities, perhaps as a result of being breast-fed by women other than their mothers, being held almost all the time, and being soothed immediately if they fuss (Hewlett, Lamb, Leyendecker, & Schöelmerich, 2000).

The cultural socialization of emotion is not a passive process. Each child contributes to it actively. Individual differences in infant fussiness, for example, may be interpreted and handled differently by different groups at particular points in their community's history. Parental beliefs about what a child of a given age can be expected to do also vary (Harkness & Super, 1996). Thus, a cultural model of the socialization of emotion must consider child influences. If there are genetic differences in cultural groups, these could lead to group differences in infant emotion that then may contribute to and explain differences in parenting practices. We begin then with a review of work on culture and infant temperament, followed by work on culture and attachment. We then turn to parenting practices that implicitly or explicitly socialize emotion.

Our summaries are limited in several important ways. First, they are based on scholarly publications in English, without the benefit of scholarly work in other languages. Second, we focus on comparative studies of two or more groups, which are needed to build evidence for the cultural socialization of emotion. We largely omit many interesting studies that focus on single cultures despite their essential importance for understanding the cultural socialization of emotion. Last, we focus on parents and children, mostly young children. Other agents of socialization—peers, siblings, other adults (e.g., teachers), the media, and the larger structure of society—are not well represented in the emotion socialization literature.

Emotional Processes in Socialization

Temperament: Individual Differences in Infant Emotionality

Differences in infant emotional reactivity and regulation are conceptualized as temperament (i.e., biological predispositions to react in particular ways; Goldsmith et al., 1987). Temperament is influenced by both genetic and pre- and postnatal environmental factors, reflecting not only stable inborn qualities but also the emergence of dispositional factors with maturation and experience (Rothbart & Bates, 1998). Temperament influences parental emotion socialization in that parents are presented with unique challenges and opportunities by each child. Those child characteristics influence the emotions caregivers express in the presence of and to the child, the practices in which caregivers engage, and the opportunities for emotional experience they provide for the child (N. Eisenberg et al., 1998).

Evidence for cross-national differences is mixed but, generally, Western European or American infants are described as approach-oriented, emotionally expressive, and easy to soothe in contrast to infants of Asian heritage, who are described as easily distressed (Gartstein et al., 2006; Russell, Hart, Robinson, & Olsen, 2003). Observations of infant behavior are also mixed, but these portray a different pattern of cross-national findings. East Asian youngsters appear to be less irritable, better at self-quieting, and easier to soothe (e.g., Caudill & Weinstein, 1969; Kagan et al., 1994; Lewis, Ramsay, & Kawakami, 1993). Interestingly, Palestinian parents describe their infants as more temperamentally negative than do Israeli parents, but observers do not detect these differences (Feldman & Masalha, 2007); as with other studies, the group that is arguably more interdependent in its orientation, the Palestinians, emphasized child compliance, quietness, and respectfulness as socialization goals, whereas Israelis focused more on child self-expression and assertiveness. Possibly, different socialization goals lead to different interpretations of infant negative affect. Finally, it is critical that we remember that there appear to be differences in temperament *among* infants from cultures that emphasize the interdependence of selves, for example, Chinese infants were less reactive to restraint and novelty than Japanese infants (Camras et al., 2002).

An elegant study of early childhood emotional expressiveness compared four groups of 3-year-old girls: Chinese girls in Mainland China, Chinese girls raised in the United States by Chinese parents, Chinese adopted girls raised in the United States by European American parents, and European American girls (Camras, Chen, Bakeman, Norris, & Cain, 2006). The study also assessed parental socialization and acculturation goals. The findings generally indicated that the less frequent, less intense displays of positive and negative emotion among children of Chinese heritage were probably due to socialization factors. Another study that assessed physiological responses indicated that less expressivity may not reflect less reactivity. Japanese infants exhibited fewer behavioral indications of stress in response to inoculation but higher cortisol responses than infants in the United States (Lewis et al., 1993). Conclusions about cultural differences in temperament will depend on continuing research that moves beyond the apparent limits of parental reports. Nonetheless, the inconsistencies between parental report and observations of Chinese infants raise additional culturally influenced questions. Possibly, Chinese parents who have a well-developed sense of interdependence, which is associated with keen sensitivity to other' needs and less expressivity, may anticipate or be sensitive to infant distress, detecting cues that research assistants do not. Parental cultural standards may also influence how critically or positively a child is described. For example, Latina mothers are said to demonstrate a positive bias, and Asian parents a negative bias, when describing their children (Marín, Gamba, & Marín, 1992; Rao, McHale, & Pearson, 2003).

The study of cultural influences on infant temperament must also not overlook the fact that prenatal environments vary in ways that may influence infant temperament. Iron deficiency, which is common in developing countries and among poorer families in industrialized countries, is associated with greater infant wariness and diminished positive emotion (Lozoff et al., 2003). Maternal stress may also affect temperament (Davis et al., 2007). In summary, the case for inborn cultural differences in infant temperament is inconclusive. If future research identifies such differences, it will be crucial to examine how they influence parent–infant interactions, including those that lead to an infant's emotional security.

Attachment: Emotional Security within Relationships with Caregivers

Theoretically, attachment is a universal feature of infant development (Bowlby, 1969). Infants form selective emotional bonds with their primary caregivers that allow them to achieve a sense of emotional security and explore their surroundings with the confidence that they can return to their "secure base." A secure attachment is regarded as a critical forerunner of emotional competence. To venture into the world while maintaining a sense of security requires a balance of independence and dependence. Cultures vary in terms of their caregiving environments in ways that may bear on the development of emotional security, such as the number of primary caregivers, nature of caregiving practices, amount of experience infants have being separated from primary caregivers, and physical risks in the infant's environment.

Most studies of infant attachment have relied on the Strange Situation, a procedure inspired by Mary Ainsworth's observations of striking similarities in mothers and infants in the United States and Uganda (Ainsworth, 1967; Ainsworth & Bell, 1970). In both settings, infants seemed distressed when left by their mothers, the distress seemed to be related to how warm and responsive the mothers were, and the ability of mother–infant dyads to regain infant security seemed related to later child adjustment. Work based on this paradigm suggests the universality of infant attachment classifications (van IJzendoorn & Sagi, 1999) and of relations between maternal sensitivity and infant security (De Wolff & van IJzendoorn, 1997). All infants may form attachments, but there appear to be cultural variations in how infant security and maternal sensitivity are defined (Grossmann, Grossmann, Spangler, Suess, & Unzner, 1985; Jin, Jacobvitz, Hazen, & Jung, 2012; Rothbaum, Weisz, Pott, Miyake, & Morelli, 2000).

Consider laboratory observations of children reunited with their mothers after separation. In terms of security, Japanese preschool-age children whined and clambered onto their mothers upon reunion, whereas U.S. children continued to play (Mizuta, Zahn-Waxler, Cole, & Hiruma, 1996). Japanese mothers felt their children had achieved security because they had acquired a sense of *amae*, or enduring emotional dependence, which was achieved by always yielding to a child's needs and never creating conflict (Rothbaum, Morelli, Pott, & Liu-Constant, 2000). U.S. mothers regarded such whining and clambering as insecure and emotionally immature (Mizuta et al., 1996). Like German mothers, U.S. mothers are responsive but try to do so in ways that foster self-sufficiency and self-discipline in their young children (Ahnert, Lamb, & Seltenheim, 2000; Grossmann, Grossmann, Huber, & Wartner, 1981; Keller, 2007).

In terms of sensitivity, German and American mothers engage in synchronized face-to-face emotional exchanges with their infants, but in other settings, mothers feel it is sensitive to keep an infant close (e.g., carried on one's back), touching the child frequently to foster well-being, and regard face-to-face interaction as unnecessary (Keller, Yovsi, et al., 2004). These variations are likely embedded in the ecology of daily routines (e.g., agrarian or farming) and in culturally distinct beliefs about infant needs and socialization goals. Finally, relations between sensitivity and attachment may vary in terms of those practices and beliefs. Middle-class Puerto Rican mothers, for example, strive to promote proper demeanor, as well as emotional security in their infants (Carlson & Harwood, 2003). They use more physical control of their infants' activity and movement than do Anglo American mothers. While early physical control may seem intrusive through one cultural lens, this maternal style predicted attachment security in Puerto Rican but not Anglo American children.

In summary, attachment is likely a universal phenomenon that fosters a young child's sense of emotional security, but the specific practices that foster a child's emotional security may vary. We next address parental socialization of children's emotions, focusing on two variables: parental emotion expressions that model and provide feedback about emotions, and parental communication about emotion, such as labeling emotion and teaching children about emotions.

Parental Socialization of Children's Emotions

In the course of socialization, parents may proactively teach children about socially acceptable behavior and respond to children's behavior. They may directly teach children about emotion (e.g., coaching), but often children's emotions are implicitly socialized as parents model behavior and react to children's behavior. Parental emotion expressions model emotional behavior, expose children to a range of different emotions and, as responses to children, provide feedback (e.g., approval or disapproval) about child emotions and behavior (Denham, 1998; N. Eisenberg et al., 1998). Parental joy, disappointment, and irritation also reflect parents' investment in their children (Dix, 1991). In addition, parental emotion expressions elicit emotional reactions in children. The emotional exchanges that accompany interaction are powerful aspects of parent–child relationships and are vehicles for communicating cultural messages that influence children's emotion understanding, emotion regulation, and emotional well-being. Cultural influences on parental emotion expression have been studied as both direct processes (e.g., observations of contingent emotional responses) and as more implicit processes (e.g., inclusion of affect in ratings of hostility).

Parental Expression of Positive Emotion

Maternal expressions of positive emotion with infants are, in some respects, universal (e.g., Bornstein, Tamís-LeMonda, et al., 1992; Carlson & Harwood, 2003; Fogel, Toda, & Kawai, 1988; Keller, Lohaus, et al., 2004). Mothers exaggerate the lilt in their voice and smile as they cuddle, soothe, and care for their infants. Parents around the world also value parental warmth and feel positively when children behave according to cultural values (Honig & Chung, 1989; Wu et al., 2002). Indeed, infants seem to expect positive expressions from their parents. Infants from both China and Canada appeared distressed by the still-face paradigm in which their mothers briefly stopped their positive emotional expressions (Kisilevsky et al., 1998).

Culture, nonetheless, may influence the *relative* emphasis caregivers place on expressing warmth and positive emotion. White mothers of European heritage from Western industrialized nations express, and value expressing, positive emotions to their children more than do mothers of African, Asian, and South and Central American heritages (e.g., Bornstein et al., 1996; Deater-Deckard, Atzaba-Poria, & Pike, 2004; Ispa et al., 2004; Keller, Voelker, & Yovsi, 2005; Wu et al., 2002; Zahn-Waxler, Friedman, Cole, Mizuta, & Hiruma, 1996). The latter groups, thought to emphasize the interdependent nature of selves, may achieve closeness without the expressiveness of groups who emphasize the independence of selves and rely on overt expression of emotion to achieve closeness (Markus & Kitayama, 1991). However, this heuristic dichotomy cannot explain all cultural variations, suggesting a need for more nuanced views. Puerto Rican mothers praise and are affectionate with their toddlers, as much as Anglo parents, except when teaching (Harwood, Schöelmerich, Schulze, & Gonzalez, 1999). Greek mothers, who are regarded as more interdependent than German mothers, smile at their infants more than German mothers do (Keller et al., 2003). Japanese mothers, who value interdependence, express less positive emotion than more independence-oriented U.S. mothers (Dennis, Cole, Zahn-Waxler, & Mizuta, 2002) but more than independence-oriented Dutch mothers (Zevalkink & Riksen-Walraven, 2001). Moreover, parents of a given ethnic group may appear less warm and positive toward their children *until* contextual factors are considered; African American mothers appeared less positive than European American mothers until neighborhood quality was taken into account (Pinderhughes, Nix, Foster, & Jones, 2001; Zevalkink & Riksen-Walraven, 2001). These interesting findings illustrate the importance of considering (1) differences among interdependent groups, (2) situational context (e.g., teaching vs. play) and child age, and (3) the conditions, values, and goals that underlie parenting practices.

Parental Expression of Negative Emotion

Parental expression of negative emotion is a risk factor for children's development (Dix, Gershoff, Meunier, & Miller, 2004; Ispa et al., 2004), but this may be qualified by cross-cultural evidence. Parents from different cultural backgrounds feel negatively if their children engage in inappropriate behavior as defined by cultural norms (e.g., Honig & Chung, 1989). They differ, however, in their inclinations to *express* such feelings. Asian parents use love withdrawal, open criticism, and shaming in response to children's inappropriate behavior more than do North American parents, and Asian parents are less concerned about negotiating with children and protecting self-esteem than North American parents from relatively advantaged circumstances (e.g., Bowes, Chen, San, & Yuan, 2004; Fung, 1999; C. Y. C. Lin & Fu, 1990; Wu et al., 2002).

Interesting cultural perspectives are revealed by research that delves more deeply into the meaning and impact of parental negative emotion expression. First, parental negative emotion can be considered in relation to positive emotions parents convey. Chinese, Japanese, and Hispanic parents, all of whom endorse practices that include communicating negative emotion (e.g., harshness, shaming), also value accepting and protecting children (Chen et al., 1998; Power, Kobayashi-Winata, & Kelley, 1992; Varela et al., 2004). Perhaps parental negative emotion in the *absence* of parental warmth and positive emotion is problematic in any culture (Chen, Wu, Chen, Wang, & Cen, 2001; Deater-Deckard & Dodge, 1997). Second, in some cultures, parental negative emotion is typical and perceived by both parents and children as legitimate parental assertion of authority (Gershoff et al., 2010). Such perceptions may have different consequences than parental negative emotion that is viewed as harmful, abusive, or harsh (Lansford et al., 2010). Confucian values, for example, morally obligate Chinese parents to train their children; open disapproval promotes a child's sense of shame in violating social standards, which then fosters greater filial piety and empathy for others—important aspects of socioemotional competence (Chao, 1994). Economically strained North American mothers, both European American and African American (e.g., Martini, Root, & Jenkins, 2004; Miller & Sperry, 1987), also engage in expressions of open disapproval and anger, but for different reasons than Chinese parents. U.S. urban, working-class mothers intend to "toughen" their children (Miller & Sperry, 1987) and some lower-income, minority-group parents use sternness to enforce compliance, a quality that they expect their children will need as they interact with members of the majority culture (Kelley, Power, & Wimbush, 1992). Third, in addition to the part played by socioeconomic and majority–minority status roles that may legitimize parental negative emotion expressions, we should also consider the physical ecology of socialization. One study indicated that neighborhood quality influenced the degree to which parents believed in yelling at or threatening children as a discipline strategy, particularly among African American and U.S.-born Latino families (Caughy & Franzini, 2005). Conditions of economic stress in neighborhoods, which are associated with weaker community and family ties, as well as a history of discrimination, are all potential factors that may influence the affective nature of parenting and parental self-efficacy. At least two studies have linked concerns about neighborhood safety to harsher parental control, although not necessarily parental affection (Hill & Herman-Stahl, 2002; Pinderhughes et al., 2001). These issues remain to be understood but clearly suggest that parenting is best investigated in its cultural and ecological contexts. Last, all negative emotion expressions are not alike. Parental stress or psychopathology can interfere with a parent's culturally appropriate expression of negative emotion, and this may predict child maladjustment even in cultures that value authoritarian parenting (Bradford et al., 2004; Chang, Lansford, Schwartz, & Farver, 2004; Chen et al., 2001; Phinney, Kim-Jo, Osorio, & Vilhjalmsdottir, 2005; Tao, Zhou, & Wang, 2010; Walker-Barnes & Mason, 2001).

In summary, culture influences the relative balance between negative and positive emotion expression in parents as they interact with their children, and the meanings attributed to those expressions. Parental emotion expression is clearly a mechanism by which children's emotions are enculturated. There is convincing evidence that future research on parental emotion expressions should include assessment of parental socialization goals, cultural values, and the social and physical ecology in which parents are raising children.

Parental Encouragement of Children's Emotions

Historically, the research literature has indicated that children's sense of self-efficacy and self-esteem is enhanced when parents value children's emotions and encourage emotion expression (e.g., Block, 1981; Gottman, Katz, & Hooven, 1997) but this may not be universal. East Asian parents, for example, prefer emotional restraint and calmness to happiness or expressiveness in children (Chen et al., 1998; C. Y. C. Lin & Fu, 1990; Tsai, Knutson, & Fung, 2006). Moreover, parents achieve these various goals for their children's emotional development in different ways. Japanese mothers strive to anticipate and prevent children from experiencing negative emotions, whereas European American mothers give children opportunity to experience and self-regulate negative emotions, and want children to try to cope before they help them (Rothbaum, Pott, et al., 2000). Japanese parents believe they should not disapprove of or set limits on young children's emotion expression because limit setting weakens parent–child *amae*, the emotional dependency that promotes later emotional restraint, empathy, and sense of filial duty (Hayashi, Karasawa, & Tobin, 2009; cf. Q. Wang, 2001). The cultural significance of indulging a child's negative emotion is evident in the contrast between Japanese caregivers' pride and Chinese and American caregivers' criticism when they see a Japanese teacher fail to set limits on poorly regulated emotion and behavior (Tobin, Wu, & Davidson, 1989). Differences in Chinese and American children's emotional responses to success and failure appear to be mediated by their parents' emotional responses to that success or failure; U.S. parents felt more positively about child success and deemphasized child failures more than Chinese parents, who were more concerned about child failure and deemphasized success.

These differences accounted for why Chinese children felt more negatively about their failures and American children felt more positively about their successes (Ng, Pomerantz, & Lam, 2007). Finally, Cameroonian Nso mothers also aim to prevent crying, but rather than anticipate or indulge children, they express disapproval to a crying youngster, with the goal that the child achieve emotional control by 3 years of age; these values and practices differ from those of German mothers, who want their children to feel free to express themselves (Keller & Otto, 2009).

In summary, all caregivers want their children to achieve emotional well-being, as well as emotional control. They vary in terms of their beliefs about what constitutes optimal well-being and emotional control. Parents' encouragement and discouragement of child emotion expression vary across cultures and appear to be a function of differing socialization goals and beliefs about how these are achieved. The method of having caregivers from different cultural heritages observing each other's behavior is particularly effective in illuminating cultural values that explain parental practices (Keller et al., 2005; Tobin et al., 1989). Observational studies are also valuable because parental self-report may fail to reflect actual practices (Bornstein, Cote, & Venuti, 2001; Hsu, Tseng, Ashton, McDermott, & Char, 1985).

Parental Conversations about Children's Emotions

Discourse is replete with cultural messages about emotion and is therefore a mechanism of emotion socialization (Dunn, 1988; Miller, Fung, & Mintz, 1996). Caregivers converse about hypothetical emotional events and actual emotional incidents with and in the presence of children, sometimes explicitly referring to emotion and often implicitly conveying the emotional significance of experiences and behavior (without using emotion terms). The ways culture influences communication begin in infancy and continue throughout childhood. For example, even before children speak, caregivers communicate in ways that focus on or away from emotional aspects of experience. Japanese mothers more often engage in "affect-salient" speech than do European American mothers (Bornstein, Tal, et al., 1992; Toda, Fogel, & Kawai, 1990). That is, they coo and use terms of endearment when interacting with their infants, in contrast to European American mothers, who direct the infant's attention elsewhere by describing objects and informing the infant about them. Japanese mothers' use of affect-salient speech may reflect the importance they place on an infant feeling content and dependent on them, whereas European American mothers' primary use of informational speech may reflect the cultural value placed on acquiring knowledge and control.

Once children acquire expressive language, parent and child can converse about emotions, an aspect of interaction that has been studied in cultures ranging from Great Britain, the United States, China, and Taiwan to communities in Micronesia and the Andes (e.g., Cervántes, 2002; Lutz, 1987; Melzi & Fernández, 2004). Culture influences how often, in what ways, and why emotional experiences are discussed with and in front of children. Chinese parents, for example, talk less about a child's emotions and more about others' emotions (Q. Wang, 2001). This may minimize emphasis on the child's emotionality and promote concern for and sensitivity toward others. This is consistent with an attitude that children should be emotionally reserved, and that children's emotions are disruptive (Q. Wang, 2001). In South Asia, Hindu parents appear to believe it is important to foster child understanding of emotions and the situations in which they occur, explaining, for example, why anger is problematic (Cole, Bruschi, & Tamang, 2002; Raval & Martini, 2011), although Buddhist parents, who agree that anger is not useful, shame and ignore child anger, more in the manner depicted by East Asian parents (Cole et al., 2002). In the United States, working-class parents responded to their toddlers' references to negative events (e.g., dangers) with reference to negative emotion, whereas middle-class parents responded by focusing on positive emotion, perhaps trying to reassure rather than prepare their children for negative events (Burger & Miller, 1999). Knowing why parents from similar backgrounds differ and focusing on the ecology of and goals for parent–child conversations will add substantively to knowledge about cultural socialization of emotion.

In addition to explaining and teaching about emotions, parents can label emotions. Comparative research on emotion talk attempts to disentangle educational and economic advantage from cultural heritage. In fact, economic status, more than culture, influences the frequency and complexity of conversations about emotional experiences among Latino and Anglo parents in the United States (A. R. Eisenberg, 1999; Flannagan & Perese, 1996; Hoff-Ginsberg, 1991). Culture, nonetheless, influences parents' discourse about emotions (Cervántes, 2002; Fung, 1999; Q. Wang, 2001). For example, Latina mothers use emotion terms more when discussing children's social experiences, and Anglo mothers use emotion terms when discussing children's learning experiences (Flannagan & Perese, 1996).

Personal storytelling is a form of discourse that involves the telling and retelling of events (Miller, Fung, Lin, Chen, & Boldt, 2012). It conveys cultural values by defining which events are worth retelling. Culture influences the frequency, form, and function of storytelling as a tool for socializing children's emotions. In Chinese society, personal storytelling is used to reinforce moral values (e.g., teaching what is wrong about selfish anger), whereas in European American homes, it occurs less frequently and is used mainly as a source of mutual enjoyment, reinforcing relationships and downplaying negative events (e.g., Miller, Wiley, Fung, & Liang, 1997). European American mothers, however, report using children's storybooks and videos to help children manage their emotions, and young children have a high interest in such stories (Alexander, Miller, & Hengst, 2001; Miller, Hoogstra, Mintz, Fung, & Williams, 1993).

Conclusions

Our review of the literature indicates that there are universal and culturally variable influences on the socialization of emotion. At one level of analysis, parents around the world strive to give their children a sense of emotional security and emotional well-being and the ability to behave emotionally in accord with cultural values. Moreover, parents feel positive emotions when their children behave according to their values and negative emotions when children fail to conform to culturally appropriate behavior. The variability is largely in terms of what child behaviors comprise child emotional well-being and control, and what caregiving behaviors foster those child outcomes. Less is known about the ecology of cultural similarities and differences. That is, there is a growing trend for studies to link differences in practices to differences in socialization goals. What is not well understood is what factors in a cultural setting, usually defined as a nation, drive differences in socialization goals. In addition, there is an ever-growing permeability in the boundaries of culture—technology, immigration, and globalization must all be considered. Child emotional competence can no longer be defined solely in terms of circumscribed geographic areas; we must now also consider what it means to be competent in a global society.

Universal and Culturally Specific Aspects of the Socialization of Emotion

One way to view the evidence is to return to the framework that emotional processes are biologically prepared capacities that motivate goal-directed behavior. Cultures are socially constructed, shared adaptations to the pressures and resources of the setting in which a community is formed, and those adaptations influence goals and how they are met. Culture influences emotional processes in the course of socializing children to become emotionally competent members of their community who can achieve goals. It is reasonable to conclude that there are some universal features to the socialization of emotion. All parents care about children's emotional well-being and self-regulation, and share the goal of raising children who will be secure as young children and emotionally competent as adults. Caregivers are tender and emotionally positive with their infants, soothing, coddling, and nurturing them, and promoting their physical and emotional well-being. Infants, as a result, form attachments to primary caregivers. Caregivers also care that children behave in socially appropriate ways and feel negatively when they do not.

There are also cultural variations in how these goals are achieved, and these are evident even within the first year of life. Even before attachment security is established, there are cultural differences in how caregiver warmth, nurturance, and positive emotion are expressed. These early practices model emotional behavior, convey messages about emotional dependence and self-reliance, and indicate which emotional states are desirable and which are not. Future research will benefit from continued focus on the pathways between cultural values and socialization goals, caregiver sensitivity or emotional expressivity, and children's later emotional competence. Moreover, future studies must appreciate that practical demands on the family and the social structure of the community, as well as cultural beliefs, influence how caregivers administer to infant distress and define infant well-being. Finally, the matter of whether cultural differences in infant temperament drive cultural differences in emotion socialization remains to be determined.

Beyond infancy, positive and negative emotion is expressed by caregivers and encouraged in children in culturally different ways. There is a reasonable amount of evidence that the goals of emotional self-reliance, emotional self-assertion, interpersonal sensitivity, cooperativeness, and respectfulness influence parents' emotional expressions with their children. Moreover, the degree to which a parent expresses negative and positive emotions may reflect cultural values, but to what degree does it really reflect the physical and social realities of the setting in which children are being raised? Concerns such as neighborhood safety, racist and discriminatory practices, majority–minority status in terms of both numbers and power, the relative diversity or homogeneity of the cultural composition of a community, and the nature of intergroup relations between different cultural groups all have a bearing on the emotional lives of parents and how they socialize their children.

Finally, little is known about cultural effects associated with children's observations of others' emotions, children's opportunities to experience a range of emotions, children's perceptions of and reactions to others' emotions, and the influences of other socializing persons such as siblings and peers (but see Chen, French, & Schneider, 2006). Schools and various media formats also differ across cultures, yet these are rarely studied in the context of emotion socialization. Our reading of the comparative literature leaves us with a remarkable sense of not only how much humans have in common but also the many subtle influences culture has on universal processes. It seems very important that future research move beyond cataloguing cultural group differences and similarities, and attempt to explain *how* and *why* culture has its influences.

Conceptualizing and Assessing Culture

To advance knowledge about the cultural socialization of emotion, we need to not only define but also assess culture. We must evaluate what culture is for each individual, in each given group, considering both the immediate and historical realities that community members share. Culturally sensitive questionnaires, interviews, and focus groups have all been used effectively to understand the context and meaning of parental and child behavior, and to determine the degree to which each member of a group ascribes to the purported cultural values and practices. As part of understanding culture within a place in time, it is essential to avoid two common limitations of the comparative literature: (1) confounding cultural group assignment with other factors that influence the emotional lives of families and communities and (2) overlooking important cultural differences within a nation and individual differences within groups. Studies that combine qualitative and quantitative methods, and those that have members of each group observe members of another group have been particularly interesting.

Culturally sensitive, developmentally oriented comparative research is needed to demonstrate that particular features of a culture influence children's emotional development and explain how and why culture influences socialization of emotion. Such an approach, however, brings with it the formidable challenge of finding culturally fair ways to conduct the research. Berry (1990) recommends a *derived etic* approach, an iterative process of scrutinizing "outside" models and measures from an "inside" perspective. For example, the definition of *emotion*, a Western concept, can be subjected to the scrutiny of the non-Westerners in a research team to determine whether there is a common understanding of such a concept and to develop culturally relevant procedures that are comparable across groups.

With increasing globalization and mobility of populations, immigration patterns are further diversifying how culture affects the socialization of emotion. Some children are experiencing separation from their primary caregivers (e.g., one or both parents move to a new country, while children remain behind), whereas others are moving with their parents (e.g., maintaining their socialization relationships but now embedded within new cultural experiences). There has been little research on the effects of such changes on the socialization of emotion.

The study of emotional processes in socialization, examined from a cultural perspective, is both challenging and exciting. The corpus of work that informed our discussion clearly indicates that comparative research is necessary for a comprehensive understanding of the universal and culturally variable aspects of socialization. The evidence we examined suggests many new hypotheses. These are best assessed with culturally relevant, developmental studies that avail themselves of multiple disciplinary expertise and techniques. The increasing capacity to conduct research in all the corners of the world bodes well for exciting advances in the years ahead.

ACKNOWLEDGMENTS

This work was supported, in part, by an award from the National Science Foundation (Grant No. 9711519) to Pamela M. Cole. We also wish to acknowledge Babu Lal Tamang, Mukta Singh Tamang, and Sara Harkness, who contributed to our understanding of culture.

REFERENCES

Ahnert, L., Lamb, M. E., & Seltenheim, K. (2000). Infant-care provider attachments in contrasting child care settings I: Group-oriented care before German unification. *Infant Behavior and Development, 23*, 197–209.

Ainsworth, M. D. S. (1967). *Infancy in Uganda: Infant care and the growth of love.* Baltimore: Johns Hopkins University Press.

Ainsworth, M. D. S., & Bell, S. M. (1970). Attachment, exploration, and separation: Illustrated by the behavior of one-year-olds in a strange situation. *Child Development, 41*, 49–67.

Alexander, K. J., Miller, P. J., & Hengst, J. A. (2001). Young children's emotional attachments to stories. *Social Development, 10*, 374–398.

Berry, J. W. (1990). Imposed etics, emics, and derived etics: Their conceptual and operational status in cross-cultural psychology. In T. N. Headland, K. L. Pike, & M. Harris (Eds.), *Emics and etics: The insider/outsider debate* (Vol. 7, pp. 84–99). Thousand Oaks, CA: Sage.

Berry, J. W., Poortinga, Y. H., Segall, M. H., & Dasen, P. R. (2002). *Cross-cultural psychology: Research and applications* (2nd ed.). New York: Cambridge University Press.

Block, J. H. (1981). *The Child Rearing Practices Report (CRPR): A set of Q items for the description of parental socialization attitudes and values.* Berkeley: University of California, Institute of Human Development.

Bohr, Y. (2010). Transnational infancy: A new context for attachment and the need for better models. *Child Development Perspectives, 3*, 189–196.

Bornstein, M. H. (2002). Toward a multicultural, multiage, multimethod science. *Human Development, 45*, 257–263.

Bornstein, M. H., Cote, L. R., & Venuti, P. (2001). Parenting beliefs and behaviors in northern and southern groups of Italian mothers of young infants. *Journal of Family Psychology, 15*, 663–675.

Bornstein, M. H., Tal, J., Rahn, C., Galperín, C. Z., Pêcheux, M., Lamour, M., et al. (1992). Functional analysis of the contents of maternal speech to infants of 5 and 13 months in four cultures: Argentina, France, Japan, and the United States. *Developmental Psychology, 28*, 593–603.

Bornstein, M. H., Tamis-LeMonda, C. S., Pascual, L., Haynes, M. O., Painter, K. M., Galperín, C. Z., et al. (1996). Ideas about parenting in Argentina, France, and the United States. *International Journal of Behavioral Development, 19*, 347–367.

Bornstein, M. H., Tamis-LeMonda, C. S., Tal, J., Ludemann, P., Toda, S., Rahn, C. W., et al. (1992). Maternal responsiveness to infants in three societies: The United States, France, and Japan. *Child Development, 63*, 808–821.

Bowes, J. M., Chen, M., San, L. Q., & Yuan, L. (2004). Reasoning and negotiation about child responsibility in urban Chinese families: Reports from mothers, father, and children. *International Journal of Behavioral Development, 28*, 48–58.

Bowlby, J. (1969). *Attachment and loss: Vol. 1. Attachment.* New York: Basic Books.

Bradford, K., Barber, B. K., Olsen, J. A., Maughan, S. L., Erickson, L. D., Ward, D., et al. (2004). A multi-national study of interparental conflict, parenting, and adolescent functioning: South Africa, Bangladesh, China, India, Bosnia, Germany, Palestine, Colombia, and the United States. *Marriage and Family Review, 35*, 107–137.

Bronfenbrenner, U. (1977). *The ecology of human development: Experiments by nature and design.* Cambridge, MA: Harvard University Press.

Burger, L. K., & Miller, P. (1999). Early talk about the past revisited: Affect in working-class and middle-class children's co-narrations. *Journal of Child Language, 26,* 133–162.

Camras, L. A., Chen, Y., Bakeman, R., Norris, K., & Cain, T. R. (2006). Culture, ethnicity, and children's facial expressions: A study of European American, Mainland Chinese, Chinese American, and adopted Chinese girls. *Emotion, 6,* 103–114.

Camras, L. A., Meng, Z., Ujiie, T., Dharamsi, S., Miyake, K., Oster, H., et al. (2002). Observing emotion in infants: Facial expression, body behavior, and rater judgments of responses to an expectancy-violating event. *Emotion, 2,* 179–193.

Carlson, V. J., & Harwood, R. L. (2003). Attachment, culture, and the caregiving system: The cultural patterning of everyday experiences among Anglo and Puerto Rican mother–infant pairs. *Infant Mental Health Journal, 24,* 53–73.

Caudill, W., & Weinstein, H. (1969). Maternal care and infant behavior in Japan and America. *Psychiatry, 32,* 12–43.

Caughy, M. O., & Franzini, L. (2005). Neighborhood correlates of cultural differences in perceived effectiveness of parental disciplinary tactics. *Parenting: Practice and Science, 5,* 119–151.

Cervántes, C. A. (2002). Explanatory emotion talk in Mexican immigrant and Mexican American families. *Hispanic Journal of Behavioral Sciences, 24,* 138–163.

Chang, L., Lansford, J. E., Schwartz, D., & Farver, J. M. (2004). Marital quality, maternal depressed affect, harsh parenting, and child externalizing in Hong Kong Chinese families. *International Journal of Behavioral Development, 28,* 311–318.

Chao, R. K. (1994). Beyond parental control and authoritarian parenting style: Understanding Chinese parenting through the cultural notion of training. *Child Development, 65,* 1111–1119.

Chen, X. (2012). Human development in the context of social change. *Child Development Perspectives, 6,* 321–325.

Chen, X., French, D., & Schneider, B. (Eds.). (2006). *Peer relationships in cultural context.* Cambridge, UK: Cambridge University Press.

Chen, X., Hastings, P. D., Rubin, K. H., Chen, H., Cen, G., & Stewart, S. L. (1998). Child-rearing attitudes and behavioral inhibition in Chinese and Canadian toddlers: A cross-cultural study. *Developmental Psychology, 34,* 677–686.

Chen, X., Wu, H., Chen, H., Wang, L., & Cen, G. (2001). Parenting practices and aggressive behavior in Chinese children. *Parenting: Science and Practice, 1,* 159–184.

Cole, P. M., Bruschi, C. J., & Tamang, B. L. (2002). Cultural differences in children's emotional reactions to difficult situations. *Child Development, 73,* 983–996.

Davis, E. P., Glynn, L. M., Schetter, C. D., Hobel, C., Chicz-Demet, A., & Sandman, C. A. (2007). Prenatal exposure to maternal depression and cortisol influences infant temperament. *Journal of the American Academy of Child and Adolescent Psychiatry, 46,* 737–746.

De Wolff, M. S., & van IJzendoorn, M. H. (1997). Sensitivity and attachment: A meta-analysis on parental antecedents of infant attachment. *Child Development, 68,* 571–591.

Deater-Deckard, K., Atzaba-Poria, P. N., & Pike, A. (2004). Mother– and father–child mutuality in Anglo and Indian British families: A link with lower externalizing problems. *Journal of Abnormal Child Psychology, 32,* 609–620.

Deater-Deckard, K., & Dodge, K. A. (1997). Externalizing behavior problems and discipline revisited: Nonlinear effects and variation by culture, context, and gender. *Psychological Inquiry, 8,* 161–175.

Denham, S. A. (1998). *Emotional development in young children.* New York: Guilford Press.

Dennis, T. A., Cole, P. M., Zahn-Waxler, C., & Mizuta, I. (2002). Self in context: Autonomy and relatedness in Japanese and U.S. mother–preschooler dyads. *Child Development, 73,* 1803–1817.

Dix, T. (1991). The affective organization of parenting: Adaptive and maladaptive processes. *Psychological Bulletin, 110,* 3–25.

Dix, T., Gershoff, E. T., Meunier, L. N., & Miller, P. C. (2004). The affective structure of supportive parenting: Depressive symptoms, immediate emotions, and child-oriented motivation. *Developmental Psychology, 40,* 1212–1227.

Dunn, J. (1988). *The beginnings of social understanding.* Cambridge, MA: Harvard University Press.

Eisenberg, A. R. (1999). Emotion talk among Mexican American and Anglo American mothers and children from two social classes. *Merrill–Palmer Quarterly, , 45,* 267–284.

Eisenberg, N., Cumberland, A., & Spinrad, T. L. (1998). Parental socialization of emotion. *Psychological Inquiry, 9,* 241–273.

Ekman, P. (1992). Are there basic emotions? *Psychological Review, 99,* 550–553.

Elfenbein, H. A., & Ambady, N. (2002). On the universality and cultural specificity of emotion regulation: A meta-analysis. *Psychological Bulletin, 128,* 203–235.

Feldman, R., & Masalha, S. (2010). Parent–child and triadic antecedents of children's social competence: Cultural specificity, shared process. *Developmental Psychology, 46,* 455–467.

Flannagan, D., & Perese, S. (1996). Emotional references in mother–daughter and mother–son dyads' conversations about school. *Sex Roles, 39,* 353–367.

Fogel, A., Toda, S., & Kawai, M. (1988). Mother–infant face-to-face interactions in Japan and the United States: A laboratory comparison using 3-month-old infants. *Developmental Psychology, 24,* 398–406.

Fung, H. (1999). Becoming a moral child: The socialization of shame among young Chinese children. *Ethos, 27,* 180–209.

García Coll, C., Lamberty, G., Jenkins, R., McAdoo, H. P., Crnic, K., Wasik, B. H., et al. (1996). An integrative model for the study of developmental competencies in minority children. *Child Development, 67,* 1891–1914.

Garner, P. W., Jones, D., & Miner, J. L. (1994). Social competence among low-income preschoolers: Emotion socialization practices and social cognitive correlates. *Child Development, 65,* 622–637.

Gartstein, M. A., Gonzalez, C., Carranza, J. A., Ahadi, S. A., Ye, R., Rothbart, M. K., et al. (2006). Studying the development of infant temperament through parent report: Commonalities and differences for the People's Republic of China, the United States of America, and Spain. *Child Psychiatry and Human Development, 37,* 145–161.

Gershoff, E. T., Grogan-Kaylor, A., Lansford, J. E., Chang, L., Zelli, A., Deater-Deckard, K., et al. (2010). Parent discipline practices in an international sample: Associations with child behaviors and moderation by perceived normativeness. *Child Development, 81,* 487–502.

Gjerde, P. F. (2004). Culture, power, and experience: Toward a person-centered cultural psychology. *Human Development, 47,* 138–157.

Goldsmith, H. H., Buss, A. H., Plomin, R., Rothbart, M. K., Thomas, A., Chess, S., et al. (1987). Roundtable: What is temperament?: Four approaches. *Child Development, 58,* 505–529.

Gottman, J. M., Katz, L. F., & Hooven, C. (1997). *Meta-emotion: How families communicate emotionally.* Hillsdale, NJ: Erlbaum.

Greenfield, P. M. (2009). Linking social change and developmental change: Shifting pathways of human development. *Developmental Psychology, 45,* 401–418.

Grossmann, K., Grossmann, K. E., Spangler, G., Suess, G., & Unzner, L. (1985). Maternal sensitivity and newborns' orientation responses as related to quality of attachment in northern Germany. *Monographs of the Society for Research in Child Development, 50,* 233–256.

Grossmann, K. E., Grossmann, K., Huber, F., & Wartner, U. (1981). German children's behavior towards their mothers at 12 months and their fathers at 18 months in Ainsworth's strange situation. *International Journal of Behavioral Development, 4,* 157–181.

Halberstadt, A. G., Denham, S. A., & Dunsmore, J. C. (2001). Affective social competence. *Social Development, 10,* 79–119.

Harkness, S., & Super, C. M. (1996). *Parents' cultural belief systems: Their origins, expressions, and consequences.* New York: Guilford Press.

Harwood, R. L., Schöelmerich, A., Schulze, P. A., & Gonzalez, Z. (1999). Cultural differences in maternal beliefs and behaviors: A study of middle-class Anglo and Puerto Rican mother–infant pairs in four everyday situations. *Child Development, 70,* 1005–1016.

Hayashi, A., Karasawa, M., & Tobin, J. (2009). The Japanese preschool's pedagogy of feeling: Cultural strategies for supporting young children's emotional development. *Journal of the Society for Psychological Anthropology, 37,* 32–49.

Hewlett, B. S., Lamb, M. E., Shannon, D., Leyendecker, B., & Schöelmerich, A. (1998). Culture and early infancy among central African foragers and farmers. *Developmental Psychology, 34,* 653–661.

Hill, N. E., & Herman-Stahl, M. A. (2002). Neighborhood safety and social involvement: Associations with parenting behaviors and depressive symptoms among African-American and Euro-American mothers. *Journal of Family Psychology, 16,* 209–219.

Hoff-Ginsberg, E. (1991). Mother–child conversation in different social classes and communicative settings. *Child Development, 62,* 782–796.

Hofstede, G. (1984). *Culture's consequences: International differences in work-related values.* Beverly Hills, CA: Sage.

Honig, A. S., & Chung, M. (1989). Child-rearing practices of urban poor mothers of infants and three-year-olds in five cultures. *Early Child Development and Care, 50,* 75–97.

Hsu, J., Tseng, W., Ashton, G., McDermott, J. F., & Char, W. (1985). Family interaction patterns among Japanese-American and Caucasian families in Hawaii. *American Journal of Psychiatry, 142,* 577–581.

Ispa, J. M., Fine, M. A., Halgunseth, L. C., Harper, S., Robinson, J., Boyce, L., et al. (2004). Maternal intrusiveness, maternal warmth, and mother–toddler relationship outcomes: Variations across low-income ethnic and acculturation groups. *Child Development, 75,* 1613–1631.

Jin, M. K., Jacobvitz, D., Hazen, N., & Jung, S. H. (2012). Maternal sensitivity and infant attachment security in Korea: Cross-cultural validation of the Strange Situation. *Attachment and Human Development, 14,* 33–44.

Kagan, J., Arcus, D., Snidman, N., Feng, W. Y., Hendler, J., & Greene, S. (1994). Reactivity in infants: A cross-national comparison. *Developmental Psychology, 30,* 342–345.

Kağitçibaşi, C. (1996). Individualism and collectivism. In J. W. Berry, M. H. Segall, & C. Kağitçibaşi (Ed.), *Handbook of cross-cultural psychology: Vol. 3. Social behavior and applications* (2nd ed., pp. 1–49). Boston: Allyn & Bacon.

Kağitçibaşi, C., & Ataca, B., (2005). Value of children and family change: A three-decade portrait from Turkey. *Applied Psychology, 54,* 317–337.

Keller, H. (2003). Socialization for competence: Cultural models of infancy. *Human Development, 46,* 288–311.

Keller, H. (2007). *Cultures of infancy.* Mahwah, NJ: Erlbaum.

Keller, H., & Lamm, B. (2005). Parenting as the expression of sociohistorical time: The case of German individualism. *International Journal of Behavioral Development, 29,* 238–246.

Keller, H., Lohaus, A., Kuensemueller, P., Abels, M., Yovis, R., Voelker, S., et al. (2004). The bio-culture of parenting: Evidence from five cultural communities. *Parenting: Science and Practice, 4,* 25–50.

Keller, H., & Otto, H. (2009). The cultural socialization of emotion regulation during infancy. *Journal of Cross-Cultural Psychology, 40,* 996–1011.

Keller, H., Papaligoura, Z., Kuensemueller, P., Voelker, S., Papaeliou, C., Lohaus, A., et al. (2003). Concepts of mother–infant interactions in Greece and Germany. *Journal of Cross-Cultural Psychology, 34,* 677–689.

Keller, H., Voelker, S., & Yovsi, R. D. (2005). Conceptions of parenting in different cultural communities: The case of West African Nso and Northern German women. *Social Development, 14,* 158–180.

Keller, H., Yovsi, R., Borke, J., Kartner, J., Jensen, H., & Papaligoura, Z. (2004). Developmental consequences of early parenting experiences: Self-recognition and self-regulation in three cultural communities. *Child Development, 75,* 1745–1760.

Kelley, M. L., Power, T. G., & Wimbush, D. D. (1992). Determinants of disciplinary practices in low-income Black mothers. *Child Development, 63,* 573–582.

Kisilevsky, B. S., Hains, S. M., Lee, K., Muir, D. W., Xu, F., Zhao, Z. Y., et al. (1998). The still-face effect in Chinese and Canadian 3- to 6- month infants. *Developmental Psychology, 34,* 629–639.

Lambert, M. C., Weisz, J. R., Knight, F., Desrosiers, M., Overly, K., & Thesiger, C. (1992). Jamaican and American adult perspectives on child psychopathology: Further exploration of the threshold model. *Journal of Consulting and Clinical Psychology, 60,* 146–149.

Lansford, J. E., Malone, P. S., Dodge, K. A., Chang, L. Chaudhary, N., Tapanya, S., et al. (2010). Children's perceptions of maternal hostility and rejection as mediators of the link between discipline and children's adjustment in five countries. *International Journal of Behavioral Development, 34,* 452–461.

LeVine, R. A. (1969). Culture, personality, and socialization: An evolutionary view. In D. Goslin (Ed.), *Handbook of socialization: Theory and research* (pp. 503–541). New York: Rand McNally.

LeVine, R. A., Dixon, S., LeVine, S., Richman, A., Leiderman, P. H., Keefer, C. H., et al. (1994). *Childcare and culture: Lessons from Africa.* New York: Cambridge University Press.

LeVine, R. A., & Norman, K. (2001). The infant's acquisition of culture: Early attachment reexamined in anthropological perspective. *Publications of Society for Psychological Anthropology, 12,* 83–104.

Lewis, M., Ramsay, D. S., & Kawakami, K. (1993). Differences between Japanese infants and Caucasian American infants in behavioral and cortisol response to inoculation. *Child Development, 64,* 1722–1731.

Lin, C. Y. C., & Fu, V. R. (1990). A comparison of child rearing practices among Chinese, immigrant Chinese, and Caucasian-American parents. *Child Development, 61,* 429–433.

Lozoff, B., DeAndraca, I., Castíllo, M., Smith, J. G., Walter, T., & Piño, P. (2003). Behavioral and developmental effects of preventing iron-deficiency anemia in healthy full-term infants. *Pediatrics, 112,* 846–854.

Lutz, C. A. (1987). Goals, events, and understanding in Ifaluk emotion theory. In N. Quinn & D. Holland (Eds.), *Cultural models in language and thought* (pp. 290–312). New York: Cambridge University Press.

Marín, G., Gamba, R. J., & Marín, B. V. (1992). Extreme response style and acquiescence among hispanics: The role of acculturation and education. *Journal of Cross-Cultural Psychology, 23,* 498–509.

Markus, H. R., & Kitayama, S. (1991). Culture and the self: Implications for cognition, emotion and motivation. *Psychological Review, 98,* 224–253.

Martini, T. S., Root, C. A., & Jenkins, J. M. (2004). Low and middle income mothers' regulation of negative emotion: Effects of children's temperament and situational emotional responses. *Social Development, 13,* 515–530.

McLoyd, V. C. (2004). Linking race and ethnicity to culture: Steps along the road from inference and hypothesis testing. *Human Development, 47,* 185–191.

Melzi, G., & Fernández, C. (2004). Talking about past emotions: Conversations between Peruvian mothers and their preschool children. *Sex Roles, 50,* 641–657.

Mesquita, B., & Frijda, N. H. (1992). Cultural variations in emotions: A review. *Psychological Bulletin, 112,* 179–204.

Miller, P. J., Fung, H., Lin, S., Chen, E. C., & Boldt, B. R. (2012). How socialization happens on the ground: Narrative practices as alternate socializing pathways in Taiwanese and European-American families. *Monographs of the Society for Research in Child Development, 77,* 1–140.

Miller, P. J., Fung, H., & Mintz, J. (1996). Self-construction through narrative practices: A Chinese and American comparison of early socialization. *Ethos, 24,* 237–280.

Miller, P. J., Hoogstra, L., Mintz, J., Fung, H., & Williams, K. (1993). Troubles in the garden and how they get resolved: A young child's transformation of his favorite story. In C. A. Nelson (Ed.), *Memory and affect in development* (pp. 87–114). Hillsdale, NJ: Erlbaum.

Miller, P. J., & Sperry, L. L. (1987). The socialization of anger and aggression. *Merrill–Palmer Quarterly, 33*, 1–31.

Miller, P. J., Wiley, A. R., Fung, H., & Liang, C. H. (1997). Personal storytelling as a medium of socialization in Chinese and American families. *Child Development, 68*, 557–568.

Mizuta, I., Zahn-Waxler, C., Cole, P. M., & Hiruma, N. (1996). A cross-cultural study of preschoolers' attachment: Security and sensitivity in Japanese and US dyads. *International Journal of Behavioral Development, 19*, 141–159.

Ng, F. F., Pomerantz, E. M., & Lam, S. (2007). European American and Chinese parents' responses to children's success and failure: Implications for children's responses. *Developmental Psychology, 43*, 1239–1255.

Phinney, J. S., Kim-Jo, T., Osorio, S., & Vilhjalmsdottir, P. (2005). Autonomy and relatedness in adolescent–parent disagreements: Ethnic and developmental factors. *Journal of Adolescent Research, 20*, 8–39.

Pinderhughes, E. E., Nix, R., Foster, E. M., & Jones, D. (2001). Parenting in context: Impact of neighborhood poverty, residential stability, public services, social networks, and danger on parental behaviors. *Journal of Marriage and the Family, 63*, 941–953.

Power, T. G., Kobayashi-Winata, H., & Kelley, M. L. (1992). Childrearing patterns in Japan and the United States: A cluster analytic study. *International Journal of Behavioral Development, 15*, 185–205.

Raval, V. V., & Martini, T. S. (2011). "Making the child understand": Socialization of emotion in urban India. *Journal of Family Psychology, 25*, 847–856.

Rao, N., McHale, J. P., & Pearson, E. (2003). Links between socialization goals and child-rearing practices in Chinese and Indian mothers. *Child Development, 12*, 475–492.

Rogoff, B. (2003). *The cultural nature of human development.* New York: Oxford University Press.

Rothbart, M. K., & Bates, J. E. (1998). Temperament. In W. Damon & N. Eisenberg (Eds.), *Handbook of child psychology: Social, emotional, and personality development* (Vol. 3, pp. 105–176). New York: Wiley.

Rothbaum, F., Morelli, G., Pott, M., & Liu-Constant, Y. (2000). Immigrant Chinese and Euro-American parents' physical closeness with young children: Themes of family relatedness. *Journal of Family Psychology, 14*, 334–348.

Rothbaum, F., Pott, M., Azuma, H., Miyake, K., & Weisz, J. (2000). The development of close relationships in Japan and the United States: Paths of symbiotic harmony and generative tension. *Child Development, 71*, 1121–1142.

Rothbaum, F., Weisz, J., Pott, M., Miyake, K., & Morelli, G. (2000). Attachment and culture: Security in the United States and Japan. *American Psychologist, 55*, 1093–1104.

Russell, A., Hart, C. H., Robinson, C. C., & Olsen, S. F. (2003). Children's sociable and aggressive behavior with peers: A comparison of the US and Australian, and contributions of temperament and parenting styles. *International Journal of Behavioral Development, 27*, 74–86.

Saarni, C. (1999). *The development of emotional competence.* New York: Guilford Press.

Super, C. M., & Harkness, S. (1986). The developmental niche: A conceptualization at the interface of child and culture. *International Journal of Behavioral Development, 9*, 545–569.

Tao, A., Zhou, Q., & Wang, Y. (2010). Parental reactions to children's negative emotions: Prospective relations to Chinese children's psychological adjustment. *Journal of Family Psychology, 24*, 135–144.

Tobin, J., Wu, D., & Davidson, D. (1989). *Preschool in three cultures: Japan, China, and the United States.* New Haven, CT: Yale University Press.

Toda, S., Fogel, A., & Kawai, M. (1990). Maternal speech to three-month-old infants in the United States and Japan. *Journal of Child Language, 17*, 279–294.

Triandis, H. C. (1989). The self and social behavior in differing cultural contexts. *Psychological Review, 96*, 506–520.

Tsai, J. L., Knutson, B., & Fung, H. H. (2006). Cultural variation in affect valuation. *Journal of Personality and Social Psychology, 90,* 288–307.

van IJzendoorn, M. H., & Sagi, A. (1999). Cross-cultural patterns of attachment: Universal and contextual dimensions. In J. Cassidy & P. R. Shaver (Eds.), *Handbook of attachment: Theory, research, and clinical applications* (pp. 713–734). New York: Guilford Press.

Varela, R. E., Vernberg, E. M., Sanchez-Sosa, J. J., Riveros, A., Mitchell, M., & Mashunkashey, J. (2004). Parenting style of Mexican, Mexican American, and Caucasian-non-Hispanic families: Social context and cultural influences. *Journal of Family Psychology, 18,* 651–657.

Walker-Barnes, C. J., & Mason, C. A. (2001). Ethnic differences of parenting on gang involvement and gang delinquency: A longitudinal, hierarchical linear modeling perspective. *Child Development, 72,* 1814–1831.

Wang, Q. (2001). Culture effects on adults' earliest childhood recollection and self-description: Implications for the relation between memory and the self. *Journal of Personality and Social Psychology, 81,* 220–233.

Weisner, T. S. (2002). Ecocultural understanding of children's developing pathways. *Human Development, 45,* 272–281.

Whiting, B. B., & Edwards, C. P. (1988). *Children of different worlds: The formation of social behavior.* Cambridge, MA: Harvard University Press.

Wood, L., Cole, P. M., Trommsdorff, G., Mishra, R., Park, S., & Niraula, S. (2014). *Cultural variations in maternal conceptions of child competence.* Manuscript submitted for publication.

Wu, P., Robinson, C. C., Yang, C., Hart, C. H., Olsen, S. F., Porter, C. L., et al. (2002). Similarities and differences in mothers' parenting of preschoolers in China and the United States. *International Journal of Behavioral Development, 26,* 481–491.

Zahn-Waxler, C., Friedman, R. J., Cole, P. M., Mizuta, I., & Hiruma, N. (1996). Japanese and United States preschool children's responses to conflict and distress. *Child Development, 67,* 2462–2477.

Zevalkink, J., & Riksen-Walraven, J. M. (2001). Parenting in Indonesia: Inter- and intracultural differences in mothers' interactions with their young children. *International Journal of Behavioral Development, 25,* 167–175.

CHAPTER 22

Acculturation

John W. Berry

Acculturation is the dual process of cultural and psychological change that takes place as a result of contact between two or more cultural groups and their individual members. At the group level, it involves changes in social structures and institutions and in cultural practices. At the individual level, it involves changes in a person's behavioral repertoire; these psychological changes come about through a long-term process. Acculturation is a process that parallels many features of the process of socialization. Acculturation may follow individuals' initial socialization into their own culture (e.g., after immigration to a new society); it may also take place at the same time (e.g., among members of ethnocultural communities that are involved with two cultures within one country). In this chapter, the processes of socialization and acculturation are considered to be distinguishable features of the general concept of *cultural transmission*.

Intercultural contact and cultural change occur for many reasons, including colonization, military invasion, migration, and sojourning (e.g., tourism, international study, and overseas posting). It continues after initial contact in culturally plural societies, where ethnocultural communities maintain features of their heritage cultures. Adaptation to living in culture–contact settings takes place over time; occasionally it is stressful, but often it results in some form of longer-term accommodation. Acculturation and adaptation are now reasonably well understood, permitting the development of some generalizations, policies, and programs that are intended to promote successful outcomes for all parties involved in the contact situation.

This chapter begins with an examination of the history of the study of acculturation, including the development of current definitions of acculturation as distinct from socialization. This examination is followed by a description of the attitudes and behaviors that together comprise various acculturation strategies and adaptations. The chapter concludes with some possible policy and program applications that may assist individuals, institutions, and cultural groups to deal more effectively with the process of acculturation.

The Concept of Acculturation

The initial interest of researchers in the process of acculturation grew out of a concern for the effects of European domination of colonial and indigenous peoples. Later, it focused on how immigrants (both voluntary and involuntary) changed following their entry and adaptation into societies of settlement. More recently, much of the work has been involved with how immigrant and ethnocultural groups relate to each other, and change, as a result of their attempts to live together in culturally plural societies (Redfield, Linton, & Herskovits, 1936). Nowadays, all these aspects of acculturation are important because globalization results in ever-larger trading and political relations: Indigenous national populations have experienced neocolonization, while new waves of immigrants, sojourners, and refugees have flowed from these economic and political changes, and large ethnocultural populations have become established in many countries (Berry, 2005; Sam & Berry, 2010).

Much of the initial research on acculturation was carried out with colonized populations in Africa and the Americas (e.g., Linton, 1940), and has continued in the traditional immigrant-receiving ("settler") countries of Australia, Canada, New Zealand, and the United States (see Chun, Balls-Organista, & Marin, 2003; Sam & Berry, 2006). Acculturation issues have become more and more important in the rest of the world (especially in Europe and Asia), where massive population contacts and cultural transfers are taking place. These concerns are usually linked to the concepts of *globalization* (Berry, 2008) and *multiculturalism* (Berry & Sam, 2013; Leong & Liu, 2013). In Asia, where half of the world's population lives in culturally diverse societies, and in Europe, where large migration flows have increased dramatically in recent years, individuals experience daily intercultural encounters and have to meet the challenges of cultural and psychological change. As a cross-cultural psychologist, I take seriously the view that findings from research in one culture area of the world (or even in a few societies) cannot be generalized to other societies. Thus, international experiences, ideologies, and sensitivities may alter the conceptions and empirical findings that are portrayed in this chapter. It is, of course, up to all societies, and their diverse residents, to assess the relevance and validity of this existing work for their own societies.

Early views about the nature of acculturation are a useful foundation for contemporary discussion. The following two formulations in particular have been widely quoted:

> Acculturation comprehends those phenomena which result when groups of individuals having different cultures come into continuous first-hand contact, with subsequent changes in the original culture patterns of either or both groups. . . . Under this definition, acculturation is to be distinguished from culture change, of which it is but one aspect, and assimilation, which is at times a phase of acculturation. (Redfield et al., 1936, p. 149)

In the other formulation, *acculturation* was defined as

> culture change that is initiated by the conjunction of two or more autonomous cultural systems. Acculturative change may be the consequence of direct cultural transmission; it may be derived from non-cultural causes, such as ecological or demographic modification induced by an impinging culture; it may be delayed, as with internal adjustments

following upon the acceptance of alien traits or patterns; or it may be a reactive adaptation of traditional modes of life. (Social Science Research Council, 1954, p. 974)

In the first formulation, acculturation is seen as one aspect of the broader concept of culture change (that which results from intercultural contact), is considered to generate change in "either or both groups," and is distinguished from assimilation (which may be "at times a phase"). These are important distinctions for psychological work and I pursue them later in this chapter. In the second definition, a few extra features are added: Change can be *indirect* (not cultural but "ecological," due to alteration in habitat); *delayed* (there can be cultural and psychological lag, which can result in change years after contact); and sometimes "reactive" (i.e., groups and individuals may reject the cultural influences and change back toward a more "traditional" way of life rather than inevitably toward greater similarity with the dominant culture).

These anthropological definitions were followed by Graves (1967), who introduced the concept of *psychological acculturation*, which refers to changes in an individual who is a participant in a culture–contact situation, being influenced both directly by the external culture, and by the changing culture of which the individual is a member. While these early definitions still serve as the basis for much work on acculturation, there are some more recent dimensions that have been proposed. First, it is no longer considered necessary for acculturation to be based on "continuous firsthand" contact. For example, research by Ferguson and Bornstein (2012) has shown that Jamaican youth are taking on U.S. cultural attributes without ever having been in direct personal contact with that society. The second new dimension examines acculturation that takes place over the long term. Rather than being a phenomenon that occurs within the lifetime of an individual or in a few generations, acculturation can take place over centuries, even millennia. This phenomenon has been examined by Gezentsvey-Lamy, Ward, and Liu (2013) with Jewish, Maori, and Chinese samples. In this study, Jewish and Maori samples (more than Chinese) showed a very high level of motivation for ethnocultural continuity and cultural persistence across generations. These attributes were related to their preference for ingroup dating and endogamy.

In the third dimension that has become prominent with the increasing cultural diversity of national societies, there is no longer a single dominant or "mainstream" group with which to be in contact (van Oudenhoven & Ward, 2012). With multiple groups available in the larger society, the pattern of intercultural contacts become more complex. As a result, more ethnographic research becomes necessary in order to understand this increasingly complex network of intercultural relations. A fourth dimension is that of contact within plural societies that results from large-scale internal migration. For example, Gui, Zheng, and Berry (2012) examined migrant worker acculturation with men moving from peasant villages to large metropolises in China. This phenomenon is also important within the Russian Federation (Lebedeva & Tatarko, 2013), where individuals from the regions are moving to the large cities and changing the cultural complexity of these metropolises.

Finally, as for other areas of psychological study, the perspective of social constructivism has begun to challenge the positivist tradition of research (Chirkov, 2009). From this perspective, behavior is considered to be "socially constructed" in day-to-day interactions with others, rather than being a "given" that is available for direct empirical observation. In my response (Berry, 2009), I argued that both the traditional positivist and the constructivist perspectives were required for a comprehensive understanding of acculturation.

Despite these new complexities, there remain two reasons for keeping the cultural and psychological levels of acculturation distinct. The first is that in cross-cultural psychology, we view individual human behavior as interacting with the cultural context within which it occurs; hence, separate conceptions and measurements are required at the two levels (Berry, Poortinga, Breugelmans, Chasiotis, & Sam, 2011). This then allows the search for systematic relationships between the two levels. Recent advances in the assessment of acculturation phenomena (e.g., van de Vijver & Celenk, 2013) permit this examination. The second reason is that not every individual enters into the contact situation, participates in the new culture, or changes in the same way; there are vast individual differences in psychological acculturation, even among individuals who live in the same acculturative arena. This allows a search for systematic relationships among psychological variables in an acculturating population.

Figure 22.1 presents a framework that displays and links cultural-level and psychological-level acculturation, and identifies the two (or more) groups in contact. This framework serves as a kind of map of those phenomena that I believe need to be conceptualized and measured during acculturation research. At the cultural level (on the left), we need to understand key features of the two (or more) original cultural groups (A and B) prior to their major contact, the nature of their contact relationships, and the resulting dynamic cultural changes in both groups and in the emergent ethnocultural groups, during the process of acculturation. The gathering of this information requires extensive ethnographic, community-level work. These changes can be minor or substantial and range from being easily accomplished to being a source of major cultural disruption. At the individual level (on the right), we need to consider the *psychological acculturation* that individuals undergo in all groups in contact, and their eventual *adaptation* to their

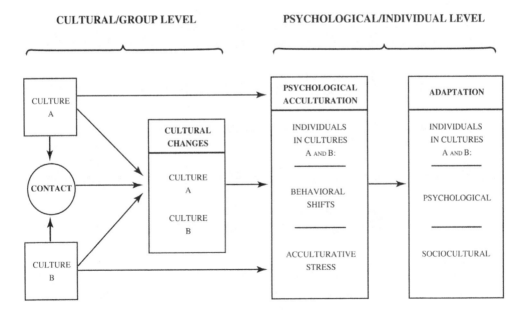

FIGURE 22.1. A general framework for understanding acculturation.

new situations. Identifying these changes requires sampling a population and studying individuals who are variably involved in the process of acculturation. These changes can be a set of rather easily accomplished *behavioral shifts* (e.g., in ways of speaking, dressing, and eating and in one's cultural identity) or they can be more challenging, even problematic.

In this latter category are changes in an individual's cultural values (Schiefer, 2013) and even in their personality (Gungor et al., 2013). In this case, the result may be an increase in *acculturative stress*, as manifested by uncertainty, anxiety, and depression (Berry, 2006b). Finally, adaptations can be primarily internal or *psychological* (e.g., a sense of well-being, or self-esteem, sometimes called "feeling well"), or *sociocultural*, linking the individual to others in the new society (sometimes called "doing well," e.g., as manifested by competence in the activities of daily intercultural living; see Ward, 1996). These italicized terms are elaborated in the following sections. First, however, it is useful to situate the concept of acculturation in the broader notion of *cultural transmission*.

Cultural Transmission

A core issue in acculturation is to understand how features of the culture become incorporated into an individual's repertoire. To assist in this examination, the concept of *cultural transmission* was introduced by Cavalli-Sforza and Feldman (1981) to parallel the notion of *genetic transmission* (see also Schönpflug, 2009). In the case of genetic transmission, certain features of a population are perpetuated across generations through genetic mechanisms. By analogy, using various forms of cultural transmission, a cultural group can perpetuate its behavioral features in subsequent generations employing teaching and learning mechanisms. Cavalli-Sforza and Feldman (1981) distinguished three forms of cultural transmission: *vertical*, *horizontal*, and *oblique*. Cultural transmission from parents to their offspring is termed *vertical transmission* because it involves the descent of cultural characteristics from the parental generation to the next generation. While vertical descent is the only possible form of genetic transmission, there is no role for genetics in the two other forms of cultural transmission (horizontal and oblique).

In vertical transmission, parents transmit cultural features (e.g., values, skills, beliefs) to their offspring. In this case, it is difficult to distinguish between cultural and genetic transmission because children typically learn most from the very people who are responsible for their conception (i.e., biological parents and cultural parents are the same). In horizontal cultural transmission, one learns from one's peers (in primary and secondary groups) during the course of development from birth to adulthood; here, there is no confounding between genetic and cultural transmission. And in the case of oblique cultural transmission, one learns from other adults (including members of one's extended family) and social institutions (including community organizations and formal schooling). When the process takes place entirely within one's own or primary culture, *socialization* (and *enculturation*) are the appropriate terms. However, if the process derives from contact with another culture, the term *acculturation* is employed. As indicated earlier, this latter term refers to the form of transmission experienced by an individual that results from contact with, and influence from, persons and institutions belonging to cultures other than one's own.

In anthropology, the concept of *enculturation* was developed and first defined by Herskovits (1948). As the term suggests, there is an encompassing or surrounding of the individual by his or her culture; the individual acquires appropriate values and behaviors by learning what the culture deems to be necessary. There is not necessarily anything deliberate or didactic about this process; often there is learning without specific teaching. The process of enculturation involves parents, other adults, and social institutions (e.g., schools and media) and peers, in a network of influences on the individual, all of which can limit, shape, and direct the developing individual. The end result (if enculturation is successful) is a person who is competent in aspects of the culture, including its language, its rituals, its values, and so on.

The concept of *socialization* was originally developed in the discipline of sociology and social psychology to refer to the process of deliberate shaping, by way of tutelage, of the individual (Child, 1954). It is generally employed in cross-cultural psychology in the same way. In developmental and social psychology, however, the concept of socialization often includes both the informal aspects of enculturation and the more deliberate aspects of socialization that have been distinguished from each other here.

The net result of both socialization and enculturation is the development of behavioral similarities within cultures and behavioral differences between cultures. They are therefore the crucial cultural mechanisms that produce the distribution of similarities and differences in psychological characteristics at the individual level. As such, they are critical to cross-cultural approaches to psychology; they provide an explanation for how features of cultural groups become features of their individual members.

As we have seen, the concept of *acculturation* also comes from anthropology and refers to cultural and psychological change brought about by contact with other peoples belonging to different cultures and exhibiting different behaviors.

Acculturation involves processes of culture shedding and culture learning (Berry, 1992, 2012). *Culture shedding* refers to the gradual process of losing some features of one's culture (e.g., attitudes, beliefs, and values), as well as some behavioral competencies (e.g., language knowledge and use). *Culture learning* refers to the process of acquisition of features of the new culture, sometimes as replacements for the attitudes and behaviors that have been lost, but often in addition to them. These two processes can create both problems and opportunities for individuals that lead to wide variability in *acculturation strategies* and acculturation outcomes (*psychological* and *sociocultural adaptations*).

The process of cultural transmission does not lead to complete replication of culture and behavior in successive generations; it falls somewhere between an exact transmission (with hardly any differences between parents, the social institutions, and offspring) and a complete failure of transmission (with offspring who are unlike their parents or others in their society). Functionally, either extreme may be problematic for a society. Exact transmission would not allow for novelty and change; the presence of variation from the parental generation enhances adaptability and provides the basis for groups and individuals to respond to new situations as they arise. In contrast, complete failure of transmission would not permit coordinated action between generations (Boyd & Richerson, 1985) and would lead to social chaos. In the case of acculturation, transmission to developing individuals comes from at least two cultural groups, sometimes creating confusion and conflict, and at other times producing new ways of living. Hence, acculturation can be seen not only in terms of loss and acquisition but also as a creative process from which new societies emerge.

The following sections of this chapter provide evidence for variations in *how* groups and individuals enter into the acculturation process, and *how well* they adapt to it. These variations in acculturation attitudes and acculturation behaviors (which together constitute *acculturation strategies*) provide the basis for adaptive responses during culture contact.

Acculturation Contexts

As for all cross-cultural psychology it is imperative that we base our work on acculturation by examining its cultural contexts (Berry, 2006a). We need to understand, in ethnographic terms, both cultures that are in contact if we are to understand the individuals that are in contact.

In Figure 22.1, there are five aspects of cultural contexts: the two original cultures (A and B), the two changing ethnocultural groups (A and B), and the nature of their contact and interactions.

Taking the immigration process as an example, one may refer to the society of origin (A) and society of settlement (B), and their respective changing cultural features following contact. A complete understanding of acculturation would need to start with a fairly comprehensive examination of the societal contexts: In the society of origin, the cultural characteristics that accompany individuals into the acculturation process need description, in part to understand (literally) where the person is coming from, and in part to establish cultural features for comparison with the society of settlement. The combination of political, economic, and demographic conditions faced by individuals in their society of origin also needs to be studied as a basis for understanding the degree of *voluntariness* in the *migration motivation* of acculturating individuals.

A distinction has been made between those groups and individuals that enter into the contact voluntarily and those who are involuntary participants. Associated with this notion are the positive ("pull") and negative ("push") motives that lead individuals to enter into contact situations. In some studies, these two motives are assessed independently, allowing examination of their separate contribution to acculturation attitudes and adaptation. In one study, it was found that those who were high on both negative and positive motives had poorer adaptation than those who had a balance between them. Groups such as indigenous peoples and refugee asylum seekers are reactive and involuntary groups, even though they may also be attracted to some aspects of the cultures with which they are in contact. However, they often experience more difficulties during acculturation than more voluntary groups (for reviews of acculturation difficulties among refugees and indigenous peoples, see Allen, Vaage, & Hauff, 2006; Dona & Ackermann, 2006; Kvernmo, 2006). In contrast, immigrants who are voluntary (in the sense that they often choose to migrate to achieve a better life for themselves and their families) typically reestablish their lives rather well and achieve levels of income, education, and well-being that are comparable to those already settled in the society (for a review of the evidence, see Beiser et al., 1988; Sam & Berry, 2006). These outcomes of the acculturation process are discussed more fully below in the section on adaptation.

In the society of settlement, a number of factors are important. First there are the general orientations that a society and its citizens have toward immigration and pluralism (see Kymlicka, 2012). With respect to immigration, some societies (those termed *settler societies*, e.g., Australia, Canada, and the United States) have been built by immigration over the centuries, and this process may be a continuing one, guided by a deliberate immigration and settlement policy. Other societies have received immigrants and refugees only reluctantly, usually without a policy to guide their entry or programs to assist in their settlement (e.g., Germany and the United Kingdom).The important issue to understand for the process of acculturation is the historical, policy, and attitudinal situation faced by immigrants in the society of settlement.

With respect to orientations toward cultural diversity, some societies are accepting of cultural pluralism resulting from immigration, and take steps to support the continuation of cultural diversity as a shared communal resource; this position represents a positive orientation to *multicultural ideology* (Berry & Kalin, 1995), which accepts the value of both diversity and equity of all cultural groups in the plural society. Of course, public attitudes and public policies do not always coincide (e.g., Sniderman & Hagendoorn, 2007). In some cases, for example, in Canada (Berry & Kalin, 2000), there is a large degree of agreement that Canada is, and should remain, a multicultural society. There is similar agreement between public attitudes and policies in the case of France (Sabatier & Boutry, 2006) and in Germany (Phalet & Kosic, 2006), where citizens and governments share more assimilationist views about how immigrants and ethnocultural groups should acculturate. In contrast, there is decreasing consensus in Australia (Sang & Ward, 2006), where the multicultural policy is increasingly challenged by public attitudes that are growing more assimilationist. Evidence across a number of societies shows that the promotion of diversity as a national policy enhances a preference for a multicultural way of living together, which in turn promotes the positive sociocultural adaptation of immigrant youth (Berry, Phinney, Sam, & Vedder, 2006).

Murphy (1965) argued that societies supportive of cultural pluralism (i.e., with a positive multicultural ideology) provide a more positive settlement context for two reasons: (1) They are less likely to enforce cultural change (assimilation) or exclusion (segregation and marginalization) on immigrants, and (2) they are more likely to provide social support both from the institutions of the larger society (e.g., culturally sensitive health care, multicultural curricula in schools), and from the continuing and evolving ethnocultural communities that usually make up pluralistic societies. However, even where pluralism is accepted, there are well-known variations in the relative acceptance of specific cultural, "racial," and religious groups (e.g., Berry & Kalin, 1995). Those groups that are less well accepted experience hostility, rejection, and discrimination, factors that are predictive of poor long-term adaptation. Numerous studies (e.g., Halpern, 1993; Noh, Beiser, Kaspar, Hou, & Rummens, 1999) of the effects of racism on personal well-being reveal that experiencing discrimination is a serious risk factor for personal well-being. More recently, in a large study of immigrant youth (Berry et al., 2006), the experience of discrimination was the most substantial predictor of poor psychological and sociocultural adaptation.

Acculturation Strategies

As noted earlier in the discussion of variations in cultural transmission, not all groups and individuals undergo acculturation in the same way; there are large variations in how people seek to engage the process. These variations have been termed *acculturation strategies* (Berry, 1997). Which strategies are used depends on a variety of antecedent factors (both cultural and psychological), and there are variable consequences (again, both cultural and psychological) of these different strategies. These strategies comprise two (usually related) components: *attitudes* and *behaviors* (i.e., a person's preferences and actual outcomes) that are exhibited in day-to-day intercultural encounters.

The centrality of the concept of acculturation strategies can be illustrated by reference to each of the components included in Figure 22.1. At the cultural level, the two groups in contact (whether dominant or nondominant) usually have some notion about what they are attempting to do (e.g., colonial policies or motivations for migration), or what is being done to them, during the contact. Similarly, the goals of the emergent ethnocultural groups are likely to influence their collective acculturation strategies. In this section, I present evidence that individual behavioral changes and acculturative stress phenomena are now known to be a function, at least to some extent, of how individuals try to acculturate. That is, *how* people acculturate is related to *how well* they adapt.

Four acculturation strategies have been derived from two basic issues facing all acculturating peoples. These issues are based on the distinction between orientations toward one's own group and those toward other groups (Berry, 1980). Since then, a number of studies have confirmed that these two dimensions are independent of each other (e.g., Berry & Sabatier, 2010; Ryder, Alden, & Paulhus, 2000). This distinction is rendered as a relative preference for maintaining one's heritage culture and identity, and a relative preference for having contact with and participating in the larger society along with other ethnocultural groups. Figure 22.2 presents this formulation.

Responses to these two issues are based on attitudinal dimensions, represented by bipolar arrows in Figure 22.2. For purposes of presentation, generally positive or negative orientations to these issues are shown; their intersection serves to define four acculturation strategies. These strategies have different names, depending on which group is being considered. The views of nondominant ethnocultural groups are shown on the left in

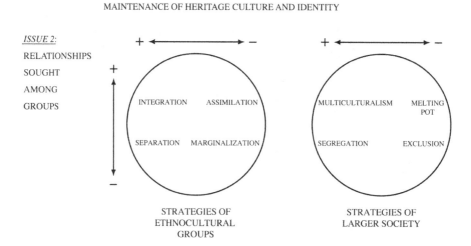

FIGURE 22.2. Four acculturation strategies based on two issues, in ethnocultural groups and in the larger society.

Figure 22.2); the views of the larger society are shown on the right. In the nondominant groups, when individuals do not wish to maintain their cultural identity and seek daily interaction with other cultures, the assimilation strategy is defined. In contrast, when individuals place a value on holding on to their original culture, and at the same time wish to avoid interaction with others, the separation alternative is defined. When there is an interest in maintaining one's original culture while engaging in daily interactions with other groups, integration is the option. In this case, there is some degree of cultural integrity maintained, while seeking, as a member of an ethnocultural group, to participate as an integral part of the larger social network. Finally, when there is little possibility or interest in cultural maintenance (often for reasons of enforced cultural loss, e.g., assimilation through enforced schooling or language change) and little interest in having relations with others (often for reasons of exclusion or discrimination), marginalization is defined (Berry, 1980, 2005). The presentation of the views of nondominant groups and their individual members assumes that they have the freedom to choose how they want to acculturate. This, of course, is not always the case. When the dominant larger society enforces certain forms of acculturation, or constrains the choices of nondominant groups or individuals, other terms need to be used (on the right of Figure 22.2). Integration can only be "freely" chosen and successfully pursued by nondominant groups when the dominant society is open and inclusive in its orientation toward cultural diversity. Thus, a mutual accommodation is required for integration to be attained, involving the acceptance by both groups of the right of all groups to live as culturally different peoples. This strategy requires nondominant groups to adopt the core values of the larger society (usually articulated in the charters of rights, or constitutions), whereas the larger society must be prepared to adapt national institutions (e.g., education, health, and labor) to better meet the needs of all groups now living together in the plural society.

Since the original anthropological definition clearly established that *both* groups in contact would become acculturated, I included the powerful role played by the dominant group in influencing the way in which mutual acculturation would take place (Berry, 1980). The views of the larger society are shown on the right side of Figure 22.2. Assimilation, when sought by the nondominant acculturating group, is termed the *melting pot*, but when it is demanded by the dominant group, it is called the *pressure cooker*. When separation is forced by the dominant group it is called *segregation*. Marginalization, when imposed by the dominant group, is *exclusion*. Finally, *integration*, which occurs when diversity is a feature accepted by the larger society as a whole, including all the various ethnocultural groups, is called *multiculturalism*. With the use of this framework, comparisons can be made between individuals and their groups, and between nondominant peoples and the larger society within which they are acculturating. The ideologies and policies of the dominant group constitute an important element of ethnic relations research (see Berry, Kalin, & Taylor, 1977; Bourhis, Moise, Perreault, & Senecal, 1997), while the preferences of nondominant people are a core feature in acculturation research (Berry, Kim, Power, Young, & Bujaki, 1989). Inconsistencies and conflicts between these various acculturation preferences are sources of difficulty for acculturating individuals.

Conceptions of these acculturation strategies have become more complex in recent years. Not only are there more groups with which to be in contact (van Oudenhoven & Ward, 2012) but also the domains of life that are subject to change have been elaborated (Navas et al., 2005; Safdar, Choung, & Lewis, 2012). These studies have shown that the preferred acculturation strategies differ according to which aspect of life in being examined (e.g., work, social relations, food, dress, and family life). Often, there is more acceptance of assimilation in the domains of work, but there is a preference for integration in the domains of social relations, food and dress, and of separation with respect to family and community life. Generally, when acculturation experiences cause problems for acculturating individuals, we observe the phenomenon of *acculturative stress* (see next section).

Evidence for the reality of these various ways of acculturating comes from a study of over 5,000 immigrant youth who had settled in 13 countries (Berry et al., 2006). The project assessed a number of concepts (including attitudes toward the four ways of acculturating, ethnic and national identities, ethnic and national language knowledge and use, and ethnic and national friends). Four distinct acculturation profiles emerged from a cluster analysis of all these attitudinal and behavioral data. The largest number of youth fell into the *integration* cluster (defined by a preference for integration, positive ethnic and national identities, knowledge and use of both languages, and a friendship network that included youth from both cultures). The second largest cluster was an *ethnic* one (defined by a preference for separation and a rejection of assimilation, a high ethnic and low national identity, predominant use of the ethnic language, and friends mainly from one's own ethnic group). A third cluster was a *national* one (defined by a pattern of attitudes and behaviors that are the opposite to the ethnic one, including a preference for assimilation, and high national and low ethnic identities, language, and friends). Finally, a *diffuse* cluster emerged that resembled marginalization. This was defined by the acceptance of three attitudes (assimilation, separation, and marginalization) and a rejection of integration (suggesting an unformed or diffuse set of acculturation attitudes), low ethnic and national identities (suggesting a feeling of nonengagement or attachment to either cultural group), high proficiency in the ethnic language (and low proficiency and use of the national language), and high contact with their own ethnic peers but low contact with national peers. Finding these four distinct ways in which youth are acculturating provides substantial evidence for the existence of the four general acculturation strategies outlined earlier. Because these include a complex set of attitudes and behaviors, they correspond well to the notion of acculturation *strategies*, which combines preferences about how to live in the new culture and daily activities that express them. Thus, there appear to be large individual differences in ways in which people seek to, and actually do, acculturate; the integrative course appears to be the most common way to do it, rather than more assimilationist or separationist courses.

Psychological Acculturation

Two ways to conceptualize *psychological acculturation* have been proposed in the literature (see Figure 22.1). The first is *behavioral shifts*, in which those changes in an individual's behavioral repertoire take place rather easily and are usually nonproblematic. As noted earlier, this process encompasses two subprocesses: *cultural shedding* and *culture learning* (Berry, 2012). These processes involve the selective, accidental, or deliberate loss of original behaviors, and either their replacement or supplementation by behaviors that allow the individual a better "fit" with the society of settlement. Most often this process has been termed *adjustment*, as virtually all the adaptive changes take place in the acculturating individual, with few changes occurring among members of the larger society (Ward, Bochner, & Furnham, 2001). These adjustments are typically made with minimal difficulty, in keeping with the appraisal of the acculturation experiences as non-problematic. The long history of successful contact and settlement of most acculturating peoples attests to this relative degree of success. Even for involuntary refugees, after an initial period of difficulty, studies show that in the longer term, their adaptation achieves psychological and social well-being on a par with those born in the country of settlement (e.g., Aycan & Berry, 1996; Beiser, 2000; Berry et al., 2006). However, for indigenous peoples (who are also involuntarily in contact), there is considerable evidence of problematic acculturation (e.g., Kvernmo, 2006).

When greater levels of conflict are experienced, and the experiences are judged to be problematic but controllable and surmountable, *acculturative stress* is the appropriate conceptualization (Berry, 2006b). In this case, individuals understand that they are facing problems resulting from intercultural contact that cannot be dealt with easily or quickly by simply adjusting or assimilating to them. Drawing on the broader stress and adaptation paradigms (e.g., Lazarus & Folkman, 1984), focusing on acculturative stress leads to the study of the processes by which individuals deal with acculturative problems on first encountering them, and over time. In this sense, acculturative stress can be defined as a stress reaction in response to life events that are rooted in the experience of acculturation. Contemporary evidence (see Berry, 2006b, for a review) shows that most people deal with such stressors effectively and reestablish their lives rather well, with health, psychological, and social outcomes that approximate those of individuals in the larger society. In a longitudinal study of Vietnamese "boat people," Beiser (2000) found that, over a period of 10 years in Canada, his sample showed an initial reduction in well-being but matched or surpassed a comparable sample of nonrefugees in psychological and social well-being after the 10 years. Similarly, Aycan and Berry (1996) found an initial decline in economic well-being (increased unemployment and underemployment) among Turkish immigrants to Canada, followed by a regaining of their economic status and psychological well-being after a period of about 7 years (also see Hayfron, 2006, for a review of the economic evidence).

Adaptation

As a result of attempts to cope with these acculturation changes, some long-term adaptations may be achieved. As mentioned earlier, *adaptation* refers to the relatively stable changes that take place in an individual or group in response to external demands. Moreover, adaptation may or may not improve the "fit" between individuals and their environments. It is therefore not a term that necessarily implies that individuals or groups change to become more like their environments (i.e., adjustment by way of assimilation), but it may involve resistance and attempts to change environments, or to move away from them altogether (i.e., by separation). In this usage, *adaptation* is an outcome that may or may not be positive in valence (i.e., meaning only well adapted). This bipolar sense of the concept of adaptation is used in the framework in Figure 22.1, where long-term adaptation to acculturation is highly variable, ranging from well to poorly adapted, and varying from a situation in which individuals can manage their new lives very well to one in which they are unable to carry on in the new society.

Adaptation is also multifaceted. The initial distinction between psychological and sociocultural adaptation was proposed and validated by Ward (1996). *Psychological adaptation* largely involves one's psychological and physical well-being, while *sociocultural adaptation* refers to how well an acculturating individual is able to manage daily life in the new cultural context. While conceptually distinct, they are empirically related to some extent (correlations between the two measures are in the .4–5 range). However, they usually have different time courses and different experiential predictors. Psychological adaptation is predicted by personality variables, social support, and various experiences in the society of settlement (particularly the experience of discrimination), while sociocultural adaptation is predicted by cultural knowledge, degree of contact with the larger society, and positive intergroup attitudes. Psychological problems often increase soon after contact, followed by a general (but variable) decrease over time; positive sociocultural adaptation, however, typically has a linear improvement with time (see Ward et al., 2001, for a comprehensive review).

Research relating adaptation to acculturation strategies allows for some further generalizations (Berry, 1997; Ward, 1996). For both forms of adaptation, those who pursue and accomplish integration appear to be better adapted, while those who are marginalized are least well adapted. And, again, the assimilation and separation strategies are associated with intermediate adaptation outcomes. For example, in research with young Chinese immigrant girls to New Zealand, Ho (1995) tracked their acculturation preferences over a period from their first arrival to between 3 and 4 years in New Zealand, using the fourfold conceptualization. Over this period, there was a persistent decline in their preference for separation, accompanied by a persistent increase in preference for integration: Both assimilation and marginalization remained constant and low over this period. These changes in acculturation preferences were accompanied by increased levels of adaptation: "The most adaptive attitude for the newly arrived Chinese immigrants is to maintain their own cultural identity and learn to participate in the new society" (Ho, 1995, p. 43).

While there are occasional variations on this pattern, it is remarkably consistent. Substantial evidence in support of this pattern comes from a study of immigrant youth (Berry et al., 2006). This project with immigrant youth found evidence for the existence of the theoretical distinction between *psychological adaptation* (having few psychological problems, and high self-esteem and life satisfaction) and *sociocultural adaptation* (good school adjustment, few behavioral problems). When these two adaptation measures were related to the four acculturation profiles, a clear and consistent pattern emerged. Those in the integrated cluster were highest on both forms of adaptation, while those in the diffuse cluster were lowest on both. Those in the ethnic cluster had moderately good psychological adaptation but lower sociocultural adaptation, while those in the national cluster had poorer scores on both forms of adaptation. These latest findings suggest that those who pursue integrative strategies (in terms of attitudes, identities, and behaviors) will achieve better adaptations than those who acculturate in other ways, especially those who acculturate in a diffuse or marginal manner.

A meta-analysis by Nguyen and Benet-Martínez (2013) examined over 80 studies with over 23,000 acculturating individuals. They found that being engaged in two cultures (what they termed *biculturalism*) was associated with greater well-being: There is a "significant, strong and positive association between biculturalism and adjustment (both psychological and sociocultural)" (p. 122).

From all this research, it is possible to conclude that the presence and use of two cultural systems provides an important basis for succeeding in the acculturation process. One possible explanation for this relationship is that those individuals who are engaged in two or more cultures have greater social capital (in the sense of having larger supportive networks). They are also likely to be able to draw upon a more diverse set of competencies when confronted with challenges of daily living in their new society (particularly with prejudice and discrimination displayed by members of the larger society).

Recently, there have been debates regarding variations in adaptation between the first and later generations, particularly between parents and youth (see Masten, Liebkind, & Hernandez, 2012). In some cases, there is evidence that the first generation has high levels of well-being, but that is lower in subsequent generations. This phenomenon may be limited to societies of settlement that have low overall health indicators (e.g., the limited availability of public health services, high rates of obesity) rather than being a general phenomenon (Sam & Berry, 2010).

Applications

There is now widespread evidence that most people who have experienced acculturation actually do survive! First, they are not destroyed or substantially diminished by it; rather, they find opportunities and achieve their goals, sometimes beyond their initial imaginings. This observation pertains more to those who are in voluntary contact situations (e.g., immigrants and sojourners) and probably less to those whose experience of acculturation is involuntary (e.g., indigenous peoples, refugees, and formerly enslaved populations).

Second, researchers often presume to know how acculturating individuals want to live and impose their own ideologies or their personal views, rather than informing themselves about culturally rooted individual preferences and differences. One key concept (but certainly not the only one) to understand this variability has been emphasized in this chapter (*acculturation strategies*). Evidence now supports the existence of large individual differences in both *how* people acculturate and *how well* they adapt. Evidence reviewed in this chapter confirms a relation between how and how well individuals deal with the process of acculturation. Given these individual differences, and the relation between these two sets of variables, researchers are on solid ground in suggesting that individuals and groups should be informed of, and encouraged to seek, the integration path during their acculturation, and to avoid marginalization. Although in some studies the two alternatives of assimilation and separation appear to promote better adaptation, these findings are less frequent.

The generalizations in this chapter on the basis of a wide range of empirical findings allow me to propose that public policies and programs that seek to reduce acculturative stress and to improve intercultural relationships should emphasize the integration or multicultural approach to acculturation. This is true of group-level action, such as national policies, institutional arrangements, and the goals of ethnocultural groups; it is equally true of individual-level action, both in the larger society and among members of nondominant acculturating groups.

There are two areas of application currently receiving considerable attention in research and policy development. One is the domain of family life (including relationships

among individuals within the family and between family members and the world outside). The other is in the area of immigration and settlement policies (including issues
of changes in the institutions of a society and the promotion of cultural diversity and
equity).

The area of family and youth acculturation has received substantial attention in
recent years, particularly from developmental psychologists (see Bornstein & Cote, 2006;
Chuang & Moreno, 2011; García Coll, 2012; Masten et al., 2012). Most of this research
is directed at understanding the acculturation and adaptation of the immigrant family as
a social unit. Issues include not only its general relationships with the new society but also
potential conflicts within the family, as different generations engage the new society with
different acculturation strategies (Sam & Berry, 2009; Sam, Vedder, Liebkind, Neto, &
Virta, 2008).

Further evidence from the study with immigrant youth (Berry et al., 2006) indicates
that parents and children sometimes have different views about parent–adolescent relationships during acculturation. For example, parents have higher scores on a measure
of family obligations (e.g., responsibility for various chores) than do their adolescent
children; in sharp contrast, immigrant youth have higher scores on a scale of adolescent
rights (e.g., independence in dating) than their parents. This pattern of discrepancy was
the case for both immigrant and national families in the study. However, the discrepancy in views about obligations between parents and adolescents was greater among
the immigrant sample than among the national sample; there was no parent–adolescent
discrepancy on rights. Moreover, the differences between parents' and adolescents' views
about family obligations varied according to which acculturation profile the youth were
in: Those in the national profile (i.e., preferring assimilation, having a stronger national
identity, and having more national friends) had greater discrepancies with the views of
their parents. Most important, these discrepancies in family obligations scores (but not
rights scores) were associated with poorer psychological and sociocultural adaptation of
the adolescents: The greater the discrepancy, the poorer the psychological and sociocultural adaptation of the adolescents.

Another project dealing with family that has been carried out in 30 countries (for
details, see Georgas, Berry, van de Vijver, Kagitçibasi, & Poortinga, 2006) examined
the similarities and differences in family structure and function, and some of their psychological correlates. This study has demonstrated both variations in family functioning
linked to ecological contexts (e.g., reliance on agriculture and general level of affluence)
and variations due to sociopolitical contexts (e.g., formal education and religion). In general, family arrangements are hierarchical and extended, and families have more conservative values (including interdependence) in high agrarian and low affluence societies,
and with Orthodox Christian or Islamic religions. In contrast, families high in affluence
and education and with a Protestant religious tradition are more nuclear, are less hierarchical, and exhibit more independence. Although not a part of this study, it may be
hypothesized that following immigration, these variations in family life are likely to set
the stage for variations in acculturation strategies, acculturative stress, and psychological
and sociocultural adaptation. The basic dimensions of variations in family and behavior
that have been established in this project will allow for their use in future studies of immigration and acculturation. When individuals migrate between the countries included in
this sample of 30 societies, their placement on these dimensions can be used to examine
discrepancies in cultural, political, and religious backgrounds that may be predictive of

how, and how well, individual immigrants will acculturate in their new societies. Differences between families and societies that are generally independent or interdependent in family values and social structure (Kagitçibasi, 2007) may well contribute to differing acculturation strategies and long-term adaptation of acculturating individuals.

A second domain of application concerns public policies with respect to cultural diversity. I have made a number of assertions in this chapter on the basis of a wide range of empirical findings. This has allowed me to propose that public policies and programs that seek to reduce acculturative stress and to improve psychological and sociocultural adaptation should emphasize the integration or multicultural approach to acculturation (see Berry, 2014, for a discussion of the social and psychological costs and benefits of multiculturalism). Recent debates in political science (e.g., Kymlicka, 2012; Sniderman & Hagendoorn, 2007) attest to the importance of dealing with these issues at both the national policy and individual psychological levels. Further research is essential, for in the absence of conceptual clarity and empirical foundations, policies may create more social and psychological problems than they solve.

In some countries (e.g., Canada and Australia; see Berry, 1984, 2013), the integrationist perspective has become legislated in policies of multiculturalism, which encourage and support the maintenance of valued features of all cultures *and* at the same time support full participation of all ethnocultural groups in the evolving institutions of the larger society. What seems certain is that cultural diversity and the resultant acculturation are here to stay in all countries. Finding a way to accommodate each other poses a challenge and an opportunity to psychologists and other social scientists everywhere. Diversity is a fact of contemporary life; whether it is the "spice of life" or the main "irritant" is probably the central question that confronts us all, citizens and social scientists alike (Berry, 2001).

REFERENCES

Allen, J., Vaage, A. B., & Hauff, E. (2006). Refugees and asylum seekers. In D. L. Sam & J. W. Berry (Eds.), *Cambridge handbook of acculturation psychology* (pp. 198–217). Cambridge, UK: Cambridge University Press.

Aycan, Z., & Berry, J. W. (1996). Impact of employment-related experiences on immigrants' psychological well-being and adaptation to Canada. *Canadian Journal of Behavioural Science, 28,* 240–251.

Beiser, M. (2000). *Strangers at the gate.* Toronto: University of Toronto Press.

Beiser, M., Barwick, C., Berry, J. W., daCosta, G., Fantino, A., Ganesan, S., et al. (1988). *After the door has been opened: Mental health issues affecting immigrants and refugees in Canada.* Ottawa: Ministries of Multiculturalism, and Health and Welfare.

Berry, J. W. (1980). Acculturation as varieties of adaptation. In A. Padilla (Ed.), *Acculturation: Theory, models and findings* (pp. 9–25). Boulder, CO: Westview.

Berry, J. W. (1984). Multicultural policy in Canada: A social psychological analysis. *Canadian Journal of Behavioural Science, 16,* 353–370.

Berry, J. W. (1992). Acculturation and adaptation in a new society. *International Migration, 30,* 69–85.

Berry, J. W. (1997). Immigration, acculturation and adaptation. *Applied Psychology: An International Review, 46,* 5–68.

Berry, J. W. (2001). A psychology of immigration. *Journal of Social Issues, 57,* 615–631.

Berry, J. W. (2005). Acculturation: Living successfully in two cultures. *International Journal of Intercultural Relations, 29,* 697–712.

Berry, J. W. (2006a). Contexts of acculturation. In D. Sam & J. W. Berry (Eds.), *Cambridge handbook of acculturation psychology* (pp. 27–42). Cambridge, UK: Cambridge University Press.

Berry, J. W. (2006b). Stress perspectives on acculturation In D. Sam & J. W. Berry, (Eds.), *Cambridge handbook of acculturation psychology* (pp. 43–57). Cambridge, UK: Cambridge University Press.

Berry, J. W. (2008). Globalization and acculturation. *International Journal of Intercultural Relations, 32*, 328–336.

Berry, J. W. (2009). A critique of critical acculturation. *International Journal of Intercultural Relations, 33*, 361–371.

Berry, J. W. (2011). Immigrant acculturation: Psychological and social adaptation. In A. Azzi, X. Chryssochoou, B. Klandermans, & B. Simon (Eds.), *Identity and participation in culturally diverse societies* (pp. 279–295). Oxford, UK: Wiley-Blackwell.

Berry, J. W. (2012). Immigration, acculturation and adaptation. In E. Tartakovsky (Ed.), *Immigration: Policies, challenges and impact* (pp. 195–212). Hauppauge, NY: Nova Science.

Berry, J. W. (2014). Multiculturalism: Psychological perspectives. In J. Jedwab (Ed.), *The multiculturalism question: Debating identity in 21st century Canada* (pp. 225–240). Kingston, Ontario, Canada: Queen's University School of Policy Studies, Queen's University.

Berry, J. W., & Kalin, R. (1995). Multicultural and ethnic attitudes in Canada. *Canadian Journal of Behavioural Science, 27*, 310–320.

Berry, J. W., & Kalin, R. (2000). Multicultural policy and social psychology. In S. Renshon & J. Duckitt (Eds.), *Political psychology in cross-cultural perspective* (pp. 263–284). New York: Macmillan.

Berry, J. W., Kalin, R., & Taylor, D. (1977). *Multiculturalism and ethnic attitudes in Canada.* Ottawa: Supply & Services.

Berry, J. W., Kim, U., Power, S., Young, M., & Bujaki, M. (1989). Acculturation attitudes in plural societies. *Applied Psychology: An International Review, 38*, 185–206.

Berry, J. W., Phinney, J. S., Sam, D. L., & Vedder, P. (2006). *Immigrant youth in cultural transition: Acculturation, identity and adaptation across national contexts.* Mahwah, NJ: Erlbaum.

Berry, J. W., Poortinga, Y. H., Breugelmans, S. M., Chasiotis, A., & Sam, D. L. (2011). *Cross-cultural psychology: Research and applications* (3rd ed.). Cambridge, UK: Cambridge University Press.

Berry, J. W., & Sabatier, C. (2010). Acculturation, discrimination, and adaptation among second generation immigrant youth in Montreal and Paris. *International Journal of Intercultural Relations, 34*(3), 191–207.

Berry, J. W., & Sam, D. L. (2013). Accommodating cultural diversity and achieving equity. *European Psychologist, 18*(3), 151–157.

Bornstein, M., & Cote, L. (Eds.). (2006). *Acculturation and parent–child relationships.* Mahwah, NJ: Erlbaum.

Bourhis, R., Moise, C., Perreault, S., & Senecal, S. (1997). Towards an interactive acculturation model: A social psychological approach. *International Journal of Psychology, 32*, 369–386.

Boyd, R., & Richerson, P. (1985). *Culture and the evolutionary process.* Chicago: University of Chicago Press.

Cavalli-Sforza, L. L., & Feldman, M. (1981). *Cultural transmission and evolution.* Princeton, NJ: Princeton University Press.

Child, I. (1954). Socialization. In. G. Lindzey (Ed.), *Handbook of social psychology* (Vol. 2, pp. 655–692). Cambridge, UK: Addison-Wesley.

Chirkov, V. (Ed.). (2009). Critical acculturation psychology [Special issue]. *International Journal of Intercultural Relations, 33*(2), 87–182.

Chuang, S., & Moreno, R. (Eds.). (2011). *Immigrant children: Change, adaptation, and cultural transformation.* New York: Lexington Books.

Chun, K., Balls-Organista, P., & Marin, G. (Eds.). (2003). *Acculturation: Advances in theory, measurement and applied research*. Washington, DC: American Psychological Association Press.

Dona, G., & Ackermann, L. (2006). Refugees in camps. In D. L. Sam & J. W. Berry (Eds.), *Cambridge handbook of acculturation psychology* (pp. 218–232). Cambridge, UK: Cambridge University Press.

Ferguson, G. M., & Bornstein, M. H. (2012). Remote acculturation: The "Americanization" of Jamaican Islanders. *International Journal of Behavioral Development, 36*, 167–177.

García Coll, C. (2012). *The impact of immigration on children's development*. Freiburg, Germany: Karger.

Georgas, J., Berry, J. W., van de Vijver, F., Kagitçibasi, C., & Poortinga, Y. H. (2006). *Families across cultures: A 30 nation psychological study*. Cambridge, UK: Cambridge University Press.

Gezentsvey-Lamy, M., Ward, C., & Liu, J. (2013). Motivation for ethno-cultural continuity. *Journal of Cross-Cultural Psychology, 44*, 1047–1066.

Graves, T. (1967). Psychological acculturation in a tri-ethnic community. *South-Western Journal of Anthropology, 23*, 337–350.

Gui, Y., Zheng, Y., & Berry, J. W. (2012). Migrant worker acculturation in China. *International Journal of Intercultural Relations, 36*, 598–610.

Gungor, D., Bornstein, M., Leersnyder, J., Cote, L., Ceulemans, E., & Mesquita, B. (2013). Acculturation of personality. *Journal of Cross-Cultural Psychology, 44*, 701–718.

Halpern, D. (1993). Minorities and mental health. *Social Science and Medicine, 36*, 597–607.

Hayfron, J. (2006). Immigrants in the labour market. In D. L. Sam & J. W. Berry (Eds.), *Cambridge handbook of acculturation psychology* (pp. 439–451). Cambridge, UK: Cambridge University Press.

Herskovits, M. J. (1948). *Man and his works: The science of cultural anthropology*. New York: Knopf.

Ho, E. (1995). Chinese or New Zealander?: Differential paths of adaptation of Hong Kong Chinese adolescent immigrants in New Zealand. *New Zealand Population Review, 21*, 27–49.

Kagitçibasi, C. (2007). *Families, self and human development across cultures: Theory and applications*. Mahwah, NJ: Erlbaum.

Kvernmo, S. (2006). Indigenous peoples. In D. L. Sam & J. W. Berry (Eds.), *Cambridge handbook of acculturation psychology* (pp. 233–250). Cambridge, UK: Cambridge University Press.

Kymlicka, W. (2012). *Multiculturalism: Success, failure and the future*. Washington, DC: Migration Policy Institute.

Lazarus, R. S., & Folkman, S. (1984). *Stress, appraisal and coping*. New York: Springer.

Lebedeva, N. & Tatarko, A. (2013). Immigration, acculturation and multiculturalism in post-Soviet Russia. *European Psychologist, 18*, 169–178.

Leong, C. H., & Liu, J. (2013). Whither multiculturalism?: Global identities at a cross-roads. *International Journal of Intercultural Relations, 38*(1), 120–132.

Linton, R. (1940). *Acculturation in seven American Indian tribes*. New York: Appleton-Century.

Masten, A., Liebkind, K., & Hernandez, D. (Eds.). (2012). *Realizing the potential of immigrant youth*. Cambridge, UK: Cambridge University Press.

Murphy, H. B. M. (1965). Migration and the major mental disorders. In M. B. Kantor (Ed.), *Mobility and mental health* (pp. 221–249). Springfield, MA: Thomas.

Navas, M., García, M., Sánchez, J., Rojas, A., Pumares, P., & Fernández, J. S. (2005). Relative acculturation extended model: New contributions with regard to the study of acculturation. *International Journal of Intercultural Relations, 29*, 21–37.

Nguyen, A.-M., & Benet-Martínez, V. (2013). Biculturalism and adjustment: A meta-analysis. *Journal of Cross-Cultural Psychology, 44*, 122–159.

Noh, S., Beiser, M., Kaspar, V., Hou, F., & Rummens, J. (1999). Perceived racial discrimination, depression and coping. *Journal of Health and Social Behaviour, 40*, 193–207.

Phalet, K., & Kosic, A. (2006). Acculturation in the European Union. In D. L. Sam & J. W. Berry (Eds.), *Cambridge handbook of acculturation psychology* (pp. 331–348). Cambridge, UK: Cambridge University Press.

Redfield, R., Linton, R., & Herskovits, M. (1936). Memorandum on the study of acculturation. *American Anthropologist, 38,* 149–152.

Ryder, A., Alden, L., & Paulhus, D. (2000). Is acculturation unidimensional or bi-dimensional? *Journal of Personality and Social Psychology, 79,* 49–65.

Sabatier, C., & Boutry, V. (2006). Acculturation in francophone European countries. In D. L. Sam & J. W. Berry (Eds.), *Cambridge handbook of acculturation psychology* (pp. 349–367). Cambridge, UK: Cambridge University Press.

Safdar, S., Choung, K., & Lewis, J. R. (2012). A review of the MIDA model and other contemporary acculturation models. In E. Tartakovsky (Ed.), *Immigration: Policies, challenges and impact.* Hauppauge, NY: Nova Science.

Sam, D., & Berry, J. W. (Eds.). (2006). *Cambridge handbook of acculturation psychology.* Cambridge, UK: Cambridge University Press.

Sam, D., & Berry, J. W. (2009). Adaptation of young immigrants: The double jeopardy of acculturation. In I. Jasinskaja-Lahti (Ed.), *Identities, intergroup relations and acculturation* (pp. 191–205). Helsinki, Finland: Helsinki University Press.

Sam, D., & Berry, J. W. (2010). Acculturation: When individuals and groups of different cultural backgrounds meet. *Perspectives on Psychological Science, 5,* 472–481.

Sam, D. L., Vedder, P., Liebkind, K., Neto, F., Virta, E. (2008). Migration, acculturation and the paradox of adaptation in Europe. *European Journal of Developmental Psychology, 5,* 138–158.

Sang, D., & Ward, C. (2006). Acculturation in Australia and New Zealand. In D. Sam & J. W. Berry (Eds.), *Cambridge handbook of acculturation psychology* (pp. 253–273). Cambridge, UK: Cambridge University Press.

Schiefer, D. (2013). Cultural values and group-related attitudes: A comparison of individuals with and without migration backgrounds across 24 countries. *Journal of Cross-Cultural Psychology, 44,* 245–262.

Schönpflug, U. (Ed.). (2009). *Cultural transmission: Developmental, psychological, social and methodological perspectives.* Cambridge, UK: Cambridge University Press.

Sniderman, P., & Hagendoorn, L. (2007). *When ways of life collide: Multiculturalism and its discontents in the Netherlands.* Princeton, NJ: Princeton University Press.

Social Science Research Council. (1954). Acculturation: An exploratory formulation. *American Anthropologist, 56,* 973–1002.

van de Vijver, F., & Celenk, Ö. (2013). Assessment of acculturation and multiculturalism: An overview of measures in the public domain. In V. Benet-Martínez & Y. Hong (Eds.), *Oxford handbook of multicultural identity: Basic and applied psychological perspectives* (pp. 168–181). Oxford, UK: Oxford University Press.

van Oudenhoven, J. P., & Ward, C. (2012). Fading majority cultures: The effects of transnationalism and demographic developments on the acculturation of immigrants. *Journal of Community and Applied Social Psychology, 23,* 81–97.

Ward, C. (1996). Acculturation. In D. Landis & R. Bhagat (Eds.), *Handbook of intercultural training* (2nd ed., pp. 124–147). Newbury Park, CA: Sage.

Ward, C., Bochner, S., & Furnham, A. (2001). *The psychology of culture shock.* London: Routledge.

PART VI

TARGETS OF SOCIALIZATION

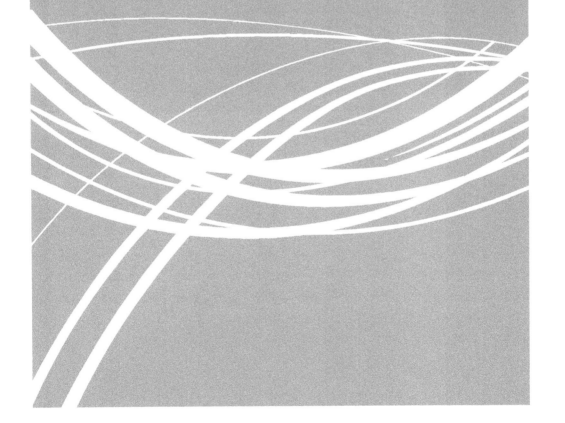

CHAPTER 23

The Socialization of Gender during Childhood and Adolescence

Campbell Leaper
Timea Farkas

From the moment of birth, a child's gender influences the opportunities she or he will experience. Within a few years of life, children begin to form their own ideas about gender that subsequently guide the types of activities they practice, what they find interesting, and the achievements they attain. As children develop, their gender self-concepts, beliefs, and motives are informed and transformed by families, peers, the media, and schools. These social contexts both reflect and perpetuate gender roles and gender inequities in the larger society (Leaper, 2000b; Wood & Eagly, 2002). However, as more individuals are able to transcend traditional gender roles, society changes (Leaper, 2000b). Our purpose in this chapter is to review the major social influences on these developments. We begin our review with a brief survey of theoretical approaches that have proven most helpful in understanding the socialization of gender.

Theoretical Frameworks

For the most part, contemporary theories of gender development are complementary rather than contradictory; that is, most theories either explicitly or implicitly acknowledge the combined influences of social–structural, cognitive–motivational, and biological influences. Theories tend to differ, however, in how much they address each of these processes in the transmission of gender (see Bussey & Bandura, 1999; Martin, Ruble, & Szkrybalo, 2002). The field could benefit from more concerted efforts aimed at integrating theoretical approaches (Leaper, 2011). Although positing an integrative theory is beyond the scope of this chapter, we highlight some explanatory constructs synthesized from contemporary theoretical approaches.

Social–Structural Processes

Children's gender development is embedded in a larger societal context. In this regard, the social–structural approach considers how people's relative status and power in society shape their personal circumstances; this perspective also addresses the constraints that these institutionalized roles impose on individuals' behavior. In addition to gender, other important social status factors include ethnicity, race, economic class, and sexual orientation. The social–structural perspective is also compatible with a feminist analysis that emphasizes the impact of gender inequities in power that exist in the home, the labor force, and political institutions (Wood & Eagly, 2002). Although a feminist social–structural approach is common in social psychology and sociology, relatively few developmental psychologists have considered gender from an explicitly feminist social–structural perspective (see Leaper, 2000b; Miller & Scholnick, 2000).

Taking into account sexist practices in the larger society when studying children's development requires linking cultural institutions to individuals situated in specific environments. As emphasized in ecological systems and sociocultural approaches (Bronfenbrenner & Morris, 2006; Rogoff, 1990), children learn cultural practices through their interactions in everyday settings. In later sections, we consider various social agents that contribute to the socialization of gender. These include the family, teachers, peers, and the media.

Cognitive–Motivational Processes

Children internalize the culture's notions of gender once they acquire a symbolic capacity (Bussey & Bandura, 1999). As children form cognitive representations of gender, or gender schemas, they begin to filter the world through a gender lens. This is a fundamental premise of cognitive-developmental theory, gender schema theory, social cognitive theory, and social identity theory (see Bussey & Bandura, 1999; Martin et al., 2002; Powlishta, 2004). As each of these theories emphasizes, children play an active role in their gender development and a process of self-socialization ensues (Tobin et al., 2010). Girls and boys make inferences about the meaning and the consequences of gender-related behaviors from their observations and social interactions. Also, children's gender schemas and attitudes influence the type of information they notice and remember. Consequently, girls and boys tend to seek out gender-typed environments that further strengthen their gender-typed expectations and interests. In these ways, children's behavior becomes increasingly regulated by internal standards, values, and perceived consequences (Bussey & Bandura, 1999).

As emphasized in social identity theory and gender schema theory, being a member of a group typically leads to an ingroup bias. Experimental studies have documented that children are more likely (1) to pay attention to objects, activities, behaviors, and social roles associated with their own gender and (2) to avoid and devalue what is specifically associated with the other gender (see Martin et al., 2002). Children's ingroup biases are further reflected in their preferences for same-gender peers and avoidance of other-gender peers (see Leaper, 1994; Maccoby, 1998). In turn, same-gender peer groups tend to promote within-group assimilation (Harris, 1995; Leaper, 1994). That is, children are typically motivated to internalize the norms of a group that is important to them.

Group socialization processes can have different degrees of impact on individuals' motives depending on the status and power of one group relative to another group (or to other groups). Two corollaries of social identity theory are relevant. First, members of high-status groups are usually more invested in maintaining group boundaries than members of low-status groups (e.g., Bigler, Brown, & Markell, 2001). Given the greater status and power traditionally accorded to males in society, boys are more likely to maintain role and group boundaries (see Leaper, 1994). Partly for this reason, gender-typing pressures tend to be more rigid for boys than for girls. A second pertinent corollary is that characteristics associated with a high-status group are typically valued more than those of a low-status group. Thus, masculine-stereotyped attributes (e.g., assertiveness) tend to be valued more than feminine-stereotyped attributes (e.g., nurturance) in highly male-dominated societies (see Hofstede, 2000). Although cross-gender-typed behavior can sometimes enhance a girl's status, it typically diminishes a boy's status (see Leaper, 1994). Accordingly, cross-gender-typed behavior tends to be more common among girls than among boys.

Biological Processes

According to Wood and Eagly's (2002) biosocial theory, the most important biologically based physical attributes that differentiate the sexes are women's reproductive capacity and men's greater strength, speed, and size. Gender-differentiated roles tend to occur in societies wherein women's nursing and infant care hinder their performance of subsistence activities that require, for example, extended time away from home. However, cultural and technological changes have weakened gender-differentiated roles and patriarchy in many postindustrial societies: Women have gained control over their reproduction, and child day care has become common. Moreover, strength, speed, and size are no longer important within these societies for most jobs (particularly those with the highest pay and status).

Sex-linked hormones may influence brain differentiation and organization during development, and this can contribute to corresponding differences in brain functioning (see Hines, 2013). For example, sex-related differences in prenatal hormones may partly contribute to average gender differences in certain play preferences. For example, this is implicated in studies of girls with congenital adrenal hyperplasia (CAH), who are exposed to high levels of androgens during prenatal development. Girls with CAH are more likely than other girls to prefer physically active forms of play later in childhood (Hines, 2013).

Socialization pressures can exaggerate the magnitude of some gender differences in behavior that initially stem from a biological disposition. For example, activity level is a temperament quality considered to have some genetic basis. In their meta-analysis, Eaton and Enns (1986) found a small average gender difference favoring boys in activity during infancy; however, the magnitude of the difference was somewhat greater in childhood.[1] Given that adults and peers typically encourage physical activity more in boys than in girls at early ages (e.g., Fagot, 1978), socialization practices may transform a small difference into a moderate one (e.g., Martin & Fabes, 2001). Conversely, biological changes can exaggerate the impact of some social influences. As reviewed later, many girls have body image concerns before puberty. Bodily changes associated with puberty can accentuate these concerns as girls evaluate their bodies in relation to cultural ideals.

Summary

Several processes are implicated in children's gender development. First, social–structural factors include the division of labor and the prevalence of patriarchy in the larger society. The social structure shapes the kinds of opportunities and incentives that children experience. Social structures are enacted in everyday interactions with family members, teachers, peers, and the media. Second, cognitive–motivational factors shape how children interpret and act on their worlds. Finally, biological factors include average physical differences between the sexes that may (or may not) be relevant for carrying out certain roles and activities, depending on the cultural context. Sex-related hormonal influences may affect the organization and activation of the nervous system.

Socialization of Gender-Related Variations in Children's Development

We next consider the socialization of a selective set of outcomes associated with children's gender development. For each topic, we consider evidence for social–structural, parental, and peer influences on gender-typed cognitive–motivational processes and behaviors. When it is especially relevant, we also address the influences of the media and teachers. To limit the chapter's length, we chose areas that we deem to be especially relevant to understanding the developmental context for some of the gender divisions and inequities often seen in adulthood. In particular, we address the childhood socialization of (1) gender self-concepts, stereotypes, and attitudes; (2) gender-typed play; (3) social norms and social interaction; (4) sports; (5) body image; (6) academic achievement; and (7) family role expectations. Another constraint on our review is that the existing research literature focuses primarily on children growing up in middle-class, Western societies (see Henrich, Heine, & Norenzayan, 2010).

Gender Self-Concepts, Stereotypes, and Attitudes

Girls and boys apply their developing representations of gender, known as gender schemas, to interpret the world around them. When considering the development of children's gender schemas, a few distinctions are worth noting. First, gender schemas are applied to different domains of gender typing such as traits, activities, and roles (Liben & Bigler, 2002). Second, individuals form schemas for the self (e.g., personal preferences, identity) and schemas for others (e.g., stereotyped beliefs, attitudes). Third, knowledge of cultural gender stereotypes does not necessitate their endorsement (Liben & Bigler, 2002). Finally, children vary in the specific ways that they see themselves as gender-typed or in the particular gender stereotypes they might endorse (Liben & Bigler, 2002; Tobin et al., 2010).

Children's acquisition and development of gender-related cognitions tend to follow a systematic pattern (see Martin et al., 2002, for a review). Children are capable of making perceptual distinctions between gender-linked physical attributes (e.g., faces, gender-typed objects) as they approach 1 year of age. Verbal indications of a gender concept appear around 2 years of age, when children begin to use gender to label other people (i.e., gender labeling). Next, around 3 years of age, children demonstrate knowledge of their own gender (i.e., gender identity). Between 3 and 6 years of age, children's concepts of other people's and their own gender become increasingly stable and consistent (i.e., gender constancy). During this age period, children also begin to form stereotypes about physical features and activities (e.g., girls wear dresses and boys play with trucks). Children around 6 years of age also tend to stereotype more abstract qualities such as social roles (e.g., men are truck drivers) and psychological attributes (e.g., women are nice). When girls and boys attach importance to their gender identity, they tend to seek consistency in their gender-related self-concepts and stereotypes (Tobin et al., 2010).

As children undergo further advances in cognitive development during middle childhood and adolescence, they typically recognize that gender roles are social conventions that can be modified (Killen & Stangor, 2001; Serbin, Powlishta, & Gulko, 1993). Many adolescents embrace these conventions and endorse traditional gender roles. However, greater cognitive flexibility allows for the possibility that they may adopt gender-egalitarian views. Between middle childhood and adolescence, children also may begin to understand and recognize sexism and other forms of discrimination (Brown & Bigler, 2005).

Social–Structural Influences

Parents' gender attitudes may differ according to education, socioeconomic status, dual- or single-parent status, sexual orientation, and race/ethnicity (see Leaper, 2013). There is also evidence of historical changes in gender attitudes and self-concepts in Western cultures. During the last three decades of the 20th century, adolescent girls' and young women's gender role self-concepts steadily became less traditional (Twenge, 1997b), and their gender attitudes steadily became more egalitarian (Twenge, 1997a). Although research suggests that men have generally become more flexible in their views about women's roles (Twenge, 1997a), they still tend to view themselves in gender-typed ways (Twenge, 1997b). A similar pattern may occur in childhood. In one study, boys scored higher on average than girls in self-perceived gender typicality and felt gender conformity pressure (Egan & Perry, 2001).

Media Influences

Content analyses of media targeting children indicate that gender stereotyping remains pervasive in children's media across the world (Diekman & Murnen, 2004; Leaper, Breed, Hoffman, & Perlman, 2002; Signorielli, 2012). Gender stereotypes are commonly observed in most media targeting children in two ways (Signorielli, 2012). First, children will likely infer that men have higher status in society than do women through the over-representation of male characters in most television cartoon series, movies, and children's book. Second, the characters typically reflect gender-stereotyped roles and attributes. Given the prevalence of gender stereotyping in popular culture, it is no surprise that children's media consumption is positively correlated with their own degree of gender stereotyping (Signorielli, 2012). Children's gender schemas may guide what they watch and read; in turn, what children watch and read may shape their gender schemas.

Family and Peer Influences

In a meta-analysis, H. R. Tenenbaum and Leaper (2002) reviewed studies testing the relation between parents' and children's gender self-concepts and attitudes. Across studies, there was a statistically significant but small association between parents' gender attitudes and children's gender schemas. The small magnitude of the correlation may be partly due to the indirect pathway between parents' attitudes and children's beliefs. Parents must communicate their attitudes in a way that their children can learn them (Leaper & Bigler, 2004). But parents' attitudes may not be apparent to children because parents' attitudes and actions are not always consistent (Friedman, Leaper, & Bigler, 2007; Gelman, Taylor, & Nguyen, 2004).

Older siblings are other family members who may influence some children's gender attitudes and self-concepts. Farkas and Leaper (2014) conducted a meta-analysis to examine whether the older sibling's gender was related to children's gender typing in self-perceived traits, interests, activities, or behaviors. A small effect size indicated that girls and boys were significantly more likely to score higher on traditionally masculine characteristics if they had an older brother rather than an older sister. There was no significant association between scores on traditionally feminine characteristics and older sibling's gender, which may reflect the higher status accorded to masculine-stereotyped than to feminine-stereotyped qualities. Due the limited number of pertinent studies, however, Farkas and Leaper advised caution when drawing inferences from their meta-analysis.

Finally, it is important to note that peers can have a strong influence on the development of children's gender self-concepts, stereotypes, and attitudes. We address their influence in subsequent sections on children's play activities and social relationships.

Play

Although there is variability across individuals, average gender differences in play preferences are reliably observed to have large effect sizes (see Hines, 2013; Leaper, 2013; Maccoby, 1998). Preferences for gender-stereotyped toys typically emerge between the ages 1 and 2 years. For example, girls are more likely than boys to prefer dolls and cooking sets, and boys are more likely to prefer trucks and building toys. Girls and boys also tend to differ in pretend play starting around 2–3 years of age. Girls' sociodramatic play commonly focuses on domestic situations; boys' fantasy play tends to involve action–adventure stories. As many boys get older, their continued interest in aggression and adventure themes is expressed through play with video games that simulate violence or sports (Cherney & London, 2006). Similar patterns of average gender difference in toy and play preferences have been observed in North America and Europe, including highly gender-egalitarian countries such as Sweden (Nelson, 2005).

Play activities are important contexts for the socialization of gender because they provide opportunities for practicing particular behaviors. With repeated practice, play behaviors are likely to have an impact on children's developing expectations, preferences, and abilities (Bussey & Bandura, 1999; Leaper, 2000b). In general, masculine-stereotyped activities allow practice in self-assertive behaviors (e.g., object mastery, competition), whereas feminine-stereotyped activities offer practice in behaviors that are simultaneously affiliative and assertive (e.g., nurturance, collaborative discourse). On average, girls are more likely than boys to participate in both kinds of activities and thereby practice a broader repertoire of skills (see Leaper, 2013).

Although most children's play activities are amenable to social influences (reviewed below), a subset of young children (perhaps especially boys) demonstrate intense interests in particular activities (DeLoache, Simcock, & Macari, 2007). Some children with intense interests may strongly prefer certain gender-typed toys even though their parents encourage interest in a broader range of toys. Other children with intense interests strongly favor cross-gender-typed toys despite sanctions from parents or peers to do otherwise (Fridell, Owen-Anderson, Johnson, Bradley, & Zucker, 2006). Thus, dispositional factors appear to take priority over cognitive and social forces during some children's gender development.

Media Influences

Television advertisements for children's toys both model and reinforce gender-typed play for girls and boys (see Signorielli, 2012). Television commercials underscore the message that certain toys are either "for boys" or "for girls." Boys in the ads tend to exhibit action-oriented and aggressive play. In contrast, girls in commercials tend to nurture dolls and take an interest in fashion and beauty. Research indicates that these images can reinforce children's gender-typed play beliefs and preferences (e.g., Pike & Jennings, 2005).

Parental Influences

In a meta-analysis of studies on North American parents' gender typing across 19 socialization areas, Lytton and Romney (1991) found that the differential encouragement of particular play and other activities is the manner whereby parents most reliably treat daughters and sons differently. Indeed, parents commonly purchase gender-stereotyped toys for their children within a few months after birth—before children express gender-typed toy preferences themselves (see Leaper, 2013). By around 2–3 years of age, children begin to plead for particular toys. In turn, parents typically reinforce children's gender-typed toy and play requests (e.g., Lindsey, Mize, & Pettit, 1997). The Lytton and Romney (1991) meta-analysis was based on studies conducted over 20 years ago; therefore, one might question whether parents in Western societies are becoming more flexible in attitudes about gender-appropriate play. There is some evidence that this might be happening in some Western countries (Blakemore & Hill, 2008; Servin & Bohlin, 1999; Wood, Desmarais, & Gugula, 2002).

There are a few factors worth noting that can moderate the likelihood of parents' gender typing of children's play (and possibly other behavioral outcomes). First, parents tend to be stricter enforcers of gender conformity in sons than in daughters (Kane, 2006; Wood et al., 2002). Second, parents with traditional gender attitudes may be more likely than parents with egalitarian attitudes to encourage gender-typed play in their young children (Blakemore & Hill, 2008). Third, in many heterosexual, two-parent families, fathers tend to be more likely than mothers to have traditional gender attitudes and to encourage gender-typed play (Kane, 2006; Lytton & Romney, 1991). Finally, young children's play may be less gender-stereotyped in families with lesbian or gay parents than with heterosexual parents (e.g., Goldberg, Kashy, Smith, 2012).

In future years, we hope to see more studies that consider whether and how historical trends toward egalitarian gender roles in society might be related to parents' differential treatment of daughters and sons. Furthermore, more research is needed to test the extent that parental encouragement or discouragement affects children's play preferences. After early childhood, girls' and boys' play preferences may depend more on peer and media influences.

Teacher Influences

Teachers contribute to the gender-typing of children's play, for example, when they label toys or activities as for one gender or the other (Bigler & Liben, 2007; Serbin, Connor, & Iler, 1979). By the same token, when teachers assign girls and boys to similar activities, gender differences in social behavior can be reduced (e.g., Carpenter, Huston, & Holt, 1986). Finally, as seen with parents, many teachers may be more tolerant of cross-gender-typed play behavior in girls than in boys (Cahill & Adams, 1997; Fagot, 1981).

Peer Influences

In many respects, peers may constitute the most important social influence on children's gender-typed play. First, same-gender peers are *role models* that children use to infer gender-normative behavior. Children are more likely to play with a gender-neutral toy— or even a cross-gender-typed toy—after observing a same-gender (vs. cross-gender) model (e.g., Bussey & Perry, 1982). In addition, many peers are vigilant *enforcers* of traditional gender norms. Peers generally disapprove of cross-gender-typed behavior (Martin, 1989), and children quickly infer what their peers consider acceptable and unacceptable. These social norms become internalized as personal standards that guide children's behavior (Bussey & Bandura, 1999).

The impact of same-gender peer groups on play preferences was documented in a short-term longitudinal study. Martin and Fabes (2001) observed what they called a *social dosage effect*: The more that preschool children played with same-gender peers from fall to spring, the more likely they showed increases in gender-typed play behavior.

Social Norms and Social Interaction

Around 3 years of age, children begin to show a preference for same-gender peers (known as *gender segregation*). This preference steadily increases until around 6 years of age, then remains stable until the onset of adolescence (Maccoby, 1998). To the extent that girls' and boys' peer groups emphasize different activities and patterns of social interaction, gendered social norms and goals tend to emerge (see Leaper, 1994; Rose & Rudolph, 2006). In particular, different norms are often seen in the expression of *affiliation* (inter-personal sensitivity, responsiveness, and closeness) and *assertion* (independence, agency, and competition). However, there is variability in social norms with each gender, and the enactment of gender-typed norms in social behavior tends to be context-specific.

Girls' gender-typed play and relationships cultivate the development of social norms emphasizing the coordination of affiliation *with* assertion. That is, contrary to some stereotypes, research does *not* support the notion that gender-typed girls' social interactions are unassertive; instead, it appears that girls are more likely than boys to coordinate affiliative and assertive goals, producing what are known as *collaborative behaviors* (see Leaper, 1991; Leaper, Tenenbaum, & Shaffer, 1999; Leman, Ahmed, & Ozarow, 2005). Examples of collaborative communication include initiatives for joint activity ("Let's play house") and elaborating on the other speaker's comments. A meta-analysis (Leaper & Smith, 2004) indicated that collaborative and other affiliative forms of speech in children's peer interactions are more likely among girls than among boys (with a small effect size).

Gender-related variations in affiliation are also seen in the expression of intimacy in children's friendships. Self-disclosure is more likely among girls than among boys during childhood and adolescence (e.g., Rose, 2002). Also, females are more likely than males to provide active listening responses to comfort friends in childhood and adolescence (Burleson, 1982; Leaper, Carson, Baker, Holliday, & Myers, 1995).

In contrast to the patterns that may be common among girls, boys' gender-typed play and social relations tend to reflect social norms stressing self-assertion *over* affiliation. According to one meta-analysis of gender differences in speech (Leaper & Smith, 2004), boys were significantly more likely than girls (with a small effect size) to use directive speech (high in assertion and relatively low in affiliation). Another meta-analysis revealed a slightly higher likelihood of verbal aggression (e.g., insults) among boys than among girls (Card, Stucky, Sawalani, & Little, 2008). The latter meta-analysis also indicated a medium effect size regarding physical aggression (e.g., hitting), which was more likely for boys than girls.

Contrary to some earlier proposals that *indirect aggression* (also known as *social aggression* or *relational aggression*) is more common among girls than boys (see Underwood, 2003, for a review), a recent meta-analysis indicated only a very slight trend in this direction (Card et al., 2008). Thus, there does not appear to be a meaningful average gender difference in rates of indirect aggression; however, indirect aggression may constitute a higher proportion of all aggressive acts among girls than among boys (see Leaper, 2013).

Gender-related aggressive behaviors sometimes involve sexual harassment (see American Association of University Women, 2011; Leaper & Robnett, 2011). Verbal forms of sexual harassment include making sexually demeaning or homophobic insults or repeatedly offering unwanted sexual comments. These messages can also be transmitted through electronic media such as text messaging and online postings. Physical forms of sexual harassment include unwanted touching or sexual coercion. Recent surveys of adolescents in the United States and other countries indicate that sexual harassment is a problem for many girls and boys. For example, in the American Association of University Women (2011) survey of American middle school and high school students, 56% of girls and 40% of boys reported experiences with sexual harassment. Repeated experience with sexual harassment is associated with socioemotional and academic difficulties, with stronger impacts seen in girls than in boys, and in sexual-minority than in heterosexual youth (see American Association of University Women, 2011; Leaper & Robnett, 2011).

Social–Structural Influences

In their cross-cultural analysis, Wood and Eagly (2002) noted an association between adult roles in the society and the socialization of affiliation and assertion. Childrearing practices tended to stress nurturance more in girls than in boys in societies where women's primary role is caregiver; in contrast, the encouragement of independence and self-assertion in girls was more common in relatively gender-egalitarian societies compared to more traditional societies. Thus, the socialization of gender-typed social interaction styles can reflect and perpetuate traditional adult gender roles (Leaper, 2000b). More research is needed to examine whether and how the gendered division of work and family roles in a culture influences gender-related variations in children's social behavior. We also need more work aimed at understanding how and why some children and adults challenge traditional gender norms and contribute to the transformation of the society.

Sexual harassment also can be seen as reflecting and maintaining gender inequalities in status and power (see American Association of University Women, 2011; Leaper, 2013). When sexual harassment is directed toward girls, it demeans them as sexual objects. When sexual harassment is directed toward boys, it often involves homophobic and misogynistic insults that reify traditional views of masculinity. In addition, the harassment of sexual minorities (gays, lesbians, bisexuals, and transgender youth) also can be seen as enforcing traditional gender roles.

Parental Influences

Researchers have noted that many parents tend to encourage self-assertion and to tolerate aggression in sons more than in daughters. Conversely, many parents tend to foster closeness and expressiveness in daughters more than in sons (see Leaper, 2013). For example, in a meta-analysis, there were significant but small average differences between mothers and fathers in affiliative and assertive speech, as well as differences in speech to daughters and sons (Leaper, Anderson, & Sanders, 1998). Overall, fathers used significantly more directive speech than did mothers, and mothers used significantly more supportive speech than did fathers. The analyses also revealed small effect sizes, indicating that mothers tended to use more supportive speech and more directive speech with daughters than with sons. (There were not enough available studies to compare fathers' speech to daughters versus sons in the meta-analysis.) In these ways, mothers tended to emphasize affiliation more with daughters, and to allow self-assertion more with sons. Sequential analyses suggest that parents' gender-typed speech can influence children's communication (Leaper, 2000a); however, longitudinal research is needed to explore more fully how parents' communication style may influence children's gender development.

Peer Influences

Gender-typed social norms in same-gender peer groups may foster the enactment of different social behaviors for many girls and boys (Maccoby, 1998). Several features of the peer context, however, can moderate the likelihood of gender differences in affiliative and assertive behavior. One of them is the type of activity in which the children are participating (Leaper & Smith, 2004). To the extent that boys and girls consistently participate in different activities, they are likely to exert affiliation and assertion differently (see the earlier section on play). The opposite of this may apply. For example, Zarbatany, McDougall, and Hymel (2000) found that adolescent boys' participation in communal activities was positively related to their friendship intimacy.

Group size is another factor that can moderate the likelihood of gender differences in social behavior. Conformity pressures are more likely to occur in groups than in dyadic relationships (Harris, 1995). Research also indicates that children (girls as well as boys) are more competitive in larger groups and less competitive in dyads (Benenson, Nicholson, Waite, Roy, & Simpson, 2001). The finding that boys are more likely than girls to congregate in larger groups may partly explain boys' greater gender-role rigidity and use of power-assertive social behaviors.

Finally, the gender composition of the dyad or group is an important moderator of gender differences in social behavior. For example, many boys (and men) are reluctant to disclose personal feelings to male peers; instead, they sometimes turn to females to meet their needs for emotional support. This was suggested in a meta-analysis (Dindia & Allen, 1992) reporting that average gender differences in self-disclosure were smaller in cross-gender than in same-gender interactions. Many boys may be averse to disclosing to male friends out of concern with appearing tough (see Tolman, Spencer, Harmon, Rosen-Reynoso, & Striepe, 2004).

Sports

Participation in sports is correlated with physical self-efficacy, positive body image, high self-esteem, peer acceptance, and academic success for both boys and girls (e.g., Daniels & Leaper, 2006; Fredricks & Eccles, 2006). However, because sports are strongly associated with cultural constructions of masculinity, girls and women have historically been excluded from athletics. Furthermore, as described below, the macho sports culture can foster sexist, misogynistic, and homophobic attitudes in boys.

Social–Structural Influences

The importance of sport in boys' lives increased over the last century in Western societies in response to changes in the male role. At the beginning of the 20th century, boys' daily activities shifted from helping on the family farm to sitting in female-headed classrooms. Also, physical strength became less relevant for most occupations. Organized sports countered some people's fear that boys and men were becoming feminized (see Messner, 1992). The strong tie between sports and masculinity contributed to the exclusion of girls and women from sports.

Coinciding with the women's movement, girls' participation in sports dramatically increased in the United States after the 1972 enactment of Title IX of the United States Civil Rights Act (requiring equal opportunities for girls and boys in publicly funded schools). From the time of Title IX's passage, girls' participation in high school sports has increased from 1 in 27 to 1 in 2.5. In comparison, boys' participation has remained 1 in 2 during the last 30 years (National Federation of State High School Associations, 2013). Similar increases in girls' and women's sport participation occurred in many other countries during recent decades. By way of illustration, women's representation at the Olympiad Games has steadily increased from 11% in 1960 to 44% in 2012 (International Olympic Committee, 2013).

Media Influences

Regardless of whether they actively follow sports themselves, most children are exposed to sports in the media through their family or friends. The media both reflect and perpetuate society's notions of sports and gender. First, the media reinforce the strong ties of sports and masculinity. Despite women's advances in professional athletics, coverage of men's sports dominates in the media (e.g., Adams & Tuggle, 2004). Furthermore, television and magazines regularly perpetuate different images of men and women in sports. Professional male athletes are commonly portrayed as physically aggressive and dominant (G. Tenenbaum, Stewart, Singer, & Duda, 1996). In contrast, when women athletes are profiled in the media, emphasis is frequently placed on their feminine side by depicting them as sexual objects or portraying their heterosexual personal lives (Knight & Giuliano, 2003). These sexualized images of female athletes may contribute to negative body image in adolescent girls and young women (Daniels, 2009)—which is ironic given that athletic participation is generally associated with positive body image.

Parental Influences

As reviewed earlier, support for girls' sports involvement has dramatically increased in the United States and other countries. It is now common for many fathers and mothers in these societies to promote physical activity in their daughters (Weiss, Amorose, & Kip, 2012). However, many parents continue to expect greater athletic achievement in their sons than in their daughters. In turn, these beliefs may become self-fulfilling prophecies that shape their children's sports-related ability beliefs and values (Fredricks & Eccles, 2002).

Peer Influences

Sports are social contexts in which children can gain a sense of belonging with teammates and obtain prestige among their peers. When surveyed, both girls and boys cited social benefits for maintaining their involvement in high school sports; however, girls were more likely than boys to point to the social costs of sports participation as motives for decreasing or ending their involvement (Patrick et al., 1999). During adolescence, female athleticism may conflict with some girls' notions of femininity and heterosexuality (Cockburn & Clarke, 2002).

For boys, athletics has typically been associated with popularity and prestige in American schools. However, there are often costs that go along with boys' sports involvement. The male sports culture has traditionally emphasized macho norms stressing aggression, dominance, sexism, and homophobia (e.g., Osborne & Wagner, 2007). The macho pose also involves hiding vulnerable feelings, which can undermine friendship intimacy (Zarbatany et al., 2000).

Body Image

Western society emphasizes a narrowly defined standard of physical attractiveness for females (e.g., thinness) and males (e.g., muscularity). Felt pressure to attain cultural body ideals can have negative consequences on the body self-images of girls and boys. The most frequently studied facets of body image are body dissatisfaction, self-objectification, internalization of the ideal body, and body change strategies (Grabe, Ward, & Hyde, 2008). Although many girls and boys experience body image problems, they tend to be more acute for girls than for boys. A meta-analysis testing for gender differences in body satisfaction found a medium effect size indicating that males reported higher average body satisfaction than did females, and that this gender difference has been increasing for the last several decades (Feingold & Mazzella, 1998). Poor body image also tends to be related to eating disorders and other adjustment difficulties (Grabe & Hyde, 2009; Slater & Tiggemann, 2002). Around 3.8% of females and 1.5% of males in the United States develop an eating disorder sometime during their lives (Merikangas et al., 2010).

Studies show that body dissatisfaction in many girls emerges by around age 8, with some reports suggesting even earlier ages of onset (Clark & Tiggemann, 2006; Ricciardelli & McCabe, 2001). During adolescence, girls' body satisfaction tends to decrease with age, whereas boys' body satisfaction tends to increase with age (Bearman, Presnell, Martinez, & Stice, 2006). Among girls (but not boys), early pubertal development tends to be related to lower body satisfaction (Petrie, Greenleaf, & Martin, 2010).

Increasing attention is being paid to body image problems among boys. Concerns about muscularity are more prevalent among boys than among girls (e.g., Muris, Meesters, van de Blom, & Mayer, 2005; Ricciardelli, McCabe, Lillis, & Thomas, 2006). Boys' dissatisfaction with muscularity tends to be related to negative psychological (e.g., self-esteem) and physical (e.g., steroid use) outcomes (Cohane & Pope, 2001).

Social–Structural Influences

There are cultural and ethnic variations in standards of beauty. For example, in the United States, girls' concerns with thinness may be less prevalent in African American communities than among other ethnic groups. On average, African American girls tend to report higher body satisfaction than European American, Asian American, or Latina girls (Grabe & Hyde, 2006); however, the effect sizes tend to be small. Moreover, girls from all ethnic groups may experience pressures to attain the dominant culture's beauty ideals. As reviewed next, the media play a powerful role in shaping these views.

Media Influences

Images of girls and women in the mass media are disproportionately idealized and sexualized (American Psychological Association Task Force on the Sexualization of Girls, 2007). A meta-analysis indicates that exposure to mass media is related to lower body satisfaction, higher internalizing symptoms, and more disordered eating in adolescent and young adult women (Grabe et al., 2008). Similar patterns have been indicated in studies of younger children (Dohnt & Tiggemann, 2006). Moreover, the effects of media exposure seem to be cumulative over time. In a study of 11- to 16-year-old girls, older girls were more likely than younger girls to have internalized cultural body ideals; in turn, this internalization was related to a downward trend with age in girls' body satisfaction (Clay, Vignoles, & Dittmar, 2005).

Although media messages about idealized bodies may not be as pervasive for boys as they are for girls, the mass media also perpetuate idealized images of the male body. Studies show that media exposure is related to preadolescent and adolescent boys' desire to gain muscle mass and to become fit (Ricciardelli et al., 2006). Also, media exposure to muscular ideals may negatively influence adolescent boys' body satisfaction (Barlett, Vowels, & Saucier, 2008) and increase their likelihood of eating disorders (Peterson, Paulson, & Williams, 2007).

Parental Influences

Parents may influence their children's body satisfaction through modeling and through direct comments about the child's body. For example, in one study, 5-year-old girls' knowledge of dieting was related to their mothers' past and current dieting behavior

(Abramovitz & Birch, 2000). In another report, preadolescent girls who had mothers with low body satisfaction were more likely to have disordered eating 2 years later (Attie & Brooks-Gunn, 1989). In some studies, parents' negative comments regarding their children's weight predicted girls' and boys' body dissatisfaction (Phares, Steinberg, & Thompson, 2004; Smolak, Levine, & Schermer, 1999). Parents may also directly encourage their children to lose weight, which has been related to dieting in adolescent girls (Wertheim, Mee, & Paxton, 1999). Perceived pressure from parents to look a certain way has also been related to more disordered eating among both girls and boys (Peterson et al., 2007). In addition, parents' comments may be more strongly related to body dissatisfaction for girls than for boys (Phares et al., 2004; Smolak et al., 1999).

Peer Influences

Peers can affect one another's body dissatisfaction through teasing and negative comments (McCabe & Ricciardelli, 2001). Furthermore, girls tend to report having more conversations about appearance with peers, and the frequency of these conversations tends to be related to girls' body dissatisfaction (Clark & Tiggemann, 2006). Research also indicates the pressure that boys feel from peers, parents, and the media influences their body dissatisfaction and their strategies to change their bodies (Ricciardelli et al., 2006).

Academic Motivation and Achievement

Understanding gender-related variations in academic achievement is important given the continued gender disparities favoring men in income and many occupations. In some respects, one might expect females to fare better than males in achievement. For example, in most industrialized countries, girls tend to show somewhat higher overall academic achievement than boys from elementary to high school (American Association of University Women, 2008; United Nations Educational, Scientific and Cultural Organization [UNESCO], 2010). A more nuanced picture is seen, however, when particular subjects are examined. Girls tend to score higher than boys on reading and writing tests, with small-to-medium effect sizes. In contrast, math and science are areas in which boys historically have done better than girls, but American girls and boys now attain comparable average test scores in mathematics and life sciences (see Halpern, 2012).

Research guided by the expectancy–value model of achievement demonstrates that children's academic motivation and aspirations are strongly related to their competence-related expectations and values (Eccles & Wigfield, 2002; Simpkins, Fredricks, & Eccles, Chapter 26, this volume). Studies have indicated average gender differences in ability expectations in some of the same subjects associated with differences in achievement such as reading, writing, and computers (Whitley, 1997; Wilgenbusch & Merrell, 1999). However, some gender differences in self-perceived competence may occur in subjects no longer associated with differences in actual achievement. For example, boys tend to have stronger ability beliefs in math than do girls despite a lack of average difference in performance (Else-Quest, Hyde, & Linn, 2010). More boys may overestimate their ability, whereas more girls may underestimate their ability (Furnham, 2001). Average gender differences in perceived competence may have consequences at later ages, when youth make career-related decisions (Eccles & Wigfield, 2002).

Boys' and girls' values also shape academic motivation and achievement (Eccles & Wigfield, 2002). For some boys, endorsement of traditional masculinity ideology may undermine engagement and success in school (Kessels & Steinmayr, 2013; Kiefer & Ryan, 2008; Santos, Galligan, Pahlke, & Fabes, 2013). That is, boys who are concerned about appearing tough may be reluctant to comply with teachers' authority or to seek help.

For many girls, interpersonal values may partly shape their academic interests and achievement. For example, girls tend to be more interested in occupations that have helping goals (Morgan, Isaac, & Sansone, 2001); perhaps partly for this reason, girls who do well in science are more likely to go into medical and health science fields than other scientific or technological areas (Tilleczek & Lewko, 2001). As they get older, girls are also more likely than boys to consider work–family balance when evaluating career options (Mahaffy & Ward, 2002).

Social–Structural Influences

Paralleling changes in Western women's roles over the last four decades, there has been a steady closing of the gender gap in children's math achievement (Lindberg, Hyde, Petersen, & Linn, 2010) and an increase in the number of women in the United States (and many other Western countries) receiving science and engineering degrees (National Science Foundation, 2008). Socioeconomic status may also account for variability in gender differences in academic achievement. Smaller average gender differences in academic achievement were seen among children in higher-income neighborhoods or among those with highly educated parents (Burkam, Lee, & Smerdon, 1997).

Parental Influences

Longitudinal studies indicate that parents' gender-related beliefs and attitudes predict gender-related variations in children's academic self-concepts and achievement (e.g., Eccles, Freedman-Doan, Frome, Jacobs, & Yoon, 2000). However, not all parents hold gender-typed expectations about their children's abilities. Research suggests that girls may be more likely to do better in math and science when they have gender-egalitarian parents (Updegraff, McHale, & Crouter, 1996).

Teacher Influences

Some teachers have stereotyped expectations about girls' and boys' abilities in particular subject areas (see Gunderson, Ramirez, Levine, & Beilock, 2012). Other teachers may consciously disavow gender stereotypes but unwittingly perpetuate them; this can occur because most teachers are not trained to recognize and to prevent the many subtle forms of gender stereotyping (Spencer, Porche, & Tolman, 2003). These potential biases are important because teachers' expectations can act as self-fulfilling prophecies that affect children's later achievement (see Jussim & Harber, 2005).

Peer Influences

Same-gender peers serve as important sources for social comparison that many children use to evaluate their own achievement and occupational aspirations (Altermatt,

Pomerantz, Ruble, Frey, & Greulich, 2002; Young et al., 1999). When children affiliate in peer groups that are supportive of academic success, they are more likely to do well in school (Wentzel, Donlan, & Morrison, 2012). Peer norms about academic success may be domain-specific, whereby peer support for particular academic subjects may influence girls' and boys' motivation to maintain their interest in those particular subjects (Robnett & Leaper, 2013; Stake & Nickens, 2005).

When the peer culture reflects a negative attitude toward school achievement, children may fare poorly. For example, in one study, most adolescent girls had heard sexist comments, most commonly from peers, about girls' abilities in math, science, or computers (Leaper & Brown, 2008). The amount that girls reported hearing these discouraging comments was negatively related to their math and science ability beliefs and values (Brown & Leaper, 2010).

The traditional male peer culture may contribute to many of boys' difficulties in school adjustment and achievement. Thus, some boys have been shown to experience a conflict between their need to maintain an image of masculinity based on power and dominance and their perceptions of academic work and success as feminine pursuits (Kessels & Steinmayr, 2013).

Family Role Expectations

Dramatic transformations in the family have occurred during the last 50 years in many industrialized and technological societies. Today, married women typically juggle both career and family work. In contrast, married men's contributions to child care and housework have shown only modest *average* increases over the years (Krantz-Kent, 2009)—although there are many men who do share equally in domestic work with their spouses. Adult women's and men's household and work participation may be related to the expectations they develop during childhood and adolescence regarding adult roles. Starting in adolescence, girls tend to report more interpersonal goals (e.g., marriage, family) and boys tend to report more career goals (see Massey, Gebhardt, & Garnefski, 2008).

Social–Structural Influences

Daughters' and sons' assignment to household work is related to the parents' socioeconomic level, marital status, employment, family size, and cultural background (Cunningham, 2001; Hilton & Haldeman, 1991). In general, when family resources are limited (e.g., low income, single parenthood, large family size), children are more likely to be assigned household chores—with daughters especially likely to be assigned child care responsibilities. Furthermore, in cultures in which there is a traditional division of labor between women and men, childrearing practices are more likely to encourage nurturance in girls than in boys (see Wood & Eagly, 2002). Thus, assigning children to gender-typed household chores both reflects and perpetuates gender-differentiated roles in society (Etaugh & Liss, 1992).

Media Influences

Children and adolescents learn about gender-typed work and family roles in part from the mass media. Content analyses of television programming indicate that gender-role stereotyping of work and family roles is prevalent, although stereotyping has become less pervasive than it was a few decades ago (see Signorielli, 2012). Women are still more likely than men to be represented in family roles. Conversely, men are represented in work roles more consistently than are women. Women are frequently portrayed in traditionally male-dominated roles (e.g., lawyers, doctors, crime investigators). However, it is less common to see men presented in traditionally female-dominated roles (e.g., primary caregivers, elementary school teachers).

Parental Influences

Studies of children's household work in North America indicate a few patterns that are pertinent to gender socialization. First, mothers and fathers typically model a traditional division of labor in their own household work (Krantz-Kent, 2009). When mothers and fathers share household work, their children may later be more likely to have positive attitudes toward equal role sharing in marriage (Cunningham, 2001).

Some research indicates that lesbian and gay couples tend to be more egalitarian in the division of household labor and child care than heterosexual couples (Peplau & Fingerhut, 2007). By contrast, heterosexual couples often become less egalitarian in their division of household labor after having children. Thus, having lesbian or gay parents may increase egalitarian role expectations in children.

Besides role modeling, another way that parents may socialize their children's family role expectations is through the gender-typed assignment of household chores. Many parents are more likely to appoint child care and cleaning to daughters than to sons; and to consign maintenance work to sons than to daughters (Antill, Goodnow, Russell, & Cotton, 1996). Girls also are more likely than boys to be assigned household tasks in general (McHale, Bartko, Crouter, & Perry-Jenkins, 1990). In these ways, women's relegation to household work begins in childhood. Through their observations of parents' division of household labor and their own assigned chores, children may form notions of entitlement and obligation regarding household work that they carry into adulthood (Emler & Hall, 1994; Wood & Eagly, 2002).

Conclusions

This review has highlighted some of the important ways that gender is socialized from infancy into adolescence. We reviewed areas of socialization during childhood that have some of the most important consequences relative to adult roles and functioning. A developmental analysis of gender similarities and differences has two important values. First, by considering gender as a moderator, we gain a better appreciation of developmental processes in general. For example, the study of gender development reveals some of the ways that self-concepts, attitudes, and social processes are interrelated and shape developmental outcomes.

A second reason for studying gender development is to understand how gender-related variations in adult roles and status emerge. For example, the traditional division of labor by gender among adults is commonly practiced in children's play. Girls are the ones who typically recreate domestic roles (e.g., caring for baby dolls). In contrast, boys are often exploring the outside world and engaging in competitive behaviors (e.g., team sports). Children may also observe that males have higher status in society, as reflected in prevalent portrayals of gender in the media and in real life. We also have reviewed how gender-typed patterns in children's academic achievement and household chores may partly pave the way for later gender imbalances in adult occupations and family roles.

Although gender-typed patterns tend to occur, they are not always inevitable. Even when there are average behavioral differences between girls and boys, there is usually much overlap between the two genders, as well as variability within each gender (Hyde, 2005). The dramatic changes in women's and men's roles and status in Western societies during the last 50 years further underscore the human capacity for flexibility (see Leaper, 2000b; Wood & Eagly, 2002). However, there have been greater increases in gender-role flexibility for girls and women than for boys and men. This is partly attributed to the higher status traditionally associated with males, whereby females' adoption of masculine-stereotyped behaviors can lead to increased status, but males' adoption of feminine-stereotyped behaviors can lead to lowered status (Feinman, 1981). Nonetheless, gender-role change is also occurring for many men.

According to the dialectical model of development (Riegel, 1976), individuals and societies change one another. Cultural pressures shape how children develop. At the same time, during the course of development, individuals shape their society. To better understand these processes, longitudinal studies of gender development need to test which kinds of socialization experiences during childhood and adolescence might be linked to adult gender roles. In addition, we need to consider whether and how certain child characteristics, such as temperament or personality, make some individuals more likely to be norm breakers that change society's notions about gender (e.g., see Curtin, Stewart, & Duncan, 2010).

ACKNOWLEDGMENT

We thank Carly Friedman for her assistance on the version of this chapter appearing in the first edition of the *Handbook of Socialization*.

NOTE

1. When comparing two groups, an *effect size* refers to the magnitude of difference between the two averages. The amount of overlap between the two groups' distributions is one way to index an effect size. According to Cohen's (1988) conventions, a group difference is considered *trivial* when there is more than 85% overlap between the distributions; *small but meaningful* when the overlap is between 66 and 85%; *medium or moderate* when the overlap is between 53 and 65%; and *large* when the overlap is less than 53%.

REFERENCES

Abramovitz, B. A., & Birch, L. L. (2000). Five-year-old girls' ideas about dieting are predicted by mothers' dieting. *Journal of the American Dietetic Association, 100*, 1157–1163.

Adams, T., & Tuggle, C. A. (2004). ESPN's Sports Center and coverage of women's athletics: "It's a boys' club." *Mass Communication and Society, 7*, 237–248.

Altermatt, E. R., Pomerantz, E. M., Ruble, D. N., Frey, K. S., & Greulich, F. K. (2002). Predicting changes in children's self-perceptions of academic competence: A naturalistic examination of evaluative discourse among classmates. *Developmental Psychology, 38,* 903–917.

American Association of University Women. (2008). *Where the girls are: The facts about gender equity in education.* Washington, DC: Author.

American Association of University Women. (2011). *Crossing the line: Sexual harassment at school.* Washington, DC: Author.

American Psychological Association, Task Force on the Sexualization of Girls. (2007). *Report of the APA Task Force on the sexualization of girls.* Washington, DC: American Psychological Association. Retrieved from *www.apa.org/pi/wpo/sexualization.html.*

Antill, J. K., Goodnow, J. J., Russell, G., & Cotton, S. (1996). The influence of parents and family context on children's involvement in household tasks. *Sex Roles, 34,* 215–236.

Attie, I., & Brooks-Gunn, J. (1989). Development of eating problems in adolescent girls: A longitudinal study. *Developmental Psychology, 25,* 70–79.

Barlett, C. P., Vowels, C. L., & Saucier, D. A. (2008). Meta-analyses of the effects of media images on men's body-image concerns. *Journal of Social and Clinical Psychology, 27,* 279–310.

Bearman, S. K., Presnell, K., Martinez, E., & Stice, E. (2006). The skinny on body dissatisfaction: A longitudinal study of adolescent girls and boys. *Journal of Youth and Adolescence, 35,* 229–241.

Benenson, J. F., Nicholson, C., Waite, A., Roy, R., & Simpson, A. (2001). The influence of group size on children's competitive behavior. *Child Development, 72,* 921–928.

Bigler, R. S., Brown, C. S., & Markell, M. (2001). When groups are not created equal: Effects of group status on the formation of intergroup attitudes in children. *Child Development, 72,* 1151–1162.

Bigler, R. S., & Liben, L. S. (2007). Developmental intergroup theory: Explaining and reducing children's social stereotyping and prejudice. *Current Directions in Psychological Science, 16,* 162–166.

Blakemore, J. E. O., & Hill, C. A. (2008). The child gender socialization scale: A measure to compare traditional and feminist parents. *Sex Roles, 58,* 192–207.

Bronfenbrenner, U., & Morris, P. A. (2006). The bioecological model of human development. In W. Damon & R. M. Lerner (Eds.), *Handbook of child psychology: Vol. 1. Theoretical models of human development* (6th ed., pp. 793–828). Hoboken, NJ: Wiley.

Brown, C. S., & Bigler, R. S. (2005). Children's perceptions of discrimination: A developmental model. *Child Development, 76,* 533–553.

Brown, C. S., & Leaper, C. (2010). Latina and European American girls' experiences with academic sexism and their self-concepts in mathematics and science during adolescence. *Sex Roles, 63,* 860–870.

Burkam, D. T., Lee, V. E., & Smerdon, B. A. (1997). Gender and science learning early in high school: Subject matter and laboratory experiences. *American Educational Research Journal, 34,* 297–331.

Burleson, B. R. (1982). The development of comforting communication skills in childhood and adolescence. *Child Development, 53,* 1578–1588.

Bussey, K., & Bandura, A. (1999). Social cognitive theory of gender development and differentiation. *Psychological Review, 106,* 676–713.

Bussey, K., & Perry, D. G. (1982). Same-sex imitation: The avoidance of cross-sex models or the acceptance of same-sex models? *Sex Roles, 8,* 773–784.

Cahill, B., & Adams, E. (1997). An exploratory study of early childhood teachers' attitudes toward gender roles. *Sex Roles, 36,* 517–529.

Card, N. A., Stucky, B. D., Sawalani, G. M., & Little, T. D. (2008). Direct and indirect aggression during childhood and adolescence: A meta-analytic review of gender differences, intercorrelations, and relations to maladjustment. *Child Development, 79,* 1185–1229.

Carpenter, C. J., Huston, A. C., & Holt, W. (1986). Modification of preschool sex-typed behaviors by participation in adult-structured activities. *Sex Roles, 14,* 603–615.

Cherney, I. D., & London, K. (2006). Gender-linked differences in the toys, television shows, computer games, and outdoor activities of 5- to 13-year-old children. *Sex Roles, 54,* 717–726.

Clark, L., & Tiggemann, M. (2006). Sociocultural and individual psychological predictors of body image in young girls: A prospective study. *Developmental Psychology, 44*, 1124–1134.

Clay, D., Vignoles, V., & Dittmar, H. (2005). Body-image and self-esteem among adolescent females: Testing the influence of sociocultural factors. *Journal for Research on Adolescence, 15*, 451–477.

Cockburn, C., & Clarke, G. (2002). "Everybody's looking at you!": Girls negotiating the "femininity deficit" they incur in physical education. *Women's Studies International Forum, 25*, 651–665.

Cohane, G. H., & Pope, H. G. (2001). Body image in boys: A review of the literature. *International Journal of Eating Disorders, 29*, 373–379.

Cohen, J. (1988). *Statistical power analysis for the behavioral sciences* (2nd ed.). Hillsdale, NJ: Erlbaum.

Cunningham, M. (2001). Parental influences on the gendered division of housework. *American Sociological Review, 66*, 184–203.

Curtin, N., Stewart, A. J., & Duncan, L. E. (2010). What makes the political personal?: Openness, personal political salience, and activism. *Journal of Personality, 78*, 943–968.

Daniels, E. A. (2009). Sex objects, athletes, and sexy athletes: How media representations of women athletes can impact adolescent girls and college women. *Journal of Adolescent Research, 24*, 399–422.

Daniels, E., & Leaper, C. (2006). A longitudinal investigation of sport participation, peer acceptance, and self-esteem among adolescent boys and girls. *Sex Roles, 55*, 875–880.

DeLoache, J. S., Simcock, G., & Macari, S. (2007). Planes, trains, automobiles—and tea sets: Extremely intense interests in very young children. *Developmental Psychology, 43*, 1579–1586.

Diekman, A. B., & Murnen, S. K. (2004). Learning to be little women and little men: The inequitable gender equality of nonsexist children's literature. *Sex Roles, 50*, 373–385.

Dindia, K., & Allen, M. (1992). Sex differences in self-disclosure: A meta-analysis. *Psychological Bulletin, 112*, 106–124.

Dohnt, H., & Tiggemann, M. (2006). The contribution of peer and media influences to the development of body satisfaction and self-esteem in young girls: A prospective study. *Developmental Psychology, 42*, 929–936.

Eaton, W. O., & Enns, L. R. (1986). Sex differences in human motor activity level. *Psychological Bulletin, 100*, 19–28.

Eccles, J. S., Freedman-Doan, C., Frome, P., Jacobs, J., & Yoon, K. S. (2000). Gender-role socialization in the family: A longitudinal approach. In T. Eckes & H. M. Trautner (Eds.), *The developmental social psychology of gender* (pp. 333–360). Mahwah, NJ: Erlbaum.

Eccles, J. S., & Wigfield, A. (2002). Motivational beliefs, values, and goals. *Annual Review of Psychology, 53*, 109–132.

Egan, S. K., & Perry, D. G. (2001). Gender identity: A multidimensional analysis with implications for psychosocial adjustment. *Developmental Psychology, 37*, 451–463.

Else-Quest, N., Hyde, J., & Linn, M. C. (2010). Cross-national patterns of gender differences in mathematics: A meta-analysis. *Psychological Bulletin, 136*, 103–127.

Emler, N. P., & Hall, S. (1994). Economic roles in the household system: Young people's experiences and expectations. In M. Lerner & G. Mikula (Eds.), *Entitlement and the affectional bond: Justice in close relationships* (pp. 281–303). New York: Plenum Press.

Etaugh, C., & Liss, M. B. (1992). Home, school, and playroom: Training grounds for adult gender roles. *Sex Roles, 26*, 129–147.

Fagot, B. I. (1978). The influence of sex of child on parental reactions to toddler children. *Child Development, 49*, 459–465.

Farkas, T., & Leaper, C. (2014). Is having an older brother or older sister related to young siblings' gender typing?: A meta-analysis. In H. Tenenbaum & P. J. Leman (Eds.), *Current issues in psychology* (pp. 63–73). New York: Psychology Press.

Feingold, A., & Mazzella, R. (1998). Gender differences in body image are increasing. *Psychological Science, 9*, 190–195.

Feinman, S. (1981). Why is cross-sex-role behavior more approved for girls than boys?: A status characteristic approach. *Sex Roles, 7*, 289–300.

Fredricks, J. A., & Eccles, J. S. (2002). Children's competence and value beliefs from childhood through adolescence: Growth trajectories in two male-sex-typed domains. *Developmental Psychology, 38*, 519–533.

Fredricks, J. A., & Eccles, J. S. (2006). Is extracurricular participation associated with beneficial outcomes?: Concurrent and longitudinal relations. *Developmental Psychology, 42*, 698–713.

Fridell, S. R., Owen-Anderson, A., Johnson, L. L., Bradley, S. J., & Zucker, K. J. (2006). The playmate and play style preferences structured interview: A comparison of children with gender identity disorder and controls. *Archives of Sexual Behavior, 35*, 729–737.

Friedman, C. K., Leaper, C., & Bigler, R. S. (2007). Do mothers' gender-related attitudes or comments predict young children's gender beliefs? *Parenting: Science and Practice, 7*, 357–366.

Furnham, A. (2001). Self-estimates of intelligence: Culture and gender differences in self and other estimates of both general (g) and multiple intelligences. *Personality and Individual Differences, 31*, 1381–1405.

Gelman, S. A., Taylor, M. G., & Nguyen, S. P. (2004). The developmental course of gender differentiation. *Monographs of the Society for Research in Children Development, 69*(1), vii–127.

Goldberg, A. E., Kashy, D. A., & Smith, J. Z. (2012). Gender-typed play behavior in early childhood: Adopted children with lesbian, gay, and heterosexual parents. *Sex Roles, 67*, 503–515.

Grabe, S., & Hyde, J. S. (2006). Ethnicity and body dissatisfaction among women in the United States: A meta-analysis. *Psychological Bulletin, 132*, 622–640.

Grabe, S., & Hyde, J. S. (2009). Body objectification, MTV, and psychological outcomes among female adolescents. *Journal of Applied Social Psychology, 12*, 2840–2858.

Grabe, S., Ward, L. M., & Hyde, J. S. (2008). The role of the media in body image concerns among women: A meta-analysis of experimental and correlational studies. *Psychological Bulletin, 134*, 460–476.

Gunderson, E. A., Ramirez, G., Levine, S. C., & Beilock, S. L. (2012). The role of parents and teachers in the development of gender-related math attitudes. *Sex Roles, 66*, 153–166.

Halpern, D. F. (2012). *Sex differences in cognitive abilities* (4th ed.). New York: Psychology Press.

Harris, J. R. (1995). Where is the child's environment?: A group socialization theory of development. *Psychological Review, 102*, 458–489.

Henrich, J., Heine, S. J., & Norenzayan, A. (2010). The weirdest people in the world? *Behavioral and Brain Sciences, 33*, 61–135.

Hilton, J. M., & Haldeman, V. A. (1991). Gender differences in the performance of household tasks by adults and children in single-parent and two-parent, two-earner families. *Journal of Family Issues, 12*, 114–130.

Hines, M. (2013). Sex and sex differences. In P. D. Zelazo (Ed.), *Oxford handbook of developmental psychology* (Vol. 1, pp. 164–201). New York: Oxford University Press.

Hofstede, G. (2000). Masculine and feminine cultures. In A. E. Kazdin (Ed.), *Encyclopedia of psychology* (Vol. 5, pp. 115–118). Washington, DC: American Psychological Association.

Hyde, J. S. (2005). The gender similarities hypothesis. *American Psychologist, 60*, 581–592.

International Olympic Committee. (2013). *Factsheet: Women in the Olympic movement.* Lausanne, Switzerland: Author. Retrieved from *www.olympic.org/documents/reference_documents_factsheets/women_in_olympic_movement.pdf).*

Jussim, L., & Harber, K. D. (2005). Teacher expectations and self-fulfilling prophecies: Knowns and unknowns, resolved and unresolved controversies. *Personality and Social Psychology Review, 9*, 131–155.

Kane, E. W. (2006). "No way my boys are going to be like that!": Parents' responses to children's gender nonconformity. *Gender and Society, 20*, 149–176.

Kessels, U., & Steinmayr, R. (2013). Macho-man in school: Toward the role of gender role self-concepts and help seeking in school performance. *Learning and Educational Differences, 23,* 234–240.

Kiefer, S. M., & Ryan, A. M. (2008). Striving for social dominance over peers: The implications for academic adjustment during early adolescence. *Journal of Educational Psychology, 100,* 417–428.

Killen, M., & Stangor, C. (2001). Children's social reasoning about inclusion and exclusion in gender and race peer group contexts. *Child Development, 72,* 174–186.

Knight, J. L., & Giuliano, T. A. (2003). Blood, sweat, and jeers: The impact of the media's heterosexist portrayals on perceptions of male and female athletes. *Journal of Sport Behavior, 26,* 272–284.

Krantz-Kent, R. (2009). Measuring time spent in unpaid household work: Results from the American Time Use Survey. *Monthly Labor Review, 132,* 46–59.

Leaper, C. (1991). Influence and involvement in children's discourse: Age, gender, and partner effects. *Child Development, 62,* 797–811.

Leaper, C. (1994). Exploring the consequences of gender segregation on social relationships. In C. Leaper (Issue Ed.) & W. Damon (Series Ed.), *Childhood gender segregation: Causes and consequences* (New Directions for Child Development, No. 62, pp. 797–811). San Francisco: Jossey-Bass.

Leaper, C. (2000a). Gender, affiliation, assertion, and the interactive context of parent–child play. *Developmental Psychology, 36,* 381–393.

Leaper, C. (2000b). The social construction and socialization of gender. In P. H. Miller & E. K. Scholnick (Eds.), *Towards a feminist developmental psychology* (pp. 127–152). New York: Routledge Press.

Leaper, C. (2011). More similarities than differences in contemporary theories of social development?: A plea for theory bridging. In J. B. Benson (Ed.), *Advances in child development and behavior* (pp. 337–378). San Diego, CA: Elsevier.

Leaper, C. (2013). Gender development during childhood. In P. D. Zelazo (Ed.), *Oxford handbook of developmental psychology* (Vol. 2, pp. 327–377). New York: Oxford University Press.

Leaper, C., Anderson, K. J., & Sanders, P. (1998). Moderators of gender effects on parents' talk to their children: A meta-analysis. *Developmental Psychology, 34,* 3–27.

Leaper, C., & Bigler, R. S. (2004). Gendered language and sexist thought. *Monographs of the Society for Research in Child Development, 69*(1), 128–142.

Leaper, C., Breed, L., Hoffman, L., & Perlman, C. A. (2002). Variations in the gender-stereotyped content of children's television cartoons across genres. *Journal of Applied Social Psychology, 32,* 1653–1662.

Leaper, C., & Brown, C. S. (2008). Perceived experiences with sexism among adolescent girls. *Child Development, 79,* 685–704.

Leaper, C., Carson, M., Baker, C., Holliday, H., & Myers, S. B. (1995). Self-disclosure and listener verbal support in same-gender and cross-gender friends' conversations. *Sex Roles, 33,* 387–404.

Leaper, C., & Robnett, R. D. (2011). Sexism. In R. J. R. Levesque (Ed.), *Encyclopedia of adolescence* (pp. 2641–2648). New York: Springer.

Leaper, C., & Smith, T. E. (2004). A meta-analytic review of gender variations in children's language use: Talkativeness, affiliative speech, and assertive speech. *Developmental Psychology, 40,* 993–1027.

Leaper, C., Tenenbaum, H. R., & Shaffer, T. G. (1999). Communication patterns of African American girls and boys from low-income, urban background. *Child Development, 70,* 1489–1503.

Leman, P. J., Ahmed, S., & Ozarow, L. (2005). Gender, gender relations, and the social dynamics of children's conversations. *Developmental Psychology, 41,* 64–74.

Liben, L. S., & Bigler, R. S. (2002). The developmental course of gender differentiation: Conceptualizing, measuring, and evaluating constructs and pathways. *Monographs of the Society for Research in Child Development, 67*(2), vii–147.

Lindberg, S. M., Hyde, J. S., Petersen, J. L., & Linn, M. C. (2010). New trends in gender and mathematics performance: A meta-analysis. *Psychological Bulletin, 136,* 1123–1135.

Lindsey, E. W., Mize, J., & Pettit, G. S. (1997). Differential pay patterns of mothers and fathers of sons and daughters: Implications for children's gender role development. *Sex Roles, 37,* 643–661.

Lytton, H., & Romney, D. M. (1991). Parents' differential socialization of boys and girls: A meta-analysis. *Psychological Bulletin, 109,* 267–296.

Maccoby, E. E. (1998). *The two sexes: Growing up apart, coming together.* Cambridge, MA: Belknap Press/Harvard University Press.

Mahaffy, K. A., & Ward, S. K. (2002). The gendering of adolescents' childbearing and educational plans: Reciprocal effects and the influence of social context. *Sex Roles, 46,* 403–417.

Martin, C. L. (1989). Children's use of gender-related information in making social judgments. *Developmental Psychology, 25,* 80–88.

Martin, C. L., & Fabes, R. A. (2001). The stability and consequences of young children's same-sex peer interactions. *Developmental Psychology, 37,* 431–446.

Martin, C. L., Ruble, D. N., & Szkrybalo, J. (2002). Cognitive theories of early gender development. *Psychological Bulletin, 128,* 903–933.

Massey, E., Gebhardt, W., & Garnefski, N. (2008). Adolescent goal content and pursuit: A review of the literature from the past 16 years. *Developmental Review, 28,* 421–460.

McCabe, M., & Ricciardelli, L. (2001). Parent, peer and media influences on body image and strategies to both increase and decrease body size among adolescent boys and girls. *Adolescence, 36,* 225–240.

McHale, S. M., Bartko, W. T., Crouter, A. C., & Perry-Jenkins, M. (1990). Children's housework and psychosocial functioning: The mediating effects of parents' sex-role behaviors and attitudes. *Child Development, 61,* 1413–1426.

Merikangas, K. R., He, J. P., Burstein, M., Swanson, S. A., Avenevoli, S., Cui, L., et al. (2010). Lifetime prevalence of mental disorders in U.S. adolescents: Results from the National Comorbidity Survey-Adolescent Supplement (NCS-A). *Journal of the American Academy of Child and Adolescent Psychiatry, 49,* 980–989.

Messner, M. A. (1992). *Power at play: Sports and the problem of masculinity.* Boston: Beacon.

Miller, P. H., & Scholnick, E. K. (Eds.). (2000). *Toward a feminist developmental psychology.* New York: Routledge Press.

Morgan, C., Isaac, J. D., & Sansone, C. (2001). The role of interest in understanding the career choices of female and male college students. *Sex Roles, 44,* 295–320.

Muris, P., Meesters, C., van de Blom, W., & Mayer, B. (2005). Biological, psychological, and sociocultural correlates of body change strategies and eating problems in adolescent boys and girls. *Eating Behaviors, 6,* 11–22.

National Federation of State High School Associations. (2013). 2011–12 High School Athletics Participation Survey results. Retrieved from *www.nfhs.org.*

National Science Foundation. (2008). *Women, minorities, and persons with disabilities in science and engineering.* Washington, DC: Author. Document available online at *www.nsf.gov/statistics/wmpd.*

Nelson, A. (2005). Children's toy collections in Sweden: A less gender-typed country? *Sex Roles, 52,* 93–102.

Osborne, D., & Wagner, W. E. (2007). Exploring the relationship between homophobia and participation in core sports among high school students. *Sociological Perspectives, 50,* 597–613.

Patrick, H., Ryan, A. M., Alfeld-Liro, C., Fredricks, J. A., Hruda, L., & Eccles, J. S. (1999). Adolescents' commitment to developing talent: The role of peers in continuing motivation for sports and the arts. *Journal of Youth and Adolescence, 28*(6), 741–763.

Peplau, L. A., & Fingerhut, A. W. (2007). The close relationships of lesbians and gay men. *Annual Psychological Review, 58,* 405–424.

Peterson, K. A., Paulson, S. E., & Williams, K. K. (2007). Relations of eating disorder symptomatology with perceptions of pressures from mothers, peers, and media in adolescent boys and girls. *Sex Roles, 57,* 629–639.

Petrie, T. A., Greenleaf, C., & Martin, S. (2010). Biopsychosocial and physical correlates of middle school boys' and girls' body satisfaction. *Sex Roles, 63,* 631–644.

Phares, V., Steinberg, A. R., & Thompson, J. K. (2004). Gender differences in peer and parent influences: Body image disturbance, self-worth, and psychological functioning in preadolescent children. *Journal of Youth and Adolescence, 33,* 421–429.

Pike, J. J., & Jennings, N. A. (2005). The effects of commercials on children's perceptions of gender appropriate toy use. *Sex Roles, 52,* 83–91.

Powlishta, K. K. (2004). Gender as a social category: Intergroup processes and gender-role development. In M. Bennett & F. Sani (Eds.), *The development of the social self* (pp. 103–133). New York: Psychology Press.

Ricciardelli, L. A., & McCabe, M. P. (2001). Children's body image concerns and eating disturbance: A review of the literature. *Clinical Psychology Review, 21,* 325–344.

Ricciardelli, L. A., McCabe, M. P., Lillis, J., & Thomas, K. (2006). A longitudinal investigation of the development of weight and muscle concerns among preadolescent boys. *Journal of Youth and Adolescence, 35,* 177–187.

Riegel, K. F. (1976). The dialectics of human development. *American Psychologist, 31,* 689–700.

Robnett, R. D., & Leaper, C. (2013). Friendship groups, personal motivation, and gender in relation to high school students' STEM career interest. *Journal of Research on Adolescence, 23,* 652–664.

Rogoff, B. (1990). *Apprenticeship in thinking: Cognitive development in social context.* New York: Oxford University Press.

Rose, A. J. (2002). Co-rumination in the friendships of girls and boys. *Child Development, 73,* 1830–1843.

Rose, A. J., & Rudolph, K. D. (2006). A review of sex differences in peer relationship processes: Potential tradeoffs for the emotional and behavioral development of girls and boys. *Psychological Bulletin, 132,* 98–131.

Santos, C. E., Galligan, K., Pahlke, E., & Fabes, R. A. (2013). Gender-typed behaviors, achievement, and adjustment among racially and ethnically diverse boys during early adolescence. *American Journal of Orthopsychiatry, 83,* 252–264.

Serbin, L. A., Connor, J. M., & Iler, I. (1979). Sex-stereotyped and nonstereotyped introductions of new toys in the preschool classroom: An observational study of teacher behavior and its effects. *Psychology of Women Quarterly, 4,* 261–265.

Serbin, L. A., Powlishta, K. K., & Gulko, J. (1993). The development of sex typing in middle childhood. *Monographs of the Society for Research in Child Development, 58*(2), v–75.

Servin, A., & Bohlin, G. (1999). Do Swedish mothers have sex-stereotyped expectations and wishes regarding their own children? *Infant and Child Development, 8,* 197–210.

Signorielli, N. (2012). Television's gender-role images and contribution to stereotyping: Past, present and future. In D. G. Singer & J. L. Singer (Eds.), *Handbook of children and the media* (2nd ed., pp. 321–339). Thousand Oaks, CA: Sage.

Slater, A., & Tiggemann, M. (2002). A test of objectification theory in adolescent girls. *Sex Roles, 46,* 343–349.

Smolak, L., Levine, M. P., & Schermer, F. (1999). Parental input and weight concerns among elementary school children. *International Journal of Eating Disorders, 25,* 263–271.

Spencer, R., Porche, M. V., & Tolman, D. L. (2003). We've come a long way—maybe: New challenges for gender equity in education. *Teachers College Record, 105,* 1774–1807.

Stake, J. E., & Nickens, S. D. (2005). Adolescent girls' and boys' science peer relationships and perceptions of the possible self as a scientist. *Sex Roles, 52,* 1–11.

Tenenbaum, G., Stewart, E., Singer, R. N., & Duda, J. (1996). Aggression and violence in sport: An ISSP position stand. *International Journal of Sport Psychology, 27,* 229–236.

Tenenbaum, H. R., & Leaper, C. (2002). Are parents' gender schemas related to their children's gender-related cognitions?: A meta analysis. *Developmental Psychology, 38,* 615–630.

Tilleczek, K. C., & Lewko, J. H. (2001). Factors influencing the pursuit of health and science careers for Canadian adolescents in transition from school to work. *Journal of Youth Studies, 4*, 415–428.

Tobin, D. D., Menon, M., Menon, M., Spatta, B. C., Hodges, E. V. E., & Perry, D. G. (2010). The intrapsychics of gender: A model of self-socialization. *Psychological Review, 117*, 601–622.

Tolman, D. L., Spencer, R., Harmon, T., Rosen-Reynoso, M., & Striepe, M. (2004). Getting close, staying cool: Early adolescent boys' experiences with romantic relationships. In N. Way & J. Y. Chu (Eds.), *Adolescent boys: Exploring diverse cultures of boyhood* (pp. 235–255). New York: New York University Press.

Twenge, J. M. (1997a). Attitudes toward women, 1970–1995: A meta-analysis. *Psychology of Women Quarterly, 21*, 35–51.

Twenge, J. M. (1997b). Changes in masculine and feminine traits over time: A meta-analysis. *Sex Roles, 36*, 305–325.

Underwood, M. K. (2003). *Social aggression among girls.* New York: Guilford Press.

UNESCO [United Nations Educational, Scientific and Cultural Organization] Institute for Statistics. (2010). *Global Education Digest 2010: Comparing education statistics across the world.* Montréal: Author.

Updegraff, K. A., McHale, S. M., & Crouter, A. C. (1996). Gender roles in marriage: What do they mean for girls' and boys' school achievement? *Journal of Youth and Adolescence, 25*, 73–88.

Weiss, M. R., Amorose, A. J., & Kipp, L. E. (2012). Youth motivation and participation in sport and physical activity. In R. M. Ryan (Ed.), *The Oxford handbook of human motivation* (pp. 520–553). New York: Oxford University Press.

Wentzel, K. R., Donlan, A., & Morrison, D. (2012). Peer relationships and social motivational processes. In A. M. Ryan & G. W. Ladd (Eds.), *Peer relationships and adjustment at school* (pp. 79–105) Charlotte, NC: Information Age.

Wertheim, E. H., Mee, V., & Paxton, S. J. (1999). Relationships among adolescent girls' eating behaviors and their parents' weight-related attitudes and behaviors. *Sex Roles, 41*, 169–187.

Whitley, B. E. (1997). Gender differences in computer-related attitudes and behavior: A meta-analysis. *Computers in Human Behavior, 13*, 1–22.

Wilgenbusch, T., & Merrell, K. W. (1999). Gender differences in self-concept among children and adolescents: A meta-analysis of multidimensional studies. *School Psychology Quarterly, 14*, 101–120.

Wood, E., Desmarais, S., & Gugula, S. (2002). The impact of parenting experience on gender stereotyped toy play of children. *Sex Roles, 47*, 39–49.

Wood, W., & Eagly, A. H. (2002). A cross-cultural analysis of the behavior of women and men: Implications for the origins of sex differences. *Psychological Bulletin, 128*, 699–727.

Young, R. A., Antal, S., Bassett, M. E., Post, A., DeVries, N., & Valach, L. (1999). The joint actions of adolescents in peer conversations about career. *Journal of Adolescence, 22*, 527–538.

Zarbatany, L., McDougall, P., & Hymel, S. (2000). Title gender-differentiated experience in the peer culture: Links to intimacy in preadolescence. *Social Development, 9*, 62–79.

CHAPTER 24

The Socialization of Cognition

Mary Gauvain
Susan M. Perez

Cognitive development is a process of socialization to the intellectual life of the community in which children are expected to become mature, competent, and contributing members. In this chapter we discuss cognitive development as a social process, concentrating on how intellectual development is organized and directed by the social world over childhood. The social context contributes to cognitive development in two ways. First, it determines what children think about and how they think. Second, it is the primary system through which children learn about the world and develop cognitive skills. In other words, cognitive development is imbued with social information, and it emerges from social experience. During social interaction and other inherently social processes, such as cultural practices, children have opportunities to participate intellectually in the world in ways they cannot generate on their own (Vygotsky, 1978). These experiences lead to fundamental changes in children's thinking.

We focus on the participants and processes involved in the socialization of cognition. The social aspects of cognitive development cover a wide spectrum of children's experiences, including direct social encounters (e.g., interpersonal interaction) and less direct but still fundamentally social processes (e.g., participation in culturally organized activities). We recognize that biological and other internal factors also contribute by defining the possibilities and boundaries of intellectual growth at any given point in development. We begin by discussing some ideas from evolutionary developmental psychology and research on the development of social cognition that provide information about the capabilities of the human organism that enable participation in and learning from social and cultural experience.

The Evolutionary Basis of Cognitive Socialization

The social nature of cognitive development is evident in contemporary understanding of human phylogenesis (Bjorklund & Pellegrini, 2002). The protracted evolution of human intelligence favored prehominids that were capable of combating problems in the environment pertinent to survival (Buss, 2012). To succeed, several social and cognitive capabilities were critical, including the ability to cooperate in groups to reach a goal and to understand conspecifics in order to learn from them (Tomasello, Kruger, & Ratner, 1993). In addition, the vast potential for learning, along with emerging neural properties, including brain plasticity (Kolb & Whishaw, 2013), provided early hominids with "a special potency" in modifying the environment to support survival (Flynn, Laland, Kendal, & Kendal, 2013).

Evolutionary developmental psychology concentrates on how *ontogenesis*, or individual development, relates to the history of the species (Bjorklund & Pellegrini, 2002). Several species characteristics have direct relevance to cognitive development, especially immaturity at birth, a long period of dependence, gradual specialization of intelligence to local circumstances, and the ability to attain high levels of cognitive functioning in a lifetime. The pattern and pace of growth necessitate a period of dependence on mature group members that requires a large parental investment in few offspring, many who may not survive. For this period of dependence to have been sustained over evolution, it must have provided substantial benefits. In addition to providing protection and nurturance, the main benefit seems to be opportunities for learning in the company of experienced group members who know much of what children need to learn. The fact that these individuals have strong emotional ties likely enhances the potential for learning. In brief, human evolution set in place a set of adaptations that enable *Homo sapiens* to learn from and with others over the course of child development in the context of culture (Konner, 2010).

The Social Cognitive Foundation of Cognitive Socialization

Social cognition covers a range of topics, including perspective taking, the comprehension and attribution of others' actions and intentions, theory of mind and mental state reasoning, and the consequences of these types of understanding for psychological development (Homer & Tamis-LeMonda, 2012). Underlying these topics are questions about when and how children come to comprehend the self and other people as psychological beings (Carpendale & Lewis, 2004) and how these capacities enable human beings to interpret and learn the behaviors of others and participate in, inherit, and transform culture (Tomasello, 1999).

Early cognitive development is organized around maturational constraints, including the timing and pace of learning, and biases toward certain types of information (Legerstee, Haley, & Bornstein, 2013). Much of what infants find of interest resonates with human social life, such as patterns that compose faces and speech, along with social interaction itself (Matheson, Moore, & Akhtar, 2013; Posner, 2012). At age 2 months, infants follow another person's line of vision (Scaife & Bruner, 1975) and respond to parental overtures by making sounds similar in pitch to the parent's voice (Snow, 1990). At 3 months, infants are sensitive to social contingencies (Striano, Henning, & Stahl, 2005), which paves the way for *intersubjectivity*, the coordinated attention of social partners to one another (Trevarthen, 1980). At 6 months, infants can engage in turn taking (Bruner & Sherwood, 1976). Later, in the first year, infants use social information to gauge their emotional reaction to an event (Feinman, 1992), understand other persons as intentional agents (Tomasello & Haberl, 2003), and participate in joint attention (Adamson & Bakeman, 1991), which supports the development of language and object knowledge. At 16 months, toddlers can learn a complex set of modeled behaviors (Carpenter, Akhtar, & Tomasello, 1998) and at 30 months, they can learn by watching peers (Brownell, Ramani, & Zerwas, 2006). In the preschool years, children's facility with symbolic systems, such as language and pretense, and their burgeoning skills at mental state reasoning enhance the ability to learn from others (Hughes, 2011) and develop complex cognitive skills (Gauvain, 2001). Children also increasingly know when and how to seek help when it is needed (Karabenick & Newman, 2006).

As these findings make clear, early experiences mark the beginning of a lifelong process of learning that is deeply entwined with the social context and flexibly adapted to specific learning opportunities. Learning is both common across social and historical circumstances (Spelke & Kinzler, 2007) and largely specialized to the unique circumstances of growth (Bjorklund & Pellegrini, 2002). Because human circumstances can change rapidly, the ability to adjust thinking to immediate or unexpected demands is a critical feature of adaptive intellectual functioning (Flynn et al., 2013). A mental system with a few basic cognitive skills that can jump-start the system once experiences occur facilitates this process more efficiently than a preprogrammed set of knowledge (Elman et al., 1996).

To summarize, the description of human development provided by contemporary research in evolutionary developmental psychology and social cognition is consistent with the view of cognitive development as a socially constituted process (Cole, 2006). Next we discuss the sociocultural approach to cognitive development, which provides a framework for studying cognitive development as a process of socialization.

The Sociocultural Approach to Cognitive Development

All human beings participate in *culture*, an organized pattern of social behavior that is shared by a group and passed across generations. Culture provides children with many opportunities to develop and practice cognitive skills. Both interpersonally direct processes, such as social interaction and instruction, and more distal processes, such as observational learning and cultural participation, convey ways of thinking that are valued in culture and provide opportunities and support for intellectual growth. As such, they function as processes or mechanisms of cognitive development (Gauvain, 2001). Many social partners serve as agents of cognitive socialization. We focus on two types of children's regular social partners: family members and peers. We also consider how one social institution, school, contributes to cognitive socialization.

Agents of Cognitive Socialization

Family Contributions to Cognitive Development

Both the sustained nature of family life and the asymmetrical relations of its members make the family a powerful context for cognitive socialization. Research has demonstrated that the quality of the family context in terms of access to resources (e.g., health care, family support), socioeconomic status (SES), maternal work status, family structure (e.g., single vs. two-parent household, number of siblings), and parenting practices (e.g., warmth and responsiveness relative to control and maturity demands) contributes to cognitive-developmental outcomes (Bradley & Corwyn, 2002; Lugo-Gil & Tamis-LeMonda, 2008; Ono & Sanders, 2010). Parents and siblings differ in the expertise, experience, and control they bring to interactions with children, making family interactions an important context of cognitive development. Family members' strong emotional bonds affect children's opportunities to engage in interactions with more skilled partners in ways that support learning (Bugental & Goodnow, 1998). Here we discuss specific family processes that contribute to cognitive development.

PARENTS

Parents influence children's emerging cognitive skills by encouraging and modeling behaviors and through the experiences they provide for their children. There are similarities and differences in the ways parents contribute to cognitive and social development. While the behavioral contingencies that parents use, such as rewards, play a greater role in social development, parenting practices, such as warmth, encouragement, and responsiveness, contribute to both cognitive and social development (Gauvain, Perez, & Beebe, 2013). Additionally, for cognitive skills, the structure that parents provide in face-to-face encounters and the activities they arrange for children are critical (Maccoby, 2002). As they participate with children in activities, parents introduce to them ideas and ways of thinking, and provide explanation and guidance.

The methods of cognitive socialization used by parents include everyday interactions and more structured learning situations. For example, the spatial language used by parents and children in everyday conversation predicts children's concurrent and subsequent spatial language, as well as their performance on nonverbal spatial tasks (Pruden, Levine, & Huttenlocher, 2011). As parents and children solve problems together, parents help children to manage the more difficult components of tasks, break down a problem into manageable subgoals, and provide overall structure and guidance (Gauvain, 2001). Parents also arrange opportunities for children to develop cognitive skills through play, help with homework, and providing lessons and activities outside school, as well as technology and other learning tools (Gauvain & Perez, 2005).

Cognitive development is a transactional process for parents and children. The psychological dynamics of their interactions and, in turn, any cognitive growth or learning that ensues, are affected by characteristics of the participants (Gauvain et al., 2013). Important parental characteristics include stress levels, personality, beliefs, emotional responsiveness, control, and expectations about child behavior (Senese, Bornstein, Haynes, Rossi, & Venuti, 2012). For instance, Guajardo, Snyder, and Petersen (2009) found that parenting reported by mothers as inconsistent, uninvolved, and high in stress predicted poorer performance on theory-of-mind tasks in 3- to 5-year-old children. Contributions of children include temperament and emotionality, cognitive and social skills, level of interest and motivation, and developmental status (Landry & Smith, 2010; Salonen, Lepola, & Vauras, 2007). Hammond, Müller, Carpendale, Bibok, and Liebermann-Finestone (2012) demonstrated that children's language ability mediated parental scaffolding and children's executive functioning at age 3.

Some characteristics that regulate parent–child cognitive interactions are not independent. Family members are related biologically and may genetically share characteristics and abilities pertinent to learning (Plomin, DeFries, Knopik, & Neiderhiser, 2013).

Parents and children share an intimate knowledge of one another that can influence interactions and learning opportunities for children (Gauvain & Perez, 2008). Parents are responsive to children's individual needs, offering a refined level of support for learning. For example, parents instruct differently depending on their child's temperament and emotional state (Dixon & Smith, 2003; Gauvain & Fagot, 1995; Perez & Gauvain, 2009). The context of the activity also influences parental instruction. Parents instruct differently during a game than during a problem-solving task, even when the underlying skill (e.g., mathematics) is the same (Bjorklund, Hubertz, & Reubens, 2004).

In addition to characteristics of the participants, aspects of parent–child interaction have been shown to relate to several areas of cognitive development (Gauvain, 2001). Maternal responsiveness to an infant's activities predicts the timing of language milestones (Tamis-LeMonda, Bornstein, & Baumwell, 2001). Parent–child conversations about the past contribute to children's recall of an event, as well as strategic memory development and understanding of the mind (Fivush, Haden, & Reese, 2006). With scaffolding and guidance from parents, children can acquire problem-solving skills in various areas that lead to improved individual performance on similar problems after the interaction (Gauvain & Rogoff, 1989). Such improvements have been found in many domains, including science and mathematics (Hyde, Else-Quest, Alibali, Knuth, & Romberg, 2006; Jipson & Callanan, 2003).

In the main, research indicates that parents can play an important and positive role in children's cognitive development. These contributions occur frequently throughout childhood, and they emerge spontaneously, often during interpersonal interaction. However, it has also been shown that parent–child interaction does not always lead to positive cognitive outcomes for children. Social interaction benefits learning when it is sensitive to the child's abilities and needs. For a number of reasons (e.g., child behavior, task difficulty), parental guidance may be unresponsive to children's learning needs (Gauvain & Fagot, 1995; Perez & Gauvain, 2005, 2009). When sensitive support does not occur, there are fewer cognitive gains for children.

SIBLINGS

Siblings have a dynamic relationship characterized by varied types of interaction, ranging from affectionate and supportive exchanges to hostility and conflict. Children learn from siblings during play (N. Howe & Bruno, 2010), caregiving situations (Maynard, 2002), and via joint problem solving or direct teaching (Budak & Chavajay, 2012; N. Howe, Recchia, Porta, & Funamoto, 2012). Siblings, other than twins, have an asymmetry of skills, experience, and control, and both younger and older siblings benefit from their interactions. Their emotional bonds and high levels of familiarity create learning opportunities for older and younger siblings. Thus, older siblings develop greater competence in the activities they demonstrate, as well as better teaching skills. Younger siblings benefit from being introduced to and learning new skills.

Research suggests that siblings engage in cognitive interactions that are meaningful to them and different than interactions with peers and parents. Accordingly, Azmitia and Hesser (1993) found that young children observe and imitate the problem-solving behaviors of their older siblings more than the behaviors of their sibling's friends, and that older siblings help their younger siblings more than their friends do. N. Howe and Bruno (2010) demonstrated that siblings engaged in play that is more creative and collaborative when mothers are absent than when mothers are present, which suggests that sibling interactions provide unique opportunities for cognitive growth in the family context. Research has also shown that the number of siblings present can contribute to cognitive development. In a study examining differences in autobiographical memory across three cultures, number of siblings was positively associated with more socially integrated memories, later ages of earliest memories, and less specificity of the autobiographical account (Bender & Chasiotis, 2011).

Research suggests that siblings may contribute to the development of children's theory of mind (Perner, Ruffman, & Leekam, 1994). Siblings are often in situations in which one child is motivated to take the perspective of the other—perhaps to figure out what the sibling is up to or to determine how to help or hinder the child in reaching a goal. McAlister and Peterson (2007) found that children with two or more siblings performed better on theory-of-mind tasks than children with no siblings, even after they controlled for age and intelligence. Other research suggests that the age differential between siblings may be crucial, however. Cassidy, Fineberg, Brown, and Perkins (2005) found that having an older sibling, but not a twin, benefited theory-of-mind development. This particular age pattern may motivate a child to strive to realize the sibling's perspective.

Overall, research suggests that experiences among siblings can support cognitive development. Interacting with an older sibling, particularly in the context of negotiating roles and responsibilities, appears to give young children a decided boost in the development of perspective-taking skills. In addition, research has shown that the frequency of inner state talk (e.g., about feelings, desires, cognition) between siblings may be important for the development of mental state reasoning, and that such talk is greater with siblings than with mothers (Brown, Donelan-McCall, & Dunn, 1996; Hughes, Fujisawa, Ensor, Lecce, & Marfleet, 2006).

Peer Contributions to Cognitive Development

Outside the family, the most important social influence on cognitive development is the peer group. Peer interaction is more open and egalitarian than interaction in the family, which can lead to unique opportunities for cognitive development. For Piaget (1926), peer interaction aids cognitive development because of its symmetrical nature (i.e., the relatively small cognitive and social distance between peers). When social power is equal, Piaget thought that peers would be more likely to learn from each other, particularly when they debated differing points of view. In contrast, Vygotsky (1978) placed greater emphasis on asymmetrical relationships, especially the assistance provided from a more experienced partner to a less experienced one.

Even though peers are not as likely as siblings and parents to vary in expertise, when differences occur, peer interaction may be a particularly fertile learning situation for children. To study the relative contributions of age and expertise to cognitive development, Duran and Gauvain (1993) observed child dyads at work on a planning task. The interactions of 5-year-old novice planners and 7-year-old expert planners were compared with interactions of 5-year-old novices and same-age experts. Novices who planned with same-age experts participated more in the task and performed better on an individual posttest than did novices who planned with an older expert. Also, participation during the interaction was positively related to posttest performance. As Vygotsky suggested, cognitive gains were achieved when children collaborated with more skilled partners, especially when there was substantial involvement by the learner. However, echoing Piaget's view, such involvement was more likely when partners were the same age rather than different ages. Thus, this research supports both theoretical positions, thereby underscoring the potentially broad range of contributions peers make to cognitive growth.

HOW DOES PEER INTERACTION BENEFIT CHILDREN'S LEARNING?

Peer interaction offers a variety of benefits for children's learning. Peers can contribute new information, define and restructure a problem in an accessible way, and generate discussions that lead to better problem solving. Through mutual feedback, evaluation, and debate, peers motivate one another to abandon misconceptions and search for better solutions to problems. Peer contributions to cognitive development have been demonstrated on a range of activities, including problem solving (Gauvain & Rogoff, 1989), spatial thinking (Golbeck, 1998), moral and causal reasoning (Kruger, 1992; Manion & Alexander, 1997), conceptual knowledge including areas in which learners' intuitive understandings are resistant to change (e.g., natural selection; Asterhan & Schwarz, 2009), and during peer tutoring (Flynn, 2010; LeBlanc & Bearison, 2004).

Enhanced learning in the context of peer interaction is a lifelong process (Berg & Strough, 2011) that first appears in early childhood. Cooperation by 3- and 4-year-olds during problem solving can improve both immediate and later task performance (Fletcher, Warneken, & Tomasello, 2012). Learning by observing peers is especially useful for young children, whereas, for older children, verbal exchange is increasingly important as children gain awareness of other people's perspectives and talk more about strategies, especially on tasks that require reasoning (Garton & Pratt, 2001; Teasley, 1995). Peer collaboration can promote the use of more advanced strategies and improved understanding of strategy choices (Fleming & Alexander, 2001).

FACTORS THAT CONTRIBUTE TO LEARNING FROM PEERS

The social processes that lead to learning and cognitive change during peer interaction are unclear. C. Howe (2009) found that *joint construction*, in which peers generate a solution that none could do alone, was useful for conceptual change measured soon after the interaction. However, *unresolved contradiction*, in which children try to account for anomalies that arose during the task, accounted for learning assessed several weeks later. This research is consistent with findings that *explanatory talk* by peers during problem solving, which is similar to joint construction, can promote learning (Mercer & Littleton, 2007). These studies suggest that improved understanding is needed about peer processes that advance learning both in the short and the long term (Rojas-Drummond, 2009).

Several other dimensions of peer interaction are also important to learning. Changes in competence following peer interaction may depend on the stage of skills acquisition and ability level. Cognitive benefits for children are more likely early in skills acquisition, suggesting that this is a point when learners are especially receptive to new ideas (Fawcett & Garton, 2005). This result is consistent with research by Hawkins, Homolsky, and Heide (1984), who observed that after achieving a basic level of expertise in group work, children benefited more from time working on their own—honing their individual skills—before reengaging with peers in group work. In terms of ability level, research has shown that children higher in task ability benefit more from peer collaboration, largely because they participate more in the task. Children with lower ability benefit when paired with children with higher ability, especially when they provide elaboration and assistance (Denessen, Veenman, Dobbelsteen, & Van Schilt, 2008).

The relationship that peers have may also affect learning. Friends offer more explanations and critiques to partners than do acquaintances (Azmitia & Montgomery, 1993), and they are more likely than nonfriends to resolve conflicts and assist one another (Jones, 2002). Mutually identified friends perform better on cognitive tasks than dyads when only one child in the dyad identifies the other as a friend, when the dyad members are not friends, or when children work alone (Andersson, 2001).

Other peer interaction factors that can affect children's learning include the child's interest, prior experience, self-confidence, and expectations for learning (Light & Littleton, 1999). Child gender is also important; girls prefer more collaborative interactions, whereas boys are more competitive (Light & Littleton, 1999). In mixed-gender groups, boys tend to dominate the interaction by controlling information flow and materials, which restricts learning opportunities for girls (Holmes-Lonergran, 2003). Friendship and gender also interact. On a scientific reasoning task, girls paired with same-sex friends performed better than boys and girls paired with acquaintances and boys paired with same-sex friends (Kutnick & Kington, 2005). These gender-related patterns may vary across ethnic groups. In a study with children of European and Asian ancestry, boys were more assertive in same-gender than mixed-gender pairs, but only in the all-Asian dyads (Leman et al., 2011). These studies indicate a need for research on how individual characteristics, including skills level, age, gender, social status, and personal relationships, regulate opportunities for children to learn when collaborating with a peer.

In summary, children's experiences in the family and with peers affect cognitive development. These social agents help children identify what to think about and how to solve problems, and each provides opportunities for cognitive development and socialization.

School Contributions to Cognitive Socialization

Formally organized settings for learning are a major part of cognitive socialization in childhood. Societies make a huge investment in educating young members in myriad ways, including schooling, apprenticeships, and indoctrination (Göncü & Gauvain, 2012). All of these methods involve (1) social processes in which some participants have knowledge or skills that others do not yet possess and (2) transfer of this knowledge to less experienced participants. Several sources are concerned with learning arrangements outside school (e.g., Grusec & Davidov, 2010; Rogoff, 2003); here, we concentrate on learning in the context of formal schooling.

Children's experience in school is sustained over a long and formative period of intellectual development. Formal education orients children's thinking toward the expectations of society. It also teaches them how their culture interprets the natural and social worlds, the values placed on certain ways of thinking, and the tools and technologies used to support thinking (Bruner, 1996).

COGNITIVE CONSEQUENCES OF FORMAL SCHOOLING

Cross-cultural research indicates that schooled children respond to cognitive tasks differently than do nonschooled children, children educated in urban schools perform differently from those in rural schools, and children educated in schools that focus on specific subject matter (e.g., religion) perform differently than children in schools with a general curriculum. Serpell and Hatano (1997) describe three approaches to formal education, the socialization goals they reflect, and their social cognitive consequences. In Western culture, the main cultural themes behind school are self-expression, technical expertise, and cognition as a personal and transforming accomplishment. Societal extensions of this view include the stigmatization of unschooled individuals and the legitimization of widespread educational efforts even beyond national borders (see Freire, 1970, on this point). The Sino-Japanese educational tradition emphasizes moral perfectability, filial piety, and emulation of models and cultural norms. Major societal challenges include how to increase personal creativity, intellectual exploration, and innovation. The Islamic tradition practiced in Qur'anic schools varies considerably, although there is common stress on the authority of the sacred text and memorization. For Wagner (1993), this emphasis helps prepare young children with skills useful in learning to read. However, Serpell and Hatano (1997) consider the large focus on prayer recitation as potentially limiting to the development of other types of cognitive skills.

Research conducted in Western settings indicates that the association between education and cognitive development is reciprocal and dynamic. Although this research suggests that cognitive skills, including executive functions, decision making, and problem solving, are enhanced by formal education, education in turn changes with advances in cognition (Baker, Salinas & Eslinger, 2012). In fact, as more people worldwide have increased access to formal education, the educational system itself has changed and intensified. This intensification is evident in increased demand by parents for education of their children, more spending on education, and changes in the schooling process (e.g., more time spent in school settings) (Baker et al., 2012). This intensification is likely to contribute to the socialization of cognition. In addition, several more proximate influences related to schooling contribute to the impact of education on cognitive development, including parents, teachers, and peers.

PARENTAL CONTRIBUTIONS TO CHILDREN'S SCHOOLING

Parents contribute to children's learning in school in many ways (Fantuzzo, Tighe, & Childs, 2000). Parents can support children's school learning through formal and informal activities, such as volunteering at school, helping with homework, and structured teaching at home (Fan & Chen, 2001). By simply asking their children about school, parents can contribute to children's interest and performance in school (Patrick, Johnson, Mantzicopoulos, & Gray, 2011). Parents' own experiences with school, and their beliefs and values about school, affect how they prepare children for formal schooling, the types of school settings they prefer for their children, and the ways they support children through school transitions (K. Miller, Dilworth-Bart, & Hane, 2011). Parents in cultures with compulsory schooling prepare their children for the classroom before school entry by engaging them in activities that resemble those in school, such as small lessons about how things work or sustained conversation on topics that are not the current focus of activity (Tudge, Odero, Hogan, & Etz, 2003).

Huntsinger and Jose (2009) observed cultural variation in parental engagement in formal schooling. Whereas European American parents were more likely to volunteer at their children's school, immigrant Chinese parents were more likely to engage in direct and structured teaching at home as a means of supporting children's academic achievement. Though these different types of school involvement were not explicitly examined in relation to child performance, the results did show that Chinese American children outperformed European American children in overall school performance and also had greater liking for school. This research does not suggest that parental teaching at home has greater benefits for children's learning than volunteering at school. However, it does raise questions about the meaning and effects of various parenting practices on children's academic achievement. More research on these relations is needed.

Research also indicates that schooling can have an impact on the family itself, particularly when parents' own beliefs about, knowledge of, or experiences with school are not aligned with children's experiences. The changes introduced to the family from the schooling context can have varying outcomes. In some cases, these may be positive; for example, Onyango-Ouma, Aagaard-Hansen, and Jensen (2005) found that when children learned health information at school, they brought it home to their families, essentially operating as agents of health change in their rural Kenyan villages. However, difficulties may arise in any cultural setting when parents lack the knowledge to help their children with homework or feel discomfort, embarrassment, or undermined when their children have more knowledge than they do (e.g., in computer skills).

OTHER SOCIAL FACTORS THAT CONTRIBUTE TO LEARNING IN SCHOOL

At school entry, children are exposed to a broad array of interactions and relationships with teachers and classmates that can influence their behavior in the classroom, motivation for school, engagement in learning, and academic achievement (Ladd, Kochenderfer-Ladd, Visconti, & Ettekal, 2012). A great deal of research indicates that the nature of the teacher–child relationship can influence learning (e.g., Hughes, Luo, Kwok, & Loyd, 2008; Sabol & Pianta, 2013). For example, children with teacher-child relationships that are high in conflict (e.g., frequent friction, negative affect) are less engaged in school and do not perform as well academically (Furrer & Skinner, 2003; Hamre & Pianta, 2001). Conversely, teacher–child relationships characterized by closeness (e.g., warmth, open communication) are positively associated with academic achievement (Birch & Ladd, 1997). Peers also influence learning in the classroom through peer tutoring and collaborative learning, whether child or teacher prescribed (Joiner, Littleton, Faulkner, & Miell, 2000; Ladd et al., 2012), and in less formal learning opportunities at school (Harris, 1995).

Educational approaches within classrooms also contribute to cognitive development. As previously discussed, what is taught and what is expected of children at school reflects cultural views regarding intelligence, social behavior, and what children need to know to become mature, contributing members of society. Many of the findings from laboratory studies of dyadic and small-group interaction are not directly applicable to classroom learning in which more participants, activities, and distractions are the norm. However, efforts to adapt these ideas to the classroom have met with success (see Bransford, Brown, & Cocking, 1999). Boaler and Greeno (2006) found improved mathematics learning when teachers and children worked together in sustained activities, peers learned together, and the teacher acted as an expert guide for the learning process. Several educational interventions have applied ideas about scaffolded learning to the classroom, in particular in the use of technology to support academics (Sawyer, 2006). Research has found that these cultural tools are most effective for learning when teachers are trained to use them in innovative ways, and when explicit connections between the tools and the abstract ideas they represent are provided (Kritt & Winegar, 2007).

To summarize, formal schooling is one method devised by cultures to standardize children's learning and socialize intelligence along desired cultural lines. Social agents outside the family, primarily teachers and peers, are central to this aspect of cognitive socialization.

Social Processes of Cognitive Development

The development of thinking relies on inherent connections between the broader socio-cultural context and the circumstances of individual growth. This context is instantiated in the ways people interact, the areas of mental functioning stressed and rewarded, the practices in which people engage, and the tools used to support and extend thinking. Interpersonal and other social processes are the primary means through which cultural understanding is conveyed to children, and participation in these processes helps to organize the developing mind in ways that fit with the needs and aspirations of the culture (Rogoff, 2003). Thus, a socialization approach to cognitive development is functional in orientation. It views the development of thinking as a socially mediated process that creates understanding of the world—understanding that connects the child's mind with the minds of others in the culture, and enables the child to carry out meaningful, goal-directed actions. Through participation in cultural activities and by developing skills using cultural thinking tools, children advance mentally in ways that would not be possible otherwise, and culture, in turn, becomes a constitutive component of human intelligence (Cole, 2006).

To elaborate on this view, we discuss three social processes that provide opportunities for the development of culturally attuned knowledge and cognitive skills: (1) interactions intended to teach the child about thinking and its applications, best illustrated by studies on collaboration in the child's zone of proximal development (ZPD; Vygotsky, 1978); (2) conversations and personal storytelling that convey significant cultural information to children, including what to remember and how to remember information about the world, about human experience, and even about the children themselves (Haden & Ornstein, 2009); and (3) less explicit but pervasive means of transmitting ways of thinking and acting to children, including participation in everyday activities (Göncü, 1999) and routine cultural practices in which children are allowed or expected to assume responsible and meaningful roles (Goodnow, Miller, & Kessel, 1995).

Interactions Intended to Instruct

One of the means by which experienced cultural members support cognitive socialization is by one-on-one instruction. Much of the research on this process is based on Vygotsky's (1978) idea that higher mental functions originate in social life as children interact with more experienced members, and the tools and symbol systems of their culture. To facilitate cognitive development, more experienced partners aim instruction at a child's ZPD, the region of sensitivity for learning, and support the child in using his or her current capabilities to reach higher levels of competence. In interactions in the child's ZPD, understanding is initially social or interpsychological, and after the child internalizes this understanding, it is individual or intrapsychological (Wertsch, 2008).

Research has shown that the structure provided in the ZPD serves as a "scaffold" for the learner, providing contact between old and new knowledge (Wood & Middleton, 1975). Scaffolding is beneficial when it is contingent on the child's learning needs and adjusted during the interaction as the child's competence changes. Support is increased if the child has difficulty and decreased as the child displays increased competence. Language plays a central role in this process because it transforms how a person understands and acts on the world, and enables the thinker to operate independently of immediate perceptual experiences and to consider the past and the future (Wertsch, 2008). More experienced partners use a variety of communicative techniques to advance children's understanding, including suggestions, prompts, hints, directives, questions, praise, and demonstration (Gauvain, 2001). Researchers are especially interested in internal or psychological processes that help children learn from others. For example, Foley and Ratner (1998) found that when young children collaborate with more experienced partners, they sometimes make a source error, that is, they remember themselves as being responsible for actions that the partner did, particularly when the action benefited task performance.

This approach to cognitive development is *microgenetic*, concentrating on change over a brief period of time; *ontogenetic* changes, that is, changes over longer periods of time, are not addressed. However, recent research has begun to examine how this microgenetic process may transpire longitudinally (see, e.g., Connor & Cross, 2003; Hammond et al., 2012). Observations of mother–child planning when children were ages 7, 8, and 9 years revealed that over these years, mothers changed their instruction as tasks increased in difficulty, but their responsiveness to children's learning needs and the level of child engagement was stable (Gauvain & Perez, 2013). Longitudinal research has also found connections between early scaffolding and later cognitive development. For example, Bernier, Carlson, and Whipple (2010) found relations between maternal scaffolding, sensitive responding, and attention to the child's inner mental states, or mind-mindedness (Meins et al., 2002) when infants were ages 12–15 months, and to children's executive functioning at ages 18–26 months.

Taken together, these studies suggest that interactions that are responsive to the child's learning needs are especially valuable. This research also links cognitive socialization with biological change in the prefrontal cortex (Fernyhough, 2010) and sheds light on the shift from other- to self-regulation (Luria, 1973). When interacting in his or her ZPD, the child, at the outset, does not share the adult's understanding of the activity. However, by partaking in the activity with the adult via other-regulation, the child comes to accept the adult's definition and eventually is able to carry out the activity as self-regulated action. As Wertsch (2008) explains, changes in the child's understanding are "largely the result of the child's efforts to establish and maintain coherence between his/her own action and the adult's speech" (p. 78).

Conversation and Personal Storytelling

Children learn much from other people during interactions that emerge in the course of ordinary social life and are not intended to teach or convey any particular skills. To study cognitive development in this type of context, researchers have examined the conversations of young children and their parents, including shared narratives, personal storytelling, and talk during shared activity such as reading books.

Parent–child conversations begin early in the child's life and play an important role in cognitive development. Experience with narratives when reminiscing about the past and during unfolding events is particularly important to the development of memory of events (Reese, 2002). Narratives contain a unique sequence of real or imaginary events that involve human beings as characters (Bruner, 1986). Shared narratives are common in sustained social groups, such as the family. Children are highly motivated to participate in these conversations because they are often about the children themselves and involve familiar people. Experience with narratives provides children with a cognitive structure for encoding, organizing, storing, and communicating memories (Haden & Ornstein, 2009). These conversations also contribute to the child's developing sense of self (Nelson, 1996) and help to establish and maintain identity and cohesion in social groups, including the family (Ochs, Taylor, Rudolph, & Smith, 1992).

The ability to participate in shared narratives appears in early childhood and is built on other cognitive capabilities. By 16 months of age, children are sensitive to the temporal and causal order of events (Bauer & Mandler, 1990). Shortly after the second birthday, they are able to reflect on their own ideas or representations (Nelson, 1996), and as the child's language skills develop, parents and children begin to co-construct narratives, along with increasingly detailed autobiographical stories (Farrant & Reese, 2000). Children's active participation in these conversations is especially important for developing memory skills. Research has shown that children's memory for an event is better when it is talked about by mother and child than when the event is only talked about by mothers or not discussed (Haden, Ornstein, Eckerman, & Didow, 2001). Also, children will use similar memory strategies, such as the elaboration they previously used with their mothers, in conversations with an unfamiliar adult (Lange & Carroll, 2003).

In addition to experience with the narrative form that improves how memories are constructed and recalled (Boland, Haden, & Ornstein, 2003), conversations about the past and unfolding events contribute to cognitive socialization. These conversations inform children about what events are worth remembering (Snow, 1990), thereby enhancing children's attention to certain types of information and experiences. They involve children as authentic participants whose contributions help to shape the focus and direction of the conversation. It is significant that these conversations are intentional cognitive acts. Unlike recognition memory, which happens without awareness that something is being remembered, shared event memory involves explicit awareness that something is being remembered, which may contribute to the development of the reflective capacities associated with executive functions.

Personal storytelling is also important to cognitive socialization. From early in life, children are told stories about themselves and their families. These stories focus on unique family characteristics, as well as the family's identification with the broader culture. To illustrate, P. J. Miller, Fung, Lin, Chen, and Boldt (2012) studied storytelling about past transgressions, in which the child violated social or moral rules, among European American and Taiwanese parents and their 2½-year-old children. Parents in both cultures told such stories to their children, but their emphases differed. While Taiwanese parents were more evaluative of the children's behaviors and promoted children's self-critical analysis, European American parents tended to characterize the transgressions more favorably and encouraged children's more positive self-evaluations. These conversations contribute to cognitive socialization in content and form through the cultural information they contain regarding social expectations and responsibilities. In addition, they engage children in cultural practices of self- and other-examination.

Parent–child conversations also contribute to children's developing understanding of the mind and mental states. The way parents talk about mental states when children are 2 years of age predicts children's own mental state talk at age 4, even when accounting for children's language abilities (Jenkins, Turrell, Kogushi, Lollis, & Ross, 2003). Research has also shown that parent–child storytelling based on a shared picture book relates to the development of children's theory of mind (Turnbull, Carpendale, & Racine, 2009). In this study, mothers' explanatory talk about emotional and conflictual elements of the story predicted children's understanding of false beliefs and of complex or mixed emotions, suggesting that during routine conversations, children can learn about human activity, and the intentions and sentiments behind it. More research is needed, however, to understand the relation between social experience and the development of social understanding in cultural context (Hughes & Leekam, 2004; Nelson et al., 2003).

To summarize, research suggests that adults, especially parents, provide guidance for cognitive development during conversations about the past, as events unfold, and in the context of interpreting actions. Such conversations seem to comprise a substantial portion of young children's time with adults and may be important to cognitive socialization in many cultural settings. Through these conversations children learn techniques for remembering, how others interpret actions, and how to understand and evaluate the beliefs and emotions of other people.

Participation in Everyday Activities

Much of cognitive socialization occurs in the midst of the daily activities of life that are not intended to be instructional (Goodnow et al., 1995; Rogoff, 2003). Children's participation in these activities, including the routines and rituals of the culture, helps them learn the behaviors and cognitive tools that are important in their community. Cultures differ in the type and frequency of these activities, the ways they are carried out, and the nature and extent of children's participation.

By participating in daily or routine activities, children have the chance to observe and practice the mature behaviors of individuals in their community. Adults support this involvement by directing the child's attention to aspects of an activity or pointing out the relation of an action to the goal, as described in the process of guided participation (Rogoff, 1990). Even children as young as age 2–3 years in some communities, such as the Efe foragers in Africa and the Maya in Guatemala, have experience in a limited but authentic fashion with the routine work activities of adults in their societies (Morelli, Rogoff, & Angelillo, 2003). Cultural variation in how children are involved in mature practices of the community leads to differences in what children learn to think about and how they learn to think (Goodnow et al., 1995). For instance, in industrialized communities, many activities in early childhood support the development of literacy, which is valued and important for preparing children for school (see Bennett, Weigel, & Martin, 2002). In general, research indicates that the socially organized nature of children's everyday activities contributes to the development of thinking and problem solving so as to meet cultural goals.

In the context of cultural participation, learning often occurs as children observe mature community members (see Rogoff, Moore, Correa-Chávez, & Dexter, Chapter 20, this volume). Opportunities to observe others, especially those who are more experienced, are important to cognitive socialization. Other people model ways of solving problems in children's presence, and experienced members of the culture allow this type of observational learning, referred to as *legitimate peripheral participation* (Lave & Wenger, 1991). Children play active roles in this process as they direct their attention in a sustained and resolute manner to what it is they want to learn, described by Rogoff, Paradise, Arauz, Correa-Chávez, and Angelillo (2003) as *intent community participation*. Such learning may be especially important in settings where explicit adult–child instruction is infrequent (Lancy, Bock, & Gaskins, 2010).

Also important to cognitive socialization is children's adoption and use of tools that are available in every culture to support and extend thinking. These include symbolic (e.g., language, numeracy) and material tools (e.g., pencil and paper, computers, established plans) (Maynard, Subrahmanyam, & Greenfield, 2005; Olson & Cole, 2006). Over development, children learn to use these tools to help them solve problems and engage with the social and physical world. These tools' diverse cognitive functions include helping people store, represent, manipulate, and communicate ideas and ways of doing things. Notably, these tools of thinking are evident even when someone is working alone.

Learning how to use these tools aligns children's thinking and behaviors with the culture, and provides ways of thinking and acting that would not be possible without the tools (Vygotsky, 1987). Consider, for example, how experience with the spatial representations in maps allows children to obtain insight about large-scale space (Liben, 2001). Children also develop skill at using symbolic representations to guide action, such as an established plan to build an object. The development of this type of skill is aided by other cultural members; however, guidance also exists in the representations themselves (e.g., numbering of steps in a plan; Gauvain, de la Ossa, & Hurtado-Ortiz, 2001). Cultural tools both extend and constrain human intellectual functioning (Cole, 2006). For example, at the same time that e-mail enables communication, it also determines much about what can be communicated. By extension, cultural tools allow for the development of certain psychological functions or behaviors, and they discourage the development of others. As Goodnow (1990) points out, cognitive socialization is not value-free; rather, it is laced with judgments, often made at the cultural level, about what to learn, how to learn it, and, sometimes, who may learn it (e.g., the gender marking of knowledge in notions such as women's or men's issues, or relative to what boys or girls can do).

In summary, the sociocultural context of development provides the core activities through which children learn about thinking. From early in life, children have the interest and some fundamental skills to learn from others. Social experiences build on these capacities and affect cognitive development in many ways. The social processes that support and guide this development are manifold and include instruction in the valued practices of the community, opportunities to talk with and observe more experienced partners both as psychological beings and as models for future action, and experience with the material and symbolic tools that support intelligent action. These opportunities for learning emerge in informal and formal arrangements, and children play active roles in this learning.

Conclusions

Children learn many things from social experience that are important for cognitive development. Learning how to use a symbolic tool, play a game, carry out a complex action, and understand social and psychological functioning are cognitive attainments.

These skills and understanding can only be obtained through social processes because they are not available through solitary activity or introspection. The reasoning behind this claim is simple: Symbolic representations and cultural practices are social constructions; rules of play are social conventions; and modes of informal and formal learning by observing and interacting with others are social processes. Many of the capabilities that define higher-level cognitive functioning entail culturally organized ways of doing things, including behavioral sequences (e.g., routines, rituals), symbolic representations and material tools, and formulations and interpretations of the world that reflect the language, values, and practices of the group (Goodnow, 1990). In short, much of what human beings know—and this is considered distinctive to the species—is cultural, and we acquire this knowledge socially.

There are many social processes that support cognitive development; we concentrated on instruction and collaboration in the ZPD, adult–child conversation and storytelling, and participation in socially organized activities. These processes account for many of the experiences that introduce children to cultural ways of thinking. Although we have discussed these processes separately for purposes of description (and because they tend to be studied independently), they are interrelated and co-occur in a person's experiences and in societies. For instance, a child may show interest in a skill by observing a more experienced person engage in it; upon noticing the child's interest, the experienced person may offer the child guidance or instruction in the skill. A goal of future research is to bring these various processes together into an overarching framework of how sociocultural experience and cognitive development inform and define each other. Better understanding is also needed about how these processes change as children develop, whether certain processes are critical for some areas of development, their occurrence across cultures, and whether their effectiveness is contingent on other social factors, including group composition, size, and dynamics (e.g., cooperative vs. competitive activity). The sheer range of social learning processes underscores the variety and richness of human social life and associated opportunities to develop cognitive skills.

A focus on the social contributions to cognitive development does not mean that internal contributions are unimportant. Social aspects of cognitive development reflect the coordination of human biology; the child's needs, abilities and interests; and the resources and goals of the community. The ability to learn also changes with development, along with the capability to encode, retain, retrieve, reproduce, and modify the information learned socially. Many social factors also regulate cognitive socialization, including the belief systems that guide parents and caregivers as they create situations in which children learn (Sigel, McGillicuddy-DeLisi, & Goodnow, 1992). Psychological and other characteristics of the people involved, such as education, ethnicity, and social class, may also influence the learning opportunities that emerge in social situations (Fisher, Busch-Rossnagel, Jopp, & Brown, 2006; Perez & Gauvain, 2005).

To learn from social experience, children need to play an active role and come to understand the meaning and intention behind what is learned (Tomasello, Carpenter, Call, Behne, & Moll, 2005). The social world does not pour knowledge and skills into children; children adopt, adapt, and reject the information and techniques or tools presented by the social world (Gauvain, 2009). These practices and tools are passed on to children through the many social experiences they have every day. Adults, especially parents, and more experienced partners play key roles in defining and modeling cultural practices and tools for children. Siblings and peers help children sharpen these skills and learn new behaviors. These experiences contain the tacit goal that children, the next leaders of the community, will develop the skills and understanding necessary for mature participation in and maintenance of the community.

To understand intellectual development, it is essential to examine cognitive socialization, that is, how, over the course of development, the social world becomes a constituent element of individual mental functioning. This process is not a simple matter of transmitting the culture into the child's mind. Children actively construct understanding of the world and of themselves through experiences with others and with the institutions and tools of the culture (Lawrence & Valsiner, 1993). The sociocultural context of development—that is, the values, goals, and practices of the community—is instantiated in local situations in the way people interact and the areas of mental functioning that are stressed and rewarded. These experiences are geared toward the skills and knowledge considered mature and competent in that setting. The aim is to foster the development of children's thinking in ways that are socially, culturally, and personally meaningful.

REFERENCES

Adamson, L. B., & Bakeman, R. (1991). The development of shared attention during infancy. In R. Vasta (Ed.), *Annals of child development* (Vol. 8, pp. 1–41). London: Kingsley.

Andersson, J. (2001). Net effect of memory collaboration: How is collaboration affected by factors such as friendship, gender and age? *Scandinavian Journal of Psychology, 42,* 367–375.

Asterhan, C. S. C., & Schwarz, B. B. (2009). Argumentation and explanation in conceptual change: Indications from protocol analyses of peer-to-peer dialog. *Cognitive Science, 33,* 374–400.

Azmitia, M., & Hesser, J. (1993). Why siblings are important agents of cognitive development: A comparison of siblings and peers. *Child Development, 64,* 430–444.

Azmitia, M., & Montgomery, R. (1993). Friendship, transactive dialogues and the development of scientific reasoning. *Social Development, 2,* 202–221.

Baker, D. P., Salinas, D., & Eslinger, P. J. (2012). An envisioned bridge: Schooling as a neurocognitive developmental institution. *Developmental Cognitive Neuroscience, 2*(Suppl. 1), S6–S17.

Bauer, P. J., & Mandler, J. M. (1990). Remembering what happened next: Very young children's recall of event sequences. In R. Fivush & J. A. Hudson (Eds.), *Knowing and remembering in young children* (pp. 9–29). Cambridge, UK: Cambridge University Press.

Bender, M., & Chasiotis, A. (2010). Number of siblings in childhood explains cultural variance in autobiographical memory in Cameroon, People's Republic of China, and Germany. *Journal of Cross-Cultural Psychology, 42,* 998–1017.

Bennett, K. K., Weigel, D. J., & Martin, S. S. (2002). Children's acquisition of early literacy skills: Examining family contributions. *Early Childhood Research Quarterly, 17,* 295–317.

Berg, C. A., & Strough, J. N. (2011). Problem solving across the life span. In K. L. Fingerman, C. A. Berg, J. Smith, & T. C. Antonucci (Eds.), *Handbook of life-span development* (pp. 239–267). New York: Springer.

Bernier, A., Carlson, S. M., & Whipple, N. (2010). From external regulation to self-regulation: Early parenting precursors of young children's executive functioning. *Child Development, 81,* 326–339.

Birch, S. H., & Ladd, G. W. (1997). The teacher–child relationship and children's early school adjustment. *Journal of School Psychology, 35,* 61–79.

Bjorklund, D. F., Hubertz, M. J., & Reubens, A. C. (2004). Young children's arithmetic strategies in social context: How parents contribute to young children's strategy development while playing games. *International Journal of Behavioral Development, 28,* 347–357.

Bjorklund, D. F., & Pellegrini, A. D. (2002). *The origins of human nature: Evolutionary developmental psychology.* Washington, DC: American Psychological Association.

Boaler, J., & Greeno, J. G. (2000). Identity, agency, and knowing in mathematics worlds. In J. Boaler (Ed.), *Multiple perspectives on mathematics teaching and learning* (pp. 171–200). Stamford, CT: Elsevier.

Boland, A. M., Haden, C. A., & Ornstein, P. A. (2003). Boosting children's memory by training mothers in the use of an elaborative conversational style as an event unfolds. *Journal of Cognition and Development, 4,* 39–65.

Bradley, R., & Corwyn, R. (2002). Socioeconomic status and child development. *Annual Review of Psychology, 53,* 371–399.

Bransford, J. D., Brown, A. L., & Cocking, R. R. (1999). *How people learn: Brain, mind, experience, and school.* Washington, DC: National Academy Press.

Brown, J. R., Donelan-McCall, N., & Dunn, J. (1996). Why talk about mental states?: The significance of children's conversations with friends, siblings, and mothers. *Child Development, 67,* 836–849.

Brownell, C. A., Ramani, G. B., & Zerwas, S. (2006). Becoming a social partner with peers: Cooperation and social understanding in one- and two-year-olds. *Child Development, 77,* 803–821.

Bruner, J. (1996). *The culture of education.* Cambridge, MA: Harvard University Press.

Bruner, J. S. (1986). *Actual minds, possible worlds.* Cambridge, MA: Harvard University Press.

Bruner, J. S., & Sherwood, V. (1976). Early rule structure: The case of "peekaboo." In R. Harre (Ed.), *Life sentences* (pp. 55–62). London: Wiley.

Budak, D., & Chavajay, P. (2012). Cultural variation in the social organization of problem solving among African American and European American siblings. *Cultural Diversity and Ethnic Minority Psychology, 18,* 307–311.

Bugental, D., & Goodnow, J. J. (1998). Socialization processes. In W. Damon (Series Ed.) & N. Eisenberg (Vol. Ed.), *Handbook of child psychology: Vol. 3. Social, emotional, and personality development* (pp. 389–462). New York: Wiley.

Buss, D. M. (2012). *Evolutionary psychology: The new science of the mind* (4th ed.). Boston: Allyn & Bacon.

Carpendale, J. I. M., & Lewis, C. (2004). Constructing an understanding of mind: The development of children's social understanding within social interaction. *Brain and Behavioral Sciences, 27,* 79–151.

Carpenter, M., Akhtar, N., & Tomasello, M. (1998). Fourteen- through 18-month-old infants differentially imitate intentional and accidental actions. *Infant Behavior and Development, 21,* 315–330.

Cassidy, K. W., Fineberg, D. S., Brown, K., & Perkins, A. (2005). Theory of mind may be contagious, but you don't catch it from your twin. *Child Development, 76*(1), 97–106.

Cole, M. (2006). Culture and cognitive development in phylogenetic, historical, and ontogenetic perspective. In W. Damon & R. M. Lerner (Series Eds.) & D. Kuhn & R. S. Siegler (Vol. Eds.), *Handbook of child psychology: Vol. 2, Cognition, perception, and language* (6th ed., pp. 636–683). New York: Wiley.

Connor, D. B., & Cross, D. R. (2003). Longitudinal analysis of the presence, efficacy and stability of maternal scaffolding during informal problem-solving interactions. *British Journal of Developmental Psychology, 21,* 315–334.

Denessen, D., Veenman, S., Dobbelsteen, J., & Van Schilt, J. (2008). Dyad composition effects on cognitive collaboration and student achievement. *Journal of Experimental Education, 76,* 363–383.

Dixon, W. E., & Smith, P. H. (2003). Who's controlling whom?: Infant contributions to maternal play behavior. *Infant and Child Development, 12,* 177–195.

Duran, R. T., & Gauvain, M. (1993). The role of age versus expertise in peer collaboration during joint planning. *Journal of Experimental Child Psychology, 55,* 227–242.

Elman, J. L., Bates, E. A., Johnson, M. H., Karmiloff-Smith, A., Parisi, D., & Plunkett, K. (1996). *Rethinking innateness: A connectionist perspective on development.* Cambridge, MA: MIT Press.

Fan, X., & Chen, M. (2001). Parental involvement and students' academic achievement: A meta-analysis. *Educational Psychology Review, 13*(1), 1–22.

Fantuzzo, J. W., Tighe, E., & Childs, S. (2000). Family Involvement Questionnaire: A multivariate assessment of family participation in early childhood education. *Journal of Educational Psychology, 92*(2), 367–376.

Farrant, K., & Reese, E. (2000). Maternal style and children's participation in reminiscing: Stepping stones in children's autobiographical memory development. *Journal of Cognition and Development, 1,* 193–225.

Fawcett, L. M., & Garton, A. F. (2005). The effect of peer collaboration on children's problem solving ability. *British Journal of Educational Psychology, 75,* 157–169.

Feinman, S. (1992). *Social referencing and the social construction of reality in infancy.* New York: Plenum Press.

Fernyhough, C. (2010). Vygotsky, Luria, and the social brain. In B. W. Sokol, U. Müller, J. I. M. Carpendale, A. R. Young, & G. Iarocci (Eds.), *Self and social regulation: Social interaction and the development of social understanding and executive functions* (pp. 56–79). New York: Oxford University Press.

Fisher, C. B., Busch-Rossnagel, N. A., Jopp, J. S., & Brown, J. (2006). Applied developmental science: Contributions and challenges for the 21st century. In C. B. Fisher, N. A. Busch-Rossnagel, J. S. Jopp, & J. Brown (Eds.), *Handbook of psychology: Developmental psychology* (Vol. 6, pp. 517–546). Hoboken, NJ: Wiley.

Fivush, R., Haden, C. A., & Reese, E. (2006). Elaborating on elaborations: Role of maternal reminiscing style in cognitive and socioemotional development. *Child Development, 77,* 1568–1588.

Fleming, V. M., & Alexander, J. M. (2001). The benefits of peer collaboration: A replication with a delayed posttest. *Contemporary Educational Psychology, 26,* 588–601.

Fletcher, G. C., Warneken, F., & Tomasello, M. (2012). Differences in cognitive processes underlying the collaborative activities of children and chimpanzees. *Cognitive Development, 27,* 136–153.

Flynn, E. (2010). Underpinning collaborative learning. In B. W. Sokol, U. Müller, J. M. Carpendale, A. R. Young, & G. Iarocci (Eds.), *Self and social regulation: Social interaction and the development of social understanding and executive functions* (pp. 312–336). New York: Oxford University Press.

Flynn, E. G., Laland, K. N., Kendal, R. L., & Kendal, J. R. (2013). Developmental niche constructions. *Developmental Science, 16,* 296–313.

Foley, M. A., & Ratner, H. H. (1998). Children's recoding in memory for collaboration: A way of learning from others. *Cognitive Development, 13,* 91–108.

Freire, P. (1970). *Pedagogy of the oppressed.* New York: Continuum.

Furrer, C., & Skinner, E. (2003). Sense of relatedness as a factor in children's academic engagement and performance. *Journal of Educational Psychology, 95*(1), 148–162.

Garton, A. F., & Pratt, C. (2001). Peer assistance in children's problem solving. *British Journal of Developmental Psychology, 19,* 307–318.

Gauvain, M. (2001). *The social context of cognitive development.* New York: Guilford Press.

Gauvain, M. (2009). Social and cultural transitions in cognitive development: A cross-generational view. In A. J. Sameroff (Ed.), *The transactional model of development: How children and contexts shape each other* (pp. 163–182). Washington, DC: American Psychological Association.

Gauvain, M., de la Ossa, J. L., & Hurtado-Ortiz, M. T. (2001). Parental guidance as children learn to use tools: The case of pictorial plans. *Cognitive Development, 16,* 551–575.

Gauvain, M., & Fagot, B. I. (1995). Child temperament as a mediator of mother–toddler problem solving. *Social Development, 4,* 257–276.

Gauvain, M., & Perez, S. M. (2005). Parent–child participation in planning children's activities outside of school in European American and Latino families. *Child Development, 76,* 371–383.

Gauvain, M., & Perez, S. M. (2008). Mother–child planning and child compliance. *Child Development, 79,* 761–775.

Gauvain, M., & Perez, S. M. (2013, April). *Stability and change in mother–child planning over middle childhood.* Presented at the biennial meetings of the Society for Research in Child Development, Seattle, WA.

Gauvain, M., Perez, S. M., & Beebe, H. (2013). Authoritative parenting and parental support for children's cognitive development. In R. E. Larzelere, A. S. Morris, & A. W. Harrist (Eds.), *Authoritative parenting: Synthesizing nurturance and discipline for optimal child development* (pp. 211–233). Washington, DC: American Psychological Association.

Gauvain, M., & Rogoff, B. (1989). Collaborative problem solving and children's planning skills. *Developmental Psychology, 25,* 139–151.

Golbeck, S. L. (1998). Peer collaboration and children's representation of the horizontal surface of liquid. *Journal of Applied Developmental Psychology, 19,* 571–592.

Göncü, A. (1999). *Children's engagement in the world: Sociocultural perspectives.* Cambridge, UK: Cambridge University Press.

Göncü, A., & Gauvain, M. (2012). Sociocultural approaches to educational psychology: Theory, research, and application. In K. R. Harris, S. Graham, T. Urdan, C. B. McCormick, G. M. Sinatra, & J. Sweller (Eds.), *APA educational psychology handbook: Vol. 1. Theories, constructs, and critical issues* (pp. 123–152). Washington, DC: American Psychological Association.

Goodnow, J. J. (1990). The socialization of cognition: What's involved? In J. W. Stigler, R. A. Shweder, & G. Herdt (Eds.), *Cultural psychology* (pp. 259–286). Cambridge, UK: Cambridge University Press.

Goodnow, J. J., Miller, P. J., & Kessel, F. (1995). *Cultural practices as contexts for development.* San Francisco: Jossey-Bass.

Grusec, J. E., & Davidov, M. (2010). Integrating different perspectives on socialization theory and research: A domain-specific approach. *Child Development, 81*(3), 687–709.

Guajardo, N. R., Snyder, G., & Petersen, R. (2009). Relationships among parenting practices, parental stress, child behaviour, and children's social-cognitive development. *Infant and Child Development, 60,* 37–60.

Haden, C. A., & Ornstein, P. A. (2009). Research on talking about the past: The past, present, and future. *Journal of Cognition and Development, 10,* 135–142.

Haden, C. A., Ornstein, P. A., Eckerman, C. O., & Didow, S. M. (2001). Mother–child conversational interactions as events unfold: Linkages to subsequent remembering. *Child Development, 72,* 1016–1031.

Hammond, S. I., Müller, U., Carpendale, J. I. M., Bibok, M. B., & Liebermann-Finestone, D. P. (2012). The effects of parental scaffolding on preschoolers' executive function. *Developmental Psychology, 48,* 271–281.

Hamre, B. K., & Pianta, R. C. (2001). Early teacher–child relationships and the trajectory of children's school outcomes through eighth grade. *Child Development, 72*(2), 625–638.

Harris, J. R. (1995). Where is the child's environment?: A group socialization theory of development. *Psychological Review, 102,* 458–489.

Hawkins, J., Homolsky, M., & Heide, P. (1984). *Paired problem solving in a computer context* (Technical Report No. 33). New York: Bank Street College of Education.

Holmes-Lonergran, H. (2003). Preschool children's collaborative problem-solving interactions: The role of gender, pair type, and task. *Sex Roles, 48,* 505–517.

Homer, B. D., & Tamis-LeMonda, C. S. (2012). *The development of social cognition and communication.* East Sussex, UK: Psychology Press.

Howe, C. (2009). Collaborative group work in middle childhood. *Human Development, 52,* 215–239.

Howe, N., & Bruno, A. (2010). Sibling pretend play in early and middle childhood: The role of creativity and maternal context. *Early Education and Development, 21,* 940–962.

Howe, N., Recchia, H., Porta, S. D., & Funamoto, A. (2012). "The driver doesn't sit, he stands up like the Flintstones!": Sibling teaching during teacher-directed and self-guided tasks. *Journal of Cognition and Development, 13,* 208–231.

Hughes, C. (2011). *Social understanding and social lives.* New York: Psychology Press.

Hughes, C., Fujisawa, K. K., Ensor, R., Lecce, S., & Marfleet, R. (2006). Cooperation and conversations about the mind: A study of individual differences in 2-year-olds and their siblings. *British Journal of Developmental Psychology, 24,* 53–72.

Hughes, C., & Leekam, S. (2004). What are the links between theory of mind and social relations?: Review, reflections, and new directions for studies of typical and atypical development. *Social Development, 13,* 590–619.

Hughes, J. N., Luo, W., Kwok, O., & Loyd, L. K. (2008). Teacher–student support, effortful engagement, and achievement: A 3-year longitudinal study. *Journal of Educational Psychology, 100*(1), 1–14.

Huntsinger, C. S., & Jose, P. E. (2009). Parental involvement in children's schooling: Different meanings in different cultures. *Early Childhood Research Quarterly, 24*(4), 398–410.

Hyde, J. S., Else-Quest, N. M., Alibali, M. W., Knuth, E., & Romberg, T. (2006). Mathematics in the home: Homework practices and mother–child interactions doing mathematics. *Journal of Mathematical Behavior, 25,* 136–152.

Jenkins, J. M., Turrell, S., Kogushi, Y., Lollis, S., & Ross, H. A. (2003). Longitudinal investigation of the dynamics of mental state talk in families. *Child Development, 74,* 905–920.

Jipson, J. L., & Callanan, M. A. (2003). Mother–child conversation and children's understanding of biological and nonbiological changes in size. *Child Development, 74,* 629–644.

Joiner, R., Littleton, K., Faulkner, D., & Miell, D. (2000). *Rethinking collaborative learning.* London: Free Association Books.

Jones, I. (2002). Social relationships, peer collaboration and children's oral language. *Educational Psychology, 22,* 63–73.

Karabenick, S. A., & Newman, R. S. (2006). *Help seeking in academic settings: Goals, groups, and contexts.* Mahwah, NJ: Erlbaum.

Kolb, B., & Whishaw, I. Q. (2013). *An introduction to brain and behavior* (4th ed.). New York: Worth.

Konner, M. (2010). *The evolution of childhood: Relationships, emotion, mind.* Cambridge, MA: Harvard University Press.

Kritt, D. W., & Winegar, L. T. (2007). *Education and technology: Critical perspectives, possible futures.* Lanham, MA: Lexington.

Kruger, A. C. (1992). The effect of peer and adult–child transactive discussions on moral reasoning. *Merrill–Palmer Quarterly, 38,* 191–211.

Kutnick, P., & Kington, A. (2005). Children's friendships and learning in school: Cognitive enhancement through social interaction? *British Journal of Educational Psychology, 75*(4), 521–538.

Ladd, G. W., Kochenderfer-Ladd, B., Visconti, K., & Ettekal, I. (2012). Classroom peer relations and children's social and scholastic development: Risk factors and resources. In A. M. Ryan & G. W. Ladd (Eds.), *Peer relationships and adjustment at school* (pp. 11–49). Charlotte, NC: Information Age.

Lancy, D. F., Bock, J. S., & Gaskins, S. (2009). *Anthropological perspectives on learning in childhood.* Lanham, MD: AltaMira Press.

Landry, S. H., & Smith, K. E. (2010). Early social and cognitive precursors and parental support for self-regulation and executive function: Relations from early childhood into adolescence. In B. W. Sokol, U. Müller, J. M. Carpendale, A. R. Young, & G. Iarocci (Eds.), *Self and social regulation: Social interaction and the development of social understanding and executive functions* (pp. 386–417). New York: Oxford University Press.

Lange, G., & Carroll, D. E. (2003). Mother–child conversation styles and children's laboratory memory for narrative and nonnarrative materials. *Journal of Cognition and Development, 4,* 435–457.

Lave, J., & Wenger, E. (1991). *Situated learning: Legitimate peripheral participation.* Cambridge, UK: Cambridge University Press.

Lawrence, J. A., & Valsiner, J. (1993). Conceptual roots of internalizations: From transmission to transformation. *Human Development, 36,* 150–167.

LeBlanc, G., & Bearison, D. J. (2004). Teaching and learning as a bi-directional activity: Investigating dyadic interactions between child teachers and child learners. *Cognitive Development, 19,* 499–515.

Legerstee, M., Haley, D. W., & Bornstein, M. H. (2013). *The infant mind: Origins of the social brain.* New York: Guilford Press.

Leman, P. J., Macedo, A. P., Bluschke, A., Hudson, L., Rawling, C., & Wright, H. (2011). The influence of gender and ethnicity on children's peer collaborations. *British Journal of Developmental Psychology, 29,* 131–137.

Liben, L. S. (2001). Thinking through maps. In M. Gattis (Ed.), *Spatial schemas and abstract thought* (pp. 45–77). Cambridge, MA: MIT Press.

Light, P., & Littleton, K. (1999). *Social processes in children's learning.* Cambridge, UK: Cambridge University Press.

Lugo-Gil, J., & Tamis-LeMonda, C. S. (2008). Family resources and parenting quality: Links to children's cognitive development across the first 3 years. *Child Development, 79,* 1065–1085.

Luria, A. R. (1973). *The working brain: An introduction to neuropsychology* (B. Haigh, Trans.). New York: Basic Books.

Maccoby, E. E. (2002). *Parenting and the child's world: Influences on academic, intellectual, and socio-emotional development.* Mahwah, NJ: Erlbaum.

Manion, V., & Alexander, J. M. (1997). The benefits of peer collaboration on strategy use, metacognitive causal attribution, and recall. *Journal of Experimental Child Psychology, 67,* 268–289.

Matheson, H., Moore, C., & Akhtar, N. (2013). The development of social learning in interactive and observational contexts. *Journal of Experimental Child Psychology, 114,* 161–172.

Maynard, A. E. (2002). Cultural teaching: The development of teaching skills in Maya sibling interactions. *Child Development, 73*(3), 969–982.

Maynard, A. E., Subrahmanyam, K., & Greenfield, P. M. (2005). Technology and the development of intelligence: From the loom to the computer. In R. J. Sternberg & D. D. Priess (Eds.), *Intelligence and technology: The impact of tools on the nature and development of human abilities* (pp. 29–53). Mahwah, NJ: Erlbaum.

McAlister, A., & Peterson, C. (2007). A longitudinal study of child siblings and theory of mind development. *Cognitive Development, 22,* 258–270.

Meins, E., Fernyhough, C., Wainwright, R., Gupta, M. D., Fradley, E., & Tuckey, M. (2002). Maternal mind-mindedness and attachment security as predictors of theory of mind understanding. *Child Development, 73,* 1715–1726.

Mercer, N., & Littleton, K. (2007). *Dialogue and the development of children's thinking: A socio-cultural approach.* London: Routledge.

Miller, K., Dilworth-Bart, J., & Hane, A. (2011). Maternal recollections of schooling and children's school preparation. *School Community Journal, 21*(2), 161–184.

Miller, P. J., Fung, H., Lin, S., Chen, E. C.-H., & Boldt, B. R. (2012). How socialization happens on the ground: Narrative practices as alternate socializing pathways in Taiwanese and European-American families. *Monographs of the Society for Research in Child Development, 77*(Serial No. 302), vii, 1–140.

Morelli, G., Rogoff, B., & Angelillo, C. (2003). Cultural variation in children's access to work or involvment in specialized child-focused activities. *International Journal of Behavioral Development, 27,* 264–274.

Nelson, K. (1996). *Language in cognitive development.* Cambridge, UK: Cambridge University Press.

Nelson, K., Shwerer, D. P., Goldman, S., Henseler, S., Presler, N., & Walkenfeld, F. F. (2003).

Entering a community of minds: An experiential approach to "theory of mind." *Human Development, 46*, 24–46.

Ochs, E., Taylor, C., Rudolph, D., & Smith, R. (1992). Storytelling as a theory-building activity. *Discourse Processes, 15*, 37–72.

Olson, D., & Cole, M. (2006). *Technology, literacy, and the evolution of society: Implications of the work of Jack Goody.* Mahwah, NJ: Erlbaum.

Ono, H., & Sanders, J. (2010). Diverse family types and out-of-school learning time of young school-age children. *Family Relations, 59*(5), 506–519.

Onyango-Ouma, W., Aagaard-Hansen, J., & Jensen, B. B. (2005). The potential of schoolchildren as health change agents in rural western Kenya. *Social Science and Medicine, 61*, 1711–1722.

Patrick, H., Johnson, K. R., Mantzicopoulos, P., & Gray, D. L. (2011). "I tell them I know how to do my ABCs!" *Elementary School Journal, 112*(2), 383–405.

Perez, S. M., & Gauvain, M. (2005). Relation of child emotionality to individual and mother–child planning. *Social Development, 14*, 250–272.

Perez, S. M., & Gauvain, M. (2009). Mother–child planning, child emotional functioning, and children's transition to first grade. *Child Development, 80*, 776–791.

Perner, J., Ruffman, T., & Leekam, S. R. (1994). Theory of mind is contagious: You can catch it from your sibs. *Child Development, 65*, 1228–1238.

Piaget, J. (1926). *The language and thought of the child.* New York: Harcourt Brace.

Plomin, R., DeFries, J. C., Knopik, V. S., & Neiderhiser, J. M. (2013). *Behavioral genetics* (6th ed.). New York: Worth.

Posner, M. I. (2012). *Attention in a social world.* New York: Oxford University Press.

Pruden, S. M., Levine, S. C., & Huttenlocher, J. (2011). Children's spatial thinking: Does talk about the spatial world matter? *Developmental Science, 14*, 1417–1430.

Reese, E. (2002). Social factors in the development of autobiographical memory: The state of the art. *Social Development, 11*, 124–142.

Rogoff, B. (1990). *Apprenticeship in thinking: Cognitive development in social context.* New York: Oxford University Press.

Rogoff, B. (2003). *The cultural nature of human development.* Oxford, UK: Oxford University Press.

Rogoff, B., Paradise, R., Arauz, R. M., Correa-Chávez, M., & Angelillo, C. (2003). Firsthand learning through intent participation. *Annual Review of Psychology, 54*, 175–203.

Rojas-Drummond, S. (2009). Rethinking the role of peer collaboration in enhancing cognitive growth. *Human Development, 52*, 240–245.

Sabol, T. J., & Pianta, R. C. (2013). Relationships between teachers and children. In W. M. Reynolds, G. E. Miller, & I. B. Weiner (Eds.), *Handbook of psychology: Vol. 7. Educational psychology* (2nd ed., pp. 199–211). Hoboken, NJ: Wiley.

Salonen, P., Lepola, J., & Vauras, M. (2007). Scaffolding interaction in parent–child dyads: Multimodal analysis of parental scaffolding with task and non-task oriented children. *European Journal of Psychology of Education, 22*, 77–96.

Sawyer, R. K. (2006). *The Cambridge handbook of the learning sciences.* New York: Cambridge University Press.

Scaife, M., & Bruner, J. S. (1975). The capacity for joint visual attention in the infant. *Nature, 253*, 265–266.

Senese, V. P., Bornstein, M. H., Haynes, O. M., Rossi, G., & Venuti, P. (2012). A cross-cultural comparison of mothers' beliefs about their parenting very young children. *Infant Behavior and Development, 35*, 479–488.

Serpell, R., & Hatano, G. (1997). Education, schooling, and literacy. In J. W. Berry, P. R. Dasen, & T. S. Saraswathi (Eds.), *Handbook of cross-cultural psychology: Vol. 2. Basic process and human development* (pp. 339–376). Boston: Allyn & Bacon.

Sigel, I. E., McGillicuddy-DeLisi, A. V., & Goodnow, J. J. (1992). *Parental belief systems: The psychological consequences for children* (2nd ed.). Mahwah, NJ: Erlbaum.

Snow, C. E. (1990). Building memories: The ontogeny of autobiography. In D. Cicchetti & M. Beeghly (Eds.), *The self in transition* (pp. 213–242). Chicago: University of Chicago Press.

Spelke, E. S., & Kinzler, K. D. (2007). Core knowledge. *Developmental Science, 10,* 89–96.

Striano, T., Henning, A., & Stahl, D. (2005). Sensitivity to social contingencies between 1 and 3 months of age. *Developmental Science, 8,* 509–518.

Tamis-LeMonda, C. S., Bornstein, M. H., & Baumwell, L. (2001). Maternal responsiveness and children's achievement of milestones. *Child Development, 72,* 748–767.

Teasley, S. D. (1995). The role of talk in children's peer collaboration. *Developmental Psychology, 31,* 207–220.

Tomasello, M. (1999). *The cultural origins of human cognition.* Cambridge, MA: Harvard University Press.

Tomasello, M., Carpenter, M., Call, J., Behne, T., & Moll, H. (2005). Understanding and sharing of intentions: The origins of cultural cognition. *Behavioral and Brain Sciences, 28,* 675–735.

Tomasello, M., & Haberl, K. (2003). Understanding attention: 12- and 18-month-olds know what is new for other persons. *Developmental Psychology, 39,* 906–912.

Tomasello, M., Kruger, A. C., & Ratner, H. H. (1993). Cultural learning. *Behavioral and Brain Sciences, 16,* 495–511.

Trevarthen, C. (1980). The foundations of intersubjectivity: Development of interpersonal and cooperative understanding in infants. In D. R. Olson (Ed.), *The social foundations of language and thought* (pp. 316–342). New York: Norton.

Tudge, J. R. H., Odero, D. A., Hogan, D. M., & Etz, K. E. (2003). Relations between the everyday activities of preschoolers and their teachers' perceptions of their competence in the first years of school. *Early Childhood Research Quarterly, 18,* 42–64.

Turnbull, W., Carpendale, J. I. M., & Racine, T. P. (2009). Talk and children's understanding of mind. *Journal of Consciousness Studies, 16,* 140–166.

Vygotsky, L. S. (1978). *Mind in society.* Cambridge, MA: Harvard University Press.

Vygotsky, L. S. (1987). Thinking and speech. In R. W. Rieber & A. S. Carton (Eds.), *The collected works of L. S. Vygotsky* (N. Minick, Trans.) (pp. 37–285). New York: Plenum Press.

Wagner, D. A. (1993). *Literacy, culture, and development: Becoming literate in Morocco.* Cambridge, UK: Cambridge University Press.

Wertsch, J. V. (2008). From social interaction to higher psychological processes: A clarification and application of Vygotsky's theory. *Human Development, 51,* 66–79.

Wood, D. J., & Middleton, D. (1975). A study of assisted problem solving. *British Journal of Psychology, 66,* 181–191.

CHAPTER 25

The Socialization of Emotional Competence

Susanne A. Denham
Hideko H. Bassett
Todd Wyatt

Emotions are ubiquitous in all our lives. The information that they afford—about ourselves and others—is invaluable. Our overarching goal in this chapter is to elucidate and comment on the state of current knowledge of the ways in which children, from toddlerhood through adolescence, learn from others about aspects of emotions—how others' emotion-related expressiveness, behaviors, and beliefs contribute to the development of their emotional competence. To meet this central goal, we must first define the boundaries of what we mean by *emotional competence*.

After detailing this central construct, we consider the role of both intra- and interpersonal contributors to the development of emotional competence. To flesh out central issues of concern, we again give attention to definitional matters: What *is* socialization *of emotion*? Finally, we evaluate the state of knowledge about this important area of development, address perceived gaps in the literature, and suggest ways to think about and investigate these phenomena in the future. Ultimately, we hope this important information will be shared outside the research community to build optimal support for the healthy development of emotional competence.

Emotional Competence and Its Role in Social Functioning

Aspects of emotional competence developing through the life span include emotional expression and experience, understanding emotions of self and others, and emotion regulation. Children become increasingly emotionally competent over time, and growing evidence suggests that such emotional competence contributes to their concurrent social competence and well-being, as well as to later social and academic outcomes (Denham et al., 2003; Denham, Brown, & Domitrovich, 2010). Even preschool-age children are surprisingly adept at several components of emotional competence, including but not limited to the following: (1) expressing emotions that are, or are not, experienced; (2) decoding these processes in others; and (3) regulating emotions in ways that are age- and socially appropriate (Halberstadt, Denham, & Dunsmore, 2001).

These elements of emotional competence require operationalization. Thus, when discussing *emotional expressiveness*, we refer to (1) the specific emotions shown, with varying purposefulness, by children (e.g., happiness, sadness, anger, fear, and empathy/love), and (2) the overall rate of such expressiveness, across emotions. Next, to define *emotion knowledge*, we refer to children's knowledge about the emotions of themselves and others, including (1) comprehension of basic emotions (e.g., happiness, sadness, and anger), their expressions, situations, causes, and consequences; (2) insight into more complicated facets of emotions (e.g., that two people can feel two different emotions in response to the same eliciting event, e.g., when one child finds an event scary, but another does not); and (3) discernment of display rule usage, mixed emotions, and more complex emotions (e.g., guilt and shame). Finally, children can *regulate their emotion* when its experience is "too much" or "too little" for their own comfort or others' expectations, by using physical, cognitive, and/or behavioral strategies to dampen or amplify internal emotional experience and/or external emotional expression.

Furthermore, the contribution of emotional skills to social competence is a key tenet of emotional competence theory (Denham, 1998; Saarni, 1999). For example, happier, less angry children and adolescents are better liked by peers; teachers see them as friendly and cooperative (Denham et al., 2003; Harker & Keltner, 2001; Isley, O'Neil, Clatfelter, & Parke, 1999). Negative expressiveness is associated with less positive outcomes (Miller et al., 2006).

Accurate interpretation of others' emotions provides important information about social situations. Hence, children's emotion knowledge often relates to peer status and lack of self-perceptions of rejection and victimization, prosocial behaviors, teacher ratings of social competence, and inhibiting aggression (see the meta-analysis by Trentacosta & Fine, 2010).

Emotion regulation also is a crucial contributor to aspects of social competence. Preschoolers who regulate their anger by venting are seen as less socially competent by kindergarten peers and teachers than those who use other emotion regulation strategies (Miller, Gouley, Seifer, Dickstein, & Shields, 2004). Similar relations hold for older children and adolescents (Murphy, Shepard, Eisenberg, & Fabes, 2004; Rydell, Berlin, & Bohlin, 2003).

Contributors to Individual Differences in Emotional Competence

Both intra- and interpersonal contributors to these aspects of children's emotional competence must be considered. Because emotional competence is intimately related to important child outcomes, such as social and even academic competence (e.g., Denham, Brown, et al., 2010), questions about its cultivation and individual differences must be answered. Both intrapersonal (within-child) and interpersonal (socialization) contributors are no doubt important.

Intrapersonal Contributors to Emotional Competence: How Within-Child Factors Affect Emotional Competence

Before the role of socialization agents in the development of emotional competence is considered, it should be noted that abilities and attributes of children themselves can either promote or hinder emotional competence. For example, some children have capacities for superior cognitive and language skills that allow them to better understand their social world, including the emotions within it, as well as communicate their own feelings, wishes, desires, and goals for social interactions and relationships (e.g., Morgan, Izard, & King, 2010). Children who can reason more flexibly probably also more readily perceive others' emotions that differ from their own (Bennett, Bendersky, & Lewis, 2005). More verbal children can ask more specific questions about their own and others' emotions, and understand the answers to these questions, giving them a special advantage in dealing with emotions (Beck, Kumschick, Eid, & Klann-Delius, 2012; Dunn, Brown, & Beardsall, 1991). A preschooler with advanced expressive language also can describe his or her own emotions more pointedly (e.g., "I don't want to go to bed! I am *mad*!"), allowing others to communicate with the child about the emotional situation.

Similarly, children with different emotional dispositions (i.e., different temperaments) are particularly well- or ill-equipped to demonstrate emotional competence. Thus, temperamental characteristics involving the expression or inhibition of emotion can be particularly important in setting the groundwork for social behavior. Especially emotionally negative children probably find that they have a greater need for emotion regulation, even though it is at the same time harder for them to do so. Conversely, children whose temperament predisposes them flexibly to focus attention on a comforting action, object, or thought and shift attention from a distressing situation are better able to regulate emotions, even intense ones. These intrapersonal factors no doubt continue to exert influence well into adolescence. They can be either foundations of or roadblocks to emotional and social competence. Moreover, they may interact with interpersonal contributors; for example, children with negative or positive temperaments may benefit most from specific emotion socialization techniques, depending on the nature of the interaction with socializers (Yap, Allen, Leve, & Katz, 2008).

Interpersonal Contributors to Emotional Competence: First Considerations of Socialization by Important Others

Adult caregivers are faced daily with children who vary in their emotional competence. How do they foster these emotional competencies that stand children in such good stead? Even given the important intrapersonal contributors already mentioned, much of the individual variation in children's emotional competence derives from experiences within the family, classroom, and peer group (Denham, 1998; Eisenberg, Cumberland, & Spinrad, 1998; Hyson, 1994).

Thus, socialization of emotional competence is likely to be very important—but how does it fit within a larger discipline of developmental science, and socialization in general? This question is deceptive in its simplicity: A desired outcome of socialization is emotion regulation (Grusec, 2002). Nonetheless, we must consider several issues before describing socialization of emotion.

First, where does one draw the line between everyday interaction with children, in which conscious socialization goals are not necessarily in mind but emotions are ever-present, and "real" socialization of emotion? Certainly, most parents do not focus consciously on the emotion socialization of their children while reprimanding them. Nonetheless, we argue that "socialization is any task or content area that is part of learning a cultural pattern. . . . affect is . . . an integral part of the ideas we hold, the practices that we follow . . . and our experiences with others" (Bugental & Goodnow, 1998, p. 441). The root of socialization about such a central set of beliefs and abilities lies within everyday interaction rather than resting solely on occasional moments of transgression followed by discipline. In short, both unintentional and intentional parental socialization processes are likely to impact emotional competence, just like any other socialization outcome. However, unintentional processes may be very dominant, or even exclusive, when other socialization agents, such as peers, are considered.

A second issue to consider when "pinning down" socialization of emotion is that many of the behaviors associated with what we consider the most adaptive of its forms are also closely related to parental "responsiveness," "warmth," or "control," which leaves one wondering whether the notion of "socialization of emotion" adds much at all (Gondoli & Braungart-Rieker, 1998). Parenting goals and values contribute not only to higher-order stylistic parenting dimensions such as warmth and control but also to more specific parenting behaviors, including those relevant to socialization of emotion. Therefore, it is quite likely that both parenting styles and specific emotion socialization practices are related, but not totally overlapping, constructs (see also Chang, Schwartz, Dodge, & McBride-Chang, 2003; Eisenberg, Zhou, et al., 2003). At times, aspects of parenting style may in fact directly contribute to emotional competence, such as when supportiveness predicts rates of growth in toddlers' emotion regulation (Bocknek, Brophy-Herb, & Banerjee, 2009). Alternatively, broader but still emotion-related aspects of parenting, such as warmth and supportiveness, may work together with more distinctly emotional aspects of socialization, such as emotional expressiveness (Brophy-Herb, Stansbury, Bocknek, & Horodynski, 2012; Chan, Bowes, & Wyver, 2009). At other times, although parenting style may predict social-emotional competence, socialization of emotion behaviors may still contribute uniquely or interact with parenting style in their contribution to social-emotional skill (Tang, Liang, Deng, Ye, & Lu, 2012). Thus, socialization of emotion practices occurs *within the context* of a higher-order parenting style, and these practices and styles are informed by parents' goals and values.

Specifically, parents and other socializers probably all hold "meta-emotion philosophies" about which emotions *should be* felt and expressed and how they *should be* felt and expressed, how salient they are, and what *should be* done in emotional situations (Gottman, Katz, & Hooven, 1997). An emotion-based set of beliefs such as the meta-emotion philosophy fits squarely within Bugental and Goodnow's (1998) definition of *socialization*: Others form (whether consciously or not) expectations about children's emotions and emotion-related behaviors. Furthermore, such beliefs about emotions and their socialization do predict parents' emotion socialization behaviors (Baker, Fenning, & Crnic, 2011; Perez Rivera & Dunsmore, 2011; Wong, Diener, & Isabella, 2008; Wong, McElwain, & Halberstadt, 2009; Yap, Allen, Leve, et al., 2008); parental beliefs about emotions may even make direct contributions to children's emotional competence (Cunningham, Kliewer, & Garner, 2009; Dunsmore & Karn, 2001). Thus, the child notices, interprets, and encodes these expressed expectations, adopts a stance toward them, and, finally, gives an indication of understanding the socialization message by reacting to it.

So, in our view, socialization of emotions is omnipresent in children's everyday contact with parents, teachers, caregivers, and peers. All people with whom children interact exhibit a variety of emotions, which the children observe. We refer to this aspect of socialization of emotion as *modeling*, whether discussing specific expressed emotions observed by children or referring to the totality of emotional expressiveness (and its valence) to which children are exposed within a context. Furthermore, children's emotions often require some kind of reaction from social partners. We refer to this aspect of socialization as *contingent reactions* to children's emotional expressiveness. Finally, *teaching* about the world of emotions is considered by many adults to be an important area of socialization (Eisenberg, Fabes, & Murphy, 1996; Eisenberg et al., 1999). Eisenberg, Cumberland, and colleagues (1998) cited evidence for all three mechanisms with regard to parents. Their conclusions suggest that each of these mechanisms influences children's emotional expression, knowledge, and regulation, as well as social functioning.

Socialization of Emotions

Modeling Mechanisms

EMOTIONAL EXPRESSIVENESS

Children are constantly viewing and processing others' emotional behavior and incorporating this learning into their own expressive behavior. By modeling various emotions, socializers give children information about how and when both positive and negative emotions are expressed. Exposure to a particular profile of emotions can promote children's experience and expression of the same emotions and may also contribute to differing patterns of overall emotional expressiveness (Halberstadt, Fox, & Jones, 1993; Valiente, Eisenberg, et al., 2004).

For example, parents' and children's positive emotional expression are significantly related (Isley et al., 1999). Conversely, when mothers are often angry and tense with them, young children are angrier and less emotionally positive (Denham, 1998; Denham, Mitchell-Copeland, Strandberg, Auerbach, & Blair, 1997; Isley et al., 1999; Newland & Crnic, 2011). Parents' intense, frequent negative emotions are also related to elementary school-age children's quick, unregulated anger (Snyder, Stoolmiller, Wilson, & Yamamoto, 2003). Well-modulated negative emotion may, however, have positive effects on preschoolers' emotional positivity (Denham & Grout, 1992).

Lack of emotional expressiveness can also impact children's expressiveness; for example, children diagnosed with anxiety disorder and their mothers are less emotionally expressive than nonanxious children and their mothers (Suveg, Zeman, Flannery-Schroeder, & Cassano, 2005). As suggested by Suveg and colleagues (2005), "truncated family emotional expressivity" (p. 145) may have definite consequences for the development of children's emotional competence.

Emotional expressiveness of parents and their offspring takes on a new appearance during adolescence. Parents' and adolescents' observed emotions may still be highly intercorrelated, suggesting that parents still model emotional expressiveness (Bronstein,

Fitzgerald, Briones, Pieniadz, & D'Ari, 1993). Yet early adolescents' expression of negative emotions increases, and negative affect reciprocity is present in many adolescent–parent interactions (Larson, Moneta, Richards, & Wilson, 2002). In particular, Kim, Conger, Lorenz, and Elder (2001) found that both parents' and adolescents' initial levels of negative emotion toward each other predicted the rate of growth and rate of change in growth of expressed negative affect.

Almost no research has examined these socialization effects with nonparents. Considering teachers as socializers of elementary school-age children, Demorat (1999) examined a kindergarten teacher's emotions in relation to the responses of four students over 3 months. The students matched her interest and happiness. Thus, elementary school-age children are learning about emotional expressiveness and display rules from important adults in both family and school contexts.

EMOTION KNOWLEDGE

Others' overall emotional expressiveness, and the particular profile of emotions that they express, also implicitly teach children about the emotional significance of differing events, how certain situations evoke specific emotions, the behaviors that may accompany differing emotions, and others' likely reactions. Thus, parents' emotions are associated with children's emotion knowledge (Denham & Grout, 1993; Denham et al., 1997; Nixon & Watson, 2001). In particular, positive expressiveness in the family seems to promote emotion knowledge, perhaps because positive feelings render children more open to learning and problem solving (Fredrickson, 1998).

Conversely, exposure to parents' negative emotions can hamper young children's emotion knowledge by making it difficult for them to address issues of emotion altogether. Specifically, although exposure to *well-regulated* negative emotion can be positively related to emotion knowledge (Garner, Jones, & Miner, 1994), parents' frequent, intense negative emotions—especially anger—may disturb children, as well as discourage self-reflection, so that little learning occurs (Denham, 1998; Denham, Zoller, & Couchoud, 1994; Raver & Spagnola, 2002).

Experience within the extremely angry, hostile emotional environment of physical maltreatment may confer on maltreated children the ability to identify angry expressions with less sensory input than nonmaltreated children (Pollak & Sinha, 2002). However, Pollak and Tolley-Schell's (2003) findings suggest that any advantage accrued by increased ability to identify valid anger cues may be counterbalanced by trouble disengaging from invalid anger cues, an identification bias. Thus, in terms of emotion knowledge, children developing under exceptional emotional circumstances may differ quantitatively *or* qualitatively from children in more normative socialization contexts.

During grade school, aspects of parents' emotions still predict emotion knowledge—for example, fathers' clear expressions of emotion are associated with children's general skill at recognizing emotional expressions (Dunsmore, Her, Halberstadt, & Perez-Rivera, 2009). However, children's observation of peers' emotions and rules about emotions are likely to grow in importance. Observations of peer emotions also might be expected to inform more sophisticated aspects of emotion knowledge, such as understanding of complex emotions such as guilt or shame, display rules, and ambivalence. Research is sorely needed into these new areas of socialization of emotion.

EMOTION REGULATION

Research with both middle- and low-income preschoolers indicates that emotion regulation is facilitated by mothers' appropriate expressiveness (Eisenberg, Gershoff, et al., 2001; Eisenberg, Valiente, et al., 2003; Garner & Spears, 2000). In contrast, exposure to parental negativity may overarouse young children who cannot yet regulate their own emotions well, and represents an emotionally hostile template for children to follow in dysregulated reactions to people and events (Newland & Crnic, 2011).

Positive and negative maternal emotion also contribute to elementary school-age children's emotion regulation (Eisenberg, Liew, & Pidada, 2001; see also Valiente, Fabes, Eisenberg, & Spinrad, 2004). Early exposure to parental emotions figures heavily in the emergence of relatively stable individual differences in emotion regulation (Eisenberg, Valiente, et al., 2003). Children with more negatively expressive mothers vent their own emotions less over time; perhaps to keep the peace with emotionally volatile mothers, they learn to "hold their tongues" (and emotions).

In fact, adults' persistent, intense negative emotional expressiveness and very non-supportive reactions to child emotions may have a more pervasive, less complex relation with development of children's emotion regulation; both 4- to 6-year-olds (Maughan & Cicchetti, 2002) and older children (Shields & Cicchetti, 2001) exposed to or at risk for maltreatment showed deficits in emotion regulation (see also Edwards, Shipman, & Brown, 2005; Shipman et al., 2007).

As is true for emotional expressiveness and emotion knowledge, limited parental expressiveness may pose a risk for children's optimal development. Bariola, Hughes, and Gullone (2012) found that maternal suppression of emotional expression was related to similar emotion regulation strategies in children and adolescents. However, almost no research has targeted the expressive modeling of teachers. The roles of socializers of emotions other than parents need to be examined.

SUMMARY

In summary, with regard to adults' modeling of emotions, exposure to parents' and other adults' broad but not overly negative emotions helps children learn about emotions and come to express similar profiles, even as they progress to middle childhood and into adolescence. Intense adult negative emotion, however, is often deleterious to young children's profiles of expressiveness, emotion knowledge, emotion regulation, and social competence. Obviously, more work is needed with socializers other than mothers.

Contingent Reactions to Emotions

EMOTIONAL EXPRESSIVENESS

Reactions to children's displays of emotion are another important way that other people influence children's emotional competence. Socializers' contingent reactions include behavioral and emotional encouragement or discouragement of specific emotions (Eisenberg et al., 1996, 1999). Adults may punish children's experience and expression of emotions, or show a dismissive attitude by ignoring the child's emotions in a well-meant effort to "make it better" (Denham, Renwick-DeBardi, & Hewes, 1994). Parents who respond to children's emotion by minimizing or dismissing the emotion are more likely to have sadder, more fearful young children (David-Vilker, 2000; Eisenberg et al., 1996). In fact, emotionally supportive *and non*supportive reactions to emotions are predictive of preschoolers' positive and negative expressiveness, respectively (Fabes, Poulin, Eisenberg, & Madden-Derdich, 2002). For some emotions, however, any type of attention—positive or negative—may contribute to later expression of that emotion (Chaplin, Cole, & Zahn-Waxler, 2005). For example, young children whose mothers endorsed controlling their children's emotion displays showed less emotion when winning or losing a challenging game (Berlin & Cassidy, 2003); they were already "getting the message" that expressing emotions was disapproved of, even when reasonable. In addition, children who receive punishing or derogatory reactions to their emotions also may suppress feelings but remain aroused, without the skills to rectify the situation or their potentially explosive emotional response (Eisenberg et al., 1996; Fabes, Leonard, Kupanoff, & Martin, 2001).

Regarding older children, mothers who used more punishing and magnifying (e.g., "making it worse") or fewer rewarding or overriding (e.g., helping change emotional focus) strategies for socializing sadness had sadder adolescents (Race & Brand, 2003). Klimes-Dougan and colleagues (2007; Garside & Klimes-Dougan, 2002) also found, with adolescents, that more punitive or dismissing parental socialization of emotion was related to negative outcomes. More research is needed to elucidate the links between these parental reactions and children's patterns of emotional expressiveness, particularly with older children.

EMOTION KNOWLEDGE

Parents' emotional reactions that are contingent on the child's emotions also may help the child in differentiating emotions (Denham & Kochanoff, 2002; Denham, Zoller, et al., 1994; Fabes et al., 2001, 2002). For example, Fabes and colleagues (2002) found that supportive reactions positively and distress reactions negatively predicted emotion knowledge. Still more work needs to be done, especially for children older than preschool and with socializers other than mother (e.g., siblings; see Sawyer et al., 2002); we must find out whether, and how, parents' reactions to children's emotions change as children grow, and how these changes affect developmentally more sophisticated emotion knowledge (e.g., understanding display rules or ambivalence). As well, friends' influence becomes more significant as children mature; how, and under what conditions, do their reactions help or hurt their peers' emotion knowledge?

EMOTION REGULATION

Positive reactions, such as tolerance or comfort, convey that emotions are manageable, even useful (Gottman et al., 1997). Parents who are positive emotion socializers, at least in Western contexts, accept children's experiences of emotion and their expression of emotions that do not harm others; they empathize with and validate emotions. Regardless of age, emotional moments are seen as opportunities for intimacy (see Denham & Kochanoff, 2002; Eisenberg, Valiente, et al., 2003; for an even more differentiated picture, see Jones, Eisenberg, Fabes, & MacKinnon, 2002).

Such optimal responses to children's emotions are a supportive breeding ground for emotion regulation (Denham & Grout, 1993; Fabes et al., 2001). Children's temperamental makeup may moderate the contribution of parental reactions to emotions, however;

Mirabile, Scaramella, Sohr-Preston, and Robison (2009) found that less reactive toddlers, in particular, used more active distraction emotion regulation (e.g., object engagement) when their mothers physically comforted them during arm restraint and waiting tasks. This interesting finding needs to be followed by longitudinal research in which socialization of emotion predicts emotion regulation and its development over time; in a similar study (Spinrad, Stifter, Donelan-McCall, & Turner, 2004), relations not moderated by temperament were found between maternal comforting of toddlers and preschoolers, and later use of distraction in a disappointing gift paradigm.

In contrast, nonsupportive parents who are either punitive or dismissive of their children's emotions are sowing the seeds of diminished emotion regulatory abilities. These effects may begin as early as toddlerhood, predicting later internalizing difficulties (Luebbe, Kiel, & Buss, 2011); Engle and McElwain (2010) found similar effects, but only for emotionally negative boys.

Parents continue as grade schoolers' primary emotional support (Rimé, Dozier, Vandenplas, & Declercq, 1996; Zeman & Shipman, 1997). Unsupportive reactions to grade schoolers' emotions are negatively associated with emotion regulation (Shaffer, Suveg, Thomassin, & Bradbury, 2012). More positive reactions, such as attention refocusing and cognitive reframing, are related to children's lessened anger and sadness in response to disappointment (Morris et al., 2011). Even adolescents are not immune to deleterious effects of dismissing socialization of emotion; they report less positive emotion regulation strategies (Yap, Allen, & Ladouceur, 2008).

Although parents' reactions to children's emotions remain important, they do change across time. From toddlerhood onward, parents change the frequency, intensity, and nature of their reactions, transferring responsibility for regulation from caregiver to child, allowing for the child's autonomy and parents' heightened expectations of their children's behavior (Grolnick, Kurowski, McMenamy, Rivkin, & Bridges, 1998). Positively reinforcing the child's emotions (e.g., listening, accepting, querying, and complying) may be more predictive of older children's emotional competence, including emotion regulation, than overindulgent helping and comforting, or even simple distraction (Morris et al., 2011). Some measure of restrictiveness may also have beneficial outcomes: teaching older children when emotions are appropriate and when they are not, and their emotions' effects on other people (Eisenberg, Spinrad, & Cumberland, 1998). Conversely, encouragement of emotional expression may not be as predictive of emotion regulation as it was for younger children. Whether or not socializers' encouragement of emotional expressiveness portends children's competence also may be a function of the emotions encouraged—acceptable or unacceptable—and whether such encouragement is accompanied by teaching children how to deal with the emotions. Such developmental changes in reactions to children's emotions—increasing complexity, emotion specificity, and interaction with other aspects of socialization—remain to be investigated.

Close friends also react to grade schoolers' emotions. Older children value being helpful to friends in need rather than ignoring or blaming them (Rose & Asher, 1999). In the horizontal relationship between friends, reactions to emotions that both comfort ("Don't worry about the test. You'll do better next time") and exhort ("Stop crying—everybody's looking at you!") may predict emotion regulation. We doubt that friends' mildly punishing socialization, such as chiding a friend who is overemotional, has deleterious effects equal to that of parents; a supportive equal's punitive reactions may have "more message" and "less fear." As echoed throughout this chapter, however, these studies remain to be performed. In one exception, Sorber (2001) examined grade school-ers' reactions to specific emotions. Happy computer characters were given the most approval; angry characters received the least; acceptance of negative emotions decreased with age. Thus, children may become less accepting of "real" peers' negative emotions over time.

A few investigations have revealed that teachers of toddlers and preschoolers social-ize children's emotions differently based on age, tailoring their reactions to children's emotions and their discussion about emotions to the developmental level of the children (Ahn, 2005a, 2005b; Ahn & Stifter, 2006; Reimer, 1996). In Ahn and Stifter's 2006 study, teachers used physical comfort and distraction in response to toddlers' negative emotions. With preschoolers, teachers more often relied on verbal mediation, helping children infer the causes of their negative emotions, and teaching them constructive ways of expressing negative emotion. Teachers of preschoolers were also less likely to match or encourage preschoolers' positive emotions and more likely to discourage emotional dis-plays of any valence. Finally, teachers did not often validate children's negative emotion—one of the tenets of optimal socialization of emotion. Reimer's work also suggests that preschool teachers are most concerned with young children's control of emotion-related behavior and situationally appropriate expression of emotions. Taken together, these studies suggest a need for teachers' professional development on socialization of emo-tion, particularly in reacting positively to children's emotions and its relation to emotion regulation.

SUMMARY

The bulk of research suggests that accepting, supportive reactions to children's emotional expressiveness patterns generally is associated with all three components of emotional competence, although the research coverage is quite uneven—with most concentrating on parents' (mostly mothers') reactions to emotions and children's emotion regulation. At the same time, much could be gained from examining friends' reactions to older chil-dren's emotions and their relation to emotional competence. Obviously, we are taking the stance that different relationships moderate the differing effects of others' reactions to children's emotions. At the same time, an intriguing alternative (or additional) hypothesis relates to context: Children need to learn different emotional competence skills for differ-ent venues. One way that the emotional norms of differing contexts (e.g., home, school, or playground) are demonstrated is via the different socializing goals and behaviors of parents, teachers, and friends.

Teaching Mechanisms

EMOTIONAL EXPRESSIVENESS

Socializers' tendencies to discuss emotions, and the quality of their communications about emotions, if nested within a warm relationship, assist the child in expressing emo-tions. Socializers may draw attention to emotions and validate or clarify the child's emo-tions, helping the child to react to emotions and express them authentically, in a regulated manner. Whether socializers use emotion talk to clarify, teach, or share rather than to modify behavior or preach also may be critical (Denham & Grout, 1992; Eisenberg,

Cumberland, et al., 1998); the former pattern is associated with more positive profiles of young children's expressiveness.

Although there are fewer studies on "talk about feelings" in middle childhood, it can be assumed that socializers' age-appropriate "emotion talk" (e.g., regarding complex or mixed emotions, masked emotions, strategies for managing emotions) may be related to children's positive profile of emotional expressiveness, with ramifications for well-being and social competence. With better understanding of the social context, older peers' emotion conversation may become especially important to children's emotional expressiveness. This area, particularly with older children, needs more investigation; see some beginnings in this direction in Suveg and colleagues (2008).

EMOTION KNOWLEDGE

In its simplest form, teaching about emotion consists of verbally explaining an emotion and its relation to an observed event or expression. Thus, what adults say, or intentionally attempt to convey through other means, may impact their children's emotion knowledge. Teaching about emotions may help to direct children's attention to salient emotional cues, helping them understand the entire social interaction and manage their own responses to it.

Parental, especially mothers', didactic techniques for discussing emotions with their children are associated with preschoolers' emotion knowledge (Denham, Zoller, et al., 1994; Garner, Jones, Gaddy, & Rennie, 1997; Kochanoff, 2001). The verbal give-and-take about emotional experience within the scaffolded context of chatting with an adult helps young children to formulate a coherent body of knowledge about emotional expressions, situations, and causes (Denham, Renwick-DeBardi, et al., 1994; Dunn et al., 1991; Dunn, Slomkowski, Donelan, & Herrera, 1995). Mothers' explanations of emotions may be particularly useful in promoting emotion knowledge (Denham, Zoller, et al., 1994; Garner, Dunsmore, & Southam-Gerrow, 2008). Furthermore, mother–preschooler emotion conversations may predict even later emotion knowledge (e.g., about emotion regulation and display rules; Garner, 1999).

These findings appear to hold across socioeconomic and ethnic variations and are even stronger within secure mother–child relationships, where both mother and child may be more comfortable about emotions (Kochanoff, 2001; Ontai & Thompson, 2002). However, in two dissertations, *fathers* who used *more* emotion language while reminiscing about past emotional experiences had children with *less* advanced emotion knowledge (Colwell, 2001; Kochanoff, 2001). In contrast to the reminiscence task, however, *both* parents' discussion of emotion during an Emotion Game were associated with preschoolers' more mature emotion knowledge (Colwell, 2001); perhaps fathers perceive reminiscence as more formal or didactic, and talk more in this context with (or "at") children whose emotion knowledge needs bolstering.

When adults' admonitions about emotions are misleading or idiosyncratic, children may enter middle childhood with distorted emotion knowledge. A particular hazard is the anger-intensifying hostile attribution bias. At the same time, the form and function of conversations about emotions *may* change during later childhood; children's input into emotion-laden conversation is apt to be more active than it was years earlier, and as parents "overdo" talk about emotions, children tune out. Again, we know of no extant research on this topic, although we advocate for it (but see Zeman, Perry-Parrish, & Cassano, 2010, for data on parent–adolescent emotion conversations without developmental comparisons).

EMOTION REGULATION

Talk about emotions also gives the child a new tool to use in modulating overt expression of emotions. With age and assistance from caregivers, regulation is transferred from external control (e.g., parents calming a crying child) to internal control (e.g., children using self-talk to calm themselves; Thompson, 1991). Emotion conversations with parents allow children to separate impulses from behavior, giving them reflective distance from feeling states themselves, and space in which to interpret and evaluate their feelings' causes and consequences. Thus, conversations about feelings are an important context for teaching children about how to regulate emotions (Brown & Dunn, 1992). The general trend of these findings also holds true for low-income, minority families (Garner, Jones, et al., 1997). For example, Garner (2006) found that maternal explanations of emotions (and not mere comments on them) during conversations at home predicted African American preschoolers' constructive emotion regulation.

This linkage of emotion discussion and emotion regulation appears to be important for older, as well as younger, children. Elementary school–age children were better regulated when mothers linked emotionally evocative slides' content with the child's own experiences while conversing about them (Eisenberg, Losoya, et al., 2001). Furthermore, elementary school–age children of both mothers and fathers who showed verbal support (e.g., helping the child to understand his or her emotions, validating them, promoting adaptive emotion regulation, or talking about their own emotions) during emotion discussions showed more adaptive emotion regulation during the conversations (Morelen & Suveg, 2012). In contrast, empirical evidence of negative effects of emotion-dismissing parents' verbalizations on grade school children's emotion regulation has been provided by Lunkenheimer, Shields, and Cortina (2007), who found that emotion-teaching verbalizations protected against such dismissing verbalizations' effects.

Finally, young children absorb not only the content but also the form and quality of emotion teaching from people other than parents. Preschoolers remembered sadness, anger and fear during child care transitions, as well as comfort given by teachers and friends (Dunn, 1994).

Friends should also be considered as potential teachers of emotion; after all, older children confide emotional experiences, especially feelings of vulnerability (Rose & Asher, 1999). Friends may use such socializing emotion talk in several ways. First, gossip may allow them to broach potential insecurities without actually naming them (similar to fantasy play during earlier years). One can imagine emotion talk in such gossip ("She's such a little cry-baby, isn't she, Erica?") or statements of group norms ("I hate it when he blows up like that, don't you?"). Second, statements of support–approval of their friend (i.e., sympathy and affection) can easily include emotion language relevant for regulation. Third, relationship talk also goes on, along with self-disclosure, and unsurprisingly, conflict processes often rear their not-necessarily-ugly heads—these aspects of conversation may be replete with emotion regulation talk. In many ways, then, peers can promote friends' emotion regulation. Conversely, in one study, relational peer victimization (which is undoubtedly full of negative emotion language) was related to dysregulation of emotions (McLaughlin, Hatzenbuehler, & Hilt, 2009). This area continues to be ripe for investigation.

SUMMARY

Discussion of emotions, particularly in an elaborative rather than coercive context, is related to children's emotion knowledge and emotion regulation, as well as their emotional positivity (although research is more scant in this area). What remains to be expanded is the role of fathers, whose discussion of emotion seems to serve different functions than that of mothers, the potential role of teachers, and, especially the role of friends' emotion talk, starting in middle childhood.

In short, there is a growing body of knowledge regarding the contributions of adults to young children's emotional competence. Knowing about the contributions of socializers' modeling, contingent reactions, and teaching to emotional competence is useful in guiding adult roles in any successful social-emotional programming for young children. Although cultural values and variations crucially require our attention, so that the unique perspectives of both adults and children may be honored, several principles seem to hold true across cultural groups (Denham, Caal, Bassett, Benga, & Geangu, 2004). The positive picture that emerges is of socializers' positive expressiveness, supportive reactions to children's emotions (although some tutelage about when to control emotions appears beneficial under certain conditions), and discussions about emotions with children. In terms of promoting emotional competence, parent and teacher–caregiver training should focus on ways to manifest these socialization behaviors.

Socialization of Emotional Competence: How Are We Progressing and Where Do We Go from Here?

The amount of published research on the topic of socialization of emotion since Eisenberg, Cumberland, and colleagues' (1998) review and the earlier edition of this volume is quite impressive. But, as noted throughout this chapter, there is still work to do. In this concluding section we sketch out our thoughts on the important new directions for the investigation of emotion socialization, as well as particular issues needing attention.

"It's (Not) All My Fault"

We also wish to leave the reader with the clear notion that socializer–child effects can be bidirectional, and that parent characteristics moderate ability to provide optimal socialization of emotion. For example, Siegel (1997) found that maternal reactions to the emotions of children diagnosed with attention-deficit/hyperactivity disorder (ADHD) are less rewarding, and more punishing and dismissing than those of mothers of children without ADHD. It is easy to envision this effect as part of a sequence in which the child's negativity plays a big role. More focused work on child contributions to socialization of emotion has occurred. For example, Morelen and Suveg (2012) found that emotion-related verbal and nonverbal behaviors of parents and children influence each other. Moreover, there has been increasing attention on how toddlers', children's, and adolescents' temperaments contribute to aspects of socialization of emotion. Findings are mixed; clearer evidence is found for toddlers and adolescents (e.g., Bryan & Dix, 2009; Davenport, Yap, Simmons, Sheeber, & Allen, 2011; Yap, Allen, Leve et al., 2008; cf. Chen, Lin, & Li, 2012; Engle & McElwain, 2010; Rubin, Burgess, Dwyer, & Hastings, 2003), although Wong and colleagues (2009) did find kindergartners' negativity related to maternal negative expressiveness and nonsupportiveness with gender partialled.

At the same time, socialization of emotion techniques is likely to stem from socializers' own personal characteristics. For example, Broth (2004) examined mothers' (of preschoolers) negative emotionality and levels of stress as predictors of socialization of emotion techniques, along with maternal emotional competence as a moderator of this relation. Mothers' negative emotionality and, to a lesser degree, stress predicted poorer-quality socialization of emotion practices; their emotional competence made both additive and interactive contributions. Teachers' emotional competence has also been isolated as a contributor to their ability to positively socialize students' emotional competence (Ersay, 2007; Swartz & McElwain, 2012).

Finally, aspects of the socialization context have been explored; for example, Nelson, O'Brien, Blankson, Calkins, and Keane (2009) found effects of marital distress (especially for fathers), home chaos (especially for mothers), and depression on supportive and nonsupportive reactions to children's emotions. Both marital distress and home chaos showed spillover effects; complex crossover effects were also found (i.e., if one parent was dissatisfied with employment, the other showed fewer supportive reactions to child emotions). A compensation effect was also found; if one parent was depressed, the other reported more supportiveness of their child's emotions.

Much more work needs to be done in each of these areas. We must try to disentangle bidirectional sequences, possibly via naturalistic, microgenetic, and longitudinal methods, and to expand study of context and personal characteristics as moderators of socialization of emotion, fully informed by knowledge of developmentally appropriate child and parent behaviors.

Beyond (or before) Preschool

What about developmental change? In this chapter we have put forward developmental progressions for socialization of emotion. One notable change since the first edition of this volume is the variety of research performed with toddlers, elementary school–age children, adolescents, and their parents. Nonetheless, a skewed age balance in favor of preschoolers and their parents, mostly mothers, still exists. So although we applaud this surge in research with nonpreschoolers, we advocate continued elaboration of our theory *and* empirical work on older children's and adolescents' emotional competence and its socialization, as well as situating the study of toddlers' developing emotional competence more clearly within the socialization of emotion framework proposed here. Moreover, longitudinal change in socialization of emotion and accompanying emotion competence, across these age epochs, is still largely unstudied.

Not Just European American Culture

Eisenberg and colleagues (1998) appropriately include cultural factors as part of their model. Nonetheless, almost all findings reported in this chapter (and this research area in general) relate to middle-income, Western, European American parents and their children. Although there may be some more universally beneficial socialization of emotion techniques, predicting positive outcomes for children, and promoting emotion socialization practices that support them, depends on an intimate knowledge of emotion-related cultural beliefs and practices (see Cole & Tan, Chapter 21, this volume, for a discussion of emotion socialization from a cultural perspective). Hence, when the correct cultural lens is in place, practices may be accurately understood and evaluated, and a more complete story can be told.

Fortunately, several organizing frameworks have been put forward since the first edition of this volume (Friedlmeier, Corapci, & Cole, 2011; Halberstadt & Lozada, 2011; Parker et al., 2012). Halberstadt and Lozada (2011) note five broad cultural frames to consider when exploring differences and similarities in various cultures' socialization of emotion: (a) issues of collectivism/individualism, (b) power distance, (c) children's place in the family and culture, (d) ways children learn, and (e) the value of emotional experience and expression.

Along these lines, Raval, Martini, and Raval (2010; Raval & Martini, 2009) have compared and contrasted mothers' beliefs about and reactions to children's emotions both within differing cultural groups in India and between such groups and American mothers. Furthermore, Wang and colleagues (e.g., Doan & Wang, 2010; Wang, 2012; Wang & Fivush, 2005) have examined emotion conversations among and between immigrant and native Chinese, and European American mothers and children. In both lines of research, cultural models of collectivism–individualism and the value of emotion, as well as specific issues related to social class, caste, and adherence to ideologies, helped explain group differences in socialization of emotion, and other emotion-related parenting behaviors, such as foci for narrative discussion and discipline. However, regardless of cultural group, socialization of emotion predicted important child outcomes, such as emotion knowledge and internalizing behavior.

He Felt, She Felt

It is inappropriate to leave the impression that gender is irrelevant to the socialization of emotion; it appears in Eisenberg and colleagues' (1998) model as a child characteristic, but gender of both child and parent must be examined. There are some child gender differences in socialization of emotion in the preschool age range; for example, both parents of preschoolers often discuss emotions more elaboratively with daughters than with sons (Fivush, Berlin, Sales, Mennuti-Washburn, & Cassidy, 2003). However, by adolescence, few such child gender differences are found (Klimes-Dougan et al., 2007).

In contrast, it may be the rule, not the exception, that gender of parents is associated with different emotion socialization practices; adolescents, for example, report that they perceive differential reactions from mother and father to their varying emotions (Klimes-Dougan et al, 2007; O'Neal & Magai, 2005). In some cases, mothers' and fathers' beliefs and practices are also dependent on their child's gender, reflected in differences between mothers' and fathers' socialization techniques (Garner, Robertson, & Smith, 1997; see also Zahn-Waxler, Klimes-Dougan, & Kendziora, 1998). For example, mothers and fathers have reported that they respond differentially to preschool-age sons' and daughters' emotions (e.g., in one study, mothers responded more positively to daughters' positive emotions than did fathers of either sons or daughters, possibly suggesting that mothers see this as their role, whereas fathers reacted with more surprise, but also comfort, to sons' anxiety than did mothers; Root & Rubin, 2010).

It is also important that specific parents' socialization of emotion techniques predict emotional competence, and this chapter is replete with evidence regarding this assertion for mothers. Aspects of fathers' socialization of emotion also figures prominently in younger and older children's emotional competence (Denham, Bassett, & Wyatt, 2010; Zeman et al., 2010). Gender issues in prediction of emotional competence may be even more complex, however (e.g., distinct roles for mother–daughter and father–son socialization of emotion may exist, with one parent's socialization of emotion predicting one gender's emotional competence (e.g., Cassano, Perry-Parish, & Zeman, 2007; Root & Rubin, 2010; Suveg et al., 2008).

In summary, overall findings still suggest that although mothers may be the "emotional gatekeeper" of the family, providing more supportive socialization of emotion (Baker et al., 2011; Cassano et al., 2007; Denham, Bassett, et al., 2010; Wong et al., 2008; Zeman et al., 2010), fathers' socialization of emotion is very important. Furthermore, the emerging literature on gender differences in socialization of emotion and its outcomes often shows complicated, and varying, relations between child gender and parental gender on observed and reported socialization of emotion practices. These differences are often dependent on the aspect of emotional competence and the age of child studied. Cataloguing these differences by gender of parent, gender and age of child, aspect of emotional competence, and socialization of emotion practice is a daunting but important task yet to be fully tackled.

Beyond the Family

Knowing how parents socialize emotion is very important, but it does not come close to telling the whole story of how emotional competence is supported by persons in each child's environment. If developmental scientists are serious about understanding the socialization of emotion, *everyone* who is important to children as they grow *must* be considered. We find it surprising that adults other than parents have yet to be frequently considered. Because positive relationships with teachers in the preschool and primary years can have long-lasting sequelae (Hamre & Pianta, 2001), it follows that these important adults would also be crucial socializers of emotion. We, as well as others cited here, have begun some of this work on teachers' socialization of emotion, but almost nothing has as yet been published. Given this dearth of information, comparisons among socializer are almost nonexistent; Denham, Grant, and Hamada (2002) did find evidence that the socialization of emotion of both preschool teachers and mothers is important for the development of children's emotion regulation; maternal expressiveness and teachers' beliefs about teaching young children about emotion were the most important predictors of emotion regulation. Finally, because much of the material presented here on friends' and peers' socialization of emotion was speculative, we encourage new research into how the important world of agemates, with whom older children and adolescents spend so much time, contributes to the elements of emotional competence.

Final Remarks

Obviously, we have merely scratched the surface of a fascinating and critical set of developmental phenomena. We have seen that parents are pivotal in modeling emotional expressiveness and display rules, teaching about a variety of emotions, and reacting contingently to emotions; across the period from toddlerhood to adolescence, these specific aspects of socialization of emotion are associated with and/or predict all aspects of emotional competence (with occasional findings of important moderation by child gender or age). Much less is known about how acquaintances, friends, and other adults socialize emotions across this period. Getting a firm grasp of the socialization of emotion within a developmental perspective (i.e., a progression from infancy to adulthood, and attending to issues of context and meaning) is the next challenge for developmental scientists.

We hope this knowledge base will increasingly be shared with parents (Havighurst, Wilson, Harley, Prior, & Kehoe, 2010; Wilson, Havighurst, & Harley, 2012), as well as schools and wider communities, particularly with at-risk children and within our juvenile justice systems. The links between emotional competence and both social and academic success make this knowledge sharing a necessity (Denham, 2005; Denham & Weissberg, 2004). We hope our comments set the stage for new ideas and a continued vitalization of research in this important area.

REFERENCES

Ahn, H. J. (2005a). Child care teachers' strategies in children's socialization of emotion. *Early Child Development and Care, 175,* 49–61.

Ahn, H. J. (2005b). Teachers' discussions of emotion in child care centers. *Early Childhood Education Journal, 32,* 237–242.

Ahn, H. J., & Stifter, C. (2006). Child care teachers' response to children's emotional expression. *Early Education and Development, 17,* 253–270.

Baker, J. K., Fenning, R. M., & Crnic, K. A. (2011). Emotion socialization by mothers and fathers: Coherence among behaviors and associations with parent attitudes and children's social competence. *Social Development, 20,* 412–430.

Bariola, E., Hughes, E. K., & Gullone, E. (2012). Relationships between parent and child emotion regulation strategy use: A brief report. *Journal of Child and Family Studies, 21,* 443–448.

Beck, L., Kumschick, I. R., Eid, M., & Klann-Delius, G. (2012). Relationship between language competence and emotional competence in middle childhood. *Emotion, 12,* 503–514.

Bennett, D. S., Bendersky, M., & Lewis, M. (2005). Antecedents of emotion knowledge: Predictors of individual differences in young children. *Cognition and Emotion, 19,* 375–396.

Berlin, L. J., & Cassidy, J. (2003). Mothers' self-reported control of their preschool children's emotional expressiveness: A longitudinal study of associations with infant–mother attachment and children's emotion regulation. *Social Development, 12,* 478–495.

Bocknek, E. L., Brophy-Herb, H. E., & Banerjee, M. (2009). Effects of parental supportiveness on toddlers' emotion regulation over the first three years of life in a low-income African American sample. *Infant Mental Health Journal, 30,* 452–476.

Bronstein, P., Fitzgerald, M., Briones, M., Pieniadz, J., & D'Ari, A. (1993). Family emotional expressiveness as a predictor of early adolescent social and psychological adjustment. *Journal of Early Adolescence, 13,* 448–471.

Brophy-Herb, H. E., Stansbury, K., Bocknek, E., & Horodynski, M. A. (2012). Modeling maternal emotion-related socialization behaviors in a low-income sample: Relations with toddlers' self-regulation. *Early Childhood Research Quarterly, 27,* 352–364.

Broth, M. R. (2004). *Associations between mothers' negative emotionality and stress and their socialization of emotion practices: Mothers' emotional competence as resiliency or risk* (Doctoral dissertation). Retrieved from ProQuest Dissertations and Theses (Accession Order No. 3103780).

Brown, J. R., & Dunn, J. (1992). Talk with your mother or your sibling?: Developmental changes in early family conversations about feelings. *Child Development, 63,* 336–349.

Bryan, A. E., & Dix, T. (2009). Mothers' emotions and behavioral support during interactions with toddlers: The role of child temperament. *Social Development, 18,* 647–670.

Bugental, D. B., & Goodnow, J. J. (1998). Socialization processes. In N. Eisenberg (Ed.), *Handbook of child psychology: Social, emotional, and personality development* (3rd ed., Vol. 3, pp. 389–462). New York: Wiley.

Cassano, M., Perry-Parrish, C., & Zeman, J. (2007). Influence of gender on parental socialization of children's sadness regulation. *Social Development, 16,* 210–231.

Chan, S. M., Bowes, J., & Wyver, S. (2009). Parenting style as a context for emotion socialization. *Early Education and Development, 20,* 631–656.

Chang, L., Schwartz, D., Dodge, K. A., & McBride-Chang, C. (2003). Harsh parenting in relation to child emotion regulation and aggression. *Journal of Family Psychology, 17,* 598–606.

Chaplin, T. M., Cole, P. M., & Zahn-Waxler, C. (2005). Parental socialization of emotion expression: Gender differences and relations to child adjustment. *Emotion, 5,* 80–88.

Chen, F. M., Lin, H. S., & Li, C. H. (2012). The role of emotion in parent–child relationships: Children's emotionality, maternal meta-emotion, and children's attachment security. *Journal of Child and Family Studies, 21,* 403–410.

Colwell, M. J. (2001). *Mother–child emotion talk, mothers' expressiveness, and mother–child relationship quality: Links with children's emotional competence* (Doctoral dissertation). Retrieved from ProQuest Dissertations and Theses (Accession Order No. 9978312).

Cunningham, J. N., Kliewer, W., & Garner, P. W. (2009). Emotion socialization, child emotion knowledge and regulation, and adjustment in urban African American families: Differential associations across child gender. *Development and Psychopathology, 21,* 261–283.

Davenport, E., Yap, M. B. H., Simmons, J. G., Sheeber, L. B., & Allen, N. B. (2011). Maternal and adolescent temperament as predictors of maternal affective behavior during mother–adolescent interactions. *Journal of Adolescence, 34,* 829–839.

David-Vilker, R. J. (2000). *The contribution of emotion socialization and attachment to adult emotion organization and regulation* (Doctoral dissertation). Retrieved from ProQuest Dissertations and Theses (Accession Order No. 9959126).

Demorat, M. G. (1999). *Emotion socialization in the classroom context: A functionalist analysis* (Doctoral dissertation). Retrieved from ProQuest Dissertations and Theses (Accession Order No. 9921584).

Denham, S. A. (1998). *Emotional development in young children.* New York: Guilford Press.

Denham, S. A. (2005). The emotional basis of learning and development in early childhood education. In B. Spodek (Ed.), *Handbook of research in early childhood education* (pp. 85–103). New York: Erlbaum.

Denham, S. A., Bassett, H. H., & Wyatt, T. M. (2010). Gender differences in the socialization of preschoolers' emotional competence. *New Directions for Child and Adolescent Development, 128,* 29–49.

Denham, S. A., Blair, K. A., DeMulder, E., Levitas, J., Sawyer, K. S., Auerbach-Major, S. T., et al. (2003). Preschoolers' emotional competence: Pathway to mental health? *Child Development, 74,* 238–256.

Denham, S. A., Brown, C. E., & Domitrovich, C. E. (2010). Plays nice with others: Social-emotional learning and academic success. *Early Education and Development, 21,* 652–680.

Denham, S. A., Caal, S., Bassett, H. H., Benga, O., & Geangu, E. (2004). Listening to parents: Cultural variations in the meaning of emotions and emotion socialization. *Cognitie Creier Comportament, 8,* 321–350.

Denham, S. A., Grant, S., & Hamada, H. A. (2002, June). *"I have two 1st teachers": Mother and teacher socialization of preschoolers' emotional and social competence.* Paper presented at the 7th Head Start Research Conference, Washington, DC.

Denham, S. A., & Grout, L. (1992). Mothers' emotional expressiveness and coping: Topography and relations with preschoolers' social–emotional competence. *Genetic, Social, and General Psychology Monographs, 118,* 75–101.

Denham, S. A., & Grout, L. (1993). Socialization of emotion: Pathway to preschoolers' affect regulation. *Journal of Nonverbal Behavior, 17,* 215–227.

Denham, S. A., & Kochanoff, A. T. (2002). Parental contributions to preschoolers' understanding of emotion. *Marriage and Family Review, 34,* 311–343.

Denham, S. A., Mitchell-Copeland, J., Strandberg, K., Auerbach, S., & Blair, K. (1997). Parental contributions to preschoolers' emotional competence: Direct and indirect effects. *Motivation and Emotion, 27,* 65–86.

Denham, S. A., Renwick-DeBardi, S., & Hewes, S. (1994). Emotional communication between mothers and preschoolers: Relations with emotional competence. *Merrill–Palmer Quarterly, 40,* 488–508.

Denham, S. A., & Weissberg, R. P. (2004). Social–emotional learning in early childhood: What we know and where to go from here? In E. Chesebrough, P. King, T. P. Gullotta, & M. Bloom (Eds.), *A blueprint for the promotion of prosocial behavior in early childhood* (pp. 13–50). New York: Kluwer Academic/Plenum Press.

Denham, S. A., Zoller, D., & Couchoud, E. A. (1994). Socialization of preschoolers' emotion knowledge. *Developmental Psychology, 30,* 928–936.

Doan, S. N., & Wang, Q. (2010). Maternal discussions of mental states and behaviors: Relations to emotion situation knowledge in European American and immigrant Chinese children. *Child Development, 81,* 1490–1503.

Dunn, J. (1994). Understanding others and the social world: Current issues in developmental research and their relation to preschool experiences and practice. *Journal of Applied Developmental Psychology, 15,* 571–583.

Dunn, J., Brown, J. R., & Beardsall, L. A. (1991). Family talk about emotions, and children's later understanding of others' emotions. *Developmental Psychology, 27,* 448–455.

Dunn, J., Slomkowski, C., Donelan, N., & Herrera, C. (1995). Conflict, understanding, and relationships: Developments and differences in the preschool years. *Early Education and Development, 6,* 303–316.

Dunsmore, J. C., Her, P., Halberstadt, A. G., & Perez-Rivera, M. B. (2009). Parents' beliefs about emotions and children's recognition of parents' emotions. *Journal of Nonverbal Behavior, 33,* 121–140.

Dunsmore, J. C., & Karn, M. A. (2001). Mothers' beliefs about feelings and children's emotional understanding. *Early Education and Development, 12,* 117–138.

Edwards, A., Shipman, K., & Brown, A. (2005). The socialization of emotional understanding: A Comparison of neglectful and nonneglectful mothers and their children. *Child Maltreatment, 10,* 293–304.

Eisenberg, N., Cumberland, A., & Spinrad, T. L. (1998). Parental socialization of emotion. *Psychological Inquiry, 9,* 241–273.

Eisenberg, N., Fabes, R. A., & Murphy, B. C. (1996). Parents' reactions to children's negative emotions: Relations to children's social competence and comforting behavior. *Child Development, 67,* 2227–2247.

Eisenberg, N., Fabes, R. A., Shepard, S. A., Guthrie, I., Murphy, B. C., & Reiser, M. (1999). Parental reactions to children's negative emotions: Longitudinal relations to quality of children's social functioning. *Child Development, 70,* 513–534.

Eisenberg, N., Gershoff, E. T., Fabes, R. A., Shepard, S. A., Cumberland, A., Losoya, S., et al. (2001). Mothers' emotional expressivity and children's behavior problems and social competence: Mediation through children's regulation. *Developmental Psychology, 37,* 475–490.

Eisenberg, N., Liew, J., & Pidada, S. U. (2001). The relations of parental emotional expressivity with quality of Indonesian children's social functioning. *Emotion, 1,* 116–136.

Eisenberg, N., Losoya, S., Fabes, R. A., Guthrie, I. K., Reiser, M., Murphy, B., et al. (2001). Parental socialization of children's dysregulated expression of emotion and externalizing problems. *Journal of Family Psychology, 15,* 183–205.

Eisenberg, N., Spinrad, T. L., & Cumberland, A. (1998). The socialization of emotion: Reply to commentaries. *Psychological Inquiry, 9,* 317–333.

Eisenberg, N., Valiente, C., Morris, A. S., Fabes, R. A., Cumberland, A., Reiser, M., et al. (2003). Longitudinal relations among parental emotional expressivity, children's regulation, and quality of socioemotional functioning. *Developmental Psychology, 39,* 3–19.

Eisenberg, N., Zhou, Q., Losoya, S. H., Fabes, R. A., Shepard, S. A., Murphy, B. C., et al. (2003). The relations of parenting, effortful control, and ego control to children's emotional expressivity. *Child Development, 74,* 875–895.

Engle, J. M., & McElwain, N. L. (2010). Parental reactions to toddlers' negative emotions and child negative emotionality as correlates of problem behavior at the age of three. *Social Development, 20,* 251–271.

Ersay, E. (2007). *Preschool teachers' emotional experience traits, awareness of their own emotions and their emotional socialization practices* (Doctoral dissertation). Retrieved from ProQuest Dissertations and Theses. (Accession Order No. 3266106).

Fabes, R. A., Leonard, S. A., Kupanoff, K., & Martin, C. L. (2001). Parental coping with children's negative emotions: Relations with children's emotional and social responding. *Child Development, 72,* 907–920.

Fabes, R. A., Poulin, R. E., Eisenberg, N., & Madden-Derdich, D. A. (2002). The Coping with Children's Negative Emotions Scale (CCNES): Psychometric properties and relations with children's emotional competence. *Marriage and Family Review, 34,* 285–310.

Fivush, R., Berlin, L. J., Sales, J. M., Mennuti-Washburn, J., & Cassidy, J. (2003). Functions of parent–child reminiscing about emotionally negative events. *Memory, 11,* 179–192.

Fredrickson, B. L. (1998). Cultivated emotions: Parental socialization of positive emotions and self-conscious emotions. *Psychological Inquiry, 9,* 279–281.

Friedlmeier, W., Corapci, F., & Cole, P. M. (2011). Emotion socialization in cross-cultural perspective. *Social and Personality Psychology Compass, 5,* 410–427.

Garner, P. W. (1999). Continuity in emotion knowledge from preschool to middle-childhood and relation to emotion socialization. *Motivation and Emotion, 23,* 247–266.

Garner, P. W. (2006). Prediction of prosocial and emotional competence from maternal behavior in African American preschoolers. *Cultural Diversity and Ethnic Minority Psychology, 12,* 179–198.

Garner, P. W., Dunsmore, J. C., & Southam-Gerrow, M. (2008). Mother–child conversations about emotions: Linkages to child aggression and prosocial behavior. *Social Development, 17,* 259–277.

Garner, P. W., Jones, D. C., Gaddy, G., & Rennie, K. (1997). Low income mothers' conversations about emotions and their children's emotional competence. *Social Development, 6,* 37–52.

Garner, P. W., Jones, D. C., & Miner, J. L. (1994). Social competence among low-income preschoolers: Emotion socialization practices and social cognitive correlates. *Child Development, 65,* 622–637.

Garner, P. W., Robertson, S., & Smith, G. (1997). Preschool children's emotional expressions with peers: The roles of gender and emotion socialization. *Sex Roles, 36,* 675–691.

Garner, P. W., & Spears, F. M. (2000). Emotion regulation in low-income preschoolers. *Social Development, 9,* 246–264.

Garside, R. B., & Klimes-Dougan, B. (2002). Socialization of discrete negative emotions: Gender differences and links with psychological distress. *Sex Roles, 47,* 115–128.

Gondoli, D. M., & Braungart-Rieker, J. M. (1998). Constructs and processes in parental socialization of emotions. *Psychological Inquiry, 9,* 283–285.

Gottman, J. M., Katz, L. F., & Hooven, C. (1997). *Meta-emotion: How families communicate emotionally.* Mahwah, NJ: Erlbaum.

Grolnick, W. S., Kurowski, C. O., McMenamy, J. M., Rivkin, I., & Bridges, L. J. (1998). Mothers' strategies for regulating their toddlers' distress. *Infant Behavior and Development, 21,* 437–450.

Grusec, J. E. (2002). Parental socialization and children's acquisition of values. In M. H. Bornstein (Ed.), *Handbook of parenting* (2nd ed., Vol. 5, pp. 143–167). Mahwah, NJ: Erlbaum.

Halberstadt, A. G., Denham, S. A., & Dunsmore, J. (2001). Affective social competence. *Social Development, 10,* 79–119.

Halberstadt, A. G., Fox, N. A., & Jones, N. A. (1993). Do expressive mothers have expressive children?: The role of socialization in children's affect expression. *Social Development, 2,* 48–65.

Halberstadt, A. G., & Lozada, F. T. (2011). Emotion development in infancy through the lens of culture. *Emotion Review, 3,* 158–168.

Hamre, B. K., & Pianta, R. C. (2001). Early teacher–child relationships and the trajectory of children's school outcomes through eighth grade. *Child Development, 72,* 625–638.

Harker, L., & Keltner, D. (2001). Expressions of positive emotion in women's college yearbook pictures and their relationship to personality and life outcomes across adulthood. *Journal of Personality and Social Psychology, 80,* 112–124.

Havighurst, S. S., Wilson, K. R., Harley, A. E., Prior, M. R., & Kehoe, C. (2010). Tuning In to Kids: Improving emotion socialization practices in parents of preschool children—findings from a community trial. *Journal of Child Psychology and Psychiatry, 51,* 1342–1350.

Hyson, M. C. (1994). *The emotional development of young children: Building an emotion-centered curriculum.* New York: Teachers College Press.

Isley, S. L., O'Neil, R., Clatfelter, D., & Parke, R. D. (1999). Parent and child expressed affect and children's social competence: Modeling direct and indirect pathways. *Developmental Psychology, 35,* 547–560.

Jones, S., Eisenberg, N., Fabes, R. A., & MacKinnon, D. P. (2002). Parents' reactions to elementary school children's negative emotions: Relations to social and emotional functioning at school. *Merrill–Palmer Quarterly, 48,* 133–159.

Kim, K. J., Conger, R. D., Lorenz, F. O., & Elder, G. H. (2001). Parent–adolescent reciprocity in negative affect and its relation to early adult social development. *Developmental Psychology, 37,* 775–790.

Klimes-Dougan, B., Brand, A. E., Zahn-Waxler, C., Usher, B., Hastings, P. D., Kendziora, K., et al. (2007). Parental emotion socialization in adolescence: Differences in sex, age and problem status. *Social Development, 16,* 326–342.

Kochanoff, A. T. (2001). *Parental disciplinary styles, parental elaborativeness, and attachment: Links to preschoolers' emotion knowledge* (Doctoral dissertation). Retrieved from ProQuest Dissertations and Theses (Accession Order No. 3015120).

Larson, R. W., Moneta, G., Richards, M. H., & Wilson, S. (2002). Continuity, stability, and change in daily emotional experience across adolescence. *Child Development, 73,* 1151–1165.

Luebbe, A. M., Kiel, E. J., & Buss, K. A. (2011). Toddlers' context-varying emotions, maternal responses to emotions, and internalizing behaviors. *Emotion, 11,* 697–703.

Lunkenheimer, E. S., Shields, A. M., & Cortina, K. S. (2007). Parental emotion coaching and dismissing in family interaction. *Social Development, 16,* 232–248.

Maughan, A., & Cicchetti, D. (2002). Impact of child maltreatment and interadult violence on children's emotion regulation abilities and socioemotional adjustment. *Child Development, 73,* 1525–1542.

McLaughlin, K. A., Hatzenbuehler, M. L., & Hilt, L. M. (2009). Emotion dysregulation as a mechanism linking peer victimization to internalizing symptoms in adolescents. *Journal of Consulting and Clinical Psychology, 77,* 894–904.

Miller, A. L., Fine, S. E., Gouley, K. K., Seifer, R., Dickstein, S., & Shields, A. (2006). Showing and telling about emotions: Interrelations between facets of emotional competence and associations with classroom adjustment in Head Start preschoolers. *Cognition and Emotion, 20*, 1170–1192.

Miller, A. L., Gouley, K. K., Seifer, R., Dickstein, S., & Shields, A. (2004). Emotions and behaviors in the head start classroom: Associations among observed dysregulation, social competence, and preschool adjustment. *Early Education and Development, 15*, 147–165.

Mirabile, S. P., Scaramella, L. V., Sohr-Preston, S. L., & Robison, S. D. (2009). Mothers' socialization of emotion regulation: The moderating role of children's negative emotional reactivity. *Child and Youth Care Forum, 38*, 19–37.

Morelen, D., & Suveg, C. (2012). A real-time analysis of parent–child emotion discussions: The interaction is reciprocal. *Journal of Family Psychology, 26*, 998–1003.

Morgan, J., Izard, C. E., & King, K. A. (2010). Construct validity of the Emotion Matching Task: Preliminary evidence for convergent and criterion validity of a new emotion knowledge measure for young children. *Social Development, 19*, 52–70.

Morris, A. S., Silk, J. S., Morris, M. D. S., Steinberg, L., Aucoin, K. J., & Keyes, A. W. (2011). The influence of mother–child emotion regulation strategies on children's expression of anger and sadness. *Developmental Psychology, 47*, 213–225.

Murphy, B. C., Shepard, S. A., Eisenberg, N., & Fabes, R. A. (2004). Concurrent and across time prediction of young adolescents' social functioning: The role of emotionality and regulation. *Social Development, 13*, 56–86.

Nelson, J. A., O'Brien, M., Blankson, A. N., Calkins, S. D., & Keane, S. P. (2009). Family stress and parental responses to children's negative emotions: Tests of the spillover, crossover, and compensatory hypotheses. *Journal of Family Psychology, 23*, 671–679.

Newland, R. P., & Crnic, K. A. (2011). Mother–child affect and emotion socialization processes across the late preschool period: Predictions of emerging behaviour problems. *Infant and Child Development, 20*, 371–388.

Nixon, C. L., & Watson, A. C. (2001). Family experiences and early emotion knowledge. *Merrill–Palmer Quarterly, 47*, 300–322.

O'Neal, C. R., & Magai, C. (2005). Do parents respond in different ways when children feel different emotions?: The emotional context of parenting. *Development and Psychopathology, 17*, 467–487.

Ontai, L. L., & Thompson, R. A. (2002). Patterns of attachment and maternal discourse effects on children's emotion knowledge from 3 to 5 years of age. *Social Development, 11*, 433–450.

Parker, A. E., Halberstadt, A. G., Dunsmore, J. C., Townley, G., Bryant, A., Thompson, J. A., et al. (2012). "Emotions are a window into one's heart": A qualitative analysis of parental beliefs about children's emotions across three ethnic groups *Monographs of the Society for Research in Child Development, 77*, 1–25.

Perez Rivera, M. B., & Dunsmore, J. C. (2011). Mothers' acculturation and beliefs about emotions, mother–child emotion discourse, and children's emotion knowledge in Latino families. *Early Education and Development, 22*, 324–354.

Pollak, S. D., & Sinha, P. (2002). Effects of early experience on children's recognition of facial displays of emotion. *Developmental Psychology, 38*, 784–791.

Pollak, S. D., & Tolley-Schell, S. A. (2003). Selective attention to facial emotion in physically abused children. *Journal of Abnormal Psychology, 112*, 323–338.

Race, E., & Brand, A. E. (2003). *Parental personality and its relationship to socialization of sadness in children*. Paper presented at the biennial meeting of the Society for Research in Child Development, Tampa, FL.

Raval, V. V., & Martini, T. S. (2009). Maternal socialization of children's anger, sadness, and physical pain in two communities in Gujarat, India. *International Journal of Behavioral Development, 33*, 215–229.

Raval, V. V., Martini, T. S., & Raval, P. H. (2007). "Would others think it is okay to express my feelings?": Regulation of anger, sadness and physical pain in Gujarati children in India. *Social Development, 16*, 79–105.

Raval, V. V., Martini, T. S., & Raval, P. H. (2010). Methods of, and reasons for, emotional expression and control in children with internalizing, externalizing, and somatic problems in urban India. *Social Development, 19*, 93–112.

Raver, C. C., & Spagnola, M. (2002). "When my mommy was angry, I was speechless": Children's perceptions of maternal emotional expressiveness within the context of economic hardship. *Marriage and Family Review, 34*, 63–88.

Reimer, K. J. (1996). *Emotion socialization and children's emotional expressiveness in the preschool context (emotional expression)* (Doctoral dissertation). Retrieved from ProQuest Dissertations and Theses (Accession Order No. 9640050).

Rimé, B., Dozier, S., Vandenplas, C., & Declercq, M. (1996). *Social sharing of emotion in children*. Paper presented at the annual conference of the International Society for Research on Emotions, Toronto, Ontario, Canada.

Root, A. K., & Rubin, K. H. (2010). Gender and parents' reactions to children's emotion during the preschool years. *New Directions for Child and Adolescent Development, 2010*(128), 51–64.

Rose, A. J., & Asher, S. R. (1999). Children's goals and strategies in response to conflicts within a friendship. *Developmental Psychology, 35*, 69–70.

Rubin, K. H., Burgess, K. B., Dwyer, K. M., & Hastings, P. D. (2003). Predicting preschoolers' externalizing behaviors from toddler temperament, conflict, and maternal negativity. *Developmental Psychology, 39*(1), 164–176.

Rydell, A.-M., Berlin, L., & Bohlin, G. (2003). Emotionality, emotion regulation, and adaptation among 5- to 8-year-old children. *Emotion, 3*, 30–47.

Saarni, C. (1999). *The development of emotional competence*. New York: Guilford Press.

Sawyer, K. S., Denham, S., DeMulder, E., Blair, K., Auerbach-Major, S., & Levitas, J. (2002). The contribution of older siblings' reactions to emotions to preschoolers' emotional and social competence. *Marriage and Family Review, 34*, 183–212.

Shaffer, A., Suveg, C., Thomassin, K., & Bradbury, L. L. (2012). Emotion socialization in the context of family risks: Links to child emotion regulation. *Journal of Child and Family Studies, 21*, 917–924.

Shields, A., & Cicchetti, D. (2001). Parental maltreatment and emotion dysregulation as risk factors for bullying and victimization in middle childhood. *Journal of Clinical Child Psychology, 30*, 349–363.

Shipman, K. L., Schneider, R., Fitzgerald, M. M., Sims, C., Swisher, L., & Edwards, A. (2007). Maternal emotion socialization in maltreating and non-maltreating families: Implications for children's emotion regulation. *Social Development, 16*, 268–285.

Siegel, H. I. (1997). *Emotion socialization and affect regulation in children with attention deficit hyperactivity disorder* (Doctoral dissertation). Retrieved from ProQuest Dissertations and Theses (Accession Order No. 9704797)

Snyder, J., Stoolmiller, M., Wilson, M., & Yamamoto, M. (2003). Child anger regulation, parental responses to children's anger displays, and early child antisocial behavior. *Social Development, 12*, 335–360.

Sorber, A. V. (2001). *The role of peer socialization in the development of emotion display rules: Effects of age, gender, and emotion* (Doctoral dissertation). Retrieved from ProQuest Dissertations and Theses (Accession Order No. 3004981).

Spinrad, T. L., Stifter, C. A., Donelan-McCall, N., & Turner, L. (2004). Mothers' regulation strategies in response to toddlers' affect: Links to later emotion self-regulation. *Social Development, 13*, 40–55.

Suveg, C., Sood, E., Barmish, A., Tiwari, S., Hudson, J. L., & Kendall, P. C. (2008). "I'd rather not talk about it": Emotion parenting in families of children with an anxiety disorder. *Journal of Family Psychology, 22*, 875–884.

Suveg, C., Zeman, J., Flannery-Schroeder, E., & Cassano, M. (2005). Emotion socialization in families of children with an anxiety disorder. *Journal of Abnormal Child Psychology, 33*, 145–155.

Swartz, R. A., & McElwain, N. L. (2012). Preservice teachers' emotion-related regulation and cognition: Associations with teachers' responses to children's emotions in early childhood classrooms. *Early Education and Development, 23*, 202–226.

Tang, X., Liang, Z., Deng, H., Ye, M., & Lu, Z. (2012). Association between parental emotion-related socialization behaviors and adolescents' peer social skills: Moderated by parenting style. *Advances in Psychology, 2*, 141–148.

Thompson, R. A. (1991). Emotional regulation and emotional development. *Educational Psychology Review, 3*, 269–307.

Trentacosta, C. J., & Fine, S. E. (2010). Emotion knowledge, social competence, and behavior problems in childhood and adolescence: A meta-analytic review. *Social Development, 19*, 1–29.

Valiente, C., Eisenberg, N., Shepard, S. A., Fabes, R. A., Cumberland, A. J., Losoya, S. H., et al. (2004). The relations of mothers' negative expressivity to children's experience and expression of negative emotion. *Journal of Applied Developmental Psychology, 25*, 215–235.

Valiente, C., Fabes, R. A., Eisenberg, N., & Spinrad, T. L. (2004). The relations of parental expressivity and support to children's coping with daily stress. *Journal of Family Psychology, 18*, 97–106.

Wang, Q. (2012). Chinese socialization and emotion talk between mothers and children in native and immigrant Chinese families. *Asian American Journal of Psychology, 4*(3), 185–192.

Wang, Q., & Fivush, R. (2005). Mother–child conversations of emotionally salient events: Exploring the functions of emotional reminiscing in European-American and Chinese families. *Social Development, 14*, 473–495.

Wilson, K. R., Havighurst, S. S., & Harley, A. E. (2012). Tuning in to Kids: An effectiveness trial of a parenting program targeting emotion socialization of preschoolers. *Journal of Family Psychology, 26*, 56–65.

Wong, M. S., Diener, M. L., & Isabella, R. A. (2008). Parents' emotion related beliefs and behaviors and child grade: Associations with children's perceptions of peer competence. *Journal of Applied Developmental Psychology, 29*, 175–186.

Wong, M. S., McElwain, N. L., & Halberstadt, A. G. (2009). Parent, family, and child characteristics: Associations with mother- and father-reported emotion socialization practices. *Journal of Family Psychology, 23*, 452–463.

Yap, M. B. H., Allen, N. B., & Ladouceur, C. D. (2008). Maternal socialization of positive affect: The impact of invalidation on adolescent emotion regulation and depressive symptomatology. *Child Development, 79*, 1415–1431.

Yap, M. B. H., Allen, N. B., Leve, C., & Katz, L. F. (2008). Maternal meta-emotion philosophy and socialization of adolescent affect: The moderating role of adolescent temperament. *Journal of Family Psychology, 22*, 688–700.

Zahn-Waxler, C., Klimes-Dougan, B., & Kendziora, K. T. (1998). The study of emotion socialization: Conceptual, methodological, and developmental considerations. *Psychological Inquiry, 9*, 313–316.

Zeman, J., Perry-Parrish, C., & Cassano, M. (2010). Parent–child discussions of anger and sadness: The importance of parent and child gender during middle childhood. *New Directions for Child and Adolescent Development, 2010*(128), 65–83.

Zeman, J., & Shipman, K. (1997). Social-contextual influences on expectancies for managing anger and sadness: The transition from middle childhood to adolescence. *Developmental Psychology, 33*, 917–924.

CHAPTER 26

Families, Schools, and Developing Achievement-Related Motivations and Engagement

Sandra D. Simpkins
Jennifer A. Fredricks
Jacquelynne S. Eccles

In this chapter, we review the impact of experiences in the family and at school on the development of achievement motivation and engagement in skills-based learning. We begin with a brief overview of achievement motivation and engagement in skills-based learning, organized around the expectancy–value model of achievement-related choices and behaviors presented in Figure 26.1. We draw on person–environment and stage–environment fit theories to discuss when and how aspects of the expectancy–value model are optimized to shape motivation. We then review the current research on how families and schools support or undermine the development of positive achievement motivation.

The Eccles et al. Expectancy–Value Model of Achievement-Related Choices and Behaviors

Over the past 30 years, Eccles-Parsons and her colleagues (1983) have studied the psychological and social factors influencing achievement-related motivation, task choice, and performance (see Figure 26.1 for the most recent version). They hypothesized that achievement-related behaviors such as educational, vocational, and leisure choices would be most directly shaped by individuals' expectations for success and task value. Eccles and her colleagues predicted that people will select achievement-related pursuits (e.g., high school courses) that they value and think they can master. Individuals' expectations for success depend on both their confidence in their abilities and their estimations of the

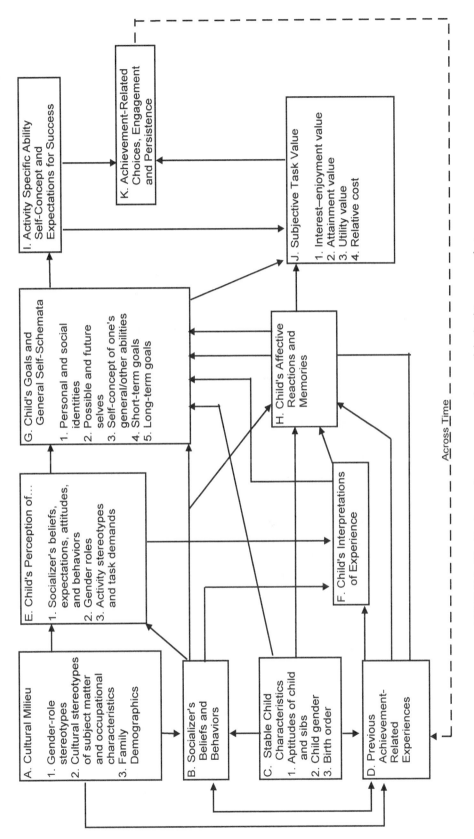

FIGURE 26.1. The Eccles et al. expectancy–value model of achievement choices.

difficulty of the various options they are considering. Subjective task value is grouped into four broad categories: interest (the enjoyment one gets from engaging in the task or activity), utility value (the instrumental value of the task or activity for helping to fulfill another short- or long-range goal), attainment value (the link between the task and one's sense of self and either personal or social identity), and cost (defined in terms of either what may be given up by making a specific choice or the negative experiences associated with each possible choice).

Person–environment fit and stage–environment fit theories are complementary to the expectancy–value theory in that these theories denote how to optimize the family and school influences on motivation. According to person–environment fit, motivation will be optimized in learning settings that meet individuals' basic needs (Hunt, 1979). For example, Deci, Ryan, and their colleagues have focused attention on three fundamental psychological needs: competence (e.g., experiencing oneself as effective in social interactions), relatedness (e.g., experiencing oneself as connected to other people), and autonomy (e.g., experiencing oneself as source of action) (Ryan & Deci, 2002). A stage–environment fit perspective expands on person–environment fit models by focusing on the match between the social context and individuals' development needs. Eccles and Midgley (1989) used stage–environment fit to explain declines in motivation during the middle school years. They argued that students will be more likely to experience motivational declines in schools that fail to meet adolescents' changing developmental needs.

Family Influences on Achievement

Figure 26.2 provides a general overview of the ways in which families, and parents in particular, can influence their children's engagement in and performance on achievement-related tasks through their influence on children's achievement-related self-perceptions and subjective task values (Eccles, 1992). Beginning at the far left, this model predicts that exogenous, cultural, and demographic characteristics of the family, in combination with specific child characteristics, influence parents' general and child-specific beliefs. In turn, these parents' beliefs influence parents' general and child-specific behaviors and practices, which in turn, influence children's motivational beliefs and actual behavior. In this section, we review the current research addressing the various paths depicted in the model.

Child and Family Demographic Characteristics

Child gender is one of the central child-level demographic characteristics that filter through the entire expectancy–value model. Gender differences in youth achievement, engagement, and motivational beliefs are evident when children begin formal schooling and often persist throughout school and even to career selection (e.g., Andre, Whigham, Hendrickson, & Chambers, 1999). The early onset of these gender differences before schooling suggests that families could be a source of influence. For example, parents rate children's math and sports abilities higher for boys than for girls (Bhanot & Jovanovic, 2005; Fredricks & Eccles, 2005b). However, it is important to note that most studies focus on mean-level gender differences and not whether gender functions as a moderator. Testing mean-level gender differences helps identify groups that may benefit from

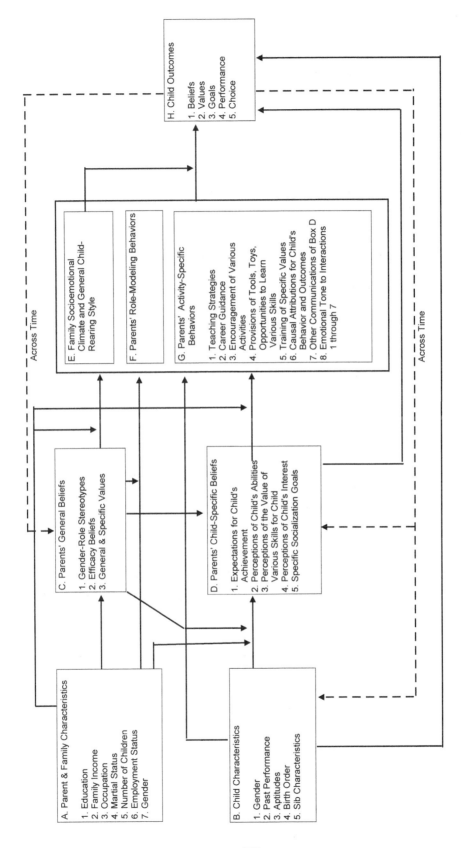

FIGURE 26.2. Model of parents' influence on children's achievement related to self-perception, values, and behaviors.

617

an intervention or points that might be amenable to an intervention. Testing gender as a moderator addresses whether similar precursors may work for girls and boys. Emerging evidence suggests that although parents' beliefs and behaviors may vary by child gender, the relations among the indicators are similar (Fredricks et al., 2005; Simpkins, Fredricks, & Eccles, 2012). In other words, boys *and* girls should have more confidence in their abilities if parents believe they are good (i.e., lack of moderation based on gender). Unless noted otherwise, the findings presented in this chapter address mean-level differences between boys and girls.

Family-level demographic characteristics also determine family socialization and youth motivation and achievement. The demographic landscape of families in many countries has become much more diverse over the last 50 years. Four key demographic indicators are socioeconomic status (SES), ethnicity/race, immigration, and culture (Quintana et al., 2006). Although these key demographic indicators are related, they are also differentially linked to indicators of family climate and general childrearing style (box E in Figure 26.2; Ceballo et al., 2008). Here, we discuss the potential influence of SES, immigration, and culture on families. Ethnicity and race are discussed in the section on schools.

By and large, studies show that children growing up in high-SES families do better academically and are involved in more organized activities and skills-based informal activities during the afterschool hours (e.g., Mahoney, Vandell, Simpkins, & Zarrett, 2009). Family SES can affect children's motivation through the opportunity structures and through parents' beliefs and practices. For children to engage and succeed in a domain, they need to have available opportunities and a family that has the knowledge and ability to take advantage of those opportunities—both of which are often limited in low-SES families (Archer et al., 2012; Simpkins, Delgado, Price, Quach, & Starbuck, 2013). Not only do parents in low-SES families have limited resources to implement whatever strategies they think might be effective, but they also have to cope with more external stressors than do middle-class families living in stable, resource-rich neighborhoods (Conger et al., 2002; Furstenberg, Cook, Eccles, Elder, & Sameroff, 1999). For example, low-SES parents' jobs are often characterized by long hours, nonstandard shifts, and high physical demands (Updegraff, Crouter, Umaña-Taylor, & Cansler, 2007) that can limit the time and energy parents have to devote to their children (Yoshikawa, 2011). Furthermore, Lareau (2003) suggested that SES differences are not simply a function of resources, but that family norms vary by social class. Middle- and upper-class families, in contrast to lower-SES families, engage in a variety of behaviors, such as enrolling their children in organized activities, because they believe such experiences help to cultivate the skills and experiences their children need to be successful.

A second demographic variable affecting children's achievement is immigration. In 2011, approximately 40 million people in the United States, for example, were immigrants (Pew Hispanic Center, 2013). Families who immigrate have many strengths, but they also experience many challenges, such as high mobility, language barriers, and poor work conditions. Many second- and third-generation ethnic/minority youth also are likely to attend schools that are overcrowded, understaffed, and have higher rates of teacher and student turnover (Suárez-Orozco, Rhodes, & Milburn, 2009). These challenges can impede families' efforts to be involved in their children's lives and can have profound implications for children's early achievement (Glick, 2010; Yoshikawa, 2011). Yet despite these challenges, many immigrant youth outperform second- or third-generation immigrant children in school, even after researchers control for differences in resources at the family and neighborhood levels. This is known as the *immigrant paradox* (e.g., Suárez-Orozco et al., 2009). Parents often move to a new country in an effort to provide a better life for their families and more opportunities for their children (Suárez-Orozco et al., 2010). Therefore, the high value that parents place on education and children's sense of obligation to the family are two mechanisms that are suggested to account for the higher academic achievement of immigrant children (Fuligni & Fuligni, 2007). In contrast, the lower academic achievement of later generations may be the result of immigrants acculturating to American values, spending more time with their peers, and losing the protective benefits of their homeland (Garcia-Coll & Marx, 2009). The third demographic indicator, culture, also shapes parents' general childrearing beliefs, theories, and goals (Rogoff, 2003). For instance, traditional gender roles and familism are two core values within Latino cultures. Latino daughters in families with strong traditional gender roles may be less likely to engage in masculine activities (e.g., sports) and often find it challenging to attend organized afterschool activities because they often are more protected and have more family duties than sons (Simpkins et al., 2013). This type of work highlights the variability in families' adherence to cultural values of their host country (if they are immigrants) and their country of origin. Furthermore, this between-family variability can influence children's development by shaping parents' behavior and the general childrearing environment (Calzada, Tamis-LeMonda, & Yoshikawa, 2013), which is shown box E in Figure 26.2.

In summary, there are many ways in which family demographic characteristics shape the development of children's achievement motivation. It is important to note, however, that even though family demographic characteristics have been linked repeatedly to children's school achievement, their effects are almost always mediated by their association with parents' beliefs, practices, and resources (Benner, Graham, & Mistry, 2008; Melby, Conger, Fang, Wickrama, & Conger, 2008). In addition, parents' beliefs and psychological and social resources can override the effects of even the most stressful circumstances (Van Horn et al., 2009).

General Childrearing Climate

Historically, researchers studying parental influence have focused on the impact of the general patterns and philosophy of childrearing on children's overall orientation toward achievement (Eccles, Wigfield, & Schiefele, 1998). Recent work has focused on support for autonomy. Drawing on self-determination theory, scholars have argued that supporting children's sense of autonomy is the key to fostering high levels of achievement motivation and engagement (e.g., Grolnick, 2003). Autonomy-supportive parents allow children to explore their own environment, to initiate their own behavior, to take an active role in solving their own problems, and to express their points of view (Raftery, Grolnick, & Flamm, 2012). Autonomy support seems to be particularly important for low-achieving children (Ng, Kenney-Benson, & Pomerantz, 2004), especially if mothers stress the importance of effort and learning strategies as they help their children with homework (Pomerantz, Grolnick, & Price, 2005). Such practices may help low-achieving children feel both competent and socially supported.

Eccles (1992) stressed the importance of the right balance among structure, control, challenge, and developmentally appropriate levels of support for autonomy. This balance depends on cultural systems, the specific context in which the family is living, the age of the child, and other individual characteristics. Although the magnitude of effects varies by race/ethnicity, gender, SES, and nationality, there is consensus that these general parental practices impact a variety of quite general indicators of children's achievement motivation and motivated achievement behavior (e.g., Benner et al., 2008; Melby et al., 2008).

The affective and motivational climate created by parents is also likely to impact the extent to which more specific parental practices and role modeling actually influence children's domain-specific ability, self-concepts, and subjective task values. Families that provide a positive emotional environment are more likely to produce children who want to internalize the parents' values and goals, and therefore want to imitate the behaviors being modeled by their parents. Parental overcontrol and excess pressure on their children to succeed at particular activities are likely to undermine children's intrinsic interest in the activity, reduce children's confidence in their ability to succeed, and lead to negative affective associations with the activity due to classical conditioning (Grolnick, 2003; Lepper & Henderlong, 2000). For example, mothers' academic support actually had negative consequences for youth with whom they did not share a warm relationship (Simpkins, Weiss, McCartney, Kreider, & Dearing, 2006), an illustration of the fact that it is important to understand *what* was conveyed as well as *how* it was conveyed.

Translating General Beliefs into Specific Beliefs and Practices

Researchers have shown that parents' general beliefs, such as the valuing of achievement and sex-typed ideologies and goals, are linked to parenting behaviors concerning school achievement (Eccles, 1992; Goodnow & Collins, 1990; Jacobs & Eccles, 2000). Two of the central pathways by which general beliefs are translated into specific beliefs are by their direct influence on parents' child-specific beliefs (see boxes C and D in Figure 26.2) and by shaping parents' interpretation of the child's previous performance and aptitude (see the moderating role of box C on the relation between boxes B and D).

As outlined in the expectancy–value model, parents' general beliefs, such as their gender-stereotypical beliefs, directly shape their child-specific beliefs. Some recent work focuses on the potential implication of mothers' gender-stereotypical beliefs in mathematics. Mothers with more traditional gender-stereotyped beliefs about math, that is, that boys are better at math than girls, had lower confidence in their daughters' math abilities than mothers with less traditional beliefs (Bleeker & Jacobs, 2004). In addition, early elementary school-age daughters of mothers with more traditional gender-stereotyped beliefs in math were more susceptible to stereotype threat, that is, anxiety when in a situation that could potentially confirm the stereotype, than daughters of mothers with less traditional beliefs (Tomasetto, Alparone, & Cadinu, 2011). Having a mother who is less likely to believe that males are better suited for math than females seems to bolster daughters' motivation.

Eccles (1992) also theorized that parents' general beliefs shape how children's characteristics (box B in Figure 26.2) influence their child-specific beliefs (box D). In a recent review, Yamamoto and Holloway (2010) argued that three general parental beliefs change the extent to which children's previous achievement predicts parents' education expectations for their children across racial/ethnic groups. Specifically, parents' educational expectations were more closely tied to children's previous achievement if parents believed the ability was innate (rather than malleable or due to hard work), trusted the school and the feedback the school provided, and believed they could influence their children's achievement. Several of these themes are reminiscent of Dweck's (1999) work on whether people believe abilities are entity-based and highly stable over time or that abilities are incremental in nature and therefore amenable to substantial change through effort.

Parents' Child-Specific Beliefs, Values, and Perceptions

According to the Eccles expectancy–value model, children's motivational beliefs, performance, and engagement are shaped by those around them. As shown in Figure 26.2, parents hold many child-specific beliefs, such as the importance of a particular domain for their child and whether their child is skilled in that domain. These beliefs are domain- and child-specific so, for example, parents may believe their child is highly skilled in math but has limited skills in reading and music. These specific beliefs are consistent, powerful predictors of youth motivation and achievement. Furthermore, these effects hold even when independent estimates of children's actual competence (e.g., teachers' ratings and scores on standardized tests) and demographic characteristics are controlled.

One of the most consistent links is that parents' educational expectations predict children's subsequent academic motivation and performance (Davis-Kean & Sexton, 2009). Although parents' general educational goals are important, their beliefs about specific academic subjects, such as science, are stronger predictors of children's outcomes in these subjects (Archer et al., 2012). Parents' perceptions of children's competence and their valuing of a subject or domain have been shown to predict children's subsequent beliefs about their ability and perceptions of the value of math, reading, and sports (e.g., Bhanot & Jovanovic, 2005; Shumow & Lomax, 2002).

Parental beliefs also predict long-term outcomes. Several studies have documented that children's confidence in their own achievement-related abilities decline from kindergarten to 12th grade, when researchers control for children's aptitude (e.g., Fredricks & Eccles, 2002; Jacobs, Hyatt, Osgood, Eccles, & Wigfield, 2002). The confidence parents have in their children's math, reading, and sport abilities in early elementary school can slow these typical declines (Fredricks & Eccles, 2002). Additionally, mothers' prediction of children's success in math-related careers when children were in seventh grade predicted children's beliefs about careers and actual career choices 12 years later (Bleeker & Jacobs, 2004). This pattern was particularly strong for female offspring who, as young adults, were 66% more likely to have a non-science-related job compared to a physical science job if their mother did not have high confidence in their math abilities in seventh grade. According to the expectancy–value model, parents convey these specific beliefs to children through their behaviors.

Parents as Socializers

Parents socialize children through direct parent–child interactions, as well as how they manage and design their children's environments (Furstenberg et al., 1999; Parke et al., 2003). Researchers have documented the benefits of active involvement with, and monitoring of, children's schoolwork and time spent on other achievement-related activities such as sports and instrumental music (e.g., Archer et al., 2012; Steinberg, Dornbusch, & Brown, 1992). For example, researchers have shown that reading to preschool children predicts children's later reading achievement and motivation (Linver, Brooks-Gunn, & Kohen, 2002). However, it is not essential that parent–child activities focus on skills instruction to have an impact. In early elementary school, playing games together that involve math, such as board games with dice, was one of the stronger, consistent family predictors of children's math knowledge and fluency (LeFevre et al., 2009). Such experiences likely influence both children's skill level and interest in doing these activities.

Parents also structure their children's learning experiences by providing specific toys, materials, and role models in the home environment, as well as by making decisions about the environments children engage in outside of the home (Eccles, 1992; Furstenberg et al., 1999; Parke et al., 2003). Such decisions expose their children to particular experiences and value systems, and restrict dangers and exposure to undesirable influences. Children who have greater access to activity-related materials in the home have more positive attitudes about those activities (e.g., athletics, music), spend more time engaging in those activities, and have higher achievement than their peers in those activities (Pugliese & Tinsley, 2007; Simpkins et al., 2012).

Much of the existing work on parental socialization has taken a limited look at parenting by focusing on one or two parental behaviors. A few researchers, however, have adopted an integrated view of family influences. One promising method to integrate a more holistic perspective is the creation of indices that include a variety of parental indicators theorized to influence a particular outcome. These indices often include a heterogeneous set of indicators that may have a low interitem reliability but should nevertheless be combined in a single construct because they are all theorized to cause the same outcome (Bradley, 2004). Classic examples include research on cumulative risk (Sameroff, Bartko, Baldwin, Baldwin, & Seifer, 1998), the Home Observation Measurement of the Environment (HOME) scales (Bradley, 2004), and family involvement in children's education (Jeynes, 2007). Recently, we have used these frameworks to study parents' beliefs and behaviors with respect to children's achievement (Fredricks & Eccles, 2005a; Fredricks, Simpkins, & Eccles, 2005). In these studies, we documented a linear relation between an index of parental beliefs and behaviors and youth achievement-related outcomes in math, science, sports, and music, suggesting that socialization factors have a cumulative positive impact on motivation. In contrast, when all family predictors were entered at the same time in a regression model, parents' expectations for child performance trumped all other potential sources of influence, suggesting that parents' behaviors did not matter. Clearly, this was not the case when using an overall index. Researchers should consider the use of indices, latent variables in structural equation modeling (Simpkins et al., 2012), or cluster analysis to provide a more holistic view of parental influences that complement the knowledge gained through a traditional regression analysis.

Summary

The studies reviewed suggest a multivariate model of the relation between antecedent childrearing variables and the development of achievement orientation that depends on the presence of several variables interacting with each other. Specifically, proper timing of achievement demands creates a situation in which children can develop a sense of competence in dealing with their environment. An optimally warm and supportive environment with the minimal necessary control should optimize the influence of parents. Hopefully, these factors coalesce to promote motivation. However, these factors may come together to discourage motivation. If parents believe math and science are inappropriate for girls and they share a warm relationship with their daughter, their daughter may be deterred from pursuing math and science. The presence of high yet realistic expectations creates a demand situation in which the child will perform in accord with the expectancies of the parents. All these factors are essential for the child to develop a positive achievement orientation.

Most studies are limited to a single area of achievement. In a recent study, Simpkins and her colleagues (2012) examined the parental correlates of children's beliefs and outcomes in math, reading, sports, and music. Inclusion of all four domains led to some interesting comparisons across domains. For instance, the relations between parenting and youth variables were stronger in the leisure (e.g., sports and music) domains than in the academic domains (e.g., reading and math). This may be because sports and music increasingly occur outside of the traditional curriculum and are therefore less influenced by school factors than are math and reading. Parents also play a large number of roles in leisure domains, such as driving children to practices and lessons; cheering at games and recitals; paying for equipment, uniforms, and camps; and watching sports and music together. Parental influence may also vary based on the extent to which a domain is gender-stereotyped (e.g., physical science as a masculine domain), and is a core academic course versus an elective (e.g., math vs. a foreign language).

School Influences on Achievement

In this section, we review the work concerning school influences on achievement-related beliefs, behaviors, and choices, including social dimensions (i.e., teacher–student relationships, and peers and belonging), instructional dimensions (i.e., task characteristics, autonomy support, level of structure), racial and ethnic context, and microsettings nested within the school environment (i.e., curricular tracking and extracurricular activities). Much of the research reviewed is directly related to the assumption that motivation is optimized in learning settings that meet individuals' basic and developmental needs, some of which are universal and others that are a function of individual differences in aptitudes, temperament, interests, and socialization histories (R. M. Ryan & Deci, 2002). Individuals will place high value on an area of achievement, will have high expectations for success, and will be optimally motivated in settings that provide opportunities for them to fulfill these needs, and they will withdraw their engagement in settings that do not provide such opportunities.

Social Dimensions

Teacher–Student Relationships

There is a growing consensus that the quality of students' relationships with their teachers plays a critical role in enhancing motivation and engagement (Eccles & Roeser, 2011; Wentzel, 2009). In both elementary and secondary school, children who believe they share a good relationship with their teacher are more motivated and engaged than their peers who believe they do not have a good relationship (Furrer & Skinner, 2003; Wang & Eccles, 2012). Students who perceive their teacher to be supportive and caring are more likely to develop positive attitudes toward school, take intellectual risks, and persist in the face of difficulty. Teachers who are trusting, caring, and respectful of students provide the kinds of socioemotional support students need to approach, engage in, and persist with academic learning tasks (Wentzel, 2009). Caring teachers are also attuned to and sensitive to the needs of students in their classroom, and adjust their instruction in response to students' needs (Pianta, Hamre, & Allen, 2012).

A close–supportive relationship with a teacher is particularly important for academically at-risk students (Pianta, Hamre, & Stuhlman, 2003). Unfortunately, students who would benefit most from positive relationships with their teachers are also those who are least likely to get this support (Baker, Grant, & Morlock, 2008). There is also evidence that teachers hold differential expectations for various individuals within the same classroom. Teachers are likely to have low expectations for African American and Hispanic children, children from low-SES family backgrounds, low achievers, and girls in math and science (Jussim & Harber, 2005). In general, the research suggests that these expectations accurately reflect children's abilities (compared to expectations based on stereotypes). An important question is, what is the potential impact of these low expectations? There is some evidence that these teacher expectations have a small negative impact over the short term (Jussim & Harber, 2005).

This link between the quality of teacher–student relationships and motivation and engagement is reciprocal over time (Skinner & Pitzer, 2012). High-quality relationships with teachers serve to bolster students' perceptions of their competence, autonomy, and relatedness, which in turn elicit further teacher support. In contrast, unsupportive interactions between teachers and students makes it more likely that students will perceive themselves as unwelcome, incompetent, and pressured. In turn, these negative self-perceptions lead to further withdrawal of support from the teacher.

Peers and Belonging

In addition to teachers, peers are an important influence on motivation for school engagement. Peers are especially important during adolescence, when youth have an increased need for relatedness outside of the family. Researchers have explored the consequences of status or acceptance by peers, having friends, and features of friendships on children's achievement motivation and engagement (Ladd, Herald-Brown, & Kochel, 2009; Wentzel, Baker, & Russell, 2009). Studies indicate that children who are accepted by their peers and have high-quality friendships display higher classroom participation and intrinsic motivation (Ladd, 2005). In contrast, negative peer experiences (e.g., rejection and bullying) and not having close friendships increases the risk for disengagement. Students who are actively disliked by classmates participate less in class and have more negative attitudes toward school because they are either ignored or actively excluded from classroom activities (Graham & Bellmore, 2007; Juvonen, Nishina, & Graham, 2006). Crosnoe (2011) theorized that feeling they do not belong to the peer group at school has a profound negative impact on adolescents' academic adjustment because adolescents use counterproductive coping strategies to deal with their feelings (e.g., using drugs, disengaging from school).

Not only does it matter whether students have friends at school and feel a sense of belonging, but it is also important to know who their friends are. Are the students on the honor role or are they students who skip class? Students self-select into peer groups that have similar motivation and engagement levels, and this clustering provides opportunities for peer socialization that strengthen existing differences in engagement over time. Affiliating with a highly engaged peer group is related to higher engagement over time, whereas spending time with peers who are disengaged and low-achievers is predictive of lower engagement over time (Kindermann, 2007).

Instructional Dimensions

Task Characteristics

Another aspect of the classroom that influences motivation, engagement, and the investment of cognitive and affective resources in learning is task characteristics. One important characteristic of tasks is whether they are relevant to children's lives. There is evidence that the curriculum to which most students are exposed is often not particularly meaningful from either a cultural or a developmental perspective, and can lead to the alienation of some group members from the educational process, sometimes leading to school dropout (Gallimore & Goldenberg, 2001). In many classrooms, students spend much of their time on tasks that require memorization and applying formulas and procedures to solve decontextualized problems (Fredricks, 2013). The lack of task meaningfulness has been exacerbated by the increasing emphasis on standardized test preparation.

Another important task dimension is the level of challenge. Classroom tasks that are challenging but can be accomplished with reasonable effort promote engagement. If the task is too easy, students do not have the opportunities to be deeply invested, and they may even disengage because they are bored. Conversely, if any of the aspects of the task are too difficult, students may give up because it is too hard (Blumenfeld, Kempler, & Krajcik, 2006). According to Csikzentimihalyi (1991), individuals experience *flow* when there is a match between task challenge and skills level. Individuals in flow merge action and awareness, lose sense of time, and have stronger concentration.

To counteract problems of low motivation and engagement, educators have focused on designing authentic learning tasks that are situated in meaningful contexts, cognitively complex, and reflect how learning happens outside of the classroom (Blumenfeld et al., 2006). In these instructional environments, students often work together collaboratively to solve real-world problems, use technology-based tools, and are guided by teachers who scaffold instruction. Although these types of tasks are not yet the norm in most classrooms, research from both motivation and cognitive psychology demonstrates their benefits for engagement and learning (Bransford, Brown, & Cocking, 1999; Fredricks, Blumenfeld, & Paris, 2004).

Autonomy Support

Instructional practices that support student autonomy are critical for fostering intrinsic motivation to learn. Support for this hypothesis has been found in both laboratory and field-based studies (Lepper & Henderlong, 2000). Closely related to this idea is work showing the negative impact of excessive use of praise and rewards for participation in school tasks on students' intrinsic interest in these tasks (Henderlong & Lepper, 2002). It is likely that such rewards undermine their sense of autonomy because students are motivated by external factors rather than their own internal motivation.

Recently, researchers have differentiated between the instructional behaviors of autonomy-supportive teachers, who create classroom environments in which students have some control over their own learning, and teachers with more controlling styles (Reeve & Halusic, 2009). Autonomy-supportive teachers use noncontrolling and informational language, allow students to work in their own ways, encourage students to take greater responsibility for their own learning, and give students opportunities to have input and make decisions (Reeve & Jang, 2006). In contrast, controlling teachers pressure students to act in a certain way by using external incentives, controlling statements, directives, and commands. Students with autonomy-supportive teachers report greater autonomy, higher classroom engagement, and higher academic achievement, than do students with controlling teachers (Reeve, Jang, Carrell, Jeon, & Barch, 2004).

Level of Structure

It is critical that teachers support student autonomy in conjunction with adequate structure. Classrooms with adequate structure have clear and consistent rules, guidelines, and expectations, so that students know how to effectively achieve desired outcomes (Skinner & Belmont, 1993). In contrast, in classrooms that lack structure, students often experience confusion about expectations and consequences of their behavior. Teachers in well-managed classrooms use behavioral management strategies and organizational strategies that encourage students to do the work and be active participants in classroom activities (Bohn, Roehrig, & Pressley, 2004). In these classrooms, students display less disruptive behavior and higher engagement in learning (Pianta et al., 2012). The optimal balance between structure and autonomy support changes as students grow older and desire more opportunities for autonomy (Eccles et al., 1993). This same balance between structure and support is what makes authoritative parenting styles optimal for the development of youth (Steinberg et al., 1992). One reason for the decline in achievement motivation over time is that many students do not experience changes in the balance between structure and opportunities for autonomy as they pass through K–12 school years.

Racial and Ethnic Context

Race and ethnicity are two demographic factors that influence development through social mechanisms, including stereotypes, discrimination, and prejudice (Garcia-Coll et al., 1996; Juvonen et al., 2006). One example of a racial stereotype is the belief that being black and male is associated with lower intelligence, aggressiveness, and violence (Krueger, 1996). In contrast, an ethnic stereotype is that Asian youth are hardworking and high achievers, especially in math and science (Kao, 1995). The work on stereotype threat suggests that reminders of people's race or ethnicity can cue such stereotypes and promote performance for some groups (e.g., Asian Americans) and depress performance for other groups (e.g., African Americans) (Aronson & Steele, 2005). An extensive body of experimental research over the last two decades has shown that in situations where race is salient, African American and Hispanic youth do worse than expected on standardized tests (Aronson & Steele, 2005; Gonzalez, Blanton, & Williams, 2002). Moreover, in situations where stereotype threat is activated, students are less likely to focus on mastery or task goals, and more likely to avoid situations where they might demonstrate low ability relative to their peers (K. E. Ryan & Ryan, 2005). This causes some African American students to dis-identify with academics as a way to protect their self-concept (Osborne, 1997). These stereotypes can also have implications beyond testing and achievement. In the case of Asian Americans, their internalization of the model minority stereotype may have some achievement boosts, but it may also have psychological costs in terms of feeling more symptoms of general distress and negative affect (Yoo, Burrola, & Steger, 2010).

Experiences of racial/ethnic discrimination from students and teachers at school are common for African American and Hispanic youth (Portes & Rumbaut, 2001). These experiences can impact students' expectations for performance and subjective task value, as well as feelings of belonging at school (Roeser, 2004; Wong, Eccles, & Sameroff, 2003). However, the impact of discrimination may depend on whether it is anticipated discrimination or actual, daily experiences with discrimination. Wong and her colleagues (2003) found that *anticipated* future discrimination was associated with increases in motivation and academic performance of African American youth, whereas *daily* experiences of racial discrimination led to declines in their school engagement and confidence in academic competence and grades, and increases in depression and anger. Scholars suggest, however, that having a strong, positive racial/ethnic identity can help to buffer the negative effects of perceived daily racial discrimination on school-related motivation and achievement (Rodriguez, Umaña-Taylor, Smith, & Johnson, 2009).

Racial and ethnic experiences of youth may be dependent on the larger school context. The transition to middle or high school can be particularly challenging for African American and Hispanic students because middle and high schools tend to be larger, more stratified by race and class, and more performance-oriented (Juvonen, 2007). One factor that may be especially relevant to this transition is the ethnic composition of the school. Benner and Graham (2007) found that African American students in schools with a lower proportion of African American students had a larger decline in feelings of belonging over time than African American students in schools with a higher proportion of same-ethnicity students. Being in a context with fewer same-ethnicity classmates may make ethnicity more salient and increase concerns about being the targets of others' prejudice.

Microsettings Nested within the School Environment

One aspect of the school context that can affect students' expectations for success is curricular tracking (e.g., college track course sequences vs. general or vocational education sequences; Oakes, 2005). The best justification for curricular tracking derives from a person–environment fit perspective. Students are more motivated to learn if the material can be adapted to their current competence level. There is some evidence consistent with this perspective for children placed in high-ability classrooms, high within-class ability groups, and college tracks (Pallas, Entwisle, Alexander, & Stluka, 1994). In contrast, adolescents placed in low-ability and non-college-bound tracks do not do well. They have been found to have less positive attitudes toward school, lower self-concepts of ability, and higher rates of problem behavior (Eccles & Roeser, 2011; Oakes, 2005). The primary explanation given for the negative effects of tracking is that students are provided with a lower-quality learning experience and are given less supports than students in high-ability tracks (Eccles & Roeser, 2011; Oakes, 2005).

A persistent concern is how students get placed into different tracks and how easy it is for them to move between tracks. Poor students, ethnic/minority non-Asian youth, and non-native speakers are more likely to be placed in low-ability classes and non-college-bound tracks than are their wealthier and European or Asian American peers (Kao & Thompson, 2003; Oakes, 2005). At this point, it is unclear whether there is bias in the assignment to tracks or whether the demographic characteristics are proxies for lower achievement. In other words, children with these demographic characteristics may be overrepresented in low-ability tracks because they have lower achievement that places them in the classes.

Another aspect of the school context that can support students' needs for relatedness and competence is the opportunity to participate in extracurricular activities such as sports, the arts, and school clubs. Extracurricular participation has been positively linked to academic outcomes including higher grades, school engagement, and educational aspirations (for a review, see Feldman & Matjasko, 2012). Furthermore, extracurricular participation has protective value in terms of reducing dropout rates and involvement in delinquent and other risky behaviors (Mahoney et al., 2009). These effects likely reflect several processes. Involvement in extracurricular contexts increases students' connections to teachers, helps them maintain friendships and make new ones at school, and connects them to a prosocial peer group that is more likely to value academics (Fredricks & Eccles, 2005a; Schaefer, Simpkins, Vest, & Price, 2011). Activity participation may also have benefits because it provides opportunities for interpersonal competence, challenging life goals, and educational success (Mahoney, Cairns, & Farmer, 2003). Indeed, engaging in an activity that is meaningful to one's identity can reverse outcomes for students who otherwise were on the road to academic failure (Crosnoe, 2011).

Family Involvement in Schools

Our focus in this chapter has been on the potential impact of two major socialization contexts on the development of children's and adolescents' achievement motivation, engagement, and performance: the family and the school. Most of the existing research has looked at these two contexts separately. Thus, despite increasing calls for more integrated, cross-context studies that allow one to investigate the full complexity of social experience on human development, very little is known about how these two contexts interact with each other over time to both influence and accommodate to that development. However, these two settings are inextricably linked. Positive and negative experiences of youth in one of these settings spill over and affect them in the other setting (Flook & Fuligni, 2008). Furthermore, how families are involved in schools is linked to academic success of youth.

In a recent meta-analysis, Hill and Tyson (2009) examined the relations among three types of parental involvement and academic achievement in middle school. They found that academic socialization (e.g., communicating expectations, discussing the value of education) was most strongly correlated with achievement, followed by school-based involvement (e.g., parent–teacher conference, PTA). Home-based involvement positively predicted achievement if the focus was on enrichment, such as visiting museums and books in the home. In contrast, helping with homework was the only aspect of parental involvement negatively associated with subsequent achievement. In some cases, this negative relation may reflect parents' increased involvement in homework when their children are struggling academically.

The positive association between family involvement and achievement seems to be fairly robust. Most types of family involvement seem to be beneficial for youth from a variety of types of families in the United States, including immigrant and ethnic/minority families, as well as youth from China (e.g., Cheung & Pomerantz, 2011; Hill & Tyson, 2009). We also know that culture plays a major role in the extent to which, and the manner in which, parents get involved with their children's schooling (Cheung & Pomerantz, 2011). Certain types of family involvement, such as attending parent–teacher conferences, are more common in mainstream American culture than in other cultures (Garcia-Coll & Marks, 2009).

The kinds of general and child-specific beliefs proposed in Figure 26.2 are likely to influence the ways in which parents choose to interact with their children's schooling (Lareau, 2003). For example, Hoover-Dempsey and colleagues (2005) found that mothers are most likely to be involved in school and at home if they believe it is part of their role as a parent, and that they can make a difference. Conversely, stereotypes that teachers and school administrators have about their children's families likely influence the ways in which the schools reach out to parents (Booth & Dunn, 1996). Parents are more likely to be involved with their children's school if they believe the teachers welcome their participation (Grolnick, Benjet, Kurowski, & Apostoleris, 1997; Patrikakou & Weissberg, 2000). However, there is evidence that some schools actively discourage parent involvement. This is especially true in schools with a high proportion of low-income and minority students, in which parents are often seen as part of the problem rather than part of the solution (Eccles & Harold, 1996). There has been an increased focus on developing home–school partnerships to increase parent involvement, especially among the most hard-to-reach families. Initial evaluations of these programs have shown some success in increasing parental involvement (Bemphecat & Shernoff, 2012; Raftery et al., 2012).

Conclusion

There is growing evidence that experiences both at home and in various school/learning contexts influence children's and adolescents' motivation to achieve, defined in terms of self- and task beliefs, and engagement. In both contexts, children learn valued skills if they feel support for their universal needs (e.g., a sense of competence) and personal needs (e.g., personal and social identity needs). Early in life, parents and other socializers play a critical role in facilitating the acquisition of general motivational orientations toward mastery, curiosity, and the self-regulation of effort and attention. The work on child gender is a case in point. Parents hold differential beliefs and provide different opportunities for their sons and daughters in gender-typed beliefs (e.g., physical science, sports). This differential socialization has implications for children's motivational beliefs. As children mature, they begin to encounter other social contexts, such as schools, peer groups, sports' and arts' programs, that also influence motivational orientation and engagement.

Finally, the central thrust of this chapter and of many theoretical perspectives is about understanding how settings influence children. Yet we know that children themselves are active agents in their own achievement-related choices and in moderating the influence of social agents on their development (Bell, 1979). Parents may value an activity more highly if that activity brings their child joy and a sense of accomplishment. Or they might, for example, lower their confidence in their child's math abilities if his or her school grades are consistently low. However, there is limited research testing the relation between children's motivation and parenting practices. For example, in sports and music, research suggests that parents may adjust their behaviors over time based on children's ability beliefs (Davison, Cutting, & Birch, 2003; Simpkins, Vest, Dawes, & Neuman, 2010). Some work in math and sports suggest that the direction of influence may flow from mothers' beliefs to children's beliefs in elementary school, but the primary causal direction might shift as children move into and through adolescence (Eccles, Freedman-Doan, Frome, Jacobs, & Yoon, 2000).

The development of children's motivation is actively shaped by children themselves and by people in their immediate environment. In this chapter, we have discussed the ways in which families and schools may influence children. These two environments are important because children spend a great deal of time in them. The work reviewed here also suggests that children's motivation can be bolstered or undermined by the feedback and information they receive in these contexts, and by the fit between the context and the child's universal and personal needs. If the fit is good, children will engage in the learning opportunities provided. If the fit is not good, children are likely either to disengage from that context altogether or to engage in counterproductive coping behaviors that make them feel better in the short term but may have long-term negative consequences (Crosnoe, 2011; Eccles, Early, Frasier, Belansky, & McCarthy, 1997). Given that humans are a very adaptive species, it is likely that youth will seek out other settings in which their needs can be met (Eccles et al., 1997). Where will these youth turn to have their needs met? Perhaps it will be to their peer groups or to other organizations and settings. If these settings provide positive developmental experiences that support healthy development, these youth may do well. But what if these settings reinforce less positive developmental trajectories—trajectories that decrease the likelihood of a successful transition into adulthood, or that increase the likelihood of very risky outcomes? It is this latter possibility that we need to avoid by providing young people with better options and more supportive developmental contexts. Supporting youth through the family is one promising avenue to help support the development of motivation.

REFERENCES

Andre, T., Whigham, M., Hendrickson, A., & Chambers, S. (1999). Competency beliefs, positive affect, and gender stereotypes of elementary students and their parents about science versus other school subjects. *Journal of Research in Science Teaching, 36,* 719–747.

Archer, L., DeWitt, J., Osborne, J., Dillon, J., Willis, B., & Wong, B. (2012). Science aspirations, capital, and family habitus: How families shape children's engagement and identification with science. *American Educational Research Journal, 49,* 881–908.

Aronson, J., & Steele, C. M. (2005). Stereotypes and the fragility of academic competence, motivation, and self-concept. In A. J. Elliot & C. S. Dweck (Eds.), *Handbook of competence and motivation* (pp. 436–456). New York: Guilford Press.

Baker, J. A., Grant, S., & Morlock, L. (2008). The teacher–student relationship as a development context for children with externalizing or internalizing behavioral problems. *School Psychology Quarterly, 23,* 3–15.

Bell, R. A. (1979). Parent, child, and reciprocal influences. *American Psychologist, 34,* 821–826.

Bemphecat, J., & Shernoff, D. J. (2012). Parental influences on achievement motivation and student engagement. In S. L. Christenson, A. L. Reschly, & C. Wylie (Eds.), *Handbook of research on student engagement* (pp. 315–342). New York: Springer.

Benner, A. D., & Graham, S. (2007). Navigating the transition to multi-ethnic urban high schools: Changing ethnic congruence and adolescents' school-related affect. *Journal of Research on Adolescence, 17,* 207–220.

Benner, A. D., Graham, S., & Mistry, R. S. (2008). Discerning direct and mediate effects of ecological structures and processes on adolescents' educational outcomes. *Developmental Psychology, 44,* 840–854.

Bhanot, R., & Jovanovic, J. (2005). Do parents' academic gender stereotypes influence whether they intrude on their children's homework? *Sex Roles, 52,* 597–607.

Bleeker, M. M., & Jacobs, J. E. (2004). Involvement in math and science: Do mothers' beliefs matter 12 years later? *Journal of Educational Psychology, 96,* 97–109.

Blumenfeld, P. C., Kempler, T., & Krajcik, J. S. (2006). Motivation and cognitive engagement in learning environments. In R. K. Sawyer (Ed.), *Cambridge handbook of the learning sciences* (pp. 950–984). New York: Cambridge University Press.

Bohn, C. M., Roehrig, A. D., & Pressley, M. (2004). The first days of school in the classrooms of two more effective and four less effective primary-grade teachers. *Elementary School Journal, 104*(4), 269–287.

Booth, A., & Dunn, J. (Eds.). (1996). *Family–school links: How do they affect educational outcomes.* Hillsdale, NJ: Erlbaum.

Bradley, R. H. (2004). Chaos, culture, and covariance structures: A dynamic systems view of children's experiences at home. *Parenting: Science and Practice, 4,* 243–257.

Bransford, J. D., Brown, A. L., & Cocking, R. R. (1999). *How people learn: Brian, mind, experience, and school.* Washington, DC: National Academy Press.

Calzada, E. J., Tamis-LeMonda, C. S., & Yoshikawa, H. (2013). Familismo in Mexican and Dominican families from low-income, urban communities. *Journal of Family Issues, 34*(12), 1696–1724.

Ceballo, R., Chao, R., Hill, N. E., Le, H., Murry, V. M., & Pinderhughes, E. E. (2008). Excavating culture: Summary of results. *Applied Developmental Science, 12,* 220–226.

Cheung, C. S., & Pomerantz, E. M. (2011). Parents' involvement in children's learning in the United States and China: Implications for children's academic and emotional adjustment. *Child Development, 82,* 932–950.

Conger, R. D., Wallace, L. E., Sun, Y., Simons, R. L., McLoyd, V. C., & Brody G. H. (2002). Economic pressure in African American families: A replication and extension of the family stress model. *Developmental Psychology, 38,* 179–193.

Crosnoe, R. (2011). *Fitting in, standing out: Navigating the social challenges of high school to get an education.* New York: Cambridge University Press.

Csikzentimihalyi, M. (1991). *Flow: The psychology of optimal experience.* New York: Harper Perennial.

Davis-Kean, P., & Sexton, H. R. (2009). Race differences in parental influences on child achievement: Multiple pathways to success. *Merrill–Palmer Quarterly, 55*(3), 285–318.

Davison, K. K., Cutting, T. M., & Birch, L. L. (2003). Parents' activity-related parenting practices predict girls' physical activity. *Medicine and Science in Sport and Exercise, 35,* 1589–1595.

Dweck, C. S. (1999). *Self-theories: Their role in motivational, personality, and development.* Philadelphia: Taylor & Francis.

Eccles, J. S. (1992). School and family effects on the ontogeny of children's interests, self-perceptions, and activity choice. *Nebraska Symposium on Motivation, 40,* 145–208.

Eccles, J. S., Early, D., Frasier, K., Belansky, E., & McCarthy, K. (1997). The relation of connection, regulation, and support for autonomy in the context of family, school, and peer group to successful adolescent development. *Journal of Adolescent Research, 12,* 263–286.

Eccles, J. S., Freedman-Doan, C., Frome, P., Jacobs, J., & Yoon, K. S. (2000). Gender-role socialization in the family: A longitudinal approach. In T. Eckes & H. M. Trautner (Eds.), *The developmental social psychology of gender* (pp. 333–360). Mahwah, NJ: Erlbaum.

Eccles, J. S., & Harold, R. (1996). Family involvement in children's and adolescents' schooling. In

A. Booth & J. Dunn (Eds.), *Family–school links: How do they affect educational outcomes?* (pp. 3–34). Hillsdale, NJ: Erlbaum.

Eccles, J. S., & Midgley, C. (1989). Stage–environment fit: Developmentally appropriate classrooms for early adolescents. In R. Ames & C. Ames (Eds.), *Research on motivation in education* (Vol. 3, pp. 139–181). New York: Academic Press.

Eccles, J. S., Midgley, C., Buchanan, C. M., Wigfield, A., Reuman, D., & MacIver, D. (1993). Developmental during adolescence: The impact of stage/environment fit. *American Psychologist, 48,* 90–101.

Eccles, J. S., & Roeser, R. W. (2011). Schools as developmental contexts during adolescence. *Journal of Research on Adolescence, 21,* 225–241.

Eccles, J. S., Wigfield, A., & Schiefele, U. (1998). Motivation to succeed. In W. Damon (Series Ed.) & N. Eisenberg (Vol. Ed.), *Handbook of child psychology* (5th ed., Vol. 3, pp. 1017–1095). New York: Wiley.

Eccles-Parsons, J., Adler, T. F., Futterman, R., Goff, S. B., Kaczala, C. M., & Meece, J. L. (1983). Expectancies, values, and academic behaviors. In J. T. Spence (Ed.), *Achievement and achievement motivations* (pp. 75–146). San Francisco: Freeman.

Feldman, A. F., & Matjasko, J. (2012). Recent advances in research on school-based extracurricular activities and adolescent development. *Developmental Review, 31,* 1–48.

Flook, L., & Fuligni, A. J. (2008). Family and school spillover in adolescents' daily lives. *Child Development, 79,* 776–787.

Fredricks, J. A. (2013). *The seven myths of student disengagement: Research-based strategies for involving all students in essential learning.* Manuscript in preparation.

Fredricks, J. A., Blumenfeld, P. C., & Paris, A. (2004). School engagement: Potential of the concept: State of the evidence. *Review of Educational Research, 74,* 59–119.

Fredricks, J. A., & Eccles, J. S. (2002). Children's competence and value beliefs from childhood through adolescence: Growth trajectories in two male sex-typed domains. *Developmental Psychology, 38,* 519–533.

Fredricks, J. A., & Eccles, J. S. (2005a). Developmental benefits of extracurricular involvement: Do peer characteristics mediate the link between activities and youth outcomes? *Journal of Youth and Adolescence, 6,* 507–520.

Fredricks, J. A., & Eccles, J. S. (2005b). Family socialization, gender, and sport motivation and involvement. *Journal of Sport and Exercise Psychology, 27,* 3–31.

Fredricks, J. A., Simpkins, S. D., & Eccles, J. S. (2005). Family socialization, gender, and participation in sports and instrumental music. In C. R. Cooper, C. Garcia Coll, W. T. Bartko, H. M. Davis, & C. Chatman (Eds.), *Developmental pathways through middle childhood: Rethinking diversity and contexts as resources* (pp. 41–62). Mahwah, NJ: Erlbaum.

Fuligni, A. J., & Fuligni, A. S. (2007). Immigrant families and the educational development of their children. In J. E. Lansford, K. D. Deater-Deckard, & M. H. Bornstein (Eds.), *Immigrant families in contemporary society* (pp. 231–249). New York: Guilford Press.

Furrer, C., & Skinner, E. (2003). Sense of relatedness as a factor in children's academic engagement and performance. *Journal of Educational Psychology, 95,* 148–162.

Furstenberg, F., Cook, T., Eccles, J., Elder, G., & Sameroff, A. (1999). *Managing to make it: Urban families in adolescent success.* Chicago: University of Chicago Press.

Gallimore, R., & Goldenberg, C. (2001). Analyzing cultural models and settings to connect minority achievement and school improvement research. *Educational Psychologist, 36,* 45–56.

Garcia-Coll, C., Crnic, K., Lamberty, G., Wasik, B. H., Jenkins, R., Garcia, H. V., et al. (1996). An integrative model for the study of developmental competencies in minority children. *Child Development, 67,* 1891–1914.

Garcia-Coll, C., & Marks, A. K. (2009). *Immigrant stories: Ethnicity and academics in middle childhood.* Oxford, UK: Oxford University Press.

Glick, J. E. (2010). Connecting complex processes: A decade of research on immigrant families. *Journal of Marriage and Family, 72,* 498–515.

Gonzales, P. M., Blanton, H., & Williams, K. J. (2002). The effects of stereotype threat and double-minority status on the test performance of Latino women. *Personality and Social Psychology Bulletin, 28*(5), 659–670.

Goodnow, J. J., & Collins, W. A. (1990). *Development according to parents: The nature, sources, and consequences of parents' ideas.* London: Erlbaum.

Graham, S., & Bellmore, A D. (2007). Peer victimization and mental health during early adolescence. *Theory into Practice, 46,* 138–146.

Grolnick, W. S. (2003). *The psychology of parental control: How well-meant parenting backfires.* Hillside, NJ: Erlbaum.

Grolnick, W. S., Benjet, C., Kurowski, C. O., & Apostoleris, N. H. (1997). Predictors of parent involvement in children's schooling. *Journal of Educational Psychology, 89,* 538–548.

Henderlong, J., & Lepper, M. R. (2002). The effects of praise on children's intrinsic motivation: A review and synthesis. *Psychological Bulletin, 128,* 774–795.

Hill, N. E., & Tyson, D. F. (2009). Parental involvement in middle school: A meta-analytic assessment of the strategies that promote achievement. *Developmental Psychology, 45,* 740–763.

Hoover-Dempsey, K. V., Walker, J. M. T., Sandler, H. M., Whetsel, D., Green, C. L., Wilkins, A. S., et al. (2005). Why do parents become involved?: Research findings and implications. *Elementary School Journal, 106,* 105–130.

Hunt, D. E. (1979). Person–environment interaction: A challenge found wanting before it was tried. *Review of Educational Research, 45,* 209–230.

Jacobs, J. E., & Eccles, J. S. (2000). Parents, task values, and real-life achievement-related choices. In C. Sansone & J. M. Harackiewicz (Eds.), *Intrinsic and extrinsic motivation: The search for optimal motivation and performance* (pp. 405–439). San Diego, CA: Academic Press.

Jacobs, J. E., Hyatt, S., Osgood, D. W., Eccles, J. S., & Wigfield, A. (2002). Changes in children's self-competence and values: Gender and domain differences across grades one through twelve. *Child Development, 73*(2), 509–527.

Jeynes, W. H. (2007). The relationship between parental involvement and urban secondary school student academic achievement: A meta-analysis. *Urban Education, 42,* 82–110.

Jussim, L., & Harber, K. D. (2005). Teacher expectations and self-fulfilling prophecies: Known and unknowns, resolved and unresolved competencies. *Personality and Social Psychology Review, 72,* 791–809.

Juvonen, J. (2007). Reforming middle schools: Focus on continuity, social connectedness, and engagement. *Educational Psychologist, 42*(4), 197–208.

Juvonen, J., Nishina, A., & Graham, S. (2006). Ethnic diversity and perceptions of safety in urban middle schools. *Psychological Science, 17*(5), 393–400.

Kao, G. (1995). Asian Americans as model minorities?: A look at their academic performance. *American Journal of Education, 103,* 121–159.

Kao, G., & Thompson, J. S. (2003). Racial and ethnic stratification in educational achievement and attainment. *Annual Review of Sociology, 29,* 417–442.

Kindermann, T. A. (2007). Effects of naturally-existing peer groups on changes in academic engagement in a cohort of sixth graders. *Child Development, 78,* 1186–1203.

Krueger, J. (1996). Personal beliefs and cultural stereotypes about racial characteristics. *Journal of Personality and Social Psychology, 71,* 536–548.

Ladd, G. W. (2005). *Children's peer relations and social competence: A century of progress.* New Haven, CT: Yale University Press.

Ladd, G. W., Herald-Brown, S. L., & Kochel, K. P. (2009). Peers and motivation. In K. R. Wentzel & A. Wigfield (Eds.), *Handbook of motivation at school* (pp. 321–348). New York: Routledge.

Lareau, A. (2003). *Unequal childhood: Class, race, and family life.* Berkeley: University of California Press.

Lee, V. E., & Smith, J. (2001). *Restructuring high schools for equity and excellence: What works.* New York: Teachers College Press.

LeFevre, J. A., Skwarchuk, S. L., Smith-Chant, B. L., Fast, L., Kamawar, D., & Bisanz, J. (2009). Home numeracy experiences and children's math performance in the early school years. *Canadian Journal of Behavioural Science, 41,* 55–66.

Lepper, M. R., & Henderlong, J. (2000). Turning "play" into "work" and "work" into "play": 25 years of research on intrinsic versus extrinsic motivation. In C. Sansone & J. M. Harackiewicz (Eds.), *Intrinsic and extrinsic motivation: The search for optimal motivation and performance* (pp. 257–307). New York: Academic Press.

Linver, M. R., Brooks-Gunn, J., & Kohen, D. E. (2002). Family processes as pathways from income to young children's development. *Developmental Psychology, 38,* 719–734.

Mahoney, J., Vandell, D. L., Simpkins, S., & Zarrett, N. (2009). Adolescent out-of-school activities. In R. M. Lerner & L. Steinberg (Eds.), *Handbook of adolescent psychology* (3rd ed., pp. 228–269). Hoboken, NJ: Wiley.

Mahoney, J. L., Cairns, B. D., & Farmer, T. (2003). Promoting interpersonal competence and educational success through extracurricular activity participation. *Journal of Educational Psychology, 95,* 409–418.

Melby, J. N., Conger, R. D., Fang, S., Wickrama, K. A. S., & Conger, K. J. (2008). Adolescent family experiences and educational attainment during early adulthood. *Developmental Psychology, 44,* 1519–1536.

Ng, F. F., Kenney-Benson, G. A., & Pomerantz, E. M. (2004). Children's achievement moderates the effects of mothers' use of control and autonomy support. *Child Development, 75,* 764–780.

Oakes, J. (2005). *Keeping track: How schools structure inequality* (2nd ed.). New Haven, CT: Yale University Press.

Osborne, J. W. (1997). Race and academic disidentification. *Journal of Educational Psychology, 89,* 728–735.

Pallas, A. M., Entwisle, D. R., Alexander, K. L., & Stluka, M. F. (1994). Ability–group effects: Instructional, social, or institutional? *Sociology of Education, 67,* 27–46.

Parke, R. D., Killian, C., Dennis, J., Flyr, M., McDowell, D. J., Simpkins, S. D., et al. (2003). Managing the external environment: The parent as active agent in the system. In L. Kuczynski (Ed.), *Handbook of dynamic in parent–child relations* (pp. 247–270). Thousand Oaks, CA: Sage.

Patrikakou, E. N., & Weissberg, R. P. (2000). Parents' perceptions of teacher outreach and parent involvement in children's education. *Journal of Prevention and Intervention in the Community, 20,* 103–109.

Pew Hispanic Center. (2013). *A nation of immigrants: A portrait of the 40 million, including 11 million unauthorized.* Retrieved from *www.pewhispanic.org/2013/01/29/a-nation-of-immigrants.*

Pianta, R. C., Hamre, B. K., & Allen, J. P. (2012). Teacher–student relationships and engagement: Conceptualizing, measuring, and improving the capacity of classroom interactions. In S. L. Christenson, A. L. Reschly, & C. Wylie (Eds.), *Handbook of research on student engagement* (pp. 365–386). New York: Springer Science.

Pianta, R. C., Hamre, B. K., Stuhlman, M. (2003). Relationships between teachers and children. In W. Reynolds & G. Miller (Eds.), *Handbook of psychology: Vol. 7. Educational psychology* (pp. 199–234). Hoboken, NJ: Wiley.

Pomerantz, E. M., Grolnick, W. S., & Price, C. E. (2005). The role of parents in how children approach achievement: A dynamic process perspective. In A. J. Elliot & C. S. Dweck (Eds.), *Handbook of competence and motivation* (pp. 259–278). New York: Guilford Press.

Portes, A., & Rumbaut, R. G. (2001). *Legacies: The story of the immigrant second generation.* Berkeley: University of California Press.

Pugliese, J. A., & Tinsley, B. J. (2007). Parental socialization of child and adolescent physical activity: A meta-analysis. *Journal of Family Psychology, 21,* 331–343.

Quintana, S. M., Aboud, F. E., Chao, R. K., Contreras-Grau, J., Cross, W. E., Hudley, C., et al. (2006). Race, ethnicity, and culture in child development: Contemporary research and future directions. *Child Development, 77*(5), 1129–1141.

Raftery, J. N., Grolnick, W. S., & Flamm, E. S. (2012). Families as facilitators of student engagement: Towards a home–school partnership. In S. L. Christenson, A. L. Reschly, &

C. Wylie (Eds.), *Handbook of research on student engagement* (pp. 343–364). New York: Springer.

Reeve, J., & Halusic, M. (2009). How K–12 teachers can put self-determination theory into practice. *Theory and Research in Education, 7,* 145–154.

Reeve, J., & Jang, H. (2006). What teachers say and do to support students' autonomy during a learning activity. *Journal of Educational Psychology, 98,* 209–221.

Reeve, J., Jang, H., Carrell, D., Jeon, S., & Barch, J. (2004). Enhancing high school students' engagement by increasing their teachers' autonomy support. *Motivation and Emotion, 28,* 147–169.

Rodriguez, J., Umaña-Taylor, A., Smith, E. P., & Johnson, D. J. (2009). Cultural processes in parenting and youth outcomes: Examining a model of racial-ethnic socialization and identity in diverse populations. *Cultural Diversity and Ethnic Minority Psychology, 15*(2), 106–111.

Roeser, R. W. (2004, July). *The diversity of selfways in school during adolescence project.* Paper presented at the annual meeting of the William T. Grant Faculty Scholars Program, Vail. CO.

Rogoff, B. (2003). *The cultural nature of human development.* Oxford, UK: Oxford University Press.

Ryan, K. E., & Ryan, A. M. (2005). Psychological processes underlying stereotype threat and standardized math performance. *Educational Psychologist, 40,* 53–63.

Ryan, R. M., & Deci, E. L. (2002). An overview of self-determination theory: An organismic-dialectical perspective. In E. L. Deci & R. M. Ryan (Eds.), *Handbook of self-determination theory research* (pp. 3–33). Rochester, NY: University of Rochester Press.

Sameroff, A. J., Bartko, T., Baldwin, A., Baldwin, C., & Seifer, R. (1998). Family and social influences on the development of child competence. In M. Lewis & C. Feiring (Eds.), *Families, risk, and competence* (pp. 161–186). Mahwah, NJ: Erlbaum.

Schaefer, D. R., Simpkins, S. D., Vest, A. E., & Price, C. D. (2011). The contribution of extracurricular activities to adolescent friendship: New insights through social network analysis. *Developmental Psychology, 47,* 1141–1152.

Shumow, L., & Lomax, R. (2002). Parenting efficacy: Predictor of parenting behavior and adolescent outcomes. *Parenting: Science and Practice, 2,* 127–150.

Simpkins, S., Fredricks, J. A., & Eccles, J. S. (2012). Charting the Eccles expectancy value model from parents' beliefs in childhood to youths' activities in adolescence. *Developmental Psychology, 48,* 1019–1032.

Simpkins, S. D., Delgado, M., Price, C., Quach, A., & Starbuck, E. (2013). Socioeconomic status, ethnicity, culture, and immigration: Examining the potential mechanisms underlying Mexican-origin adolescents' organized activities. *Developmental Psychology, 49*(4), 706–721.

Simpkins, S. D., Vest, A. E., Dawes, N. P., & Neuman, K. I. (2010). Dynamic relations between parents' behaviors and children's motivational beliefs in sports and music. *Parenting: Science and Practice, 10,* 97–118.

Simpkins, S. D., Weiss, H., McCartney, K., Kreider, H. M., & Dearing, E. (2006). Mother–child relationship as a moderator of the relation between family educational involvement and child achievement. *Parenting: Science and Practice, 6,* 49–57.

Skinner, E. A., & Belmont, M. J. (1993). Motivation in the classroom: Reciprocal effects of teacher behavior and student engagement across the school year. *Journal of Educational Psychology, 85,* 571–581.

Skinner, E. A., & Pitzer, J. R. (2012). Developmental dynamics of student engagement, coping, and everyday resilience. In S. L. Christenson, A. L. Reschly, & C. Wylie (Eds.), *Handbook of research on student engagement* (pp. 21–45). New York: Springer.

Steinberg, L., Dornbusch, S., & Brown, B. (1992). Ethnic differences in adolescents achievements: An ecological perspective. *American Psychologist, 47,* 723–729.

Suárez-Orozco, C., Gaytan, F., Bang, H. J., Pakes, J., O'Conner, E., & Rhodes, J. (2010). Academic trajectories of newcomer immigrant youth. *Developmental Psychology, 46*(3), 602–618.

Suárez-Orozco, C., Rhodes, J., & Milburn, M. (2009). Unraveling the immigrant paradox: Academic engagement and disengagement among recently arrived immigrant youth. *Youth and Society, 41*(2), 151–185.

Tomasetto, C., Alparone, F. R., & Cadinu, M. (2011). Girls' math performance under stereotype threat: The moderating role of mothers' gender stereotypes. *Developmental Psychology, 47,* 943–949.

Updegraff, K. A., Crouter, A. C., Umaña-Taylor, A. J., & Cansler, E. (2007). Work–family linkages in the lives of families of Mexican origin. In J. E. Lansford, K. D. Deater-Deckard, & M. H. Bornstein (Eds.), *Immigrant families in contemporary society* (pp. 250–267). New York: Guilford Press.

Van Horn, M. L., Jaki, T., Masyn, K., Ramey, S. L., Smith, J. A., & Antaramian, S. (2009). Assessing differential effects: Applying regression mixture models to identify variations in the influence of family resources on academic achievement. *Developmental Psychology, 45,* 1298–1313.

Wang, M. T., & Eccles, J. S. (2012). Social support matters: Longitudinal effects of social support on three dimensions of school engagement from middle to high school. *Child Development, 83,* 877–895.

Wentzel, K. (2009). Students' relationships with teachers as motivational contexts. In K. R. Wentzel & A. Wigfield (Eds.), *Handbook of motivation at school* (pp. 301–322). New York: Routledge.

Wentzel, K. R., Baker, S. A., & Russell, S. (2009). Peer relationships and positive adjustment at school. In R. Gillman, S. Huebner, & M. Furlong (Eds.), *Promoting wellness in children and youth: A handbook of positive psychology in the schools* (pp. 229–244). Mahwah, NJ: Erlbaum.

Wong, C. A., Eccles, J. S., & Sameroff, A. J. (2003). The influence of ethnic discrimination and ethnic identification on African-Americans adolescents' school and socioemotional adjustment. *Journal of Personality, 71,* 1197–1232.

Yamamoto, Y., & Holloway, S. D. (2010). Parental expectations and children's academic performance in sociocultural context. *Educational Psychological Review, 22,* 189–214.

Yoo, H. C., Burrola, K. S., & Steger, M. F. (2010). A preliminary report on a new measure: Internalization of the Model Minority Myth Measure (IM4) and its psychological correlates among Asian American college students. *Journal of Counseling Psychology, 57*(1), 114–127.

Yoshikawa, H. (2011). *Immigrants raising citizens: Undocumented parents and their young children.* New York: Russell Sage Foundation.

CHAPTER 27

Making Good
The Socialization of Children's Prosocial Development

Paul D. Hastings
Jonas G. Miller
Natalie R. Troxel

Kind, caring, compassionate attitudes and helpful, comforting, altruistic behaviors characterize what are considered by many to be the finest qualities of human nature. Historically, social scientists have given more attention to antisocial and problematic behaviors than to prosocial and positive behaviors. This picture has been progressively changing as recent years have seen increasing interest in understanding the origins and developmental course of positive other-oriented emotions, cognitions, and actions. In this chapter we consider the research on the contributions of socialization agents and processes to prosocial development.

Included within the *prosocial* category are proactive and reactive responses to the needs of others that serve to promote others' well-being (Hastings, Miller, Kahle, & Zahn-Waxler, 2014). This broad definition includes empathy, sympathy, compassion, altruism, comforting, helping, sharing, cooperating, volunteering, and donating. *Empathy*, the (cognitive) recognition and (affective) sharing of another's emotional state, has been posited as providing the foundation for prosocial development and the primary motivation for engaging positively with others who are in need. *Sympathy* and *compassion* are emotional expressions of that positive, other-oriented focus that conveys the actor's concern for the well-being of the other person. There are many behaviors that also express this prosocial orientation because the specifics of a given situation call for a particular set of actions as the appropriate responses. *Altruism*, which involves sacrificing one's own gain in order to promote another's well-being, has garnered particular attention from many sociobiologists and social scientists, but prosocial behavior toward others does not necessarily require self-sacrifice. It can also benefit the actor, or come with neither cost nor gain, which is one of the reasons developmental scientists have generally preferred the broader term *prosocial behavior* to the narrower category of altruism. Displays of concern for others may occur in the form of proactive efforts to prevent another coming to harm, spontaneous reactions to events that place someone in need, reparative actions after having been the cause of some distress to another, or compliant responses to directives or solicitations for assistance. The motivations for prosocial behavior are similarly diverse because the actor may expect rewards or reciprocity, may fear repercussions for not being prosocial, or may purely want to alleviate another's distress. These motivations and manifestations may comprise important distinctions for understanding prosocial behavior.

Perspectives on the Socialization of Prosocial Development

Many theoretical frameworks for understanding the ontogeny, socialization, and development of empathy and prosocial behavior put a primary emphasis on parents, including evolutionary theory, psychoanalytic theory, social learning theory, social cognitive theory, and domains of socialization theory (de Waal, 2008; Eisenberg, Fabes, & Spinrad, 2006; Grusec & Davidov, Chapter 7, this volume; Grusec, Hastings, & Almas, 2011; Hastings, Zahn-Waxler, & McShane, 2006; Hoffman, 2000). Empathic engagement with their infants' cues and needs serves to motivate parents' caregiving efforts that meet the infant's needs, model an other-oriented approach to relationships, and reinforce the nascent caregiving behavioral system that is at the core of the attachment relationship (Hastings et al., 2014; Mikulincer & Shaver, 2005). In early childhood, parents' use of nonpunitive discipline techniques, including limit setting and inductive reasoning, has been seen as optimal for engaging children's attention toward the prosocial socialization message being delivered by parents. As active agents in the socialization process, children reflect upon, evaluate, and ultimately accept, reject, or modify parents' socialization messages (Grusec & Goodnow, 1994), such that the prosocial lessons or principles they internalize may closely match, or depart from, the messages parents intended to convey. When children subsequently encounter others in distress or need, their empathy motivates their engagement, and the ways in which their parents' prosocial lessons have been internalized then shape their expressions of empathic arousal, such as showing sympathy and compassion, or providing assistance and resources. Thus, empathy and internalization may mediate the links between socialization experiences and prosocial development.

Recognition of children's active role in socialization and internalization parallels the growing interest in bidirectional, transactional, and interactional processes of development (Ellis, Boyce, Belsky, Bakermans-Kranenburg, & van IJzendoorn, 2011; Sameroff, 2010; see Bates & Pettit, Chapter 16, and Kuczynski, Parkin, & Pitman, Chapter 6, this volume). Children's actions and reactions are both shaped by and, in turn, shape the environment, and the forces of biology and environment conjointly affect children's development. Behavioral indicators of the biological roots of prosocial development are evident very early in life. Neonates cry when they hear the cries of other newborns, infants express facial sympathy to others' distress by 8 months, and toddlers engage in sharing and helping by 14–18 months (Brothers, 1989; Roth-Hanania, Davidov, & Zahn-Waxler, 2011; Warneken & Tomasello, 2009). Yet there are large individual differences in infants' prosocial tendencies, stemming, at least in part, from varying dispositional propensities or capacities to feel empathy and engage in other-oriented caring actions

(Hastings et al., 2014). Parents and other agents of socialization respond to individual differences in the early-emerging emotional and social tendencies of infants and toddlers, tailoring their own actions in ways that foster or redirect dispositional traits. In turn, different children vary in their responsiveness to a given socialization event, leading to diverse dynamic exchanges between children and their parents, siblings, peers, teachers, and culture. Although it is not always possible to discern the interplay of nature and nurture, their interacting influences can lead to complex patterns of development. For example, the same features of parental socialization have been found to predict different expressions of prosocial behavior by girls and boys (Hastings, McShane, Parker, & Ladha, 2007; Padilla-Walker & Nelson, 2010). Thus, children's dispositional and psychological traits may both affect the socialization experiences they receive and moderate how those experiences contribute to prosocial development.

Outline and Scope of this Chapter

In this chapter, we consider the advances in our understanding of the socialization of prosocial development that have emerged through recent investigations. It continues to be the case that the majority of this research has focused on maternal socialization of prepubertal children. However, the past decade has seen marked increases in the amount of empirical attention turned to three other socialization agents—fathers, peers, and teachers—and the beginning of a literature on the contributions of grandparents to prosocial development. Extending beyond specific agents, the roles played by media, culture, and socioeconomic context in prosocial development have been the subject of several studies. And across these sources of influence, there has been more consideration of prosocial development beyond the childhood years.

Several other emergent patterns characterize the recent literature. Some researchers have considered whether socialization agents or actions have differential influences on the many aspects of prosocial development, such as cognitive empathy/emotional perspective taking versus affective empathy/sympathy, or the direction of prosocial actions toward varied targets such as family members, friends or strangers (Padilla-Walker & Carlo, 2014). There also has been greater consideration of moderating factors that could affect how or for whom socialization shapes prosocial development, and mediating processes that could illustrate the mechanisms or pathways by which socialization exerts its effects. Related to this, there has been examination of children's roles as active evaluators and interpreters of socialization messages, and of bidirectional processes by which children's prosocial characteristics shape the actions of parents and other agents, as well as the converse.

We focus this review in particular on longitudinal studies, in which measures of socialization temporally precede measures of children's prosocial characteristics. Increasingly, researchers are implementing designs with repeated assessments of socialization and prosocial measures that, with the application of careful statistical modeling, can provide stronger evidence for the direction of socializing effects and the lasting influence of socialization on development. Non-longitudinal studies that are informative about mediating and moderating processes also are considered. Single time point, correlational studies that do not consider mediating or moderating processes are only examined closely when other sources of insight are lacking.

The Roles of Parents

We begin with what constitutes the lion's share of the research: parents as socializers of prosocial development. The more extensive research on maternal socialization is examined first. There have been many recent reviews of the literature on the contributions of parental socialization to children's prosocial development (e.g., Grusec et al., 2011; Padilla-Walker, 2014). In the previous edition of this handbook (Hastings, Utendale, & Sullivan, 2007), we provided the following summary:

> Children are more prosocial when they have formed more secure attachment relationships with their parents; when their mothers and fathers are more authoritative than authoritarian in their style; when parents avoid punitive and strict discipline in favor of gentler control techniques; when they use reasoning and provide explanations; when they are sensitive to their children's needs and are warm with their children; and when they support their children's experience and regulation of emotions. . . . All these associations have been documented in longitudinal studies, in which the socializing event or action temporally preceded the observation of prosocial behavior. Most of these associations have been replicated across at least two independent investigations. (p. 655)

To what extent has the past decade of research sustained, refined, or refuted this characterization of the aspects of parental socialization that are effective for promoting prosocial development? We consider the more substantial body of research on maternal socialization first, then turn to the links between prosocial development and parenting by fathers.

Maternal Socialization of Prosocial Development

Parenting Styles

The dominant paradigm for studying parental socialization in the last 25 years of the 20th century was through examination of parenting styles, or the usual patterns of control, responsiveness, warmth, and punishment that parents use most often, across contexts and over time, to manage their children's behavior. Authoritative parenting may support prosocial development by modeling other-oriented behavior and emotion that children may emulate, encouraging children to be more considerate and caring, and eliciting affection and connectedness that make children more receptive to efforts to foster empathic concern for others (Hastings, Zahn-Waxler, Robinson, Usher, & Bridges, 2000). An authoritarian style of parenting may undermine children's prosocial behavior by modeling a lack of concern for the needs of others, or engendering hostility and the rejection of parental socialization efforts.

Although examination of parenting styles is no longer the dominant framework for studies of the socialization of prosocial development, knowing the broad or general approach to childrearing taken by parents continues to be useful. Hastings, McShane, and colleagues (2007) reported that the extent to which mothers endorsed a more authoritative parenting style predicted their preschool-age children's sharing and turn taking during play with unfamiliar peers 6 months later. However, maternal authoritative style did not predict teachers' reports of similar behaviors with familiar peers at preschool, despite significant correspondence of preschoolers' prosocial behaviors across these contexts.

Two studies of adolescents indicated that youth who perceived their mothers to be more authoritative also were more empathic and engaged in more prosocial behavior in subsequent years. Characterizing "needs-supportive parenting" as a pattern of socialization that was responsive, warm, and respectful of autonomy, while avoiding manipulative and intrusive control, Miklikowska, Duriez, and Soenens (2011) collected reports by youth on perceived socialization experiences, perspective taking, and sympathy annually over three years, beginning in the 10th grade. Daughters' perception of their mothers as needs-supportive predicted increases in their self-reported sympathy from grades 10 to 11, and from grades 11 to 12; maternal parenting was unrelated to sympathy for sons or perspective taking for sons and daughters. For two consecutive years, Padilla-Walker, Carlo, Christensen, and Yorgason (2012) had young adolescents and their parents report on the parents' authoritative parenting and the adolescents' prosocial behavior toward family members; adolescents' prosocial engagement with their parents also was observed during parent–child conversations. Youth who saw their mothers as more authoritative were also more respectful, sensitive, and sympathetic toward them during their conversations 1 year later. This did not extend to the questionnaire measures of prosocial behavior, nor did mother-reported authoritative parenting predict adolescents' prosocial development.

These analyses indicate that mothers' authoritative parenting styles can make lasting contributions to prosocial development. The two studies of adolescent development are in accord with hypothesized processes of internalization of parental expectations and values, in which the adolescents' evaluations of their mothers' parenting as appropriate and fair increase the likelihood that they will accept the positive socialization messages being delivered (Grusec & Goodnow, 1994; Grusec, Goodnow, & Kuczynski, 2000). At the same time, each study indicated that maternal authoritative parenting was limited with regard to which children or which behaviors appeared to be subject to influence. Parenting styles are complex and multifaceted, and a given parent will not always behave in ways that match with a single, defined style, such that it can be difficult to infer the likely processes or mechanisms that explain associations between parenting styles and child outcomes (Hastings & Grusec, 1998). Increasingly, researchers have examined more specific parenting practices as the means by which parents socialize desired outcomes.

Control and Discipline

Researchers have examined aspects of parental control to determine which appear to foster, or to undermine, prosocial development. Most of this research has focused on what Barber, Olsen, and Shagle (1994) call *behavioral control*, which encompasses the "rules and consequences" at the traditional core of parents' management of children's behavior. This range of actions includes establishing regulations, monitoring activities, supervising, recommending behaviors, issuing directives, threatening, and meting out nonphysical (e.g., withdrawal of privileges) and corporal punishment.

Parents' use of control is associated with the socialization goals they hold for their children, with strict and punitive control reflecting their desires for children's compliance and obedience (Hastings & Grusec, 1998). Garner (2012) found that mothers who reported using more power assertive and punitive discipline with their preschoolers also described their children as less empathic and comforting 4 years later. However, other researchers failed to find links between Chinese mothers' demanding and disapproving management of toddlers and the children's prosocial behavior toward peers 2 years later

(Wang, Chen, Chen, Cui, & Li, 2006). In a study by Mounts (2011), young adolescents with mothers who had stronger beliefs in their authority over their children's peer relationships reported decreasing levels of cooperativeness with peers over 7 months. Carlo, Mestre, Samper, Tur, and Armenta (2011) asked young adolescents to report on their sympathy, prosocial behavior, and experiences of parental behavior annually over 3 years. Youth who reported that their mothers used more strict control in the first year tended to report feeling less sympathy in the second year; in turn, those reports of less sympathy predicted fewer prosocial behaviors in the third year. Thus, strict and punitive control by mothers may act against the development of sympathetic responsiveness in childhood and adolescence, and thereby indirectly work against children's development of prosocial behavior.

This does not appear to be the case for less forceful, more gentle means of exercising parental control, such as suggesting appropriate behavior, providing structure, establishing standards or guidelines, and supervising or monitoring children. With young children, mothers' use of such low-power techniques has been found to predict more prosocial acts toward unfamiliar peers in daughters (Hastings, McShane, et al., 2007), and more cooperative and helpful behavior with peers in toddlers with affectively positive temperaments (Wang et al., 2006). Lindsey and colleagues (2010) found that mutual compliance between mothers and 15-month-olds during play (which involved mothers both initiating play activities and accepting children's initiations) predicted the children's cooperative and prosocial behaviors with peers at daycare at 24 months. However, Garner (2012) did not find mothers' lower-power parenting to predict children's empathic responsiveness 4 years later. Together, these studies suggest that low-power control might be particularly effective for fostering toddlers' and preschoolers' prosocial behaviors rather than their empathy or sympathy.

The picture is somewhat more complex in studies of older children and adolescents. Following a sample of youth from preadolescence into mid-adolescence, Yoo, Feng, and Day (2013) found that the quality of the parent–child relationship mediated the link between parental monitoring and empathic development. Youth who, at age 11 years, reported that their parents monitored them by regularly asking about their activities subsequently reported, at 14 years, that they felt closer and more connected to their parents. In turn, youth with closer connections to their parents reported greater increases in their empathic development from 11–15 years. In a 1-year longitudinal study, Bebiroglu, Pinderhughes, Phelps, and Lerner (2013) found more limited support for the benefits of monitoring. In grades 8 and 9, youth who reported more parental monitoring also reported more civic engagement concurrently, which included sensitivity to societal problems and engaging in helping activities. However, when adolescents' initial levels of civic engagement were controlled, earlier monitoring did not predict later engagement. Even less encouragingly, Mounts (2011) found that mothers' intentions and actions were differentially associated with their children's prosocial development over 7 months in the seventh grade. Children of mothers with more strongly held goals of improving their children's peer relationships subsequently reported more cooperative and empathic behaviors toward peers. However, for mothers who reported that they had many conflicts with their children about peer relationships, engaging in more consulting and problem-solving predicted decreases in youth-reported empathy for peers. Similarly, mothers who provided more advice and guidance about peer relationships also characterized their children as less cooperative with peers 7 months later.

This suggests that, particularly in a context of frequent disagreements, young adolescents may experience their mothers' active engagement in their social lives as an unjustified intrusion into their friendships, a domain over which many youth feel they should have personal control (see Smetana, Robinson, & Rote, Chapter 3, this volume). This is consistent with self-determination theory (Deci & Ryan, 1991; see Grusec & Davidov, Chapter 7, this volume): If youth feel that their parents intrude into their friendship choices and therefore undermine their autonomy, they are likely to reject their parents' efforts to foster more positive social engagement. Presumably, though, there was some aspect of the socializing behavior of parents that effectively translated their goals of facilitating good peer relationships into greater empathy and cooperativeness (Mounts, 2011). If not direct guidance and consultation, then what?

A recent study of "proactive parenting" by Padilla-Walker, Fraser, and Harper (2012) identified one possibility. Whereas reactive parenting involves parental responses to child behaviors that have already occurred, proactive parenting reflects anticipatory actions before events occur, such as shielding children from certain experiences, prearming children with strategies prior to events, or deferring to children's autonomy to make choices. They found that mothers of 12-year-olds primarily used shielding, prearming, or deferential approaches, and that their children reported valuing honesty and generosity at 13 years. They also collected parent and child reports of prosocial behaviors of youth toward family members at 14 years, and found the greatest congruence of prosocial values and prosocial behaviors in children of mothers who reported more deferent and trusting forms of proactive parenting.

The cumulative story of these studies of discipline and control appears to unfold developmentally. Although overly controlling, strict, and punitive parenting is disadvantageous for prosocial development across childhood and adolescence, the implementation of low-power parenting may need to be tailored to a child's developmental stage in order to foster prosocial growth. Young children benefit from more direct involvement through guidance and encouragement, which may be necessary to teach them appropriately prosocial values. By late childhood or early adolescence, when their offspring increasingly want and expect to make their own decisions, parents may need to trust that those values have been internalized. While maintaining an available presence for youth to turn to when they choose to seek advice, parents can allow their maturing children to have choices and make decisions. Effectively socialized children should (for the most part) make prosocial choices as adolescents. Of course, studies have yet to map out fully this hypothesized sequence, and it will be interesting to see whether future work supports this model of the development of effective parental control.

Psychological Control

Distinct from behavioral control, psychological control reflects parents' attempts to regulate their children's behavior by manipulating their emotions, thereby undermining their independence, self-esteem, and security within the parent–child relationship. Strong expressions of psychological control include criticism, derision, and rejection, whereas more subtle forms include love withdrawal, guilt induction, and intrusive micromanagement that is smothering, overprotective and infantilizing (Barber, Stolz, & Olsen, 2005; McShane & Hastings, 2009).

Longitudinal investigations generally indicate that parents' psychological control does not support children's prosocial development. Although, Garner (2012) found that mothers' reports of love withdrawal were positively associated with preschoolers' concurrent empathic responses to a vignette-based interview, love withdrawal did not predict mother-reported empathy 4 years later. In a 10-year study of boys, Hyde, Shaw, and Moilanen (2010) observed that mothers who were more rejecting of their toddlers had sons who were less empathic and prosocial at 12 years, according to mother and child reports. The previously discussed study by Yoo and colleagues (2013) also examined young adolescents' reports of their parents' psychological control, and found that lower parent–child connectedness at 14 years mediated the negative associations between psychological control and the development of empathy and prosocial behavior from 11 to 15 years. These findings are generally consistent with earlier literature on psychological control and prosocial development (Hastings, Utendale, & Sullivan, 2007), and suggest that the more explicit or less subtle expressions of psychological control might be the most maladaptive. Parents' rejecting, demeaning, or domineering actions may model the showing of low regard for others' feelings, decrease children's confidence in the dependability of parental nurturance, and engender resentment that may undermine empathy across relationships.

Induction and Reasoning

Parents use inductive reasoning to inform children of norms and principles, to explain why rules are necessary, to highlight the needs or well-being of others, and to illuminate the effects of children's actions. Parents' other-oriented inductions may promote children's prosocial behavior through both cognitive and affective mechanisms. Being told the needs of another person could clarify a child's understanding of another's state, which is an important component of the socialization of emotional competence (see Denham, Bassett, & Wyatt, Chapter 25, this volume). Especially for infants and very young children characterized by egocentrism and limited perspective-taking abilities, this may give necessary support for children's ability to identify others' distress and be aware of when their help might be effective. Because inductions may clarify cause-and-effect relations, such as the adverse effects of hurtful acts, children may also increase in their understanding of their own agency, responsibility to avoid harm, and ability to make reparations.

Somewhat surprisingly, relatively few prospective longitudinal studies have specifically examined parents' use of induction in relation to prosocial development, and those few studies offer a mixed picture. Hastings, McShane, and colleagues (2007) found that, for boys only, mothers' discussions of nice behavior predicted more prosocial and compassionate behaviors with familiar and unfamiliar peers 6 months later. However, Garner (2012) did not find associations between mothers' other-oriented reasoning with preschoolers and their children's empathy 4 years later. Finally, Scrimgeour, Blandon, Stifter, and Buss (2013) found that cooperative coparenting by mothers and fathers moderated the links between maternal reasoning with toddlers and their children's prosocial behavior 2 years later. Preschoolers were the least prosocial when their mothers had used little reasoning and their parents had not coparented cooperatively. Preschoolers with mothers who used more reasoning (regardless of coparenting style) or with more cooperative parents (regardless of maternal reasoning) were all comparable in their higher levels of prosocial behavior.

Generally, mothers' use of induction and reasoning with young children appears to be favorable for prosocial development, although this may vary across family contexts, child characteristics, and specific aspects of prosocial behavior. Clearly, more longitudinal studies are needed to properly evaluate the developmental effects of reasoning. Including assessments of children's affective and social cognitive functioning could assist with understanding children's active part in the internalization process.

Sensitivity, Responsiveness, Warmth, and Attachment

Parents' sensitive responses to children's distress cues and emotional needs generally are thought to facilitate children's prosocial development. Sensitive, responsive parenting addresses an array of infant needs, soothes distress, and fosters safety and comfort. Thus, it may both support the development of early emotional self-regulation and serve as a model for compassionate other-oriented behavior. Recent evidence for this was reported by Narvaez and colleagues (2013). Mothers' overall responsiveness to their young infants was assessed in home visits through interviews and observations, and children's cooperative, engaged, and positive responses to mothers were observed at 18 and 30 months. Mothers who were more responsive at 4 months had toddlers who were more prosocial during interactions at 18 and 30 months. Maternal responsiveness also predicted fewer behavior problems and greater cognitive ability, although Narvaez and colleagues did not examine whether these effects may have accounted for the links between maternal responsiveness and children's prosocial engagement. Similarly, they did not consider whether maternal responsiveness to infant distress cues versus nondistress cues were differentially associated with children's prosocial development, as some research has indicated (Leerkes, Blankson, & O'Brien, 2009; see Grusec & Davidov, Chapter 7, this volume).

There has been considerable debate around whether parental warmth and affection contribute to prosocial development (see Grusec & Davidov, 2007; also see Chapter 7, this volume), and recent studies have done little to resolve the issue. Lindsey, Cremeens, and Caldera (2010) found that shared positive affect during play between mothers and their 15-month-old children predicted more prosocial behavior with peers at child care at 24 months. However, Hastings, McShane, and colleagues (2007) found that mothers' reported affectionate responses to preschoolers' prosocial behavior was not related to the children's prosocial behavior with peers 6 months later. Bebiroglu and colleagues (2013) found that youth who reported more parental warmth also concurrently reported more civil engagement in grades 8 and 9, but as with parental monitoring, when the stability of civic engagement was controlled, earlier warmth did not predict later engagement. In their study of young adolescents' reported experiences of parenting, Carlo, Mestre, and colleagues (2011) found an interesting transactional pattern. On the one hand, adolescents who initially were more prosocial saw their mothers as warmer in subsequent years; on the other hand, earlier perceived maternal warmth was positively predictive of later sympathy. Thus, raising a nicer youth may help a mother to engage more positively with her child, which in turn fosters the youth's ability to feel compassionate toward others. Warmth also negatively predicted later prosocial behavior, but this was attributed to a suppressor effect due to the strongly positive relation between sympathy and prosocial behavior.

Rather than being a parent characteristic, warmth might be more effectively treated as a relationship quality. In addition to parents expressing warmth, children may need to experience and reciprocate that warmth as an ongoing component of their shared lives together in order for it to support their internalization of prosocial norms. Consistent with this idea, warmth and affection, along with sensitivity and responsiveness, and the provision of a safe and secure caregiving context, are key factors for facilitating infants' formation of secure attachment relationships. Children's internalization of secure relationship qualities may provide a basis for effective self-regulation of arousal and empathic engagement with others in need, which prepares children to act on the behalf of others (Mikulincer & Shaver, 2005). Most studies of the links between the security of infants' or toddlers' attachment relationships with their parents and the children's prosocial behavior have shown that early attachment security predicts stronger prosocial development (Hastings, Utendale, et al., 2007). Consistent with this, Murphy and Laible (2013) recently reported that children with more secure attachment at 42 months showed more empathic concern in response to the sound of an infant crying at 48 months, even when controlling for the children's earlier levels of concerned responding. Conversely, earlier empathic concern did not predict the development of attachment security over this period.

Recent examinations of prosocial development in adolescence offer some support for the continued importance of attachment relationships beyond the early childhood period. As described earlier, Yoo and colleagues (2013) found that parent–child emotional closeness in mid-adolescence predicted youths' empathy and prosocial behavior, and mediated links between earlier parenting and later prosocial development. Carlo, Padilla-Walker and Day (2011) also found that youths' and mothers' reports of more connected relationships predicted subsequent prosocial behaviors by the youth toward family, peers, and strangers. In another sample, however, Carlo, Crockett, Randall, and Roesch (2007) found that despite positive associations between close parent–child relationships and prosocial behavior in repeated assessments of adolescent reports, changes in parent–child relationship quality over time were not related to changes in prosocial behavior. Similarly, Yorgason and Gustafson (2014) found that adolescents' perceptions of closer attachments were positively associated with their initial levels of prosocial behavior toward family and strangers, but did not predict the development of prosocial behavior toward any targets over subsequent years.

Some of the inconsistency across studies might be attributable to the varying measures of attachment quality or emotional closeness that have been used to assess parent–adolescent relationships. At a minimum, though, adolescents appear to be more prepared to behave prosocially toward others when they have a close and connected relationship with their parents, and there is some evidence that such relationships provide a platform for further prosocial growth. As is thought to be the case with younger children, a secure attachment relationship in adolescence may help to provide youth with the emotional and cognitive skills that support their ability to engage positively with others. Of course, it is likely that the same individuals who share close, connected relationships with their parents in adolescence are the ones who, in infancy, had established secure attachments. It remains to be seen whether the quality of adolescents' attachments to parents contributes to prosocial development, above and beyond the affective and social cognitive foundations established by secure attachments in early childhood.

Emotion Socialization

Emotion socialization involves fostering children's understanding of their own and others' emotional experiences and their ability to regulate emotions effectively, and is reflected in practices such as explaining and discussing emotions, and being open to and encouraging emotional expressivity. Several cross-sectional studies have indicated that parents who effectively support their children's competent emotional functioning have children who are more sympathetic, helpful, and kind (Hastings, Utendale, et al., 2007), and some longitudinal studies have linked parental emotion socialization to children's emotional competence, of which empathy is a component (see Denham, Bassett, & Wyatt, Chapter 25, this volume). There have been fewer longitudinal studies specifically examining the roles of emotion socialization for prosocial development.

In two cross-sectional studies, Brownell, Svetlova, Anderson, Nichols, and Drummond (2012) looked at the relations between mothers' emotion language during storytelling and their toddlers' prosocial and sympathetic responses to examiners. They found that it was not simply mothers' labeling or describing emotions, but rather their elicitation and encouragement of toddlers' talking about emotions that was associated with the children's helping, sharing, and empathy. Conversely, Taumoepeau and Ruffman (2008) did not find significant associations between mothers' emotion language and toddlers' cognitive empathy between 15 and 33 months, but perhaps that was because they looked at maternal production of emotion words rather than the elicitation of emotion language from children. Taylor, Eisenberg, Spinrad, Eggum, and Sulik (2013) examined mothers' encouragement and acceptance of negative affect (when situations warranted it) when children were 18 months and the development of empathy and prosocial behavior between 2 and 7 years. Mothers' acceptance of toddlers' negative affect was correlated with mothers' reports of the children's empathy at five assessments between 24 and 54 months. In modeling analyses, openness to their children's negative emotions predicted empathy at 24 months but not its growth over time. Furthermore, the empathy at 24 months significantly mediated the link between mothers' expressive acceptance and teachers' reports of the children's prosocial behavior at 72 and 84 months.

Thus, both direct and indirect links between emotion socialization and empathic and prosocial development have been documented. Eliciting children's production of emotion words may promote their attentiveness toward, and understanding of, others' emotions. Accepting children's distressed and upset feelings, rather than dismissing or condemning them, may provide an example of a sympathetic orientation toward others. Further research into these proposals clearly is warranted, and it will be important for future studies to move beyond early childhood and consider emotion socialization and prosocial development in older children and adolescents (Klimes-Dougan & Zeman, 2007).

Paternal Socialization of Prosocial Development

A striking advance in the broader socialization literature over the past decade has been the concerted effort to consider the influences of socialization agents other than mothers. This is particularly true for research on paternal socialization. Several of the studies of prosocial development examined thus far included assessments of fathers' parenting, as well as that of mothers. They provide mixed evidence of fathers' contributions to their children's prosocial development, with a possible shift toward an increasing role for paternal socialization in adolescence.

Considering young children first, Lindsey and colleagues (2010) observed fathers playing with their toddlers at 18 months. Father–child mutual compliance, and to a lesser extent shared positive emotion, predicted toddlers' prosocial behaviors toward peers 6 months later. Mothers' and fathers' behaviors were weakly to nonsignificantly correlated, suggesting that the associations between fathers' parenting and toddlers' prosocial behavior were independent of those of mothers. Conversely, although Garner (2012) found that fathers' low-power teaching behavior was associated with preschoolers' sympathetic responses to vignettes, no aspect of paternal control or induction predicted children's mother-reported empathy 4 years later. Similarly, Hastings, McShane, and colleagues (2007) did not find significant associations between fathers' authoritative style or parenting behaviors and preschoolers' prosocial behavior toward peers 6 months later.

Rather than focusing on parenting behaviors, Scrimgeour and colleagues (2013) observed the extent to which mothers and fathers engaged in cooperative coparenting during triadic interactions with their children. More cooperative coparenting predicted mother-reported empathy 6 months later and also buffered children from the adverse effects of mothers not using much induction. However, two other studies failed to show that interparental conflict at early elementary school age predicted lowered levels of empathy or prosocial behavior in early adolescence (Hyde et al., 2010; Kouros, Cummings, & Davies, 2010).

Three investigations provided evidence for paternal influences on prosocial development in adolescence. Adolescents' perceptions that fathers used a needs-supportive style of parenting—akin to being authoritative—predicted the subsequent development of their self-reported cognitive empathy (perspective taking), but not their sympathy (concern for others) (Miklikowska et al., 2011). Young adolescents had more congruent prosocial values and prosocial behaviors when their fathers reported using "reason deferred" proactive parenting—a combination of using induction methods and allowing youth to make their own decisions—than did youth with fathers who were more protective, or who deferred decision making to their children without also discussing matters (Padilla-Walker, Fraser, et al. 2012). And, youth who reported more emotionally close, connected relationships with their fathers subsequently reported more prosocial behavior, although this did not hold for fathers' reports of connectedness (Carlo, Padilla-Walker, et al., 2011). However, in a fourth study (Carlo, Mestre, et al., 2011), neither perceived paternal control nor warmth predicted the development of adolescents' sympathy and prosocial behavior over the following 2 years; nor did positive characteristics of youth predict later perceived paternal parenting.

There are several factors that may contribute to a pattern of increased paternal influences on prosocial development as children move into adolescence. The nature of fathers' involvement changes from infancy to early adolescence, becoming less playful and more educational and task-related (Parke et al., 2005), which may provide distinct opportunities for positive socialization. The tendency for men to be more agentic and instrumental, and less expressive of or engaged with emotions (Miklikowska et al., 2011), might be reflected in paternal behaviors that are less relevant for young children's empathy and sympathy than for older children's effective engagement of these affective motivators in the production of prosocial actions. It also should be noted that researchers often obtain adolescents' perspectives on their socialization experiences, whereas most studies of younger children rely on parent reports or direct observations of parenting. To the extent that children's interpretations and evaluations of their fathers' parenting provide a clearer picture of the socialization messages that have been internalized, youth reports of paternal socialization should be expected to be more closely tied to their prosocial development.

Other Agents and Sources of Socialization

Sibling Relationships and Prosocial Development

Sibling relationships are often portrayed as a training ground for children to learn about social behavior, for good or for ill. The contributions of siblings to social development are dealt with extensively elsewhere (see Dunn, Chapter 8, this volume), but one recent report warrants particular attention here. Between late childhood and early adolescence, Lam, Solmeyer, and McHale (2012) collected three annual measures of relationship warmth and conflict between firstborn and second-born siblings, as well the children's self-reported empathy. When the authors controlled for factors such as parental responsiveness and parents' marital quality, greater warmth and less conflict in the sibling relationship predicted greater empathy in the subsequent year, and the predictive link between sibling warmth and empathic development strengthened with age. Thus, although many consider the transition to adolescence to be a period in which children turn away from family and toward peers as their preferred social partners, this study suggests that siblings may play increasingly important roles in shaping each other's empathic development at this critical stage.

Grandparents and Prosocial Development

While there has long been interest in the intergenerational relationships between grandparents and their grandchildren (Bengtson & Roberts, 1991), consideration of the contributions grandparents might make to their grandchildren's empathy and prosocial behavior is a relatively recent development. In a large sample of British adolescents, Attar-Schwartz, Tan, Buchanan, Flouri, and Griggs (2009) found that youth reported more prosocial behavior when their grandparents were more involved in their lives. In a 1-year longitudinal study of young adolescents, Yorgason, Padilla-Walker, and Jackson (2011) examined how the grandparent–grandchild relationship predicted the development of prosocial behavior. Youth who felt closer (more affectionate, warmer) with their grandparents reported more kindness and generosity to strangers 1 year later, even controlling for initial prosocial behavior and attachment to parents. Most recently, Yorgason and Gustafson (2014) examined adolescents' descriptions of their relationships with their grandparents, and their reports of prosocial behavior toward family, friends, and strangers over the next 4 years. Overall, prosocial behavior toward all targets increased over time. Youth who reported emotionally closer relationships with their grandparents had higher intercepts of prosocial behavior, and less steep slopes of change. In other words, they were initially more mature or advanced in their prosocial development, but over time, youth with less warm or affectionate relationships to their grandparents caught up. Intriguingly, the grandparent–parent relationship showed parallel associations with the grandchild's prosocial development: youth with parents and grandparents who were closer also had initially higher levels of prosocial behavior and less steep slopes of growth over time.

Peers, Friends, and Prosocial Development

Peer influences on social development are the focus of another chapter in this handbook (see Bukowski, Castellanos, Vitaro, & Brendgen, Chapter 10); here, we consider the recent evidence for peers' contributions to prosocial development. Past research on children's friendships and peer relationships indicated that more prosocial children are more popular and well liked, receive more positive responses from peers, and are more likely to have close friends, and that having prosocial friends fosters children's further prosocial development (Hastings, Utendale, et al., 2007). More recent studies suggest that the picture is not quite so straightforward.

In a single time point, sociometric study of children's friendships in fourth grade, Peters, Cillessen, Riksen-Walraven, and Haselager (2010) found that having a highly popular best friend was associated with girls not only being more prosocial but also using more relational aggression. They suggested that girls might selectively direct their prosocial behaviors toward their friends, while using relational aggression to maintain the dominant status of themselves and their friends relative to others. Consistent with this was the observation by Carlo and colleagues (2007) that although friend relationship quality was initially positively associated with prosocial behavior in young adolescents, increases in girls' relationship closeness over subsequent years was predictive of decreases in their prosocial behavior. Bowker, Rubin, Buskirk-Cohen, Rose-Krasnor, and Booth-LaForce (2010) used classroom sociometric ratings to examine how children's perceived popular status among their peers was related to their perceived prosocial behavior and other characteristics over the transition from fifth grade to middle school. Although children who were seen by their classmates as more prosocial also were considered to be more popular, when children's prosocial behavior increased over this period, their popular status was likely to decrease. Children who became more aggressive and arrogant, as well those who developed better leadership skills, gained greater popularity status. It would appear that in the period of early adolescence, nice kids really might finish last.

In a brief longitudinal study of young adolescents, Ellis and Zarbatany (2007) found that whether having a peer group that included many prosocial children fostered a given child's own prosocial development depended on the social status of that peer group. Being in a highly prosocial peer group that had central status (i.e., that was highly visible and well known to other children) predicted increases in children's prosocial behavior. However, for more peripheral groups, a group norm of high prosociality actually tended to predict decreases in individual children's prosocial behavior. Thus, children were likely to conform to a group norm of prosociality when that went along with reinforcing attention from other peers, but to reject that same norm when the prosocial group was relatively overlooked.

Both the Bowker and colleagues (2010) and Ellis and Zarbatany (2007) studies can be understood in terms of the strong motivations of young adolescents simultaneously to connect with their peers and display their autonomy from their parents, and to establish positions of acceptance and respect within the peer hierarchy. If prosocial behavior is an aspect of the social repertoire that the peer community expects and supports, then youth are likely to take on more prosocial characteristics (Pozzoli, Gini, & Vieno, 2012). However, when the local culture or norms of peers do not prioritize being prosocial, or when new classrooms of pre-adolescents are first being assembled in middle school and the group's norms are still being defined, being compassionate rather than domineering might entail some social costs for youth, at least in the short term.

Teachers and Prosocial Development

Teachers and educational contexts have marked impacts on children's cognitive and social development (see Wentzel, Chapter 11, this volume), and increasing evidence shows that this extends to their prosocial development as well. Although Merritt, Wanless, Rimm-Kaufman, Cameron, and Peugh (2012) did not find that emotionally supportive teacher–child interactions in the first grade were correlated with teacher-reported prosocial behavior, Arbeau, Coplan, and Weeks (2010) found that when teachers reported closer relationships with first graders, they also characterized the children as more prosocial with peers a few months later. Luckner and Pianta (2011) looked at concurrent associations between prosocial behavior of children in fifth grade with supportive teacher–child relationships and degree of classroom organization, while controlling for the stability of children's prosocial behavior assessed in earlier years. Children in more organized classrooms were observed to be more prosocial with peers, and teachers who were observed to have more emotionally supportive relationships with children reported that those children engaged in more prosocial behavior with peers. Finally, Batanova and Loukas (2012) found that the degree to which young adolescents felt positively connected to their school predicted boys' development of empathy and perspective taking over 1 year, and it buffered the negative link between conflicted parent–daughter relationships and the development of girls' perspective taking.

These studies may indicate that, with regard to promoting students' prosocial development, teachers and school systems can establish a relationship context that in many ways parallels the parent–child attachment relationship. Teachers who sensitively and responsively engage with their students' needs, while providing a predictable and consistent classroom setting, likely foster the extent to which children feel secure, safe, and respected within their classrooms and schools. The teachers also provide a model for a positive approach to classroom interactions. Feeling connected to their teachers and schools, children would be better able to cope with other stressors, such as tensions at home, and also would be likely to emulate their teachers' considerate and compassionate style in their own interactions with peers.

Community Involvement and Prosocial Development

Volunteerism and involvement in community-minded activities are thought to promote the development of prosocial characteristics in children and youth (Hastings, Utendale, et al., 2007). In effect, children and youth might become good by doing good. Two recent cross-sectional studies of youth that examined mediating processes offer some support for this proposal. With a diverse group of youth enrolled in a summer sports program that focused on providing supportive coaching in order to promote positive participation, Gano-Overway and colleagues (2009) examined adolescents' confidence in their abilities to regulate their emotions and engage empathically with others as mediating factors. Modeling analyses supported both aspects of affective efficacy as mediators: Perceiving the camp context as more caring predicted greater efficacy in positive affect regulation, which predicted greater empathic efficacy, which predicted reports of more prosocial behaviors directed toward the other campers. McGinley, Lipperman-Kreda, Byrnes, and Carlo (2010) also found evidence for a multi-step chain of mediation in a large group of Israeli youth enrolled in a first-aid and disaster-relief volunteer program. They found that adolescents' perceptions of their parents' encouragement to volunteer predicted their sympathy and perspective taking, which predicted their "dire" prosocial behavior (readiness to help when others are in desperate situations), which predicted their intentions to continue volunteering.

Thus, these studies again point to the essential roles played by affective empathy, cognitive empathy, sympathy, and self-regulation in linking socializing experiences to prosocial actions. One of the ways in which parents can promote this positive path of development is by engaging their children in activities outside of the home that provide novel opportunities to learn and practice a caring orientation toward others. This might be particularly important in adolescence, when youth are invested in exploring and forging their own identities. By finding alternative social contexts and effective mentors who share the values and messages they want to confer, parents can simultaneously respect the autonomy of their adolescents and achieve their parenting goal of rearing kind, compassionate, and helpful youth.

Social Media and Prosocial Development

The contributions of a variety of media to prosocial development are considered extensively in another chapter of this handbook (see Prot et al., Chapter 12, this volume). Here, we only consider an additional pair of recent studies by Coyne and colleagues (Coyne, Padilla-Walker, Harper, Day, & Stockdale, 2014; Coyne & Smith, 2014) on social media, family processes, and prosocial development. They found that adolescents who spent more time on cell phones and social networks felt less connected to their parents and, subsequently, engaged in less prosocial behavior—*unless* their parents were involved in these activities. Adolescents who spent more time with their parents on these new media felt closer to their parents and engaged in more prosocial behavior. As argued by Coyne and Smith (2014), this shared activity might reflect an effective method of parental monitoring of adolescents' activities and relationships, and it also could provide a developmentally appropriate venue for parents to discuss prosocial values. In addition, by sharing enjoyable activities that foster a closer parent–child relationship, their mutual use of social media might make adolescents more receptive to such socialization messages from their parents (Grusec & Goodnow, 1994).

Socioeconomic Status, Culture, and Prosocial Development

Past research has indicated that children from adverse family backgrounds, characterized by lower incomes or job status, younger and less educated parents, and non-intact families, are less prosocial than children from more privileged homes (Hastings, Utendale, et al., 2007). More recent developmental studies continue to show that being raised under conditions of relative socioeconomic hardship is not conducive to prosocial development.

In one study, Carlo and colleagues (2007) found that adolescents had smaller increases in prosocial behavior over repeated assessments when their mothers had completed fewer years of formal education. In another, they found that greater economic strain on the family was weakly associated with less prosocial behavior by youth 1 year later, and that two mediating factors accounted for this association (Carlo, Padilla-Walker, et al., 2011). Parents under greater economic strain reported more depression, parents with more depression had less close relationships with their adolescent children, and youth who were less close with their parents were less prosocial. This mediated path of influence was stronger for the mother–child than for the father–child relationship, but similar processes were identified across parents.

In a third longitudinal study, Hyde and colleagues (2010) found that living in more impoverished neighborhoods in middle to late childhood, as indicated through census tract data, weakly predicted lower empathy, sympathy, and guilt in early adolescence. More strikingly, Bandy and Ottoni-Wilhelm (2012) used a birth cohort of more than 1,000 participants in the Panel Study of Income Dynamics (PSID) to show that family income during childhood and adolescence predicted volunteering and charitable giving in adulthood, at ages 25–33 years. Adults who had been raised in lower income families were less likely to make a charitable gift, and their average gift was smaller. They also were less likely to engage in volunteer work, although those who did volunteer contributed more hours on average than adult volunteers from more affluent backgrounds. These findings held when the researchers controlled for the adults' current income, which suggests the results were not simply due to adults from lower income families having fewer resources to give to others.

Thus, across four prospective longitudinal studies that varied widely in their sample populations, assessments of family socioeconomic status, and prosocial measures, there was consistent evidence that individuals raised in families with fewer resources were less likely to engage in various kinds of prosocial behavior, although there was only weak evidence that they also felt less empathic engagement with others. In accord with the family stress model of economic hardship (Conger & Dogan, 2007), it appears that the adverse effects of economic hardship on prosocial development may be partially mediated by chronic stress eroding parents' well-being and ability to provide effective parenting and supportive relationships for their children.

Curiously, recent work with adult samples points to an opposite pattern, wherein more affluent adults are more self-focused, and less considerate and compassionate toward others compared to adults with more modest means (Kraus, Piff, & Keltner, 2011; Stellar, Manzo, Kraus, & Keltner, 2012). These two literatures are difficult to reconcile, although their differences might be related to both sampling and measurement. The prospective longitudinal studies cited here have utilized representative epidemiological samples (PSID) or targeted community samples that are overrepresented for risk or hardship, whereas many of the adult studies have used undergraduate student populations. Young adults from impoverished backgrounds who overcame their families' hardships and earned admittance to universities showed evidence of resilience (Masten & Wright, 2010), and may have benefited from atypically strong personal (e.g., self-regulation) or social (e.g., relationships and support systems) resources that fostered their compassionate orientations toward others, as well as their abilities to succeed academically. With regard to measurement, the prospective longitudinal studies showed stronger and more consistent effects of economic hardship on prosocial behavior than on sympathy and compassion. Perhaps impoverishment undermines the ability of some individuals to act on their empathic concern for others in easily observable ways.

In cross-cultural comparisons of prosocial development, past research has pointed to a pattern of greater empathy and prosocial behavior in children from more collectivist cultures than in children from more individualist cultures (Hastings, Utendale, et al., 2007), although findings have varied across samples and measures (Grusec et al., 2011). Findings in recent studies have been less consistent, suggesting that the collectivist–individualist distinction often drawn in cross-cultural studies might be less strongly associated with prosocial behavior than previously thought. Comparing toddlers in Berlin and Delhi, Kärtner, Keller, and Chaudhary (2010) found no differences in prosocial responses to examiners' simulations of distress. Trommsdorff, Friedlmeier, and Mayer (2007) also looked at responses to examiners' distress and sadness, and found that preschoolers in Germany and Israel showed more prosocial behavior and less personal distress than preschoolers in Indonesia and Malaysia. Examining mother-reported, teacher-reported, and observed sympathetic and prosocial behavior of preschoolers, Yagmurlu and Sanson (2009) found no differences between Anglo Australian and Turkish Australian samples. French, Chen, Chung, Chen, and Li (2011) observed Canadian and Chinese elementary school-age children in playgroups, and noted that the Chinese children engaged in more spontaneous giving of toys but less sharing or turn taking than the Canadian children. Li, Xie, and Shi (2012) examined how Chinese and American children in fifth grade thought of the relations between prosocial behavior and popularity. In both groups, children perceived more prosocial children to be more popular, and (in what might be considered a self-serving bias) the most popular children were particularly likely to think that being prosocial led to popularity (although the previously discussed research by Bowker and colleagues (2010) might suggest that they would soon be dissuaded of this belief). Finally, Telzer, Masten, Berkman, Lieberman, and Fuligni (2010) found that Latino and European American late adolescents were equally likely to allocate financial rewards to their families, rather than themselves, in a financial decision-making task administered in a magnetic resonance imaging (MRI) study. Latino youth, however, showed greater activation of reward regions (dorsal striatum and ventral tegmental) during costly donations, which suggests that they may have experienced their altruistic acts more positively.

Overall, then, there is not consistent evidence for differences in the prosocial responsiveness of children raised in more individualistic or collectivistic cultures. Countries and cultures develop and change (see Chen, Fu, & Zhao, Chapter 19, this volume), and it is possible that with increasing globalization of media, communications, and travel, there are now fewer or weaker broad differences in the national values and belief systems that matter for prosocial development. Parental socialization that predicts prosocial development in Western countries, such as low-power discipline, also has been found to predict prosocial development in Eastern countries (Wang et al., 2006). On the other hand, some cross-cultural studies have shown that different socialization measures predict similar levels of prosocial behavior across groups (e.g., Yagmurlu & Sanson, 2009), and some studies conducted within specific cultural groups have shown that traditional cultural values predict at least some aspects of prosocial development (e.g., Brittian et al., 2013; Calderón-Tena, Knight, & Carlo, 2010). To the extent that raising kind, caring, and helpful children is a parenting goal that is shared across diverse cultures, there may be subtly different socializing mechanisms within cultures that lead to commonly desired outcomes across cultures.

Conclusions

The past decade has witnessed an impressive expansion of the efforts by developmental scientists to understand the contributions of multiple socialization agents, experiences, and processes to prosocial development. Several consistent findings across studies have both bolstered past evidence for socialization effects and extended the scope of knowledge.

Mothers' overly strict, punitive, and psychologically controlling discipline undermines children's empathic concern, sympathy, and compassion, whereas management practices that are less directive and, increasingly as children mature, more respectful of autonomy serve to promote prosocial values and behaviors. Encouraging young children's consideration of others' emotions and experiences, and accepting children's own emotions as valid, promote affective and cognitive empathy and sympathetic orientations toward others. Establishing responsive, closely connected, and securely attached parent–child relationships facilitates emotion regulation and emotional competence that support children's abilities to engage positively with others. The socialization patterns are similar for paternal parenting and father–child relationships, although the contributions of fathers may increase with children's age, and may shape the development of cognitive empathy and prosocial behavior more than affective empathy, sympathy, and compassion. (Although it was not the focus here, similar actions by caregivers in family configurations other than those with two opposite-sex parents also promote prosocial development; see Patterson, Farr, & Hastings, Chapter 9, this volume; Scheib & Hastings, 2012.)

Children and youth actively evaluate and interpret the legitimacy and meaning of the socialization experiences they have with their parents. Parenting practices that are fair and respectful, and relationships that are close and trustworthy, increase the likelihood that children will accept and internalize the prosocial lessons that parents try to teach, and act in accord with their empathy and prosocial values. Simultaneously, when children show that they are considerate and kind, they elicit even more of the parental socialization experiences that foster their prosocial development, perhaps establishing a transactional cycle that helps to maintain a positive trajectory of development over time.

These patterns of socialization are more likely to occur in stable homes with adequate resources than in economically disadvantaged homes where parents have fewer resources and may be too stressed and distraught to put their energies toward prosocial socialization. As well, they appear to be evident across cultures and countries given that fostering prosocial development is a widely held parenting goal, and children from many lands and backgrounds typically display similar levels of empathy, sympathy and prosocial behavior.

Across the spectrum of children's relationships, including their siblings, grandparents, and teachers, there is evidence for the promotion of prosocial development through warmth, support, and respect. The one relationship type for which this was not as clearly evident was in the peer context of early adolescence. Pressures to establish social status and influence, and to distinguish the members of close friendships and cliques from other, less intimate peers can act against a general pattern of being compassionate and helpful. However, youth who affiliate with peers who are both prosocial and hold prominent status are themselves likely to emulate those positive interpersonal patterns. Analogously, youth who gain experience making empathy and altruism a part of their daily practice through volunteer work or supportive mentorship in group contexts are more likely to see "prosocial" as part of their character and future goals or activities.

It may be easier to establish some of these socialization influences in some children than in others. There are hints that affective empathy, sympathy, and compassion are fostered more readily in girls and in children with positive emotional traits, whereas prosocial behavior and altruism may be more readily socialized in boys. It may be important to socialize empathic engagement with others and prosocial values in young children, as elements of their early emotional development, in order to establish the basis for soliciting prosocial behavior from older children and youth.

Many of these conclusions are, of course, tentative inferences from a science that is continuing to advance. Overall, though, the recent research on the socialization of prosocial development is very heartening. If kind, caring, compassionate attitudes and helpful, comforting, altruistic behaviors are indeed the finest qualities of human nature, then we are making great progress in learning how we help our children to become finer humans.

REFERENCES

Arbeau, K. A., Coplan, R. J., & Weeks, M. (2010). Shyness, teacher–child relationships, and socio-emotional adjustment in grade 1. *International Journal of Behavioral Development, 34*, 259–269.

Attar-Schwartz, S., Tan, J.-P., Buchanan, A., Flouri, E., & Griggs, J. (2009). Grandparenting and adolescent adjustment in two-parent biological, lone-parent, and step-families. *Journal of Family Psychology, 23*, 67–75.

Bandy, R., & Ottoni-Wilhelm, M. (2012). Parental, social and dispositional pathways to Israeli adolescents' volunteering. *Journal of Adolescence, 35*, 1023–1034.

Barber, B. K., Olsen, J. E., & Shagle, S. C. (1994). Associations between parental psychological and behavioral control and youth internalized and externalized behaviors. *Child Development, 65*, 1120–1136.

Barber, B. K., Stolz, H. E., & Olsen, J. A. (2005). Parental support, psychological control, and behavioral control: Assessing relevance across time, culture, and method. *Monographs of the Society for Research in Child Development, 70*(4), 1–137.

Batanova, M. D., & Loukas, A. (2012). What are the unique and interacting contributions of school and family factors to early adolescents' empathic concern and perspective taking? *Journal of Youth and Adolescence, 41*, 1382–1391.

Bebiroglu, N., Pinderhughes, E. E., Phelps, E., & Lerner, R. M. (2013). From family to society: The role of perceived parenting behaviors in promoting youth civic engagement. *Parenting, 13*, 153–168.

Bengtson, V. L., & Roberts, R. E. (1991). Intergenerational solidarity in aging families: An example of formal theory construction. *Journal of Marriage and the Family, 53*, 856–870.

Bowker, J. C., Rubin, K. H., Buskirk-Cohen, A., Rose-Krasnor, L., & Booth-LaForce, C. (2010). Behavioral changes predicting temporal changes in perceived popular status. *Journal of Applied Developmental Psychology, 31*, 126–133.

Brittian, A. S., O'Donnell, M., Knight, G. P., Carlo, G., Umana-Taylor, A. J., & Roosa, M. W. (2013). Associations between adolescents' perceived discrimination and prosocial tendencies: The mediating role of Mexican American values. *Journal of Youth and Adolescence, 42*, 328–341.

Brothers, L. (1989). A biological perspective on empathy. *American Journal of Psychiatry, 146*, 10–19.

Brownell, C. A., Svetlova, M., Anderson, R., Nichols, S. R., & Drummond, J. (2012). Socialization of early prosocial behavior: Parents' talk about emotions is associated with sharing and helping in toddlers. *Infancy, 18*, 91–119.

Calderón-Tena, C. O., Knight, G. P., & Carlo, G. (2011). The socialization of prosocial behavioral tendencies among Mexican American adolescents: The role of familism values. *Cultural Diversity and Ethnic Minority Psychology, 17*, 98–106.

Carlo, G., Crockett, L. J., Randall, B. A., & Roesch, S. C. (2007). A latent growth curve analysis of prosocial behavior among rural adolescents. *Journal of Research on Adolescence, 17*, 301–324.

Carlo, G., Mestre, M. V., Samper, P., Tur, A., & Armenta, B. E. (2011). The longitudinal relations among dimensions of parenting styles, sympathy, prosocial moral reasoning, and prosocial behaviors. *International Journal of Behavioral Development, 35*, 116–124.

Carlo, G., Padilla-Walker, L. M., & Day, R. D. (2011). A test of the economic strain model on adolescents' prosocial behaviors. *Journal of Research on Adolescence, 21*, 842–848.

Conger, R. D., & Dogan, S. J. (2007). Social class and socialization in families. In J. E. Grusec & P. D. Hastings (Eds.), *Handbook of socialization* (pp. 433–460). New York: Guilford Press.

Coyne, S. M., Padilla-Walker, L. M., Harper, J., Day, R. D., & Stockdale, L. (2014). A friend request from dear old dad: Associations between parent/child social networking and adolescent outcomes. *Cyberpsychology, Behavior, and Social Networking, 17*(1), 8–13.

Coyne, S. M., & Smith, N. J. (2014). Sweetness on the screen: A multidimensional view of prosocial behavior in media. In L. M. Padilla-Walker & G. Carlo (Eds.), *Prosocial development: A multidimensional approach* (pp. 156–178). New York: Oxford University Press.

Deci, E. L., & Ryan, R. M. (1991). A motivational approach to self: Integration in personality. In R. Dienstbier (Ed.), *Nebraska Symposium on Motivation: Vol. 38. Perspectives on motivation* (pp. 237–288). Lincoln: University of Nebraska Press.

de Waal, F. B. M. (2008). Putting the altruism back into altruism: The evolution of empathy. *Annual Review of Psychology, 59*, 279–300.

Eisenberg, N., Fabes, R. A., & Spinrad, T. L. (2006). Prosocial development. In W. Damon, R. M. Lerner, & N. Eisenberg (Eds.), *Handbook of child psychology: Vol. 3. Social, emotional, and personality development* (6th ed., pp. 646–718). Hoboken, NJ: Wiley.

Ellis, B. J., Boyce, W. T., Belsky, J., Bakermans-Kranenburg, M. J., & van IJzendoorn, M. H. (2011). Differential susceptibility to the environment: An evolutionary–neurodevelopmental theory. *Development and Psychopathology, 23*, 7–28.

Ellis, W. E., & Zarbatany, L. (2007). Peer group status as a moderator of group influence on children's deviant, aggressive, and prosocial behavior. *Child Development, 78*, 1240–1254.

French, D. C., Chen, X., Chung, J., Li, M., Chen, H., & Li, D. (2011). Four children and one toy: Chinese and Canadian children faced with potential conflict over a limited resource. *Child Development, 82*, 830–841.

Gano-Overway, L. A., Newton, M., Magyar, T. M., Fry, M. D., Kim, M., & Guivernau, M. R. (2009). Influence of caring youth sport contexts on efficacy-related beliefs and social behaviors. *Developmental Psychology, 45*, 329–340.

Garner, P. W. (2012). Children's emotional responsiveness and sociomoral understanding and associations with mothers' and fathers' socialization practices. *Infant Mental Health Journal, 33*, 95–106.

Grusec, J. E., & Davidov, M. (2007). Socialization in the family: The role of parents. In J. E. Grusec & P. D. Hastings (Eds.), *Handbook of socialization* (pp. 284–308). New York: Guilford Press.

Grusec, J. E., & Goodnow, J. J. (1994). Impact of parental discipline methods on the child's internalization of values: A reconceptualization of current points of view. *Developmental Psychology, 30*, 4–19.

Grusec, J. E., Goodnow, J. J., & Kuczynski, L. (2000). New directions in analyses of parenting contributions to children's acquisition of values. *Child Development, 71*, 205–211.

Grusec, J. E., Hastings, P. D., & Almas, A. (2011). Helping and prosocial behavior. In C. Hart & P. Smith (Eds.), *Handbook of childhood social development* (2nd ed., pp. 549–566). Malden, MA: Wiley-Blackwell.

Hastings, P. D., & Grusec, J. E. (1998). Parenting goals as organizers of responses to parent–child disagreement. *Developmental Psychology, 34*, 465–479.

Hastings, P. D., McShane, K. E., Parker, R., & Ladha, F. (2007). Ready to make nice: Parental socialization of young sons' and daughters' prosocial behaviors with peers. *Journal of Genetic Psychology, 168*, 177–200.

Hastings, P. D., Miller, J. G., Kahle, S., & Zahn-Waxler, C. (2014). The neurobiology of empathic concern for others. In M. Killen & J. Smetana (Eds.), *Handbook of moral development* (2nd ed., pp. 411–434). Mahwah, NJ: Erlbaum.

Hastings, P. D., Utendale, W., & Sullivan, C. (2007). The socialization of prosocial development.

In J. E. Grusec & P. D. Hastings (Eds.), *Handbook of socialization* (pp. 638–664). New York: Guilford Press.

Hastings, P. D., Zahn-Waxler, C., & McShane, K. (2006). We are, by nature, moral creatures: Biological bases of concern for others. In M. Killen & J. G. Smetana (Eds.), *Handbook of moral development* (pp. 483–516). Mahwah, NJ: Erlbaum.

Hastings, P. D., Zahn-Waxler, C., Robinson, J., Usher, B., & Bridges, D. (2000). The development of concern for others in children with behavior problems. *Developmental Psychology, 36,* 531–546.

Hoffman, M. L. (2000). *Empathy and moral development: Implications for caring and justice.* New York: Cambridge University Press.

Hyde, L. W., Shaw, D. S., & Moilanen, K. S. (2010). Developmental precursors of moral disengagement and the role of moral disengagement in the development of antisocial behavior. *Journal of Abnormal Child Psychology, 38,* 197–209.

Kärtner, J., Keller, H., & Chaudhary, N. (2010). Cognitive and social influences on early prosocial behavior in two sociocultural contexts. *Developmental Psychology, 46,* 905–914.

Klimes-Dougan, B., & Zeman, J. (2007). Introduction to the special section of *Social Development*: Emotion socialization in childhood and adolescence. *Social Development, 16,* 203–209.

Kouros, C. D., Cummings, M. E., & Davies, P. T. (2010). Early trajectories of interparental conflict and externalizing problems as predictors of social competence in preadolescence. *Development and Psychopathology, 22,* 527–537.

Kraus, M. W., Piff, P. K., & Keltner, D. (2011). Social class as culture: The convergence of resources and rank in the social realm. *Current Directions in Psychological Science, 20,* 246–250.

Lam, C. B., Solmeyer, A. R., & McHale, S. M. (2012). Sibling relationships and empathy across the transition to adolescence. *Journal of Youth and Adolescence, 41,* 1657–1670.

Leerkes, E. M., Blankson, A. N., & O'Brien, M. (2009). Differential effects of maternal sensitivity to infant distress and nondistress on social–emotional functioning. *Child Development, 80,* 762–775.

Li, Y., Xie, H., & Shi, J. (2012). Chinese and American children's perceptions of popularity determinants: Cultural differences and behavioral correlates. *International Journal of Behavioral Development, 36,* 420–429.

Lindsey, E. W., Cremeens, P. R., & Caldera, Y. M. (2010). Mother–child and father–child mutuality in two contexts: Consequences for young children's peer relationships. *Infant and Child Development, 19,* 142–160.

Luckner, A. E., & Pianta, R. C. (2011). Teacher–student interactions in fifth grade classrooms: Relations with children's peer behavior. *Journal of Applied Developmental Psychology, 32,* 257–266.

Masten, A. S., & Wright, M. O. (2010). Resilience over the lifespan: Developmental perspectives on resistance, recovery, and transformation. In J. W. Reich, A. J. Zautra, & J. S. Hall (Eds.), *Handbook of adult resilience* (pp. 213–237). New York: Guilford Press.

McShane, K. E., & Hastings, P. D. (2009). The New Friends Vignettes: Measuring parental psychological control that confers risk for anxious adjustment in preschoolers. *International Journal of Behavioral Development, 33,* 481–495.

Merritt, E. G., Wanless, S. B., Rimm-Kaufman, S. E., Cameron, C., & Peugh, J. L. (2012). The contribution of teachers' emotional support to children's social behaviors and self-regulatory skills in first grade. *School Psychology Review, 41,* 141–159.

McGinley, M., Lipperman-Kreda, S., Byrnes, H. F., & Carlo, G. (2010). Parental, social and dispositional pathways to Israeli adolescents' volunteering. *Journal of Applied Developmental Psychology, 31,* 386–394.

Miklikowska, M., Duriez, B., & Soenens, B. (2011). Family roots of empathy-related characteristics: The role of perceived maternal and paternal need support in adolescence. *Developmental Psychology, 47,* 1342–1352.

Mikulincer, M., & Shaver, P. R. (2005). Mental representations of attachment security: Theoretical foundation for a positive social psychology. In M. W. Baldwin (Ed.), *Interpersonal cognition* (pp. 233–266). New York: Guilford Press.

Mounts, N. S. (2011). Parental management of peer relationships and early adolescents' social skills. *Journal of Youth and Adolescence, 40,* 416–427.

Murphy, T. P., & Laible, D. J. (2013). The influence of attachment security on preschool children's empathic concern. *International Journal of Behavioral Development, 37,* 436–440.

Narvaez, D., Gleason, T., Wang, L., Brooks, J., Lefever, J. B., Cheng, Y., et al. (2013). The evolved developmental niche: Longitudinal effects of caregiving practices on early childhood psychosocial development. *Early Childhood Research Quarterly, 28,* 759–773.

Padilla-Walker, L. M. (2014). The study of prosocial behavior: Past, present, and future. In L. M. Padilla-Walker & G. Carlo (Eds.), *Prosocial development: A multidimensional approach* (pp. 131–155). New York: Oxford University Press.

Padilla-Walker, L. M., & Carlo, G. (2014). The study of prosocial behavior: Past, present, and future. In L. M. Padilla-Walker & G. Carlo (Eds.), *Prosocial development: A multidimensional approach* (pp. 3–16). New York: Oxford University Press.

Padilla-Walker, L. M., Carlo, G., Christensen, K. J., & Yorgason, J. B. (2012). Bidirectional relations between authoritative parenting and adolescents' prosocial behaviors. *Journal of Research on Adolescence, 22,* 400–408.

Padilla-Walker, L. M., Fraser, A. M., & Harper, J. M. (2012). Walking the walk: The moderating role of proactive parenting on adolescents' value-congruent behaviors. *Journal of Adolescence, 35,* 1141–1152.

Padilla-Walker, L. M., & Nelson, L. J. (2010). Parenting and adolescents' values and behaviour: The moderating role of temperament. *Journal of Moral Education, 39,* 491–509.

Parke, R. D., Dennis, J., Flyr, M. L., Morris, K. L., Leidy, M. S., & Schofield, T. J. (2005). Fathers: Cultural and ecological perspectives. In T. Luster & L. Okagaki (Eds.), *Parenting: An ecological perspective* (2nd ed., pp. 103–144). New York: Routledge.

Peters, E., Cillessen, A. H. N., Riksen-Walraven, J. M., & Haselager, G. J. T. (2010). Best friends' preference and popularity: Associations with aggression and prosocial behavior. *International Journal of Behavioral Development, 34,* 398–405.

Pozzoli, T., Gini, G., & Vieno, A. (2012). The role of individual correlates and class norms in defending and passive bystanding behavior in bullying: A multilevel analysis. *Child Development, 83,* 1917–1931.

Roth-Hanania, R., Davidov, M., & Zahn-Waxler, C. (2011). Empathy development from 8 to 16 months: Early signs of concern for others. *Infant Behavior and Development, 34,* 447–458.

Sameroff, A. (2010). A unified theory of development: A dialectic integration of nature and nurture. *Child Development, 81,* 6–22.

Scheib, J. E., & Hastings, P. D. (2012). Donor-conceived children raised by lesbian couples. In D. Cutas & S. Chan (Eds.), *Families—beyond the nuclear ideal* (pp. 64–83). London: Bloomsbury Academic.

Scrimgeour, M. B., Blandon, A. Y., Stifter, C. A., & Buss, K. A. (2013). Cooperative coparenting moderates the association between parenting practices and children's prosocial behavior. *Journal of Family Psychology, 27,* 506–511.

Stellar, J. E., Manzo, V. M., Kraus, M. W., & Keltner, D. (2012). Class and compassion: Socioeconomic factors predict response to suffering. *Emotion, 12,* 449–459.

Taumoepeau, M., & Ruffman, T. (2008). Stepping stones to others' minds: Maternal talk relates to child mental state language and emotion understanding at 15, 24, and 33 months. *Child Development, 79,* 284–302.

Taylor, Z. E., Eisenberg, N., Spinrad, T. L., Eggum, N. D., & Sulik, M. J. (2013). The relations of ego-resiliency and emotion socialization to the development of empathy and prosocial behavior across early childhood. *Emotion, 13,* 822–831.

Telzer, E. H., Masten, C. L., Berkman, E. T., Lieberman, M. D., & Fuligni, A. J. (2010). Gaining while giving: An fMRI study of the rewards of family assistance among White and Latino youth. *Social Neuroscience, 5,* 508–518.

Trommsdorff, G., Friedlmeier, W., & Mayer, B. (2007). Sympathy, distress, and prosocial behavior of preschool children in four cultures. *International Journal of Behavioral Development, 31,* 248–294.

Wang, L., Chen, X., Chen, H., Cui, L., & Li, M. (2006). Affect and maternal parenting as predictors of adaptive and maladaptive behaviors in Chinese children. *International Journal of Behavioral Development, 30,* 158–166.

Warneken, F., & Tomasello, M. (2009). The roots of human altruism. *British Journal of Psychology, 100,* 455–471.

Yagmurlu, B., & Sanson, A. (2009). Parenting and temperament as predictors of prosocial behavior in Australian and Turkish Australian children. *Australian Journal of Psychology, 61,* 77–88.

Yoo, H., Feng, X., & Day, R. D. (2013). Adolescents' empathy and prosocial behavior in the family context: A longitudinal study. *Journal of Youth and Adolescence, 42,* 1858–1872.

Yorgason, J. B., & Gustafson, K. B. (2014). Linking grandparent involvement with the development of prosocial behavior in adolescents. The study of prosocial behavior: Past, present, and future. In L. M. Padilla-Walker & G. Carlo (Eds.), *Prosocial development: A multidimensional approach* (pp. 201–217). New York: Oxford University Press.

Yorgason, J. B., Padilla-Walker, L. M., & Jackson, J. (2011). Non-residential grandparents' financial and emotional involvement in relation to early adolescent grandchild outcomes. *Journal of Research on Adolescence, 21,* 552–558.

CHAPTER 28

Cultivating the Moral Personality
Socialization in the Family and Beyond

Michael W. Pratt
Sam A. Hardy

Moral Development and Socialization: An Orientation

All societies must find effective ways to teach moral values and behaviors to children, and have enlisted key social institutions to foster such learning, including the family, the peer group, schools, religions, and the local community. Humans have innate potential for both goodness and evil (de Waal, 1996), but socialization can have a salient effect on which path is taken. The past century was replete with examples of successes in moral socialization (Mother Theresa, Martin Luther King, Nelson Mandela) and dreadful failures (Adolph Hitler, Joseph Stalin). In this chapter, we aim to examine evidence on the socialization of the child toward the moral adult, grounding much of the review in cognitive-developmental theory (Kohlberg, 1969), social domain theory (Turiel, 1983), and personality approaches to morality (Lapsley & Hill, 2009).

A Brief History of Theory and Research on Moral Development

For much of the latter half of the 20th century, research and theory on moral development was dominated by Kohlberg's (1969) cognitive developmental framework. This stage model described the development of reasoning about moral dilemmas involving conflicts relative to core issues of rights and welfare (Kohlberg, 1969), and grew to incorporate issues of the self and the welfare of others. Kohlberg's work was the catalyst that sparked increased scholarly interest in moral development and functioning. Nevertheless, over time, a number of salient criticisms of his stage theory emerged, leading to new directions in moral development theory and research.

One critique came from Turiel (1983), who argued that Kohlberg failed to make distinctions among the types of reasoning people use in various situations. Turiel developed a structural–developmental theory known as *social domain theory*, which holds that

661

even young children make distinctions between different domains of social knowledge. The most fundamental distinctions made are between the moral, social conventional, and personal domains (Smetana, 1999; Turiel, 1983). The *moral domain* hinges on universal moral principles of welfare and justice. Rules in this domain are understood as obligatory and unalterable. The *social conventional domain* refers to rules that facilitate and regulate communication and orderly interactions among people, but are relatively arbitrary, changeable, and dependent on social conventions (Smetana, 1999). The *personal domain* is less regulated and comprises prudential concerns about the self's own welfare, and personal preferences, which are not regulated at all.

Children become aware of these domain distinctions early, and they persist throughout development. The learning of these distinctions is aided by peers and adults who provide distinctive feedback to children relative to these domains (Nucci & Turiel, 1978). In particular, moral violations elicit to a child perpetrator feedback from both the victim and adult and peer observers that focuses on harm and/or unfairness to the victim. Social conventional violations evoke feedback that focuses on the need for order and effective organization of social and interactive systems, and is much more commonly provided by adults than by peers.

Whereas Kohlberg and Turiel both focused largely on moral reasoning as the heart of moral development and functioning, others saw a more central role for moral emotions. Hoffman (2000) argued that cognitions are "cold" and do not provide much of a motivating spark for action; motivation comes from emotions, while cognitions guide the particular course of action. Thus, emotions such as empathy and guilt may help us be sensitive to moral situations and motivated to take the moral action. Hastings, Miller, and Troxel (Chapter 27, this volume) provide an overview of the socialization of empathy, so we discuss moral emotions only briefly here.

The previously discussed approaches to moral development are somewhat narrow in focus, attending largely to moral reasoning or moral emotions. Others have tried to outline integrative frameworks for morality. Rest's (1983) model puts moral reasoning and emotion in the larger context of four components necessary to produce moral action: (1) sensitivity to moral situations, (2) moral reasoning, (3) motivation to act morally, and (4) capacities to follow through with moral intentions. Thus, for moral action to ensue, people must engage in informational processes such as empathy and perspective taking that inform them about the moral stakes of a situation, effectively reason about the most moral course of action, possess the motivation to take the moral course of action, and have the capacity to carry out the moral action (e.g., self-control).

Inspired by Rest's model (1983), as well as work by Blasi (1984) and others, many scholars now move toward viewing moral development through a broader personality lens. While there is still an acknowledgment that moral reasoning and moral emotions are important to morality, there is also interest in the role of the self (Hardy & Carlo, 2011a, 2011b), traits (Walker & Hennig, 2004), social cognitions (Lapsley & Hill, 2009), life narratives (Pratt, Arnold, & Lawford, 2009), and other personality constructs, as well as understanding moral exemplars (i.e., people known for high levels of moral commitment; Walker & Frimer, 2007) and lay conceptions of moral personhood (Hardy, Walker, Skalski, Olsen, & Basinger, 2011).

Another part of personality approaches to morality is the understanding that the socialization and development of morality are lifelong processes. Traditional moral stage theories viewed the young child as largely incompetent and amoral. However, research has demonstrated that young children possess fledgling capacities regarding conscience, moral emotions, and moral self-concept (e.g., Kochanska & Aksan, 2006). Furthermore, there is evidence that various domains of morally relevant functioning, such as *generativity* (i.e., care and concern for future generations) (Erikson, 1968; McAdams, 2009), continue to develop into mature adulthood. Nevertheless, most work on moral socialization has involved older children, adolescents, and young adults. Thus, we focus on those life phases in this review, and only briefly touch on early childhood (see Thompson, 2012) and later adulthood (see Pratt, Diessner, Pratt, Hunsberger, & Pancer, 1996).

An additional aspect of personality approaches to morality is appreciation for the role of narrative research, which focuses on recall of personal stories of particular life experiences (Pratt & Fiese, 2004). There are three ways in which narratives help elucidate moral socialization: as a method of study (e.g., in the recall of specific socialization or learning experiences); as a medium of everyday socialization and teaching of values to the child; and as a process by which the self makes sense of personal, morally relevant experiences (Pratt & Fiese, 2004).

Contexts of Socialization: The Family

The parent–child relationship is arguably the most influential and widely studied context for learning ethical values and behaviors. Darling and Steinberg (1993) suggested that parenting patterns are oriented around three broad features: parenting goals, parenting practices, and parenting styles. Parents' goals vary in terms of their time focus (short vs. long term) and orientation (e.g., parent- or child-centered; Hastings & Grusec, 1998). Parents adapt their parenting practices based on their goals, from the use of punishment and rewards to reasoning and discussion. Finally, parenting styles entail broad variations on the dimensions of warmth, structure, and autonomy–support (Baumrind, 1991; Steinberg, 2001), and describe the family climate in which parenting goals and practices operate. Authoritative parenting, characterized by high levels on all three of these style dimensions, is typically the most adaptive.

More recently, Grusec and Davidov (2010; Chapter 7, this volume) distinguished different aspects of the parent–child relationship that have distinct functions, learning mechanisms, and child outcomes. Their five domains include the protection domain (parent as caretaker and attachment figure), the mutual reciprocity domain (parent as reciprocal play partner), the control domain (parent as disciplinarian, both rewarder and punisher), the guided learning domain (parent as teacher/instructor), and the group identification domain (parent as cultural model). Importantly, parents may vary in the quality of their socialization across these distinct domains.

Socialization Contexts Beyond the Family

As highlighted by Bronfenbrenner (1979), socialization involves many extrafamily contexts increasingly over development, including the peer group, the school, the church, the community, the media, and so on. At the most distal level, cultural differences impact the child indirectly through their shaping of values and behaviors that guide interactions in the more proximal, face-to-face contexts such as the family or the peer group.

The Socialization of Moral Reasoning and Domain Distinctions

The Cognitive-Developmental Approach to Moral Reasoning

Family Influences on Moral Reasoning Development

Research in the cognitive-developmental tradition on moral reasoning has examined the process of stimulating development of reasoning in children through short-term intervention studies with adults and peers designed to raise reasoning levels (e.g., Walker, 1980), and in longitudinal studies of different family background experiences (e.g., Speicher, 1992). In general, Kohlberg (1969) and others suggested that children's relations with parents are less democratic than those with peers, and therefore not as stimulating for moral reasoning development. Less hierarchical relations among peers should produce more egalitarian contexts for discussion, critique, and perspective taking to fuel moral reasoning development. Studies examining relations of family interaction patterns to development of moral reasoning have tested these assumptions (Walker, Hennig, & Krettenauer, 2000; Walker & Taylor, 1991). One finding was that parents often lower their reasoning toward the level of their child's reasoning in parent–child discussions, in an attempt to make their arguments more comprehensible, while children show more advanced reasoning during these moral discussions with parents than they do during individual interview assessments with the experimenter (Walker & Taylor, 1991). These findings are what might be expected based on the idea of a *zone of proximal development* (Vygotsky, 1978): Children are able to perform more effectively with scaffolding support provided by adults (Pratt, Kerig, Cowan, & Cowan, 1988). Such teaching and discussion might be seen as representative of working within the guided learning domain in the parent–child relationship (Grusec & Davidov, 2010).

A second important finding from these studies is that parent–child interactions most facilitative of moral reasoning development involved fewer argumentative transactions that critiqued the child's reasoning and more frequent encouraging, representational interactions (Walker & Taylor, 1991). In fact, the most productive parent–child interactions focus on children's own real-life issues, use more interactions that solicit and clarify (re-present) the child's ideas, and involve less critical and informational "lecturing" (Walker et al., 2000).

These findings are further buttressed by longitudinal research on authoritative parenting. For example, Pratt, Skoe, and Arnold (2004) found that authoritative parenting during adolescence is predictive of more advanced moral reasoning at age 20, as assessed by levels of reasoning focused on care of others and the self. Parent socialization goals that emphasize caring values, as well as their autonomy-granting practices (both measured by narratives), also uniquely predict increases in care reasoning from ages 16 to 20. These findings indicated that parental emphasis on specific goals, practices, and styles all appear to foster the development of moral reasoning during late adolescence, in line with Darling and Steinberg's (1993) model.

Nonfamily Influences on Moral Reasoning

Cognitive developmentalists have long seen peers as important facilitators of moral reasoning development (Kohlberg, 1969). Studies of discussions between unacquainted college students have shown that peer critiques of target positions framed at a modestly higher level of reasoning boosted target reasoning level (Berkowitz & Gibbs, 1983). In contrast, Walker and colleagues (2000) compared adolescents' discussions with friends and those with their parents; when adolescents interacted with their friends, challenging operational critiques were predictive of stagnation in development, whereas representational comments that solicited the adolescents' ideas were predictive of gains in moral reasoning, similar to patterns in discussions with parents. Walker and colleagues argued that critical commentary on the other's reasoning may be less successful in close friend relationships (compared to critiques from strangers) because it may provoke more distressing and distracting emotional responses, especially at younger ages. Overall, parents and peers can play positive roles in moral reasoning development by helping to explore the child's viewpoint. In fact, this may even carry over into adulthood; a longitudinal study of adult moral reasoning indicated that those reporting more social cognitive support and advice on a variety of topics were less likely to show declines in moral reasoning over 4 years (Pratt et al., 1996).

Schools, religious institutions, and other face-to-face contexts also provide important opportunities for moral reasoning development. For example, Kohlberg and colleagues conducted considerable research on school-based interventions for developing moral reasoning (see Oser, Althof, & Higgins-D'Alessandro, 2008), with evidence of at least short-term effects. Findings from research on religiousness and moral reasoning have been complex, but people do commonly discuss religious and spiritual values when responding to real-life moral dilemmas (Walker & Reimer, 2005). Finally, it should be noted that work on the socialization of moral reasoning has declined in recent years, likely due to its demands in terms of data collection, as well as lessening theoretical interest in the Kohlbergian paradigm.

Social Domain Theories of Reasoning

Family Influences on Domain Reasoning

Social domain theorists have sought to understand the role parents play in developing children's abilities to make appropriate distinctions between domains of social knowledge. Smetana (1995, 1999) examined how variations in parenting styles are reflected in the distinctions and feedback that parents provide to adolescents about different types of rules. Such variations help explain why authoritative parenting typically provides more effective moral socialization. Authoritative parents more clearly distinguished the boundaries among moral, conventional, and personal rules in their feedback to adolescents (Smetana, 1995, 2011). Authoritative parents may have a clearer sense of their appropriate authority within these different domains than do authoritarian parents, who seem to confuse the moral domain with the conventional and personal domains, and permissive parents, who insufficiently regulate adolescents in all three domains (Smetana, 2011). Authoritative parents are also more likely to provide explicit explanations and feedback to children about the bases of domain reasoning. Conflict in more authoritarian families is engendered by overregulation of the conventional and personal domains, and in turn may lead to more ineffective parent socialization processes. For example, Smetana, Campione-Barr, and Daddis (2004) conducted a longitudinal study with families of African American youth from ages 13 to 18. Too much adolescent autonomy over the personal and mixed (multifaceted) domains early on—a permissive pattern—led to poorer

adjustment at most ages (including more deviant behaviors). Too little youth input—
an authoritarian pattern—also predicted long-term problems in adolescent adjustment.
However, increasing input and involvement in these domains for youth across this
developmental period—a joint decision-making pattern typical of authoritativeness—
predicted better outcomes for adolescents by age 18.

Warm and supportive parents may also encourage their children to be more responsive to their parental views (Smetana, 1999). Indeed, authoritative parenting invites
more openness to parental influence, partly via positive affect (Darling & Steinberg,
1993). Thus, both cognitive and affective processes are involved in fostering development
toward effectively and appropriately made domain distinctions.

Nonfamily Influences on Domain Reasoning

Peers also provide feedback regarding interactions within distinct domains, and such
feedback helps children learn to distinguish these domains and develop reasoning that
underlies these distinctions (Smetana, 1999). Peers tend to provide as much information
as adults within the moral domain when their rights or welfare are violated, but they
provide much less feedback than adults in conventional domains (Smetana, 1999).

Cultural differences may also influence how domain reasoning develops. For instance,
issues in the personal domain are understood to be the individual's choice (Nucci &
Turiel, 1978), and so may come to ground a conception of individual rights. Across cultures, youth may therefore vary in how they differentially conceptualize rights in the personal domain compared to the conventional domain, particularly when contrasting more
or less authority-centered cultures. Interestingly, however, children's and adolescents'
conceptions of individual rights in China (more authority-centered) largely paralleled
those of youth in Canada (less authority-centered; Helwig, Arnold, Tan & Boyd, 2003).
Indeed, Chinese students were surprisingly more critical of authority-oriented decision
making in matters such as school curriculum, which Canadian children had been more
willing to accept in previous studies, based on the justification that children would have
limited competence to address these issues (Helwig et al., 2003). Overall, this evidence
suggests that cultural differences in reasoning and choice regarding personal issues may
be less important and more complex than is often thought (see also Wainryb, 2006).

Summary of Work on the Socialization of Moral Reasoning

In short, research on moral reasoning from the cognitive-developmental and social
domain perspectives highlights the roles of both parents and peers as socialization agents.
Opportunities for role taking and consideration of the perspectives of others in everyday
life, as well as the presentation of arguments regarding issues of fairness and caring, are
key developmental factors in each of these contexts. However, parents and peers have
different authority roles and tend to provide different types of feedback to the child, so
the processes of moral reasoning socialization may differ as a function of the nature of
the socializing agent (Smetana, 1999; Walker et al., 2000). Moral reasoning development within the family quite likely takes place substantially within the guided learning
domain, which involves the provision of adaptive cognitive stimulation (Grusec & Davidov, 2010). But it is also fostered by positive affective relations between parent and child

(Walker et al., 2000), which make children and adolescents more open and responsive to parent interventions (therefore also engaging the protection and control domains).

The Socialization of Moral Personality

The integration of work on moral development and personality is gaining momentum (Narvaez & Lapsley, 2009). McAdams and Pals (2006) outlined a three-level framework for summarizing the field of personality that provides a useful way of organizing work on moral personality (McAdams, 2009). The first level of personality involves *traits*, which are general tendencies to react to the world in particular ways that help account for behavioral consistencies across time and context (McCrae & Costa, 1997). The second level entails *characteristic adaptations*, which are motivational and social cognitive aspects of personality (e.g., emphasis on moral values) that are more tailored to the context or particular developmental tasks than traits, and change dynamically. For example, stages of personality development as characterized by Erikson (1968), such as identity and generativity, represent characteristic adaptations with particular motivational foci at different points in the life cycle. The third level of personality is the *life story* (McAdams, 2008), a narrative developing in late adolescence and emerging adulthood that expresses the sense of personal identity by giving meaning to the individual's past, present, and future self. We discuss each of these levels in turn as they relate to moral development.

Morality and Personality Traits

Research on traits has focused on the Big Five traits of Extraversion, Neuroticism–Emotional Stability, Conscientiousness, Agreeableness, and Openness to Experience (McCrae & Costa, 1997). These traits are reasonably stable across situations and time, and have considerable heritability; nevertheless, they are still subject to socialization effects. For example, Roberts and Mrozcek (2008) noted that emerging adults who entered into stable, successful careers showed increases in conscientiousness over adulthood. In contrast, young adults who engaged in negative activities at work, such as stealing, aggression and malingering, tended over time to show declines in conscientiousness (Roberts, Walton, Bogg, & Caspi, 2006).

There are two key lines of research on trait-level aspects of moral development: studies of lay conceptions of moral personhood, and studies of people known for lives of moral exemplarity. A first study on folk conceptions of morality by Walker and Pitts (1998) explored everyday language used to describe what it means to be a moral person. Six clusters of moral trait terms were identified: principled–idealistic, dependable–loyal, has integrity, caring– trustworthy, fair, and confident. A study by Hardy and colleagues (2011) using the same procedures found that adolescents' conceptions of moral personhood were similar to those of adults, with some movement toward more sophisticated and differentiated views of morality across adolescence into adulthood. Walker and Hennig (2004) more specifically examined lay conceptions of what it means to be someone who is highly just, caring, or brave. Participants were asked to think of examples of actors who engaged in great just, caring, or brave behaviors. Using standard measures of personality traits and several different methods, they found that general conceptions of exemplars of just behavior were seen as higher on conscientiousness, rationality, and openness, while exemplars of caring behavior were rated higher on agreeableness and empathy for others, and exemplars of bravery were seen as more extraverted, intrepid, and self-sacrificing. Thus, in contrast to narrow theoretical and philosophical depictions of morality, these studies suggest a more expansive and nuanced picture of moral personhood.

Another useful approach to examining moral personality at the trait level has involved studies of moral exemplars. Matsuba and Walker (2004) investigated exemplary emerging and young adults (ages 18–30) nominated by leaders in their organizations (e.g., Big Brothers, crisis centers, churches) based on their strong commitments to these civic organizations. Nonexemplars were university students matched on age, gender, education, and ethnicity. Exemplars differed from nonexemplars on only one of the Big Five traits, Agreeableness, with exemplars scoring higher. Since this sample could be considered care-oriented exemplars due to their nomination from community service organizations, these findings were consistent with the folk conceptions of the moral person prototype described earlier. Walker and Frimer (2007) reported on samples of brave and caring adults, awarded Canadian national medals of honor either for exemplary heroism or service to others, contrasting these groups with each other and with matched nonexemplar comparisons on Extraversion and Agreeableness. Agreeableness was higher for caring than for brave exemplars, consistent with Matsuba and Walker (2004), with no clear differences in Extraversion. Overall, then, research on patterns of moral personality at the trait level suggests some consistency regarding the positive roles of Agreeableness, Conscientiousness, and Openness.

Family and Nonfamily Influences on Moral Personality Traits

Kochanska and colleagues investigated how temperament interacts with socialization processes in the family to shape the development of early moral conscience and moral behavior (e.g., Kochanska & Aksan, 2006). For instance, fearful preschoolers responded well to parents' gentle discipline that avoided harsh, power-assertive techniques, and this type of discipline led to more mature moral conduct and better self-regulation. However, fearless children could not be socialized as effectively through this route. Instead, they responded better to socialization processes based on mutual responsiveness in the parent–child dyad and enjoyment of parental interaction, which in turn led to mature patterns of conscience and self-regulation. Although we know a great deal about interactions between temperament and socialization among young children (see, e.g., Belsky & Pluess, 2009), more work is needed to understand how these interactive processes play out later in adolescent and adult moral development (Thompson, 2012).

Empirical evidence suggests that mean-level increases in major traits, particularly conscientiousness, agreeableness and emotional stability, are greatest during the period from ages 20 to 40 (Roberts & Mrozcek, 2008). These traits are key elements of moral personality. Such changes in these traits may be accounted for by the socializing effects of investing in key social roles (e.g., work, stable romantic partnerships, and family and community life) that guide and deepen commitments to the social world beyond the self. Roberts, Wood, and Caspi (2008) call this pattern of effects the "social investment" principle, suggesting that it also accounts in part for individual variability in moral development.

Summary of Research on Socialization of Moral Personality Traits

Parenting and children's temperament interact in complex ways to shape the socialization of morality in the family (Kochanska & Aksan, 2006). Kochanska's extensive body of work provides evidence of how the domains of parenting described by Grusec and Davidov (2010) may be part of such moral socialization. Furthermore, investment in important normative, young adult roles involving responsibility to others shows consistent positive relations to development in the moral traits of Conscientiousness and Agreeableness (Roberts & Mrozcek, 2008). There is clearly a need in this area for more systematic research across the life span investigating how socialization processes, temperament, and personality jointly ground moral development.

Morality and Characteristic Adaptations

At a level of personality more proximal to behaviors than to broad traits, and more variable across context and time, are characteristic adaptations (McAdams & Pals, 2006). Various developmental models that describe changes in social cognitions and motivations are located at this level, including the moral reasoning levels of Kohlberg and others already reviewed earlier, as well as the personality and ego developmental stages of Erikson and Loevinger (McAdams, 2009). Here we focus on reviewing the socialization of moral values and moral identity, which are major areas of existing research, as well as emerging work on Eriksonian generativity.

Moral Values as Characteristic Adaptations

Moral values and other social cognitive facets of moral motivation are characteristic adaptations in the McAdams (2009) model of personality, and are part of the third component of morality in Rest's (1983) framework of moral action. An interesting example of research on moral motivation with younger children is a longitudinal study by Malti, Gummerum, Keller, and Buchmann (2009). They assessed moral motivation by asking 6-year-olds to respond to rule violations in hypothetical dilemmas—for example, not sharing a pencil or stealing another child's chocolate—and then assessing their reactions to the appropriateness of these actions, and their feelings about, and reasons for, their reactions. Moral motivation, assessed by prioritizing moral choices, feelings, and reasons over nonmoral responses, evidences variations in the child's evaluation of a sense of a moral self, which may later grow into a moral identity. Moral motivation generally predicted observed and teacher-reported moral behaviors concurrently and 1 year later.

Studies of moral values endorsement with adolescents and adults have also shown links to moral outcomes. Among university students, questionnaire ratings of a set of values that showed a relative predominance of moral value endorsement (e.g., kind), as compared to endorsements of positive, nonmoral values (e.g., ambitious), were associated with lower levels of antisocial behaviors (Barriga, Morrison, Liau, & Gibbs, 2001). A similar measure of moral value predominance predicted greater prosocial community participation among adolescents (Pratt, Hunsberger, Pancer, & Alisat, 2003). Furthermore, Schwartz (1994) developed a circumplex measure of values that evidences comparable value structures across cultures. Two of these value dimensions involved other-oriented moral domains (benevolence values of caring for other individuals, universalism values of caring for the wider society). Studies using this measure on a university sample in the United States indicated that higher moral values endorsement predicted higher prosocial behavior ratings as assessed by self, partners, and peers (Bardi & Schwartz, 2003).

Family Influences on Moral Values

Research on values transmission within the family is mounting. Padilla-Walker (2007), following the theorizing of Grusec and Goodnow (1994), showed that more accurate perception and greater acceptance of parent values by teens are linked to more prosocial behaviors. Relatedly, an authoritative parenting climate is associated with generally greater openness to parental influences (Darling & Steinberg, 1993). Pratt and colleagues (2003) found that more authoritative parenting is predictive of greater congruence between adolescents' own values and the values they think their parents want them to have. Patrick and Gibbs (2012) found that adolescents preferred inductive parental discipline (similar to an authoritative style in its focus on explanation and discussion) over power assertion or love withdrawal, and that greater endorsement of moral values for the self was associated with such an inductive style. Malti and Buchmann (2010) investigated the moral motivation of participants ages 15 and 21 years, assessing moral motivation as moral choices, attributed emotions, and reasons for these choices and feelings. These youth reported on both parenting quality (support) and friendship quality (support and intimacy). Parent supportiveness predicted higher moral motivation among the 15-year-olds but not the 21-year-olds, while close friendship relations did not predict moral motivation for 15-year-olds but did for 21-year-olds. Thus, parents continue to be important agents for value learning at least during adolescence, though peers may become relatively more important in emerging adulthood.

In a study utilizing a narrative methodology, Mackey, Arnold, and Pratt (2001) reported that adolescents' stories of important parental influences on their moral values showed stronger integration or appropriation of the parent's "voice" or perspective in families that were described by the adolescents as more authoritative. Such appreciation of the parents' views reflects greater and more genuine convergence between parent and adolescent perspectives.

Similarly, Hardy, Padilla-Walker, and Carlo (2008) found that components of authoritative parenting, particularly responsiveness and autonomy–support, positively predicted moral values internalization. The values studied included fairness, honesty, and kindness, as measured by questionnaires grounded in self-determination theory (Deci & Ryan, 1990).

In a different narrative study, Pratt, Norris, Hebblethwaite, and Arnold (2008) examined relations between mothers' and fathers' self-reports of generativity (a focus on care for the next generation's needs) and adolescent memories of the parents' value teaching; generative parents are more authoritative in their parenting styles (see Peterson, Smirles, & Wentworth, 1997). Adolescents with more generative parents recalled stories of parent value teaching with greater emphasis on care-oriented moral values (e.g., kindness), were more likely to be accepting of parent values, and had more vivid recollections of these teaching events. Such results fit with Grusec and Goodnow's (1994) argument that socialization requires accurate perception and acceptance of parental messages.

Interestingly, most of these late adolescents' memories of parents focused around interactive episodes during which the parent had either rewarded or punished the child, which are within the control domain of Grusec and Davidov (2010). Stories of grandparent value socialization were also readily recalled by participants in the Pratt and colleagues (2008) study but were more likely to describe how the grandparent had served as a model for adolescent values (e.g., hard work), more directly representing the group participation domain (Grusec & Davidov, 2010). This is not surprising, since noncustodial grandparents rarely have responsibility for directly regulating the child's behavior; thus, control episodes were much less commonly recalled for them than for parents.

The role of young siblings' interaction and disputes in the family, and the ways in which parents deal with these, has also received attention (e.g., Ross, Filyer, Lollis, Perlman, & Martin, 1994). Parents and siblings negotiate a sense of justice within the context of family rules and values in complex but important ways. Campione-Barr and Smetana (2010) recently found that younger adolescent siblings reported higher levels of conflict over issues of equality and fairness, whereas older adolescents reported more conflict regarding interference in the personal domain. A recent longitudinal study by Padilla-Walker, Harper, and Jensen (2010) indicated that sibling closeness and warmth predicted greater kindness and generosity in young adolescents, independently of parent relations with the target child. Earlier cross-cultural work also showed that older siblings' involvement in the "minder" role with infant siblings fostered stronger care-oriented behaviors and values in these minder boys in particular (Whiting & Whiting, 1975).

Overall, then, authoritative, autonomy-granting parents (at least in North America) may operate more effectively in the control domain than their less authoritative compatriots, in that their children show greater acceptance and internalization of parental values. However, it is unclear whether such parenting styles are more effective in other cultural contexts (Rudy, Grusec, & Wolfe, 1999). An example of cultural differences in moral socialization of young children is provided by the ethnographic research of Miller, Wiley, Fung, and Liang (1997). Chinese families made more spontaneous use of past child transgressions as a resource for narrating in the context of present child misbehaviors. American parents' spontaneous narratives about the child were commonly told for entertainment and enjoyment. Both narrative types were present in both cultures, but one was more predominant than the other, depending on the culture.

Nonfamily Influences on Moral Value Socialization

Other socialization contexts outside the family can also play a role in value socialization. For instance, greater levels of adolescent community involvement predicted increases in moral value emphasis 2 years later (Pratt et al., 2003). Furthermore, parents may encourage their children to engage in community activities, participation in which might then lead to increases in moral values through the experience of such helping activity (Hart, Atkins, & Ford, 1999; Pancer & Pratt, 1999). Similarly, community involvement may be fostered through school programs (Yates & Youniss, 1996), which in turn may increase moral value endorsement. As well, Hardy and Carlo (2005) showed that adolescent religious involvement was linked to greater endorsement of kindness as a value, which in turn predicted more helping behaviors.

Moral Identity as a Characteristic Adaptation

Hardy and Carlo (2011a, 2011b) reviewed two ways of approaching moral identity: conceptions that emphasize moral identity as the unity of self and morality, and those focused around the role of sociocognitive schemata. Blasi's (2004) theory provides a foundation for the unity of self and morality framework, stressing that moral action is more likely to be consistent with moral reasoning when accompanied by a sense of obligation to implement the action. Such a judgment of responsibility is frequently grounded in a sense of moral identity, which characterizes how central and important the moral domain is to one's sense of self. Thus, a stronger moral identity leads to more consistent follow-through on moral decisions, as individuals are driven to act consistently with their overall sense of self (Blasi, 2004).

Blasi's model is consistent with research on moral exemplars. Colby and Damon (1992) carried out a qualitative interview study of 23 adult moral exemplars (individuals well known for their dedication to morality). They document evidence of exceptional unity and little conflict between the exemplars' own personal interests and their understanding of what was morally right. Hart and Fegley (1995) compared adolescent moral and caring exemplars (nominated by community leaders) to matched nonexemplars and found greater use of moral descriptors of the self by exemplars, though no differences on moral reasoning. Furthermore, Frimer, Walker, Lee, Riches, and Dunlop (2012) analyzed the speeches and interviews of well-known moral exemplars of the 20th century versus a corresponding group of well-known negative exemplars. The exemplars (e.g., Nelson Mandela) produced a structure of value chains in their available writings or speeches in which self-focused values were integrated with final goals involving communal values focused on the betterment of others. In contrast, well-known negative figures (e.g., Adolph Hitler) produced self-oriented values in the service of self-oriented final aims. Frimer and colleagues argued that moral exemplars' speeches express personal identity, while focusing ultimately on benefiting others. For example, negative exemplars spoke of "working hard to gain respect and power," whereas exemplars spoke of "working hard in order to protect the innocent" (p. 1134).

The second approach to moral identity described by Hardy and Carlo (2011a) focuses on the role of social cognitive moral schemata that may be activated by the individual more or less readily for processing social information. These models describe cognitive processing differences that explain variations in moral engagement and behavior under different circumstances (e.g., Narvaez, Lapsley, Hagele, & Lasky, 2006). Narvaez and colleagues found that moral "chronics" (those who more habitually accessed moral frameworks in thinking about issues on a separate task) were more likely to recall sentences relevant to moral traits on a computer task than were "nonchronics" (who rarely accessed moral frameworks in thinking).

Similarly, Aquino and colleagues (Aquino, Freeman, Reed, Lim, & Felps, 2009; Aquino, McFerran, & Laven, 2011) explored how situational factors influenced the activation of the moral identity schema and thereby differentially influenced moral behaviors and emotional reactions to various morally relevant situations. Aquino and colleagues (2009) demonstrated that the accessibility of moral identity can be manipulated, and that such activation is more important for people whose moral identity is less central to the self. For example, a simple priming manipulation that required trying to recall the Ten Commandments led to higher moral intentions in response to a business scenario among those lower in moral identity, but it did not influence intentions in those higher in moral identity (who presumably did not require this priming boost). Aquino and colleagues (2011) found that those higher in self-reported moral identity were more likely to recall acts of uncommon goodness from their own personal memories and expressed greater intentions to help others in the future. Relatedly, Johnston, Sherman, and Grusec (2013) assessed moral identity implicitly, by measuring latency to respond to moral terms regarding the self. Higher levels of implicit (though not explicit) moral identity predicted greater levels of physiological responses indicative of moral outrage, such as increased heart rate when listening to taped statements that violated moral principles (e.g., the people of Haiti deserved the recent earthquake that struck them). This body of research suggests that as moral identity becomes more salient, it interacts with contexts to shape moral motivations and behaviors.

Family Influences on Moral Identity

The family context is important for socializing moral identity. For instance, Hart and Fegley's (1995) adolescent moral exemplars' self-concepts incorporated stronger representations of parents and of the self with one's parents than did those of the comparison sample, whose self-concepts instead incorporated stronger references to the best friend. Furthermore, recent studies support relations between authoritative parenting and moral identity. Hardy, Bhattacharjee, Aquino, and Reed (2010) found that parent responsiveness, demandingness, and autonomy-granting positively predicted adolescent moral identity. Other studies also found adolescent moral identity to be predicted by parent demandingness (Pratt et al., 2003) or parent support of teens (Hart et al., 1999).

There has been little research to date on the socialization of social cognitive schemata of moral identity. Nevertheless, Narvaez and colleagues (2006) suggested that a plausible account of the development of these schemata might begin from the idea of processing expertise. Children whose families encourage them to develop and use moral frameworks to think about personal experiences should more readily show activation and use of such schemata. Parenting approaches such as moral induction, as well as moral character attributions, should therefore encourage more use of moral schemata by the child. Such parental encouragement of the child's processing of daily experiences in appropriate moral terms may be reflected in the use of representational interactions with the child (Walker & Taylor, 1991), and in the sort of Vygotskian scaffolding of the child's reasoning in the guided learning domain (Grusec & Davidov, 2010).

Nonfamily Influences on Moral Identity

Research on community involvement has indicated that greater participation in prosocial activities fosters moral identity formation (Pratt et al., 2003; Yates & Youniss, 1996). More specifically, Larson, Hansen, and Moneta (2006) found that youth reported that involvement in faith-based organizations provided greater opportunities for identity development and positive relationship development than other contexts (e.g., sports, the arts, or academic clubs), while involvement in service activities encouraged greater prosocial concern. Hence, it seems likely there is a bidirectional dynamic between moral identity and engagement in moral action.

Generativity as a Characteristic Adaptation

Another important, morally relevant characteristic adaptation is *generativity*, which entails a concern for supporting and guiding the next generation (Erikson, 1968). McAdams (2009) argues that Erikson's description of generativity is highly moralized in nature and frames the issue of care for succeeding generations as a moral imperative for adults. Consistent with this, adolescents higher on moral identity were more likely to express generativity in emerging adulthood (Pratt et al., 2009). Similarly, Walker and Frimer (2007) found that adult care exemplars (those who had received "Caring Canadian" national awards) were higher on generative strivings than adult brave exemplars (recipients of the Canadian Medal of Bravery). Last, Pratt and Lawford (2014) reported that higher levels of generative concern assessed at age 23 predicted moral behaviors at age 32, such as greater community and proenvironmental activities and involvement.

Family and Nonfamily Influences on Generativity

Evidence relevant to the socialization of generativity points to the role of at least three potential factors—parental modeling, authoritative parenting, and involvement in prosocial activities. First, regarding modeling, generativity in youth is positively related to generativity in their parents (Peterson, 2006; Pratt, Alisat, Bisson, & Norris, 2013). While this does not indicate the mechanism underlying this association, modeling is one possible explanation. Second, authoritative parenting positively predicted generativity in teens and emerging adults (Lawford, Pratt, Hunsberger, & Pancer, 2005; Peterson et al., 1997; Pratt & Lawford, 2014). In fact, authoritative parenting might itself provide a model of positive caregiving and relationships. Finally, both positive parenting and community engagement in late adolescence uniquely predicted generativity in young adulthood (Pratt & Lawford, 2014), and adolescent caregiving activities with friends predicted generative concern 1 year later (Lawford, Doyle, & Markiewicz, 2013).

Summary of Research on the Socialization of Moral Adaptations.

Socialization research on moral characteristic adaptations suggests the involvement of a wide range of contexts, including the family, peers, and religious and civic experiences. Regarding the family, authoritative parents demonstrated more effective socialization of moral values, moral identity, and generativity. Many of the parental domains of socialization described by Grusec and Davidov (2010) may be relevant, including attachment processes that encourage empathy, control processes that foster stronger moral action and value development, mutual reciprocity, and even cultural modeling of appropriate patterns of responding. Positive engagement in contexts beyond the family provides additional opportunities for developing expertise and competence, as well as identity growth and development of generative care. Families themselves often help to link the child to these other socialization contexts.

Morality and the Life Story

The third level of personality in the McAdams model (McAdams & Pals, 2006) is the life story. This aspect of personality emerges during late adolescence or young adulthood, when abstract cognitive capacities are sufficient to enable the connection of features of the self across time and situations through more integrative underlying representations (Habermas & de Silveira, 2008). It also represents the most unique aspects of personality (McAdams & Pals, 2006) and contains key episodes of one's life experiences, which are selected and organized into a story that provides a sense of unity and purpose. The emergence of this life story is closely coordinated with identity development (McLean & Pratt, 2006). In the domain of religion, for example, those more advanced in identity status development told stories of personal religious high points that were more meaningful and elaborated (Alisat & Pratt, 2012).

Moral identity may represent another specific domain of the life story (Pratt et al., 2009). McAdams, Diamond, de St. Aubin, and Mansfield (1997) identified positive assets that were part of the life stories of highly generative adult exemplars, such as early life benefits (e.g., attachments to important others in the family), early concern for the suffering of others, a strong emphasis on redemption or turning bad events into good, and contemporary experiences of moral steadfastness and commitment to future social goals. It is also noteworthy that Walker and Frimer's (2007) study of Canadian caring and national award recipients found that these adult moral exemplars differed from comparison adults more in terms of their life stories than in terms of traits or characteristic adaptations. The life stories of these adult moral exemplars, in particular, showed salient redemptive themes and strong early attachments. Matsuba and Walker (2005) reported similar findings on the life stories of young adult moral exemplars.

In terms of developmental progression, Krettenauer and Mosleh (2013) asked younger adolescents, emerging adults, and midlife adults to tell stories about times when they had done something moral about which they felt good, and times when they had done something immoral about which they felt bad. Those individuals who had more strongly internalized moral norms (as assessed by a questionnaire derived from self-determination theory; Deci & Ryan, 1990) were more likely to coherently integrate both positive and negative past moral events into their narrative identity. In general, attempting to integrate disconfirming or contradictory memories into a coherent self-narrative is often seen as an important engine in promoting identity development (McLean & Pasupathi, 2012). Similarly, Soucie, Lawford, and Pratt (2012) found that emerging adults were more likely than midadolescents to be able to tell personal stories about a time when they took the perspective of others, and that the empathic stories of emerging adults were more meaningful and salient than those of adolescents. Thus, a distinctive sense of the self in the moral domain can develop during emerging adulthood (McAdams, 2008).

The Life Story, Moral Identity, and Family and Nonfamily Socialization Influences

The family, as well as communities and cultures, plays an important role in socialization of the life story. McAdams and colleagues (1997) conducted a seminal study of adult generative exemplars, identified from a pool of excellent teachers and unpaid volunteers who worked with children and families, all of whom scored high on a standard measure of generative concern. Several of the distinctive features of exemplars' life stories focused on early socialization experiences, such as early family benefits, feeling concern for others, and the presence of many helpers and few enemies compared to the stories of nonexemplars. This maps onto research evidence regarding actual positive moral socialization experiences, and indicates that exemplars found such early socialization experiences important in making sense of their own life stories. McAdams (2004) also reported that exemplars were more likely than matched nonexemplars to tell "favorite stories" of their family lives that referred to episodes of kindness and caring.

It also seems that authoritative parenting is associated with a number of positive benefits for emerging life stories. For instance, the narrative study by Soucie and colleagues (2012) assessed family experiences. Adolescents who reported being raised by authoritative parents were more likely to tell life stories with salient empathic themes. Additionally, positive views of parenting during adolescence (more support, greater discussion) were predictive of more coherent resolution of life challenges ("low points") in the life story and greater identity achievement in emerging adulthood (Dumas, Lawford, Tieu, & Pratt, 2009). Parents' supportiveness in discussions of difficult life events may foster more adaptive coping strategies and resolutions in young adult children. It would be interesting to compare the role of peer interactions in this same context given that peers surely become central listeners to the life stories of adolescents and young adults as well (e.g., Pasupathi & Wainryb, 2010), and their support may be as important as that of parents. Thorne (2000) argued that the life story is best thought of as a co-construction of both author and listener, and both parents and peers can be important audiences for the adolescent and emerging adult in narrative identity development.

In terms of broader socialization contexts, Nelson and colleagues (2012) studied the turning point stories of emerging adults from at-risk communities who had experienced a long-term intervention involving families, schools, and community organizations as a way of improving children's adult outcomes (the Better Beginnings, Better Futures project). Compared to nonintervention youth from comparable communities, the stories of intervention youth showed greater coherence and meaning, and more themes of personal growth and redemption. Increased opportunities for involvement and success in school and community may have mediated a stronger sense of self-efficacy among the intervention youth, as reflected in their identities and life stories, and interestingly, in their greater involvement in community helping as well.

There is also evidence for the role of culture in the life story. McAdams (2008) has stressed that individuals appropriate their life stories in large part from salient culturally based themes. For example, Wang and Conway (2004) have indicated differences in the way Chinese and North American adults construe experiences in their personal narratives, consistent with themes of more interdependent versus independent selves across these two cultures, respectively. Variations in these themes are likely mediated through experiences with the family and peer group, as well as the media and wider cultural models (McAdams, 2008). As one morally relevant example, Adams (2005) found in an interview study that Ghanaian young adults, whose culture portrays a more interdependent self than is typical in the United States, were also more likely than their U.S. counterparts to perceive themselves to have unknown but personal enemies, and to believe that one must be watchful regarding the dangers of these enemies in one's life. As noted, the limited role of enemies was a distinctive feature in the generative life story in American exemplars (McAdams et al., 1997).

Last, as identity is formed and the life story takes shape in late adolescence and early adulthood, there is also a critical role for the self as agent in socialization, in constructing and reflecting on the meaning of life experiences and integrating them into the self. Identity formation is a constructive and self-regulated process. The life story represents the self's active attempt to select key elements from the array of autobiographical memories and anticipation of the future (McAdams, 2008). This highlights the self-as-author's efforts to fashion a "me" that makes a coherent account of who I was, am, and will be in the future. This process of "making the self through stories" (Matsuba & Walker, 2005, p. 275) is thus an exercise in the self's agency.

Interestingly, Pasupathi and Wainryb (2010) have discussed how this story construction challenges the developing self in the moral domain to integrate difficult and negative episodes of immoral actions in a way that makes moral identity coherent, or at least tolerable. As they point out, this process of dealing with the self's complexities can challenge people to move toward a more sophisticated view of themselves, but it may also lead to efforts to distance the self from these prior actions in a defensive way. The process of narrating the self can therefore provide a key context for the experience and expression of moral agency and its development.

Summary of Socialization Influences on the Life Story and Narrative Identity

The limited set of findings on socialization and the life story to date suggests possible evidence for the roles of family and peers, as well as experiences in the wider community. The protection and guided learning domains may be implicated in parental influences on the life story, through the parent's role as a supportive and engaged listener (Dumas et al., 2009). Also, the group identification domain of socialization in the family (Grusec & Davidov, 2010) may be particularly salient in cultural differences (e.g., Wang & Conway, 2004).

Summary and Conclusions

Commonalities and Differences in Socialization Agents across Moral Personality

We have reviewed features of the developing moral personality, following the three-level framework of McAdams (2009), including moral traits, moral reasoning, moral values, moral identity, generativity, and the life story. Across these levels, there was quite consistent evidence for the role of the family in influencing moral personality development. The family has influence earliest and most often across the life course, and has been the most widely studied context with regard to moral development. Parents were the most salient family agents, but grandparents (Pratt et al., 2008) and siblings (Padilla-Walker et al., 2010) were found to be influences as well.

Social contexts outside the family are also important. Peers come to play a larger role as children mature, and the evidence of their impact is well documented in the area of moral reasoning, moral values, and prosocial and antisocial behaviors. They likely influence the development of the life story and moral identity in adolescence and emerging adulthood as well (e.g., Pasupathi & Wainryb, 2010). Research has also supported the role of community and civic involvement in shaping moral values, moral identity, and generativity (Pratt & Lawford, 2014; Yates & Youniss, 1996). The parent or peer systems may also shape the child's patterns of experiencing other face-to-face contexts (e.g., community, church or school) through differences in how the child's or adolescent's involvement is supported (or not) by these key groups.

Culture differences were also apparent for many of these moral features, moral values, moral identity, and the life story. Effects of these broader factors are likely mediated through the face-to-face groups of the child's direct experience, such as varying family value socialization patterns in the home across different cultures (e.g., Miller et al., 1997). Although there is research on the role of culture in moral reasoning, research examining culture and moral personality is still limited, as are studies of how different levels of these contexts interact.

Finally, many of the facets of moral development we have discussed strongly highlight the role of the self as agent in selecting and shaping the role of personal experiences (Pasupathi & Wainryb, 2010), constructing the impact of socialization agents, and shaping how these socialization agents interact with the child (Kuczynski, 2003). The active role of the self in the socialization process becomes steadily more salient during late adolescence and early adulthood.

Future Directions for Research on Moral Socialization

We see a number of promising areas for future research on the socialization of morality. First, more research on parent goals and practices is needed in order to understand clearly the processes of moral socialization. Although Grusec and Davidov (2010) have argued for the importance of distinguishing the various socialization roles in which parents engage, most research on moral (or other) socialization processes has not clearly distinguished these domains. Studies on family socialization of moral development have examined the role of clear cognitive explanation and feedback, as well as a supportive affective climate (e.g., Smetana, 1999; Walker et al., 2000). These patterns are labeled *inductive parenting* in the moral domain (Hoffman, 2000) and have been contrasted with more power-assertive disciplinary patterns (with inductive parenting being similar to authoritative parenting). Our review of the literature on moral socialization supports the positive impact of authoritative parenting on moral development as well. Yet it may be that effective socialization within different parenting domains is mediated by specific goals and practices only loosely correlated with such general parenting styles (Grusec & Davidov, 2010). As discussed, moral reasoning may be most susceptible to interventions in the guided learning domain. In contrast, moral value adherence and moral emotion may be more strongly socialized within the control domain, for example, by experiences of reward and punishment (Pratt et al., 2008). With regard to the socialization of moral personality, we have noted that moral traits, while substantially influenced by heredity, also may be strongly shaped by the performance of adult social roles (Roberts & Mrozcek, 2008). The cultural norms for these roles are likely influenced by observational learning processes in the group participation domain, related to culturally-shaped performance (Grusec & Davidov, 2010). Similarly, our review suggested that the life story is strongly shaped by cultural resources, which may be modeled within the family (Miller et al., 1997), again in the group participation domain. Narrative studies that focus on experiences of different types of learning might help to test how acquisition differs across the various components of morality.

Second, moral socialization research might benefit in general from greater use of narrative theoretical frameworks and research methods (Pratt & Fiese, 2004). Across several moral exemplar studies, the life story has been the most salient aspect of personality that has served to distinguish moral exemplars from comparisons (e.g., McAdams et al., 1997; Walker & Frimer, 2007). Research on the life story and moral identity is just beginning. It shows promise as a way of richly understanding the processes of self-construal in adolescence and emerging adulthood (Pasupathi & Wainryb, 2010), and how these may be linked to socialization in cultural context.

Third, much of the research on parenting has focused on the discipline context, concerning itself with what Grusec and Davidov (2010) term the *control domain*, and with the socialization of negative behaviors. Thus, more work on the socialization of prosocial behaviors is needed, although such work has been advancing recently (see Hastings et al., Chapter 27, this volume). In particular, research that systematically compares moral behaviors and emotions, and their socialization, in both antisocial and prosocial contexts, is needed (Malti & Krettenauer, 2013).

Fourth, moral socialization in the family has largely positioned parents as agents and children as passive recipients, despite arguments for the dynamic nature of parent–child interactions (Kuczynski, 2003), and interesting work on early moral socialization (Kochanska & Aksan, 2006). Conceptualizing socialization in more dynamic and multifaceted terms is needed. The distinctive roles of siblings and grandparents in moral development, as compared with parents and peers, similarly need more research (Padilla-Walker et al., 2010). More studies comparing the socialization effects of mothers and fathers are also needed.

Fifth, at several points in the review, we have noted how parents interact with other microsystems in which the child is embedded, such as peers, schools, churches, the community, and so on, in fostering adolescents' caring and generative engagement (Pratt et al., 2013). Yet such work is very unsystematic to date. More research on these "mesosystem" processes (Bronfenbrenner, 1979) is needed, assessing links between different socialization contexts.

Last, several brief points should be made about research designs in the moral socialization literature. Most research to date has been cross-sectional, and more longitudinal research is needed in order to follow the development of individual differences in moral constructs and to begin to disentangle causal ordering. Important transition periods should be studied in this manner to connect individual development and socialization across the life span, including the transition from childhood to adolescence, and the transition to adulthood (Hardy & Carlo, 2011a; Thompson, 2012). Time series research on socialization events over short periods is also needed to understand intraindividual processes, as well as day-to-day socialization dynamics (e.g., in parent–child dyads). Evidence of possible recent cohort-linked changes in morally relevant variables such as dispositional empathy among youth (Konrath, O'Brien, & Hsing, 2011) suggests that more work is needed to disentangle cohort and developmental effects in the field. Indeed, long-term historical changes in moral socialization in society must be important (Pinker, 2011) and should be investigated as possible using appropriate data. There is also a need for more research using behavior genetics to elucidate gene–environment interactions in moral socialization because such research has been helpful in the related areas of antisocial behavior and psychpathology (e.g., Moffitt & Caspi, 2007). Finally, research on social neuroscience has begun to identify interesting intersections between behavior and brain function that have educational and socialization implications, and should be pursued in moral development as well (Narvaez, 2013). One interesting topic that might merit examination is the distinction often made between automatic and controlled processing in moral responding (Haidt, 2001), which is argued to characterize rapid emotional responding to everyday moral situations versus careful reasoning about moral conflicts. An understanding of the neural substrate underlying these differing patterns of responses may elucidate the boundaries and complex features of such contexts more precisely.

REFERENCES

Adams, G. (2005). The cultural grounding of personal relationship: Enemyship in North American and West African worlds. *Journal of Personality and Social Psychology, 88,* 948–968.

Alisat, S., & Pratt, M. W. (2012). Emerging adults' religious high point stories and their relations to adolescent identity status and religiosity: A longitudinal analysis. *Identity, 12,* 29–52.

Aquino, K., Freeman, D., Reed, A., II., Lim, V. K. G., & Felps, W. (2009). Testing a social cognitive model of moral behavior: The interactive influence of situations and moral identity centrality. *Journal of Personality and Social Psychology, 97,* 123–141.

Aquino, K., McFerran, B., & Laven, M. (2011). Moral identity and the experience of moral elevation in response to acts of uncommon goodness. *Journal of Personality and Social Psychology, 100,* 703–718.

Bardi, A., & Schwartz, S. H. (2003). Values and behavior: Strength and structure of relations. *Personality and Social Psychology Bulletin, 29,* 1207–1220.

Barriga, A. Q., Morrison, E. M., Liau, A. K., & Gibbs, J. C. (2001). Moral cognition: Explaining the gender difference in antisocial behavior. *Merrill–Palmer Quarterly, 47,* 532–562.

Baumrind, D. (1991). Effective parenting of adolescents. In P. Cowan & M. Hetherington (Eds.), *The effects of transitions on families* (pp. 111–163). Hillsdale, NJ: Erlbaum.

Belsky, J., & Pluess, M. (2009). Beyond diathesis stress: Differential susceptibility to environmental influences. *Psychological Bulletin, 135,* 885–908.

Berkowitz, M. W., & Gibbs, J. (1983). Measuring the developmental features of moral discussion. *Merrill–Palmer Quarterly, 29,* 399–410.

Blasi, A. (1984). Moral identity: Its role in moral functioning. In W. L. Kurtines & J. L. Gewirtz (Eds.), *Morality, moral behavior, and moral development* (pp. 129–139). New York: Wiley Interscience.

Blasi, A. (2004). Moral functioning: Moral understanding and personality. In D. K. Lapsley & D. Narvaez (Eds.), *Moral development, self, and identity* (pp. 189–212). Mahwah, NJ: Erlbaum.

Bronfenbrenner, U. (1979). *The ecology of human development.* Cambridge, MA: Harvard Press.

Campione-Barr, N., & Smetana, J. (2010). "Who said you could wear my sweater?": Adolescent siblings' conflicts and associations with relationship quality. *Child Development, 81,* 464–471.

Colby, A., & Damon, W. (1992). *Some do care: Contemporary lives of moral commitment.* New York: Free Press.

Darling, N., & Steinberg, L. (1993). Parenting style as context: An integrative model. *Psychological Bulletin, 113,* 487–496.

Deci, E. L., & Ryan, R. M. (1990). A motivational approach to self: Integration in personality. *Nebraska Symposium on Motivation, 38,* 237 –288.

de Waal, F. (1996). *Good natured: The origins of right and wrong in humans and other animals.* Cambridge, MA: Harvard University Press.

Dumas, T. M., Lawford, H. L., Tieu, T., & Pratt, M. W. (2009). Positive parenting in adolescence and its relation to low point life story narration and identity status in emerging adulthood: A longitudinal analysis. *Developmental Psychology, 45,* 1531–1544.

Erikson, E. H. (1968). *Identity: youth and crisis.* Oxford, UK: Norton.

Frimer, J., Walker, L. J., Lee, B. H., Riches, A., & Dunlop, W. L. (2012). Hierarchical integration of agency and communion: A study of influential moral figures. *Journal of Personality, 80,* 1117–1145.

Grusec, J. E., & Davidov, M. (2010). Integrating different perspectives on socialization theory and research: A domain specific approach. *Child Development, 81,* 687–709.

Grusec, J. E., & Goodnow, J. (1994). Impact of parent discipline methods on the child's internalization of values: A reconceptualization of current points of view. *Developmental Psychology, 30,* 4–19.

Habermas, T., & de Silveira, C. L. (2008). The development of global coherence in life narratives across adolescence. *Developmental Psychology, 44,* 707–721.

Haidt, J. (2001). The emotional dog and its rational tail: A social intuitionist approach to moral judgment. *Psychological Review, 108,* 814–834.

Hardy, S. A., Bhattacharjee, A., Aquino, K., & Reed, A., II. (2010). Moral identity and psychological distance: The case of adolescent parental socialization. *Journal of Adolescence, 33,* 111–123.

Hardy, S. A., & Carlo, G. (2005). Religiosity and prosocial behaviours in adolescence: The mediating role of prosocial values. *Journal of Moral Education, 34,* 231–249.

Hardy, S. A., & Carlo, G. (2011a). Moral identity: What is it, how does it develop, and is it linked to moral action? *Child Development Perspectives, 5,* 212–218.

Hardy, S. A., & Carlo, G. (2011b). Moral identity: Where identity formation and moral development converge. In S. J. Schwartz, K. Luyckx, & V. L. Vignoles (Eds.), *Handbook of identity theory and research* (pp. 495–514). New York: Springer.

Hardy, S. A., Padilla-Walker, L. M., & Carlo, G. (2008). Parenting dimensions and adolescents' internalization of moral values. *Journal of Moral Education, 37,* 205–223.

Hardy, S. A., Walker, L. J., Skalski, J., Olsen, J. A., & Basinger, J. C. (2011). Adolescent naturalistic conceptions of morality. *Social Development, 20,* 562–586.

Hart, D., Atkins, R., & Ford, D. (1999). Family influences on the formation of moral identity in adolescence: Longitudinal analyses. *Journal of Moral Education, 28,* 375–386.

Hart, D., & Fegley, S. (1995). Prosocial behavior and caring in adolescence: Relations to self-understanding and social judgment. *Child Development, 66,* 1346–1359.

Hastings, P. D., & Grusec, J. E. (1998). Parenting goals as organizers of responses to parent–child disagreement. *Developmental Psychology, 34,* 465–479.

Helwig, C. C., Arnold, M. L., Tan, D., & Boyd, D. (2003). Chinese adolescents' reasoning about democratic and authority-based decision making in peer, family, and school contexts. *Child Development, 74,* 783–800.

Hoffman, M. L. (2000). *Empathy and moral development: Implications for caring and justice.* New York: Cambridge University Press.

Johnston, M., Sherman, A., & Grusec, J. E. (2013). Predicting moral outrage and religiosity with an implicit measure of moral identity. *Journal of Research in Personality, 47,* 209–217.

Kochanska, G., & Aksan, N. (2006). Children's conscience and self-regulation. *Journal of Personality, 74,* 1587–1617.

Kohlberg, L. (1969). Stage and sequence: The cognitive developmental approach to socialization. In D. A. Goslin (Ed.), *Handbook of socialization theory and research* (pp. 347–480). Chicago: Rand McNally.

Konrath, S. H., O'Brien, E., & Hsing, C. (2011). Changes in dispositional empathy in American college students over time: A meta-analysis. *Personality and Social Psychology Review, 15,* 180–198.

Krettenauer, T., & Mosleh, M. (2013). Remembering your (im)moral past: Autobiographical reasoning and moral identity development. *Identity, 13,* 140–158.

Kuczynski, L. (2003). *Parent–child relationships as a dyadic process.* Thousand Oaks, CA: Sage.

Lapsley, D. K., & Hill, P. L. (2009). The development of the moral personality. In D. Narvaez & D. Lapsley (Eds.), *Personality, identity, and character: Explorations in moral psychology* (pp. 185–213). New York: Cambridge University Press.

Larson, R. W., Hansen, D. M., & Moneta, G. (2006). Differing profiles of developmental experiences across types of youth activities. *Developmental Psychology, 42,* 849–862.

Lawford, H., Pratt, M. W., Hunsberger, B., & Pancer, S. M. (2005). Adolescent generativity: A longitudinal study of two possible contexts for learning concern for future generations. *Journal of Research on Adolescence, 15*, 261–273.

Lawford, H. L., Doyle, A. B., & Markiewicz, D. (2013). The association between early generative concern and caregiving with friends from early to middle adolescence. *Journal of Youth and Adolescence, 42*(12), 1847–1857.

Mackey, K., Arnold, M. L., & Pratt, M. W. (2001). Adolescents' stories of decision-making in more or less authoritative families: Representing the voices of parents in narrative. *Journal of Adolescent Research, 16*, 243–268.

Malti, T., & Buchmann, M. (2010). Socialization and individual antecedents of adolescents' and young adults' moral motivation. *Journal of Youth and Adolescence, 39*, 138–149.

Malti, T., Gummerum, M., Keller, M., & Buchmann, M. (2009). Children's moral motivation, sympathy, and prosocial behavior. *Child Development, 80*, 442–460.

Malti, T., & Krettenauer, T. (2013). The relation of moral emotion attributions to prosocial and antisocial behavior: A meta-analysis. *Child Development, 84*(2), 397–412.

Matsuba, M. K., & Walker, L. J. (2004). Extraordinary moral commitment: Young adults involved in social organizations. *Journal of Personality, 72*, 413–436.

Matsuba, M. K., & Walker, L. J. (2005). Young adult moral exemplars: The making of self through stories. *Journal of Research on Adolescence, 15*, 275–297.

McAdams, D. P. (2004). Generativity and the narrative ecology of family life. In M. W. Pratt & B. H. Fiese (Eds.), *Family stories and the life course: Across time and generations* (pp. 235–257). Mahwah, NJ: Erlbaum.

McAdams, D. P. (2008). Personal narratives and the life story. In O. P. John, R. W. Robins, & L. A. Purvin (Eds.), *Handbook of personality: Theory and research* (3rd ed., pp. 241–261). New York: Guilford Press.

McAdams, D. P. (2009). The moral personality. In D. Narvaez & D. Lapsley (Eds.), *Personality, identity, and character: Explorations in moral psychology* (pp. 11–29). New York: Cambridge University Press.

McAdams, D. P., Diamond, A., de St. Aubin, E., & Mansfield, E. D. (1997). Stories of commitment: The psychosocial construction of generative lives. *Journal of Personality and Social Psychology, 72*, 678–694.

McAdams, D. P., & Pals, J. (2006). A new Big Five: Fundamental principles for a new integrative science of personality. *American Psychologist, 61*, 204–217.

McCrae, R. R., & Costa, P. T. (1997). Personality trait structure as a human universal. *American Psychologist, 52*, 509–516.

McLean, K. C., & Pasupathi, M. (2012). Processes of identity development: Where I am and how I got there. *Identity, 12*, 8–28.

McLean, K. C., & Pratt, M. W. (2006). Life's little (and big) lessons: Identity development and the construction of meaning in the turning point narratives of emerging adulthood. *Developmental Psychology, 42*, 714–722.

Miller, P. J., Wiley, A., Fung, H., & Liang, C.-H. (1997). Personal storytelling as a medium of socialization in Chinese and American families. *Child Development, 68*, 557–568.

Moffitt, T. E., & Caspi, A. (2007). Evidence from behavioral genetics for environmental contributions to antisocial conduct. In J. E. Grusec & P. D. Hastings (Eds.), *Handbook of socialization theory and research* (pp. 96–123). New York: Guilford Press.

Narvaez, D. (2013). The future of research in moral development and education. *Journal of Moral Education, 42*, 1–11.

Narvaez, D., & Lapsley, D. (Eds.). (2009). *Personality, identity, and character: Explorations in moral psychology*. New York: Cambridge University Press.

Narvaez, D., Lapsley, D. K., Hagele, S., & Lasky, B. (2006). Moral chronicity and social information processing: Tests of a social cognitive approach to moral personality. *Journal of Research in Personality, 40*, 966–985.

Nelson, G., Van Andel, A., Curwood, S. E., Hasford, J., Love, N., Pancer, S. M., et al. (2012). Exploring outcomes through narrative: The long-term impacts of Better Beginnings, Better Futures on the turning point stories of youth at ages 18–19. *American Journal of Community Psychology, 49,* 294–306.

Nucci, L. P., & Turiel, E. (1978). Social interactions and the development of social concepts in preschool children. *Child Development, 49*(2), 400–407.

Oser, F., Althof, D., & Higgins-D'Alessandro, A. (2008). The Just Community approach to moral education: System change or individual change? *Journal of Moral Education, 37,* 395–415.

Padilla-Walker, L. M. (2007). Characteristics of mother–child interactions related to adolescents' positive values and behaviors. *Journal of Marriage and Family, 69,* 675–686.

Padilla-Walker, L. M., Harper, J. M., & Jensen, A. C. (2010). Self-regulation as a mediator between sibling relationship quality and early adolescents' positive and negative outcomes. *Journal of Family Psychology, 24,* 419–428.

Pancer, S. M., & Pratt, M. W. (1999). Social and family determinants of community service involvement in Canadian youth. In M. Yates & J. Youniss (Eds.), *Community service and civic engagement in youth* (pp. 32–55). Cambridge, UK: Cambridge University Press.

Pasupathi, M., & Wainryb, C. (2010). Developing moral agency through narrative. *Human Development, 53,* 55–80.

Patrick, R., & Gibbs, J. C. (2012). Inductive discipline, parental expression of disappointed expectations, moral identity in adolescence. *Journal of Youth and Adolescence, 41,* 973–983.

Peterson, B. E. (2006). Generativity and successful parenting: An analysis of young adult outcomes. *Journal of Personality, 74,* 847–870.

Peterson, B. E., Smirles, K. A., & Wentworth, P. A. (1997). Generativity and authoritarianism: Implications for personality, political involvement, and parenting. *Journal of Personality and Social Psychology, 72,* 1202–1216.

Pinker, S. (2011). *The better angels of our nature: Why violence has declined.* New York: Penguin Books.

Pratt, M. W., Alisat, S., Bisson, E., & Norris, J. E. (2013). Earth mothers (and fathers): Generativity and environmental concerns in adolescents and their parents. *Journal of Moral Education, 42,* 12–27.

Pratt, M. W., Arnold, M. L., & Lawford, H. L. (2009). Growing towards care: A narrative approach to prosocial moral identity and generativity of personality in emerging adulthood. In D. Narvaez & D. Lapsley (Eds.), *Moral self, identity and character: Prospects for a new field of study* (pp. 295–315). New York: Cambridge University Press.

Pratt, M. W., Diessner, R., Pratt, A., Hunsberger, B., & Pancer, S. M. (1996). Moral and social reasoning and perspective-taking in later life: A longitudinal study. *Psychology and Aging, 11,* 66–73.

Pratt, M. W., & Fiese, B. H. (2004). Family stories and the life course: An ecological context. In M. W. Pratt & B. H. Fiese (Eds.), *Family stories and the life course: Across time and generations* (pp. 1–24). Mahwah, NJ: Erlbaum.

Pratt, M. W., Hunsberger, B., Pancer, S. M., & Alisat, S. (2003). A longitudinal analysis of personal value socialization: Correlates of a moral self-ideal in adolescence. *Social Development, 12,* 563–585.

Pratt, M. W., Kerig, P., Cowan, P., & Cowan, C. (1988). Mothers and fathers teaching three year-olds: Authoritative parenting and adults' scaffolding of young children's learning. *Developmental Psychology, 24,* 732–739.

Pratt, M. W., & Lawford, H. L. (2014). Early generativity and civic engagement in adolescence and emerging adulthood. In L. M. Padilla-Walker & G. Carlo (Eds.), *Prosocial development: A multidimensional approach* (pp. 410–432). New York: Oxford University Press.

Pratt, M. W., Norris, J. E., Hebblethwaite, S., & Arnold, M. L. (2008). Intergenerational transmission of values: Family generativity and adolescents' narratives of parent and grandparent value teaching. *Journal of Personality, 76,* 171–198.

Pratt, M. W., Skoe, E. E., & Arnold, M. L. (2004). The development of care reasoning in later adolescence. *International Journal of Behavioral Development, 28,* 139–147.

Rest, J. R. (1983). Morality. In P. Mussen, J. Flavell, & E. Markman (Eds.), *Handbook of child psychology: Vol. 3. Cognitive development* (pp. 556–628). New York: Wiley.

Roberts, B. W., & Mrozcek, D. (2008). Personality trait change in adulthood. *Current Directions in Psychological Science, 1,* 31–35.

Roberts, B. W., Walton, K., Bogg, T., & Caspi, A. (2006). De-investment in work and non-normative personality trait change. *European Journal of Personality, 20,* 461–474.

Roberts, B. W., Wood, D., & Caspi, A. (2008). The development of personality traits in adulthood. In O. P. John, R. W. Robins, & L. A. Pervin (Eds.), *Handbook of personality: Theory and research* (3rd ed., pp. 375–398). New York: Guilford Press.

Ross, H. S., Filyer, R. E., Lollis, S. P., Perlman, M., & Martin, J. L. (1994). Administering justice in the family: Siblings, family relationships, and child development. *Journal of Family Psychology, 8,* 254–273.

Rudy, D., Grusec, J. E., & Wolfe, J. (1999). Implications of cross-cultural findings for a theory of family socialization. *Journal of Moral Education, 28,* 299–310.

Schwartz, S. H. (1994). Are there universal aspects in the content and structure of values? *Journal of Social Issues, 50,* 19–45.

Smetana, J. G. (1995). Parenting styles and conceptions of parental authority during adolescence. *Child Development, 66,* 299–316.

Smetana, J. G. (1999). The role of parents in moral development: A social domain analysis. *Journal of Moral Education, 28,* 311–321.

Smetana, J. G. (2011). *Adolescents, families and social development: How teens construct their worlds.* West Sussex, UK: Wiley-Blackwell.

Smetana, J. G., Campione-Barr, N., & Daddis, C. (2004). Developmental and longitudinal antecedents of family decision-making. *Child Development, 75,* 1418–1434.

Soucie, K., Lawford, H. L., & Pratt, M. W. (2012). Personal stories of empathy in adolescence and emerging adulthood. *Merrill–Palmer Quarterly, 58,* 141–158.

Speicher, B. (1992). Adolescent moral judgment and perceptions of family interaction. *Journal of Family Psychology, 6,* 128–138.

Steinberg, L. (2001). We know some things: Parent–adolescent relationships in retrospect and prospect. *Journal of Research on Adolescence, 11,* 1–19.

Thompson, R. A. (2012). Whither the preconventional child?: Toward a lifespan moral development theory. *Child Development Perspectives, 6,* 423–429.

Thorne, A. (2000). Personal memory telling and personality development. *Personality and Social Psychology Review, 4,* 45–56.

Turiel, E. (1983). *The development of social knowledge: Morality and convention.* Cambridge, UK: Cambridge University Press.

Vygotsky, L. (1978). *Mind in society: The development of higher psychological processes.* Cambridge, MA: Harvard University Press.

Wainryb, C. (2006). Moral development in culture: Diversity, tolerance, justice. In M. Killen & J. Smetana (Eds.), *Handbook of moral development* (pp. 211–240). New York: Taylor & Francis.

Walker, L. J. (1980). Cognitive and perspective taking prerequisites for moral development. *Child Development, 51,* 131–139.

Walker, L. J., & Frimer, J. A. (2007). Moral personality of brave and caring exemplars. *Journal of Personality and Social Psychology, 93,* 845–860.

Walker, L. J., & Hennig, K. H. (2004). Differing conceptions of moral exemplarity: Just, brave and caring. *Journal of Personality and Social Psychology, 86,* 629–647.

Walker, L. J., Hennig, K. H., & Krettenauer, T. (2000). Parent and peer contexts for children's moral reasoning development. *Child Development, 71,* 1033–1048.

Walker, L. J., & Pitts, R. C. (1998). Naturalistic conceptions of moral maturity. *Developmental Psychology, 34,* 403–419.

Walker, L. J., & Reimer, K. (2005). The relationship between moral and spiritual development. In E. C. Roehlkepartain (Ed.), *The handbook of spiritual development in childhood and adolescence* (pp. 224–238). Thousand Oaks, CA: Sage.

Walker L. J., & Taylor, J. H. (1991). Family interactions and the development of moral reasoning. *Child Development, 62,* 264–283.

Wang, Q., & Conway, M. A. (2004). The stories we keep: Autobiographical memory in American and Chinese middle-aged adults. *Journal of Personality, 72,* 911–938.

Whiting, B., & Whiting, J. (1975). *Children of six cultures.* Cambridge, MA: Harvard University Press.

Yates, M., & Youniss, J. (1996). A developmental perspective on community service in adolescence. *Social Development, 5,* 85–111.

Author Index

Subject Index

Page numbers followed by *f* indicate figure, *t* indicate table

709

HANDBOOK OF SOCIALIZATION